HEMODYNAMIC MONITORING

HEMODYNAMIC MONITORING

Evolving Technologies and Clinical Practice

MARY E. LOUGH PhD, RN, CNS, CCRN, CNRN, CCNS

Critical Care Clinical Nurse Specialist
Stanford Health Care
Clinical Assistant Professor
Stanford University
Stanford, California

ELSEVIER

MOSBY

3251 Riverport Lane
St. Louis, Missouri 63043

HEMODYNAMIC MONITORING: EVOLVING TECHNOLOGIES
AND CLINICAL PRACTICE

ISBN: 978-0-323-08512-0

Executive Content Strategist: Lee Henderson
Content Development Manager: Jean Sims Fornango
Senior Content Development Specialist: Tina Kaemmerer
Publishing Services Manager: Julie Eddy
Project Manager: Sara Alsup
Senior Book Designer: Amy Buxton

Printed in the United States of America

Last digit is the print number: 9 8 7 6 5 4 3 2 1

To my wonderful family
Jim, Madeleine, Michael

Contributors

Nancy M. Albert, PhD, CCNS, CHFN, CCRN, NE-BC, FAHA, FCCM
Associate Chief Nursing Officer – Nursing Research & Innovation and Clinical Nurse Specialist - Heart Failure
Cleveland Clinic
Cleveland, Ohio

Roy Ball, MS, RN, ACNP-BC, CCNS
Trauma Program Manager
Legacy Emanuel Medical Center
Portland, Oregon

Patricia A. Blissitt, PhD, RN, CCRN, CNRN, CCNS, CCM, ACNS-BC
Neuroscience Clinical Nurse Specialist
Harborview Medical Center;
Neuroscience Clinical Nurse Specialist
Swedish Medical Center-Cherry Hill;
Assistant Professor, Clinical Faculty
University of Washington School of Nursing
Seattle, Washington

John J. Gallagher, MSN, RN, CCNS, CCRN, RRT
Clinical Nurse Specialist, Trauma Program Manager, Hospital of the University of Pennsylvania
Philadelphia, Pennsylvania

Annette Haynes, MS, RN, CNS, CCRN, CCNS
Cardiology Clinical Nurse Specialist
Stanford Health Care
Stanford, California

Jan M. Headley, BS, RN
Director, Strategic Alliances & Professional Education
Edwards Lifesciences
Irvine, California

Jonathan Judy-del Rosario, MS, RN, ACNP-BC
Director of Nursing
California Pacific Medical Center
Assistant Clinical Professor
University of California, San Francisco
San Francisco, California

Bhavani Shankar Kodali, MD
Associate Professor, Vice Chair of Clinical Affairs
Anesthesiology
Brigham & Women's Hospital, Harvard Medical School
Boston, Massachusetts

Barbara "Bobbi" Leeper, MN, RN-BC, CNS M-S, CCRN, FAHA
Clinical Nurse Specialist, Cardiovascular Services
Baylor University Medical Center
Dallas, Texas

S. Jill Ley, MS, RN, CNS, FAAN
Clinical Nurse Specialist, Cardiac Surgery
California Pacific Medical Center;
Clinical Professor
University of California, San Francisco
San Francisco, California

Barbara McLean, MN, RN, CCNS-BC, NP-BC, CCRN, FCCM
Critical Care Clinical Specialist and
    Independent Critical Care Consultant
Division of Critical Care Nursing
Grady Memorial Hospital
Atlanta, Georgia

Michael Petty, PhD, RN, CCNS, ACNS-BC
Cardiothoracic Clinical Nurse Specialist
University of Minnesota Medical Center
Minneapolis, Minnesota

Rob Phillips, PhD, MPhil, FASE, DMU
The School of Medicine
The University of Queensland
Brisbane, Australia;
Chief Scientist, Uscom Limited
Sydney, Australia

Sagarika Ponnuru, MD
Staff Anesthesiologist
Excel Anesthesia
Dallas, Texas

Nitin Kumar Puri, MD
Assistant Professor of Medicine
Virginia Commonwealth University
Department of Medicine
Falls Church, Virginia;
Medical Director
Cardiovascular Intensive Care Unit
Department of Medicine
Inova Fairfax Hospital
Falls Church, Virginia

Amy Salgado, MS, RN, ACNP-BC
Nurse Practitioner
Cardiovascular Critical Care
Stanford Health Care
Stanford, California

Julie A. Shinn, MA, RN, CNS, CCRN, FAHA, FAAN
Cardiovascular Clinical Nurse Specialist
Stanford Health Care
Stanford, California

Kathleen M. Stacy, PhD, RN, CNS, CCRN, PCCN, CCNS
Critical Care Clinical Nurse Specialist
Clinical Associate Professor
Hahn School of Nursing and Health Science
University of San Diego
San Diego, California

Yasir Tarabichi, MD
Fellow Physician
Pulmonary and Critical Care Medicine
University of California, Los Angeles
Los Angeles, California

Paul Thurman, MS, RN, ACNPC, CCNS, CCRN
Clinical Nurse Specialist
R. Adams Cowley Shock Trauma Center
University of Maryland Medical System
Baltimore, Maryland

Rosemary A. Timmerman, MSN, RN, CCRN-CSC-CMC, CCNS
Clinical Nurse Specialist
Adult Critical Care
Providence Alaska Medical Center
Anchorage, Alaska

Deborah Tuggle, MN, APRN, CCNS, FCCM
Critical Care Clinical Nurse Specialist,
    Norton Healthcare
Founder and President, Critical Care
    Curriculum
Louisville, Kentucky

Elizabeth E. Turner, MD
UCLA Division of Pulmonary and Critical Care
Assistant Clinical Professor, Director of
    Bedside Ultrasound
Los Angeles, California

**Kathryn Truter Von Rueden, RN, MS,
    ACNS-BC, FCCM**
Associate Professor and Clinical Nurse
    Specialist
Adult/Gerontology CNS/ACNP Trauma/
    Critical Care/ED Program and R Adams
    Shock Trauma Center
University of Maryland School of Nursing
University of Maryland Medical Center
Baltimore, Maryland

Reviewers

Thomas Ahrens, PhD, RN, FAAN
Research Scientist
Barnes-Jewish Hospital
St. Louis, Missouri

Marie Arnone, MA, RN, CCRN
Professional Development Specialist
Cardiovascular Services
Swedish Medical Center
Seattle, Washington

Bryan Boling, RN, CCRN-CSC, CEN
DNP Student, Acute Care Nurse Practitioner
    Program
Cardiothoracic and Vascular ICU
University of Kentucky
Lexington, Kentucky

**Marylee Bressie, DNP, RN, CCNS,
    CCRN, CEN**
Core Faculty/Nurse Planner
Capella University
Minneapolis, Minnesota

**Margaret Carno, PhD, RN, D, ABSM,
    PNP, FAAN**
Associate Professor of Clinical Nursing
University of Rochester School of Nursing
Rochester, New York

**Dawn M. Christensen, MS, FNP-BC,
    ACNP-BC**
Innovative Program Solutions, LLC
Pine Grove, Pennsylvania

Erin Cox, MS, ACNS-BC, CCRN
Clinical Nurse Specialist, Vascular Surgery
Massachusetts General Hospital
Boston, Massachusetts

**Robert J. Dorman, BSN, RN-BC,
    CCRN, C-NPT**
Senior Teaching Associate
University of Rochester School of Nursing
Rochester, New York

Charles A. Downs, PhD, ACNP-BC
Assistant Professor
Nell Hodgson Woodruff School of Nursing
Emory University
Atlanta, Georgia

Maureen P. Flattery, MS, RN, ANP, CCTC
Heart Transplant Coordinator
Virginia Commonwealth University Health
    System
Richmond, Virginia

**Rhonda Fleischman, MSN, RN-BC, CNS,
    CCRN-CMC**
CCU Clinical Education Specialist
Aultman Hospital
Canton, Ohio

David Goede, DNP, ACNP-BC
Assistant Professor of Clinical Nursing
University of Rochester School of Nursing
Rochester, New York

Shannon Johnson Bortolotto, MS, RN, APN, CCNS
Critical Care Clinical Nurse Specialist
University of Colorado Hospital
Aurora, Colorado

Christopher Junker, MD
Assistant Professor Anesthesiology, Critical Care and Neurosurgery
George Washington University
Washington, D.C.

Thelma K. Lasko, RDCS (AE, PE), RT, FASE
Lead Sonographer for Echocardiography
Aultman Hospital
Canton, Ohio

Catherine McCoy-Hill, MSN, RN, CCRN, CNS, ANP-C
Assistant Professor, School of Nursing
Azusa Pacific University
Azusa, California

Michael R. Pinsky, MD, CM, Dr hc, MCCM, FCCP
Professor of Critical Care Medicine, Bioengineering, Cardiovascular Disease and Anesthesiology
University of Pittsburgh
Pittsburgh, Pennsylvania

Patricia Radovich, PhD, RN, CNS, FCCM
Director of Nursing Research
Loma Linda University Medical Center
Loma Linda, California

Karsten Roberts, MS, RCP, RRT-ACCS
Clinical Education Coordinator
Respiratory Care Services
Stanford Health Care
Stanford, California

Tracee Rose, MSN, APRN, CCRN, CCNS-BC
Critical Care Clinical Nurse Specialist
United States Army
San Antonio, Texas

Laura D. Rosenthal, DNP, ACNP
Assistant Professor
University of Colorado
Aurora, Colorado

Mary Russell, MSN, RN, CCRN, ACNS-BC, FNP-C
Clinical Nurse Specialist
Palomar Health
Escondido, California

Jonathan C. Sague, MSN, ACNP-BC
Acute Care Nurse Practitioner
Cleveland Clinic, Critical Care Transport
Cleveland, Ohio

Sandra Schutz, MSN, RN
Clinical Nurse Specialist Cardiology/Critical Care, Clinical Educator
Overlake Hospital & Medical Center
Bellevue, Washington

Helina Somervell, DNP, CRNP
Lead Nurse Practitioner, Department of Surgery
John Hopkins Hospital
Baltimore, Maryland

Joshua Squiers, PhD, ACNP-BC, AGACNP-BC
Assistant Professor of Nursing
Director of the Acute Care Nurse Practitioner
    Program (AGACNP)
Oregon Health & Science University School
    of Nursing
Assistant Professor of Anesthesiology
Division of Cardiac and Surgical Subspecialty
    Critical Care
Department of Anesthesiology and
    Perioperative Medicine
Portland, Oregon

Brenda Tousley, MS, RN, CNS, CCRN
Staff Nurse, Critical Care Float Pool
North Colorado Medical Center
Greeley, Colorado

Jean-Louis Vincent, MD, PhD
Professor of Intensive Care Medicine,
    Université Libre de Bruxelles
President, World Federation of Intensive and
    Critical Care Societies
Department of Intensive Care, Erasme
    University Hospital
Brussels, Belgium

**Theresa Wadas, PhD, DNP, FNP-BC,
    ACNP-BC, CCRN**
Assistant Professor
University of Alabama Capstone College
    of Nursing
Tuscaloosa, Alabama

**Sharon Walicek, MSN, RN, CNS,
    CCRN, ANP-BC**
Adult Nurse Practitioner (Cardiology),
    Professor of Nursing Cardiac and Vascular
    Specialists
Elgin Community College
Elgin, Illinois

Brian Wessman, MD, FACEP
Co-Director, Critical Care Medicine Fellowship
Assistant Professor of Anesthesiology and
    Emergency Medicine
Washington University School of Medicine
St. Louis, Missouri

Susan L. Woods, PhD, RN, FAAN
Professor Emerita, Biobehavioral Nursing and
    Health Systems
University of Washington
Seattle, Washington

Preface and Acknowledgments

This book is for anyone who wants to understand hemodynamic monitoring as practiced now and in the future. Hemodynamic monitoring is transitioning away from invasive vascular catheters toward less-invasive monitoring technologies. The learning curve is steep, with the variety of new monitoring technologies requiring a deeper understanding of physiologic and pathophysiologic mechanisms. The intent of this book is to provide useful knowledge with practical applications in a highly visual format.

The book is divided into three parts. The first section discusses established monitoring methods, the second section describes emerging technologies, and the third section explores application of hemodynamic monitoring technologies in clinical practice. The chapters contain several features to assist with knowledge application, including historical milestones, normal values tables, hemodynamic case studies, clinical reasoning pearls, and strategies for ensuring patient comfort, patient education, and patient safety.

The chapter authors are all experts in their field who have combined their clinical knowledge with relevant literature. I am immensely grateful for the huge time commitment and effort they have given to writing these chapters and to developing original illustrations. Writing a first edition chapter from a blank sheet of paper is challenging, and this book would not be possible without the generosity of these expert clinicians.

I have received tremendous support from my editors at Elsevier. Special thanks to Maureen Iannuzzi who first proposed the idea for this book, to Tamara Myers for making sure I had the editorial support to make it happen, and to Lee Henderson for keeping me on track with deadlines to get it published. I also owe an enormous thank you to Savannah Davis for her skill and good humor in juggling manuscripts and hundreds of art drawings for 22 chapters.

This book could not have been written without the emotional support of my family. The time and commitment required to write and edit a first edition was unexpected in its highs and lows. Our son and daughter have followed the ups and downs closely. My husband has brought me endless cups of tea as I typed at my computer, read journal articles, and reviewed manuscripts. I am originally from England, and I am irrationally sure that tea fuels the creative process.

I hope you will learn as much reading this book as I have learned as its editor.

Mary E. Lough

Contents

Physiologic Principles of Hemodynamic Monitoring

1

Mary E. Lough

Hemodynamic monitoring involves the measurement of blood flow and pressure dynamics based on cardiac and circulatory physiologic principles.

Circulation of the Blood and the Birth of Hemodynamics

In 1628, William Harvey published "Du Mortis Cordis" and thus began the field of hemodynamics. Harvey carefully documented his experiments in anatomy, physiology, and mathematics to theorize correctly that blood continuously circulates from arteries to veins with the heart as the central pump.[1] Harvey also measured the volume of the left ventricle and calculated the amount of blood flowing through the heart in 30 minutes. This represented a radical departure from the medieval belief that blood was created from digested food and circulated by the lungs.[1] Fortunately, hemodynamics is a discipline where debate is welcomed. Almost 400 years later, anatomy, physiology, and mathematics are still important, and ways to achieve the most accurate measurements are continuously being investigated. Comprehension of the basic physiologic mechanisms helps identify the benefits and limitations of existing and emerging hemodynamic technologies.

Cardiac Cycle

The term *cardiac cycle* describes blood flow through the heart during one cardiac contraction. It encompasses atrial and ventricular systole and diastole and normally lasts for less than 1 second. The different mechanical components of the cardiac cycle are represented graphically in Figure 1-1. These five phases include the following:

1. Atrial systole
2. Isovolumetric contraction
3. Ventricular systole and ejection
4. Isovolumetric relaxation
5. Passive atrial and ventricular filling

The use of five phases effectively demonstrates the time-sequence of cardiac events. Within each phase, subphases exist, as explained below.

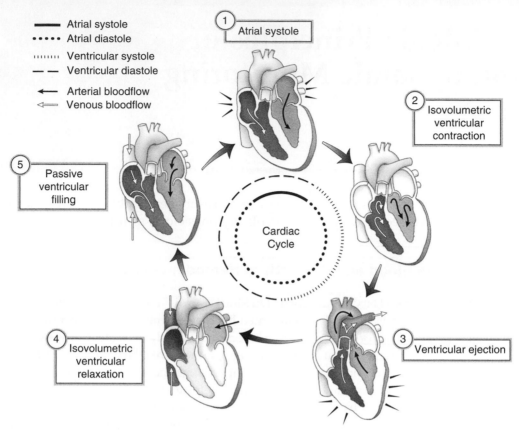

FIGURE 1-1 Phases of the cardiac cycle.

Electrocardiography

Electrocardiography (ECG) is the procedure that produces the electrocardiogram, which is a representation of the electrical events of the cardiac cycle (Figure 1-2). The electrical stimuli initiate the mechanical events of the cardiac cycle, resulting in intracardiac pressure changes that are observable on an associated pressure waveform. For example, the electrical *P wave* instigates atrial contraction, which raises the atrial chamber pressure and creates an *a wave* on the atrial pressure waveform. The electrical QRS stimulates ventricular contraction raising the ventricular chamber pressure, which is visualized as a rise in left ventricular (LV) pressure and subsequently by the upstroke of the arterial pressure waveform. The QRS signals the onset of systole (see Figure 1-2). In all cases, electrical stimulation precedes the mechanical contractile event. The *T wave* denotes electrical repolarization, which results in relaxation of the ventricular myocardium.

Cardiac Cycle Diagram

The cardiac cycle diagram is a visual representation of the electrical, mechanical, pressure, and flow elements of one full cardiac contraction (Figure 1-3). Because all of the events are

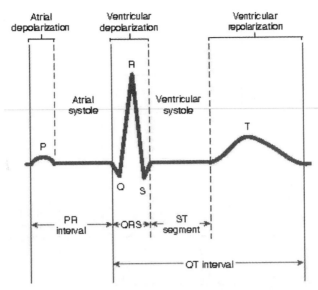

FIGURE 1-2 Electrocardiogram: electrical events and waves. (From Urden LD, Stacy KM, Lough ME: *Critical care nursing: diagnosis and management*, ed 7, St. Louis, 2014, Mosby.)

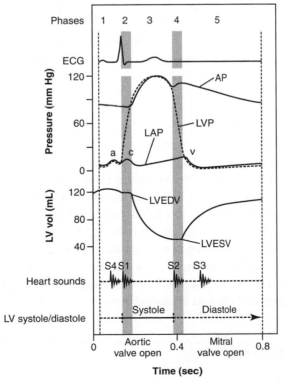

FIGURE 1-3 Cardiac cycle: left-side pressures, waveforms, and volumes. The vertical shaded areas in the cardiac cycle identify isovolumetric ventricular contraction (phase 2) and isovolumetric ventricular relaxation (phase 4). *AP*, Arterial pressure; *LAP*, left atrial pressure; *LVEDV*, left ventricular end-diastolic volume; *LVESV*, left ventricular end-systolic volume; *LVP*, left ventricular pressure.

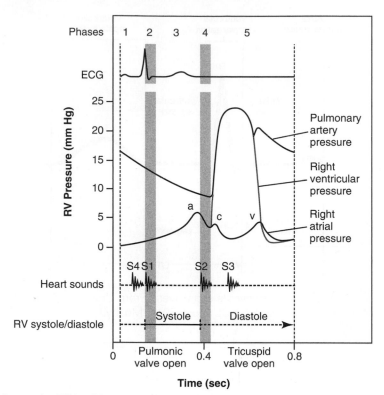

FIGURE 1-4 Cardiac cycle: Right-side pressures and waveforms. The vertical shaded areas denote right ventricular (RV) isovolumetric ventricular contraction (phase 2) and RV isovolumetric ventricular relaxation (phase 4).

time coordinated and interconnected, the vertical line drawn from the top to the bottom of the diagram connects all of the events occurring at a specific time point. This format is sometimes described as a *Wiggers diagram* after Carl Wiggers, a medical physiologist, who was the first to publish the visual representation of the cardiac cycle in 1921.

The cardiac cycle includes ECG waves, waveforms for left atrial pressure (LAP), LV pressure, and LV volume. Because the right and left sides of the heart are intricately linked, similar waveforms can be measured on the right side of the heart (Figure 1-4). Although the morphology of the waves is very similar, right-sided pressures are much lower.

To facilitate understanding of this complex interplay, the cardiac cycle is summarized in Table 1-1 in five phases. The table includes descriptions of the hemodynamic waveforms used for clinical measurements.

Cardiac Valve Movements

The cardiac valves are designed to ensure unidirectional blood flow through the heart. Each phase of the cardiac cycle begins and ends with a valve movement (open or close).

TABLE 1-1 Cardiac Cycle: Diastolic and Systolic Phases

PHASE	DESCRIPTION	FIGURE
1	**ATRIAL FILLING** Throughout the cardiac cycle, the atria are passively filling with blood. No valves exist to impede flow from the large thoracic veins to the atria. This holds equally true for venous blood flowing from the vena cava to the right atrium (RA), and for arterial blood flowing from the pulmonary vasculature via the pulmonary veins to the left atrium (LA). **ATRIAL SYSTOLE** The P wave on the electrocardiogram (ECG) signifies electrical depolarization of the atria (see Figure 1-2). Depolarization stimulates contraction of the thin atrial walls raising the pressure within each atrial chamber. Atrial contraction is known as *atrial systole* and colloquially described as the *atrial kick*. This increase in atrial pressure is identified on the atrial waveform as the "a" wave. As the flow subsides, the pressure in the atria falls, seen as the "x" descent on the atrial waveform. On the right side of the heart, atrial pressure is graphically represented by the central venous pressure (CVP) or right atrial pressure (RAP) waveform. Left atrial pressure (LAP) is graphically represented as the pulmonary artery occlusion pressure (PAOP) or "wedge" pressure waveform. In some conditions such as heart failure, atrial contraction may result in a sound that can be auscultated, known as S4 (see Figure 1-3).	**ATRIAL SYSTOLE** 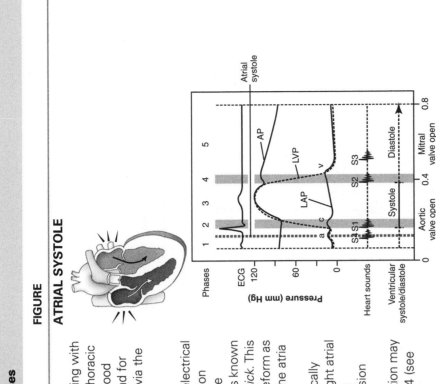

Continued

TABLE 1-1 Cardiac Cycle: Diastolic and Systolic Phases—cont'd

PHASE	DESCRIPTION	FIGURE
2	**CLOSURE OF THE ATRIOVENTRICULAR VALVES (MITRAL AND TRICUSPID)** As blood flow from the atria to the ventricle slows, the atrioventricular (AV) valves passively close. On the ECG, the isoelectric P–R interval corresponds in time to the closure of the AV valves. Just prior to valve closure, the pressure within each atrium is equal to the corresponding ventricular chamber; that is, the intraventricular pressure is low. The closure of the AV valve leaflets produces a low-pitched sound that can be auscultated with a stethoscope and is known as the first heart sound, or S1 (see Figures 1-3 and 1-6). The blood volume within each ventricle just before AV valve closure is described as the *end-diastolic volume (EDV), or preload.* *AV valve closure marks the end of diastole.* **ISOVOLUMETRIC CONTRACTION** During isovolumetric contraction, all four of the heart valves are closed. This includes the two AV valves (mitral and tricuspid), and the two semilunar vales (aortic and pulmonic). The vertical shaded area under phase 2 indicates isovolumetric ventricular contraction. On the ECG, the appearance of the QRS wave indicates that electrical depolarization of the ventricles has occurred. *The QRS signals the onset of ventricular systole.* Ventricular depolarization initiates contraction of the muscular ventricular walls and produces an increase in pressure within each ventricle without any change in the volume within the chamber, hence the name *isovolumetric contraction.* This pressure increase is sometimes reflected by a small rise in the atrial waveform known as the *C wave.* The pressure changes in the ventricular waveforms are much greater and differ between the right and left sides of the heart. Contraction of the muscular left ventricular (LV) wall raises the internal LV pressure to over 100 mm Hg (see Figure 1-3). Contraction of the thinner-walled right ventricle raises the internal right ventricular (RV) pressure to about 25 mm Hg) as shown in Figure 1-4. The pressures cited here are normal for a healthy heart. Ventricular pressures may rise above these values in disease states such as hypertension and heart failure.	**ISOVOLUMETRIC CONTRACTION**

VENTRICULAR SYSTOLE AND EJECTION

When the pressure within the ventricular chambers exceeds the pressure in the associated arterial outflow vessels, the aortic and pulmonic valve leaflets are thrust wide open. Blood is ejected at high speed and pressure from the left ventricle into the aorta, and simultaneously (at a lower pressure) from the right ventricle into the pulmonary artery. This outflow of blood is registered as an arterial pressure waveform. The systemic arterial pressure waveform is measured from the arterial waveform seen in the figure as the top part of the corresponding ventricular waveform (see Figure 1-3). The pulmonary artery pressure waveform can also be measured and reflects the lower pressures expected on the right side of the heart as shown in Figure 1-4.

The atrial waveforms (CVP/RAP and PAOP or "wedge") register a rise in pressure during ventricular systole, producing a wave known as a *V wave*. Once the semilunar valves (aortic and pulmonic) open and blood rapidly exits the ventricles, pressure in the aria is reduced. This fall in atrial pressure is seen as the "y" descent on the atrial waveform.

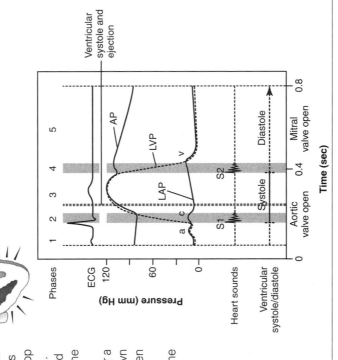

Continued

3

TABLE 1-1   Cardiac Cycle: Diastolic and Systolic Phases—cont'd

PHASE	DESCRIPTION	FIGURE
4	**CLOSURE OF THE SEMILUNAR VALVES (AORTIC AND PULMONARY)** On ECG, the appearance of the T wave signals that the ventricular muscle is starting to repolarize and relax causing a decrease in the speed and pressure of the ejected blood volume. As ventricular chamber pressures fall below the pressures in the great vessels, the semilunar valves are forced to close by backflow of blood in the aorta. As the leaflets touch, this makes a sound that can be auscultated with a stethoscope, known as the second heart sound, or S2 (see Figures 1-3 and Figure 1-5). A notch on the downward arc of the arterial waveform, called *incisura* or *dicrotic notch*, signals closure of the semilunar valves. ***Semilunar valve closure represents the end of systole.*** **ISOVOLUMETRIC RELAXATION** When all four valves are closed, the volume inside the ventricle cannot change, as the ventricular muscle relaxes to baseline. The volume within represents the ventricular end-systolic volume (ESV) (see Figure 1-3). The vertical shaded area under phase 4 identifies isovolumetric ventricular relaxation.	**ISOVOLUMETRIC RELAXATION** 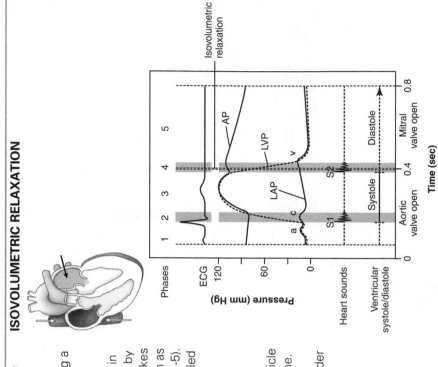

VENTRICULAR DIASTOLE AND FILLING

VENTRICULAR DIASTOLE AND FILLING

The opening of the AV valves (mitral and tricuspid) signals the start of ventricular diastole.

Once the AV valves open, the blood that has passively collected in the atria gushes into the ventricles.

In specific conditions such as heart failure, it is at this point in the cardiac cycle that an S3 heart sound may be auscultated (see Figures 1-3 and 1-5).

The sequence now loops back to atrial filling and atrial systole (see Figure 1-1).

5

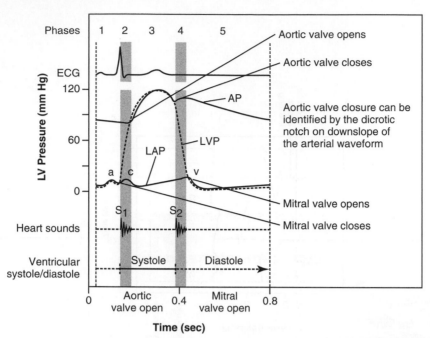

FIGURE 1-5 Cardiac cycle and cardiac valve movements. *AP*, Arterial pressure; *LAP*, left arterial pressure; *LVP*, left ventricular pressure.

The actions of the valves relative to the events of the cardiac cycle are shown in Figure 1-5.

Pressure Volume Loops

Pressure volume loops examine the cardiac cycle from a different perspective. The format is standardized and consists of LV pressure on the vertical (y) axis, and LV volume on the horizontal (x) axis. The loop is normally plotted for the left ventricle. The mitral valve and aortic valve movements anchor the four "corners" of the loop. In Figure 1-6, *A*, the letters ABCD mark the valve movements:

- Mitral valve closes (A)
- Aortic valve opens (B)
- Aortic valve closes (C)
- Mitral valve opens (D)

The four vertical "sides" of the LVP volume loop reflect the cardiac cycle. The two vertical sides represent the isovolumetric phases, during which a major change occurs in pressure but not in volume. The top and bottom sides of the loop symbolize the major volume changes in both diastole (bottom) and systole (top). The movement of

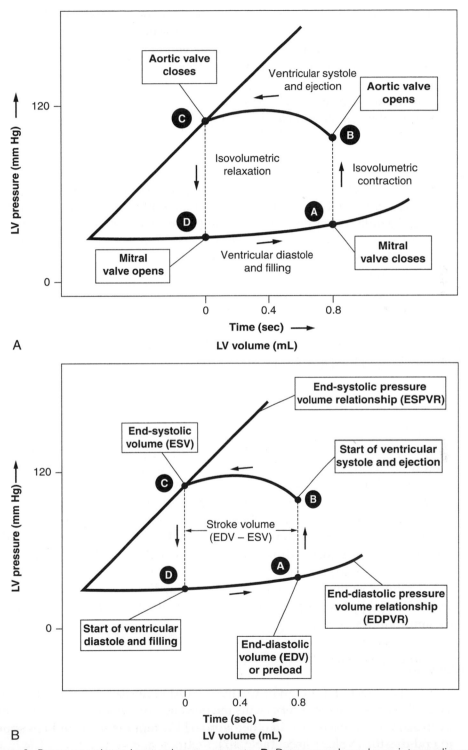

FIGURE 1-6 A, Pressure volume loop: valve movements. **B,** Pressure volume loop: intracardiac volumes.

the loop is anticlockwise, as indicated by the direction of the arrows. The space between the two vertical lines represents stroke volume as indicated in Figure 1-6, *B*. Stroke volume is the difference between end-systolic volume and end-diastolic volume.

The letters ABCD are also used to describe the loop sides (see Figure 1-6, *B*):

- Isovolumetric contraction (A-B)
- Ventricular systole and ejection (B-C)
- Isovolumetric relaxation (C-D)
- Ventricular diastole and filling (D-A)

Two other hemodynamic indices are displayed with the pressure volume loop. The two longer lines that are outside the loop, represent the pressure–volume relationship during diastole (lower line), and systole (upper line). The lower line, called the end-diastolic pressure–volume relationship, reflects the end-diastolic volume or preload volume. The upper line, called the end-systolic pressure–volume relationship, reflects the contractile state of the ventricle.[2] The shape of the loop changes in the presence of cardiac dysfunction caused by valve disorders and heart failure. In heart failure, the pressure volume loop moves to the right compared with a normal pattern.

Stroke Volume and Ejection Fraction

Stroke Volume

The volume of blood ejected during systole is known as the *stroke volume*. It is measured in milliliters (mL). Stroke volume multiplied by heart rate is a common measure of cardiac output. Stroke volume is influenced by preload, afterload, and contractility (Figure 1-7). Stroke volume is precisely calculated as the difference between end-diastolic volume (preload) and end-systolic volume. This is shown conceptually in the pressure volume loop in Figure 1-6, *B*. In clinical practice, stroke volume can be computed during LV cardiac catheterization, as shown in Figure 1-8.

Alternatively, if the cardiac output (in milliliters per minute [mL/min]) and heart rate are known, stroke volume can be calculated using the equation: stroke volume = cardiac output ÷ heart rate, or SV = CO ÷ HR (Table 1-2). For example, CO = 5 liters per minute (L/min; 5000 mL/min) divided by HR of 72 beats per minute (beats/min), approximates a stroke volume of 70 mL. See Table 1-3 for normal hemodynamic values.

Ejection Fraction

The ejection fraction (EF) can be calculated during cardiac catheterization or with bedside echocardiography. It represents the percentage of available preload that is ejected as stroke volume each beat. In other words, EF% represents the ratio of stroke volume to end-diastolic volume (see Table 1-2).

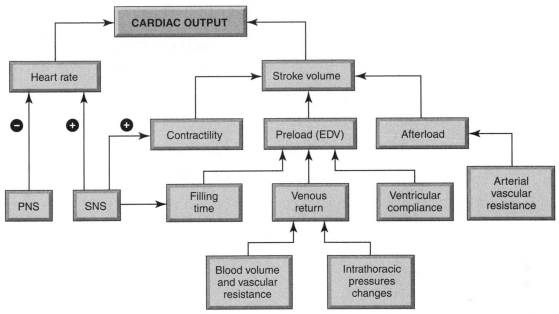

FIGURE 1-7 Determinants of cardiac output. *EDV*, End-diastolic volume; *PNS*, parasympathetic nervous system; *SNS*, sympathetic nervous system.

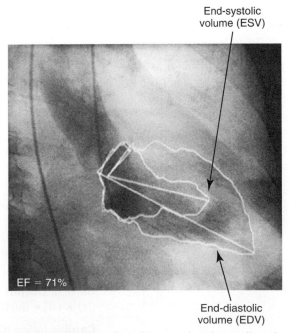

FIGURE 1-8 Cardiac catheterization: end-diastolic volume and end-systolic volume.

TABLE 1-2   Physiologic Equations

PHYSICS EQUATIONS	CLINICAL EQUATIONS
Resistance $\text{Resistance (R)} = \dfrac{\text{Pressure Difference}}{\text{Flow (Q)}}(\Delta P)$ $R = \dfrac{P1 - P2}{Q}(\Delta P)$ *This equation can also be rearranged as:* $\text{Flow (Q)} = \dfrac{\text{Pressure Difference}}{\text{Resistance (R)}}(\Delta P)$ $Q = \dfrac{P1 - P2}{R}(\Delta P)$	**Vascular Resistance** **Pulmonary Vascular Resistance (PVR)** $PVR = 80 \bullet \text{Mean PAP} - \text{LAP (PAOP)}/CO$ *Can also be written as:* $PVR = 80 \bullet \dfrac{\text{Mean PAP} - \text{LAP (PAOP)}}{CO}$ **Systemic Vascular Resistance (SVR)** $SVR = 80 \bullet \text{MAP} - \text{RAP (CVP)}/CO$ *Can also be written as:* $SVR = 80 \bullet \dfrac{\text{MAP} - \text{RAP (CVP)}}{CO}$
Poiseuille's Law $R = 8L\eta / \pi r^4$	*Related clinical concept is described in the text; a clinical equivalent equation does not exist.*
Poiseuille's Equation $Q = \Delta P\, \underline{8L\eta} / \pi r^4$	*Related clinical concept is described in the text; a clinical equivalent equation does not exist.*
Laplace's Law $P = 2\, T/r$	*Related clinical concept is described in the text; a clinical equivalent equation does not exist.*
	Mean Arterial Pressure (MAP) $MAP = SBP + (2 \bullet DBP)/3$ *The MAP equation is also written as:* $MAP = DBP + (\tfrac{1}{3})(SBP - SDP)$
	Stroke Volume (SV) $SV = CO/HR$ (multiply by 1000 to convert from milliliters to liters)
	Mean Pulmonary Artery Pressure (mPAP) $mPAP = PAS + (2 \bullet PAD)/3$ *The mPAP equation is also written as:* $mPAP = PAS + (\tfrac{1}{3})(PAS - PAD)$
	Cardiac Output (CO) in liters* $CO = HR \bullet SV/1000$
	Cardiac Index (CI)* $CI = CO/BSA$

TABLE 1-2 **Physiologic Equations—cont'd**	
PHYSICS EQUATIONS	**CLINICAL EQUATIONS**
	Ejection Fraction (EF) EF = SV/EDV *EF is reported as a %.*
	Arterial Pulse Pressure (PP) PP = SBP − DBP

*All equations that include Cardiac Output can be converted to indexed values by substituting the Cardiac Index for Cardiac Output in the equation.

—, Minus; +, plus; /, divided by; •, multiplied by. **Physics Equations Legend:** ΔP, Delta P, a change in pressure along a length of tube; η, Greek letter *eta* signifies fluid viscosity; *L*, length of a tube; *P1 – P2*, pressure difference between inflow and outflow ends of a tube; π, Greek letter *pi*; *Q*, flow rate measured as volume ÷ time; *r*, internal radius of a tube; *R*, resistance to flow measured as mm Hg × time ÷ volume; r^A, radius raised to the fourth power. **Clinical Equations Legend:** *BSA*, Body surface area; *CO*, cardiac output; *CVP*, central venous pressure; *DBP*, diastolic blood pressure; *EDV*, end-diastolic volume; *EF*, ejection fraction; *HR*, heart rate; *LAP*, left atrial pressure (PAOP or wedge is used as a surrogate for LAP); *MAP*, mean arterial pressure; *PAD*, pulmonary artery diastolic pressure; *PAOP*, pulmonary artery occlusion pressure; *PAP*, pulmonary artery pressure (mPAP=mean); *PAS*, pulmonary artery systolic pressure; *PVR*, pulmonary vascular resistance; *RAP*, right atrial pressure (CVP is used as a surrogate for RAP); *SBP*, systolic blood pressure; *SV*, stroke volume.

TABLE 1-3 **Hemodynamic Normal Value Ranges**	
HEMODYNAMIC PARAMETER	**NORMAL RANGE**
Heart rate (HR)	60–100 beats/min
Arterial blood pressure (ABP)	ABP Systolic: 90–140 mm Hg ABP Diastolic: 60-80 mm Hg
Mean arterial pressure (MAP)	70–100 mm Hg
Central venous pressure (CVP) Right atrial pressure (RAP)	2–6 mm Hg
Right ventricular pressure (RVP)	RV Systolic: 15–30 mm Hg RV Diastolic: 2–8 mm Hg
Pulmonary artery pressure (PAP)	PAP Systolic (PAS): 15–30 mm Hg PAP Diastolic (PAD: 8–15 mm Hg
Mean pulmonary artery pressure (mPAP)	9–18 mm Hg
Pulmonary artery occlusion pressure (PAOP) also known as "wedge" pressure or left atrial pressure (LAP)	4–12 mm Hg
Cardiac output (CO)*	4.0–8.0 L/min

Continued

TABLE 1-3 Hemodynamic Normal Value Ranges—cont'd	
HEMODYNAMIC PARAMETER	**NORMAL RANGE**
Cardiac index (CI)*	2.5–4.0 L/min/m^2
Stroke volume (SV)	60–100 mL
Systemic vascular resistance (SVR)	800–1200 dynes·sec/cm^5
Pulmonary vascular resistance (PVR)	<250 dynes·sec/cm^5
Pulmonary vascular resistance in Wood units	<3

*All equations that include Cardiac Output can be converted to indexed values by substituting the Cardiac Index for Cardiac Output in the equation.

beats/min, Beats per minute; *cm*, centimeter; *L/min*, liters per minute; *L/min/m^2*, liters per minute per square meter; *mL*, milliliters; *mm Hg*, millimeters of mercury; *sec*, seconds.

A healthy heart at rest ejects about 55% to 70% of the preload volume and ejects a higher percentage during exercise. An injured ventricle ejects considerably less. In severe heart failure, the ejection fraction is less than 30%. Another consequence of a low ejection fraction is that a larger amount of blood remains in the ventricle at the end of systole with a higher end-systolic volume.

Cardiac Output

Blood flow through the cardiac cycle depends on continual blood supply (venous return), pressure adaptability within the vascular tree, pumping force, and a heart pacemaker. These characteristics are more commonly described as preload, afterload, contractility, and heart rate (see Figure 1-7). Working synchronously, these factors influence both stability and variation in cardiac output. These four components provide the foundation for hemodynamic intervention in clinical practice.

Preload

The definition of preload is the volume in the ventricle at end-diastole. This end-diastolic volume is illustrated in Figure 1-3. End-diastolic volume or preload is the volume in the ventricles just before the semilunar valves close and ventricular filling is complete. Preload can be described for both the right ventricle (RVEDV) and the left ventricle (LVEDV). Logically, venous return volume must ultimately equal the cardiac output volume because the cardiovascular system is a closed double-loop, as shown in Figure 1-9.

Right Atrial Preload and Venous Return

The right atrial preload volume is influenced by multiple physiologic factors, including venous pressure, venous return, and right atrial pressure (see Figure 1-7).

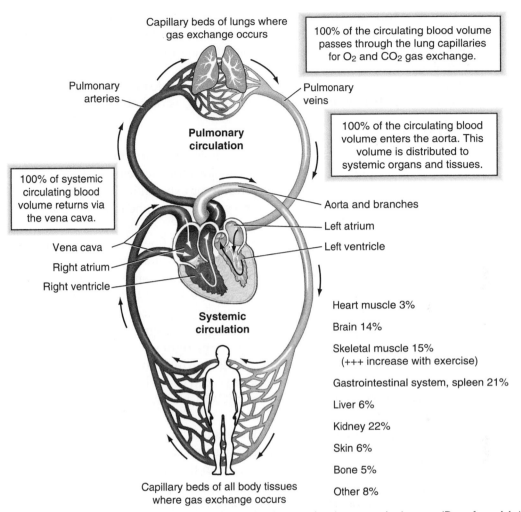

Capillary beds of lungs where gas exchange occurs

100% of the circulating blood volume passes through the lung capillaries for O_2 and CO_2 gas exchange.

Pulmonary arteries

Pulmonary veins

Pulmonary circulation

100% of the circulating blood volume enters the aorta. This volume is distributed to systemic organs and tissues.

100% of systemic circulating blood volume returns via the vena cava.

Aorta and branches

Left atrium

Left ventricle

Vena cava

Right atrium

Right ventricle

Systemic circulation

Heart muscle 3%

Brain 14%

Skeletal muscle 15% (+++ increase with exercise)

Gastrointestinal system, spleen 21%

Liver 6%

Kidney 22%

Skin 6%

Bone 5%

Other 8%

Capillary beds of all body tissues where gas exchange occurs

FIGURE 1-9 Blood circulation by percentage distribution in a resting (not exercise) state. (Data from Mohrman DE, Heller LJ: *Cardiovascular physiology*, ed 8, New York, 2014, McGraw Hill Medical.)

A small pressure gradient of 4 to 8 mm Hg exists between the venous system and the right atrium. This pressure difference drives venous blood flow toward the lower-pressure right atrium. Because 70% of the total blood volume lies within the venous system, not all of this volume can return to the right heart at the same time. Several liters of blood are always in reserve in the large sinuses of the spleen, the liver, and the veins and venules. The storage capacity of the venous system is remarkable. A systemic vein is 24 times more compliant than its corresponding artery.[3] A vein is eight times more distensible (can expand or enlarge) and is able to hold three times the volume of a similar artery.[3] This reserve volume is sometimes referred to as the venous "unstressed" volume. Reserve volume may be converted to a "stressed" volume when an increase in venous return is required. This concept is also discussed in the chapter on the hemodynamics of mechanical ventilation (see Chapter 14).

Venous return and, thus, preload are managed by well-calibrated physiologic mechanisms. Atrial stretch receptors—the arterial baroreceptors (aortic and carotid)—are responsive to hypovolemia and stimulate the sympathetic nervous system to increase arterial and venous vascular tone to augment venous flow. A healthy right ventricle is compliant and adapts easily to sudden changes in preload volume. Venous return is also influenced by changes in intrathoracic pressures, as described in the following section.

Right Ventricular Preload

Right ventricular end-diastolic volume is clinically referred to as right ventricular preload. It is dependent on flow from the major thoracic veins and is facilitated by the mechanics of venous return and inspiration or exhalation. The right ventricular end-diastolic volume is important, as it represents the volume that is available for ejection from the right side of the heart.

The effect of the respiratory mechanics on blood flow is sometimes described as the thoracic pump. During spontaneous breathing, inspiratory pleural pressure becomes more negative than the surrounding atmospheric pressure to draw air into the lungs. All thoracic structures, including the veins, are subject to this decrease in inspiratory pressure. The hemodynamic effect of negative inspiratory pressure is to facilitate venous blood flow from areas of slightly higher pressure, for example, the abdominal and cerebral vessels, via the vena cava into the right side of the heart.[4,5] No valves are present between the vena cava and the right atrium, so blood flow is continuous and unimpeded. For decades, clinicians have placed central venous catheters into the vena cava to measure central venous pressure (CVP), which is similar to right atrial pressure (RAP), as a surrogate for RV preload volume.

It is now well understood that CVP measured in millimeters of mercury (mm Hg) is an indirect and inexact estimate of right ventricular (RV) preload volume and that the relationship between volume and pressure in the vena cava or the right atrium is not linear.[6] Because it is clinically useful to estimate RV preload volume, clinicians continue to search for the most effective clinical measurement techniques.[7] Some of the physiologic reasons that contribute to the inherent difficulty in using pressure to measure central volume are described below.

Normal intrathoracic pressures are dramatically altered by the use of positive pressure mechanical ventilation and positive end-expiratory pressure (PEEP). Positive pressure ventilation raises intrathoracic pressure above atmospheric pressure during the inspiratory phase. PEEP increases intrathoracic pressure throughout the entire ventilator cycle. This increase in intrathoracic pressure may decrease venous return and reduce RV preload volume.[5,8] The positive pressure from mechanical ventilation and PEEP may artificially elevate the measured CVP value. Efforts have always been made to avoid undue influence of intrathoracic pressure fluctuations on hemodynamic pressures. CVP or RAP measurements are taken at the end of expiration at a stable or "static" point in the respiratory cycle.[9]

Newer assessment methods use "dynamic" indices. These incorporate the effects of pressure fluctuations associated with breathing on CVP and arterial pressure waveforms to assess the patient's fluid volume status.[10] Several chapters in this text address the challenges of accurately assessing RV preload at the bedside. Chapter 4 describes the challenges of obtaining an accurate CVP measurement; Chapter 12 explains the effects of respiratory variation on vena cava volume assessed with bedside echocardiography, and Chapter 14 describes the effects of mechanical ventilation on venous return.

Left Ventricular Preload

Left ventricular end-diastolic volume is also known as LV preload and is the volume in the left ventricle at end diastole just before the mitral valve closes. LV preload volume (end-diastolic volume) can be visually assessed in the cardiac catheterization laboratory from the contours of the ventricular wall. Ventricular end-systolic volume can be estimated as shown in Figure 1-8. LV preload is also measured indirectly using the pulmonary artery occlusion pressure (PAOP) or "wedge" pressure. The PAOP is obtained using a right-sided pulmonary artery catheter as described in Chapter 5.

Because the left ventricle is the major pumping chamber for the systemic circulation, the LV preload volume is an essential precursor of cardiac output. However, LV preload is far from being the only factor that determines the cardiac output, as described below.

Starling's Law of the Heart

Alterations in preload may alter cardiac output. At end diastole, an increase in preload volume, will cause the cardiac muscle to be stretched, which, in a healthy heart, increases the force of the following cardiac contraction. This is known as Starling's law of the heart. However, Starling's law also holds that if the cardiac muscle is overstretched and the ventricle is overdistended, cardiac output will decrease. This concept is visually represented as the Starling curve shown in Figure 1-10. The Startling curve's vertical axis represents ventricular volume output, and the horizontal axis represents ventricular pressure (mm Hg).

The invasive pressure catheter systems measuring static CVP and RAP or PAOP have fallen out of favor, although dynamic indices that conceptually incorporate changes in the slope of the Starling curve are used increasingly. Clinical applications of dynamic indices are described in detail in the chapter on arterial waveform and pressure-based hemodynamic monitoring (see Chapter 12).

Pressure–Volume Relationships and the Starling Curve

The underlying principle that supports pressure–volume relationships is that higher ventricular preload volumes are associated with higher intraventricular pressures. It is important to emphasize that pressure–volume relationships are not linear. According to Starling's law, if the volumetric load becomes too great, cardiac muscle fibers become overdistended and are less contractile, intraventricular pressures will be unusually high, and cardiac output decreases (see Figure 1-10). The classic example is heart failure with a dilated ventricle where the preload end-diastolic volume is much higher than normal, but limited contractility means the ejected stroke volume and

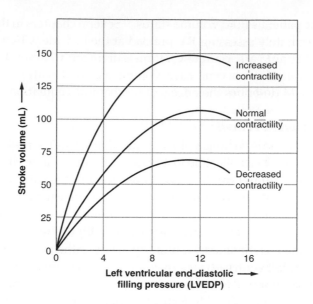

FIGURE 1-10 The Starling curve.

ejection fraction are lower than normal. This low ejection produces a higher end-systolic volume than would be expected in a healthy heart. Decreased LV compliance is an impediment to filling of the left ventricle.

Afterload

Resistance to ejection from the ventricles is often described as *afterload*. This resistance is the pressure load that the contracting ventricular chamber must overcome to open the semilunar valve and eject blood into the associated great vessel (aorta or pulmonary artery). The greater the afterload pressure, the greater is the wall stress on the contracting myocardial fibers. Calculating wall stress directly is not possible at the bedside, so a clinical surrogate value of vascular resistance is used. Resistance across the vascular bed can be calculated for both the right ventricle and the left ventricle.

Pulmonary Vascular Resistance

Right ventricular afterload is calculated as pulmonary vascular resistance (PVR) using data obtained from a pulmonary artery catheter. The equation uses pressure measurements into and out of the right side of the heart and pulmonary vasculature divided by flow: Mean pulmonary artery pressure – left atrial pressure (measured by PAOP) divided by cardiac output. The result is referred to as a Wood unit.[11] The Wood unit is converted to a metric resistance unit by multiplying the value by 80. The equation for calculating PVR is shown in Table 1-2. The clinical equations for calculating vascular resistance are derived from the physics of fluid dynamics, reviewed later in the chapter (see the section on Blood Vessel Pressure, Flow, and Resistance). Pressures in the pulmonary vascular system are normally low, as much as one sixth of systemic pressures as shown in Figure 1-4. The low RV afterload is reflective of the thin walls of that chamber. Normal PVR is <250 dynes $\cdot$ sec/cm^5 (see Table 1-3).

Systemic Vascular Resistance

LV afterload is calculated as systemic vascular resistance (SVR) by using data obtained by a pulmonary artery catheter. The equation is based on the physics of fluid dynamics and measures pressure into and out of the left side of the heart divided by flow: Mean inflow pressure (P_1) in the left atrium $-$ mean outflow pressure (P_2) in the aorta; clinically, a radial or femoral mean arterial pressure (MAP) are often used. The numerical difference between inflow and outflow pressure ($P_1 - P_2$) is divided by the measured blood flow (cardiac output) as listed in Table 1-2. The higher systemic vascular pressure is reflected in the larger muscle mass of the LV chamber wall. The units of measurement for SVR were originally reported as pressure (mm Hg) divided by flow (cardiac output in mL/min), written as mm Hg $\cdot$ min $\cdot$ mL^{-1}. In the present day, SVR values are reported using the metric system of measurement, as dynes $\cdot$ sec/cm^5.[2] Normal SVR is 800–1200 dynes $\cdot$ sec/cm^5 (see Table 1-3).

Contractility

The force of ventricular contraction is also known as *inotropy*. Ventricular contractility is the amount of muscle shortening required to create the force of contraction. No specific number corresponds to contractility, so it is inferred from other clinical variables such as preload volumes and cardiac output.

Heart Rate

Electrical depolarization from the sinus node stimulates the heart rate in sinus rhythm. Heart rate is a determinant of cardiac output as shown in Figure 1-7.

Blood Circulation

Hemodynamic structures are generally not drawn as they anatomically exist in the body but in a way that illustrates function. This is certainly true when describing blood circulation, as shown in Figure 1-9, where organs are schematically illustrated to demonstrate an arterial entry via the aorta and a venous exit via the vena cava. All of the major systemic organs receive arterial blood of a very similar oxygenation quality, although the quantity depends on the organ's requirements. Abdominal organs that have major blood cleansing functions (kidney, spleen, liver) receive much larger arterial flows than are needed to supply their own metabolic needs. This excess flow means that these organs are well protected in times of low cardiac output. It also ensures that tissue ischemia is minimized.[12] In contrast, the brain and heart muscle only receive arterial blood supply sufficient for their tissues' metabolic needs and no extra flow; consequently, these organs are vulnerable to ischemia in times of low cardiac output or low oxygenation.[12]

Arterial Vascular Dynamics

Arterial vessels are not static tubes. Vasodilation and vasoconstriction constantly adjust vascular tone to alter blood flow. All vessel walls, except capillaries, contain smooth muscle. Dynamic changes in the vascular lumen are influenced by physiologic stimuli that may be neural, local, or hormonal.[12] Vascular smooth muscle cells are 5 to 50 micrometers (mcm) in size, and use myosin and actin as cross-bridges to create force and shortening of the space between thick and thin filaments. This means that arterioles always have intrinsic tone, also known as *basal tone*, which maintains a partially constricted state even without other physiologic influences.[12] Neural, local, and hormonal influences act on this intrinsic tone to either dilate or constrict target vessels.

The primary conductor of this delicate physiologic orchestra is the autonomic nervous system. Autonomic functions describe physiologic actions that are not under conscious control. The autonomic nervous system is composed of two complementary neural systems, named sympathetic and parasympathetic. These systems innervate the same organs but exert different effects. Organs and vessels innervated by the autonomic nervous system are shown in Figure 1-11.

Sympathetic Nervous System

The sympathetic nervous system is one division of the autonomic nervous system. Neural fibers from the sympathetic nervous system innervate arterioles in the major systemic organs, as illustrated in Figure 1-11, *A*. In response to physiologic stress, an increase in electrical neural discharge causes the sympathetic nerve endings to release the catecholamine *norepinephrine*, which targets the alpha-1 adrenergic receptor on vascular smooth muscle cells. Norepinephrine causes arteriolar vasoconstriction by stimulating the release of intracellular calcium. A massive sympathetic nervous system discharge produces the phenomenon commonly known as the "fight or flight" reflex.

Parasympathetic Nervous System

The parasympathetic nervous system is the other division of the autonomic nervous system shown in Figure 1-11, *B*. The parasympathetic nerve endings discharge *acetylcholine*, but because the parasympathetic system does not innervate arterioles, it has less impact on vascular dynamics and blood pressure. Although, the parasympathetic nervous system has a big effect on heart rate through the actions of the vagus nerve on the atrial sinus node. Increased vagal stimulation leads to an increase in neural firing that decreases sinoatrial node depolarization producing a lower heart rate.

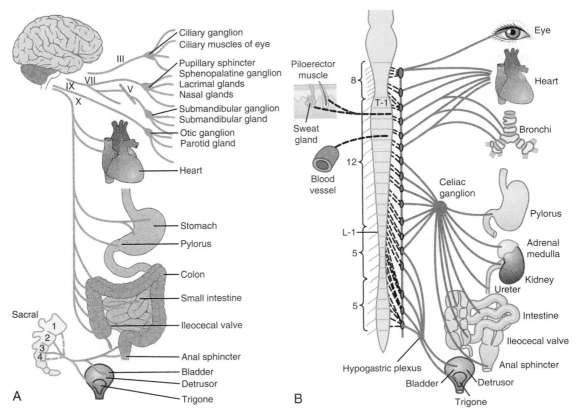

FIGURE 1-11 A, Autonomic nervous system: sympathetic. **B,** Autonomic nervous system: parasympathetic. (From Guyton AC, Hall JE: *Textbook of medical physiology*, ed 12, Philadelphia, 2011, Saunders.)

Alpha- and Beta-Adrenergic Receptors

The autonomic nervous system functions via neural discharge of compounds that target specific cell receptors.[13,14] Through the actions of the receptors, the autonomic nervous system exerts control over cardiac output and vascular tone. The major classes of adrenergic receptors are designated alpha and beta, with subunits in each class with specific actions. Both alpha-1 receptors and beta-2 receptors are located in peripheral vascular smooth muscle cell membranes. Under different physiologic conditions, or in response to pharmacologic stimulation, either vasoconstriction (alpha-1) or vasodilation (beta-2) effects may predominate. Presynaptic alpha-2 receptors inhibit the actions of norepinephrine. Beta-1 receptors are located in the cardiac myocytes and increase cardiac contractility when stimulated (Table 1-4).

Oxygen

Oxygen levels impact vascular tone. Tissue hypoxia lowers the partial pressure of oxygen (PO_2) in the interstitial fluid surrounding blood vessels; this decreases arteriolar

TABLE 1-4	**Vasoactive Receptors and Hemodynamic Effects***	
RECEPTOR (ABBREVIATION)	**LOCATION**	**ACTION WHEN STIMULATED**
Alpha-1 (α_1)	Vascular smooth muscle (arteries and veins)	Stimulation of alpha-receptor in peripheral arteries causes vasoconstriction and raises blood pressure and SVR
Alpha-2 (α_2)	Central nervous system: Cerebral cortex Brainstem Spinal column	Alpha-2 receptors in the CNS mediate SNS feedback and inhibit release of: • Norepinephrine • Acetylcholine
Beta-1 (β_1)	Myocardium Atria Ventricles	Increase • Heart Rate • Contractility
Beta-2 (β_2)	Vascular smooth muscle (arteries and veins) Bronchioles (lung)	Beta-2 receptors vasodilate arteries and veins, thus impacting BP and CO. Widens bronchioles
Dopaminergic	Kidney Mesenteric vessels	Vasodilation
Vasopressin 1 (V_1)	Vascular smooth muscle	Vasoconstriction
Vasopressin 2 (V_2)	Kidney	Re-absorbs water from the kidney tubules

*Many of the listed receptors have multiple subtypes. Only the receptors with documented hemodynamic effects are listed.
BP, Blood pressure; *CNS*, central nervous system; *CO*, cardiac output; *SNS*, sympathetic nervous system; *SVR*, systemic vascular resistance.

tone, which results in vasodilation. Conversely, high oxygen levels around the microvasculature cause an increase in vascular tone, leading to vasoconstriction.[12]

Nitric Oxide

Nitric oxide is synthesized within the endothelial cells that cover the interior vessel walls. It is a small lipid-soluble molecule that diffuses rapidly into the arteriolar smooth muscle cells, decreasing vascular tone with resultant vasodilation. Nitric oxide is made from the amino acid *L-arginine* and the enzyme nitric oxide synthase. The potent intravenous (IV) vasodilators nitroprusside and nitroglycerin both exert their vasodilator effects through increased nitric oxide production. These vasoactive medications impact venous tone as well as arterial tone and are discussed further in Chapter 9.

Venous Vascular Dynamics

The anatomy of veins is different from the anatomy of arteries. Veins have thin walls with minimal smooth muscle. The smooth muscle present in venules and larger veins is innervated by the sympathetic nervous system. Veins also respond to the release of norepinephrine, which activates alpha-1 receptors so that venoconstriction can occur.[12] Veins are described as the *capacitance vessels* of the body because over 70% of the blood volume resides within the venous system.[4] Veins are much more compliant than arteries and easily expand to accommodate volume changes.[3]

Blood Vessel Pressure, Flow, and Resistance across the Vasculature

The pressure difference between the arterial and venous vessels in a normotensive person is about 100 mm Hg. This large pressure difference helps propel blood through the vascular system from arteries to arterioles to capillaries to venules to veins as shown in Figure 1-12.[3] Blood pressure is highest in the aorta and then disperses to numerous arteries and arterioles with smaller diameters. Blood pressure is sustained throughout the arterial tree because of the intrinsic tone of vascular smooth muscle in the arteriolar walls. Arterioles always maintain some intrinsic tone.[12]

Blood flow through vessels is facilitated by the interplay among pressure, flow, and resistance. The physiology of flow derives from the physics of fluid dynamics. The tube shown in Figure 1-13 could represent any blood vessel in the body. Blood will flow through the vessel only when a sufficient pressure difference exists between inflow pressure (P_1) and outflow pressure (P_2). This pressure difference is also described as delta P (ΔP). All components are dynamic.[3] The rate of flow (Q) may be altered by pressure changes between the two ends of the tube and by changes in resistance (R).[4] The equations are listed in Table 1-2.

These principles are applied on a daily basis in operating rooms and critical care units, where vasoactive medications are administered to patients to alter vascular resistance and to alter blood flow across vascular beds. Vasodilators decrease vascular resistance and increase blood flow. Vasopressors increase arterial tone and increase systemic vascular resistance. Vasopressors may also constrict small venules.[4]

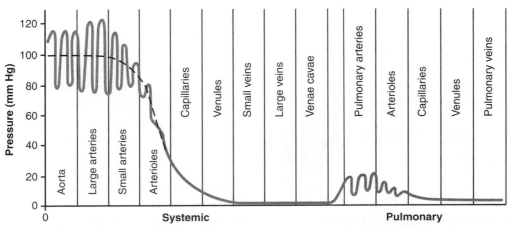

FIGURE 1-12 Pressure changes across the arterial and venous vascular systems. (From Guyton AC, Hall JE: *Textbook of medical physiology*, ed 12, Philadelphia, 2011, Saunders.)

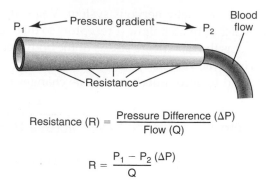

$$R = \frac{P_1 - P_2 \ (\Delta P)}{Q}$$

FIGURE 1-13 Blood vessel pressure, flow and resistance across the vasculature.

Poiseuille's Law

In 1846, Jean Leonard Marie Poiseuille published the results of a series of experiments about rates of water flow (Q) through small glass capillary tubes. He identified factors that alter resistance (R). Poiseuille listed three key factors: (1) the internal radius (r) of the tube, where the radius × 2 equals the internal diameter, (2) the tube length (L), and (3) the fluid viscosity (η).

The resultant equation is shown in Table 1-2. This law states that fluid flow through a system is related to the pressure difference across the system divided by the resistance to flow.[4] Because in this equation, the internal radius of the tube is raised to the fourth power (πr^4), even a small change in the radius has a huge impact on resistance to flow.[4] The clinical relevance is that a twofold increase in vessel radius allows vascular resistance to decrease 16-fold in that vessel.[2] This is illustrated in Figure 1-14. Note that the radius is half the diameter of a circle. These factors were later applied to the hemodynamics of blood circulation.

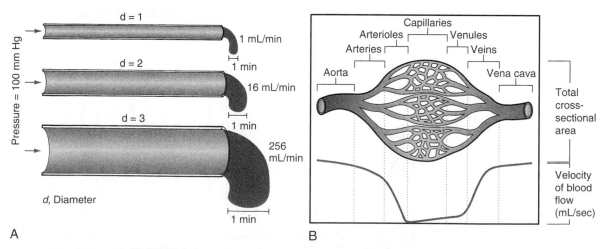

FIGURE 1-14 Poiseuille's law effect of vessel diameter on blood flow. (**A**, From McCance KL, Huether SE, eds. *Pathophysiology: the biologic basis for disease in adults and children*, ed 6, St. Louis, 2010, Mosby; **B**, from Thibodeau G, Patton K: *Anatomy and physiology*, ed 8, St. Louis, 2013, Mosby.)

LaPlace's Law

Vascular flow dynamics are also affected by transmural pressure. LaPlace's law describes the relationship between the pressures inside the vessel and the pressures outside the vessel wall, otherwise described as *transmural* pressure. The wall tension (T), vessel radius (r), and thickness of the vessel wall (M) each influence the transmural pressure (P). High transmural pressure is usually associated with a thin vessel wall, a small radius, and higher wall tension. Low transmural pressure is associated with a thicker vessel wall, a larger radius, and lower wall tension. As with other vascular fluid dynamics principles, this law is described by an equation, as listed in Table 1-2.

Laminar and Turbulent Flow

Blood flow is faster in the middle of the vessel, where the drag from the vessel wall is less, as illustrated in Figure 1-15. Turbulence is caused by vessel bifurcation and also pathologic vessel wall irregularities such as atherosclerotic plaque. Other factors that influence laminar flow include blood viscosity and blood volume.

Regulation of Blood Pressure

Arterial blood pressure is regulated by the autonomic nervous system (composed of sympathetic and parasympathetic nerves) and the vasomotor center located in the lower third of the brainstem within the lower pons and the medulla oblongata. Both sympathetic and parasympathetic fibers traverse the brainstem and communicate with specialized vasomotor tissues that regulate vasoconstriction and vasodilation. Incoming information is relayed by the parasympathetic system, predominantly by the vagus and glossopharyngeal cranial nerves, and output action is relayed via the sympathetic nervous system.

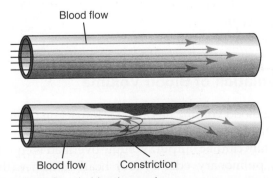

FIGURE 1-15 Laminar and turbulent flow in blood vessels.

Arterial Baroreceptors

Arterial pressure sensors, called *baroreceptors*, relay information about central arterial pressure back to the vasomotor center in the brainstem. Baroreceptors have sensory nerve endings situated in the tunica adventitia of the arterial wall of the aortic arch, and at the bifurcation of the carotid artery, a location described as the carotid sinus (Figure 1-16, *A*). These receptors are sensitive to changes in pressure and stretch and communicate changes in vessel pressure via the autonomic nervous system. Higher arterial pressures trigger faster neural firing rates. Within a single cardiac cycle, baroreceptors depolarize more rapidly during systole compared with diastole.

Baroreceptors, in combination with the autonomic nervous system (sympathetic and parasympathetic) precisely regulate blood pressure in a highly responsive feedback loop (Figure 1-16, *B*). In hypertensive states, baroreceptors depolarize more quickly to inhibit sympathetic nerve activity; this response also allows greater parasympathetic outflow. In hypotension, slower baroreceptor depolarization rates stimulate sympathetic nerve activity and the release of norepinephrine from the sympathetic nerve endings to increase blood pressure

The most important arterial baroreceptor site is the carotid sinus located at the bifurcation of the internal and external carotid arteries. Carotid baroreceptors connect to the medulla oblongata via branches of the glossopharyngeal nerve (cranial nerve IX). Carotid sinus baroreceptors respond to arterial pressures within a range of 60 to 180 mm Hg. The second baroreceptor site is located in the aortic arch (see Figure 1-16, *A*). Arterial baroreceptor signals are transmitted to the medulla oblongata via branches of the vagus nerve (cranial nerve X).

Baroreceptor responsiveness is important for short-term adjustments needed to manage sudden changes in arterial blood pressure. The baroreceptors work in tandem with the neurohormonal mechanisms used to regulate venous return and circulating blood volume, as described below.

Stretch Receptors

The junction between the right atrium and the vena cava contains stretch receptors that are sensitive to changes in preload volume. The parasympathetic vagus nerve relays information about the volumetric stretch from the right atrium to the medulla oblongata in the brainstem.

Neurohormonal Regulation of Blood Volume

The circulating blood volume has a major impact on hemodynamic stability. If the circulating volume is inadequate, hypovolemia results in hypotension and reflex tachycardia to maintain cardiac output. Volume overload is equally problematic, as it causes hypertension, pulmonary edema, and heart failure with reduced cardiac output.

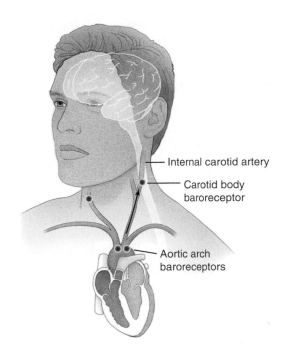

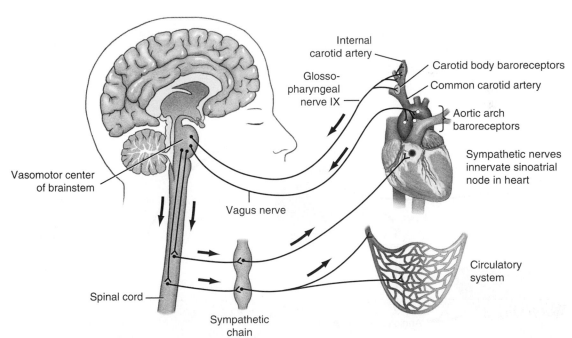

FIGURE 1-16 Arterial baroreceptors.

Several neurohormonal mechanisms involving multiple organs act in concert to optimize circulating volume, as described below.

Renin–Angiotensin–Aldosterone System

The kidneys, in conjunction with the renin–angiotensin–aldosterone system (RAAS) are major regulators of circulating fluid volume. The kidney is sensitive to decreases in both flow and pressure. Hypotension and low cardiac output stimulate the renal sympathetic nerves and the beta-1 adrenergic receptors.[13] The adrenergic receptors are located in the juxtaglomerular apparatus (JGA) situated close to the afferent and efferent arterioles of the kidney glomerulus. JGA cells produce the enzyme renin, which acts on angiotensin, a circulating peptide synthesized by the liver. Renin converts angiotensin to angiotensin I. The vascular endothelium of the lung releases angiotensin-converting enzyme (ACE), which cleaves two amino acids from angiotensin I to form angiotensin II (Figure 1-17). Angiotensin II has powerful effects on blood pressure and circulating volume. Other tissues and organs may also produce renin as well as ACE, but the kidneys and lungs are the most important organs to do so. The actions of angiotensin II include vasoconstriction, which causes an increase in systemic vascular resistance; stimulation of the sympathetic nervous system to increase norepinephrine release; and stimulation of the adrenal cortex to release aldosterone, which subsequently acts on the kidneys to retain sodium and water. Once an arcane physiologic pathway, renin and ACE are now well known because of the ubiquitous use of ACE inhibitors and angiotensin receptor blockers (ARBs). Both ACE inhibitors and ARBs interrupt the neurohormonal RAAS pathway to manage symptoms of heart

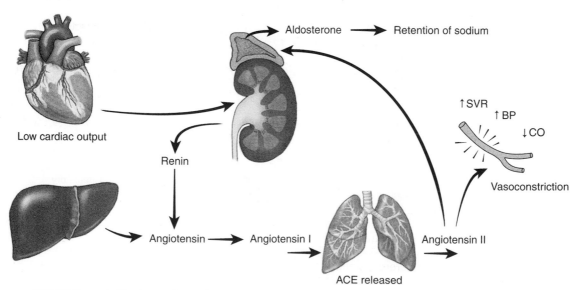

FIGURE 1-17 Renin–angiotensin–aldosterone system (RAAS). *ACE*, Angiotensin converting enzyme; *BP*, blood pressure; *CO*, cardiac output; *SVR*, systemic vascular resistance.

failure. Acting at the end of this pathway, aldosterone inhibitors are also prescribed to patients with heart failure.

Natriuretic Peptides

In response to volume overload and atrial distention, atrial and ventricular cells synthesize natriuretic peptides that rise in uncompensated heart failure. These are generally referred to as A-type (atrial) and B-type (ventricular) natriuretic peptides. The actions of the natriuretic peptides are the direct opposite of the RAAS pathway. They decrease renin release, decrease aldosterone secretion by the adrenal cortex, and increase glomerular filtration and diuresis. Natriuretic peptides have been described as a counter-regulatory mechanism to the RAAS pathway.[2]

Antidiuretic Hormone (Vasopressin)

Antidiuretic hormone (ADH), also known as *arginine vasopressin*, is released from the posterior pituitary gland in response to increased serum osmolality. The two terms accurately describe the actions of this hormone. It acts on the distal tubules of the kidney to increase the amount of water returned from the tubules back to the bloodstream (the antidiuretic effect) via V-2 receptors (see Table 1-4). It also acts on smooth muscle receptors in arteries to stimulate vasoconstriction and raise blood pressure (the vasopressin effect) via V-1 receptors (see Table 1-4). Vasopressin can be pharmacologically administered as a continuous IV infusion to increase blood pressure in the treatment of sepsis.

Conclusion

The science of hemodynamic monitoring is based on the physiologic principles of flow, pressure, and resistance. These fundamental concepts have been presented in a variety of formats for better understanding. The clinician who understands this physiology is more likely to be able to interpret clinical values and apply critical thinking to individual clinical situations.

References
1. Ribatti D: William Harvey and the discovery of the circulation of the blood, *J Angiogenes Res* 1(3), 2009.
2. Klabunde RE: *Cardiovascular physiology concepts*, ed 2, Philadelphia, 2012, Lippincott Williams & Wilkins, Wolters Kluwer.
3. Hall JE: *Guyton and Hall's textbook of medical physiology,* ed 12, Philadelphia, 2010, Elsevier.
4. Funk DJ, Jacobsohn E, Kumar A: The role of venous return in critical illness and shock-part I: physiology, *Crit Care Med* 41(1):255–262, 2013.
5. Broccard AF: Cardiopulmonary interactions and volume status assessment, *J Clin Monit Comput* 26(5):383–391, 2012.

6. Marik PE, Baram M, Vahid B: Does central venous pressure predict fluid responsiveness? A systematic review of the literature and the tale of seven mares, *Chest* 134(1):172–178, 2008.
7. Marik PE, Monnet X, Teboul JL: Hemodynamic parameters to guide fluid therapy, *Ann Intensive Care* 1(1):1, 2011.
8. Magder S: Hemodynamic monitoring in the mechanically ventilated patient, *Curr Opin Crit Care* 17(1):36–42, 2011.
9. Nahouraii RA, Rowell SE: Static measures of preload assessment, *Crit Care Clin* 26(2):295–305, 2010.
10. Enomoto TM, Harder L: Dynamic indices of preload, *Crit Care Clin* 26(2):307–321, 2010.
11. McLaughlin VV, Archer SL, Badesch DB, et al.: ACCF/AHA 2009 expert consensus document on pulmonary hypertension: a report of the American College of Cardiology Foundation Task Force on Expert Consensus Documents and the American Heart Association: developed in collaboration with the American College of Chest Physicians, American Thoracic Society, Inc., and the Pulmonary Hypertension Association, *Circulation* 119(16):2250–2294, 2009.
12. Mohrman DE, Heller LJ: *Cardiovascular physiology*, ed 8, New York, 2014, McGraw Hill Medical.
13. Thomas GD: Neural control of the circulation, *Adv Physiol Educ* 35(1):28–32, 2011.
14. Wachter SB, Gilbert EM: Beta-adrenergic receptors, from their discovery and characterization through their manipulation to beneficial clinical application, *Cardiology* 122(2):104–112, 2012.

Physical Assessment and Hemodynamic Monitoring

Kathleen M. Stacy

2

All body systems rely on adequate tissue perfusion to ensure optimal performance. Tissue perfusion is dependent on the balance between cellular oxygen supply and cellular oxygen demand. Adequate tissue perfusion depends on sufficient oxygen being transported to the tissues and the cell's ability to use it. Any imbalance between the two may result in cellular dysfunction and cell death. Cellular oxygen supply is dependent on cardiac output, oxygen, and hemoglobin for transport. Cellular oxygen demand is influenced by the internal metabolic environment and mitochondrial function.[1] Any alteration in cardiac function, pulmonary gas exchange, or hemoglobin levels in blood may disrupt oxygen supply to the cells, and this will alter the patient's hemodynamics. Often, the patient with hemodynamic dysfunction exhibits a variety of signs and symptoms that are evident during physical assessment. This chapter presents the clinical manifestations of altered hemodynamics commonly found during the physical assessment of an acutely ill patient.

Key Physiologic Concepts

The major determinants of oxygen delivery are cardiac output, oxygen, and hemoglobin.[1] Understanding the basic physiology of these determinants assists with identifying the physical manifestations of impaired tissue perfusion and altered hemodynamics.

Cardiac Output

The heart is a muscular pump whose primary function is to transport oxygen and other nutrients to different organs of the body for metabolism and to return carbon dioxide and other waste products to the lungs and kidneys for excretion. The amount of blood ejected from the ventricle with each heart beat is known as the stroke volume. The amount of blood pumped from the left ventricle each minute is known as the cardiac output. The cardiac output is calculated by multiplying the patient's heart rate by the stroke volume. A normal cardiac output at rest is 4 to 6 liters per minute (L/min). The main factors affecting cardiac output are heart rate, preload, afterload, and contractility (Figure 2-1).[2]

Preload is the end volumetric pressure that stretches the ventricle just prior to systole. Volumetric pressure is created by the quantity of blood in the ventricle and the

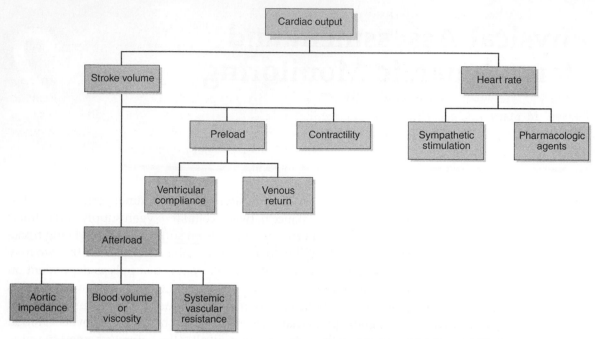

FIGURE 2-1 Determinants of cardiac output. (From Urden LD, Stacy KM, Lough ME: *Critical care nursing: diagnosis and management*, ed 7, St. Louis, 2014, Mosby.)

tension it exerts on the ventricular wall at the end of diastole. Depending on the chamber, it is commonly referred to as left ventricular end-diastolic pressure or right ventricular end-diastolic pressure.[1] Preload is determined by venous return and myocardial fiber stretch and is a major influence on the heart's ability to pump. In accordance with Starling's law, the more the ventricle fills during diastole, the greater is the myocardial fiber stretch (within limits), resulting in a stronger ventricular contraction during systole. As volume in the ventricle increases, the myocardial fibers stretch to accommodate the increasing volume. When ventricular contraction occurs, contractility is increased as a result of the increased stretch. However, if the volume is excessive, it causes the myocardial fibers to be stretched beyond their limits, and contractility decreases. Preload is a major influence on myocardial oxygen consumption.[2] Signs and symptoms of increased right ventricular preload include increased jugular venous pressure, peripheral edema, ascites, and hepatojugular reflux. Signs and symptoms of increased left ventricular preload include the presence of third and fourth heart sounds and pulmonary crackles.[3]

Afterload is the pressure against which the heart has to pump to eject blood from the ventricles during systole. Afterload is a function of arterial pressure.[1] Pressure in the aorta and larger arteries presents resistance to the left ventricle, and pressure in the pulmonary arteries presents resistance to the right ventricle. Afterload is commonly referred to as *systemic vascular resistance* (afterload of the left ventricle) and pulmonary vascular resistance (afterload of the right ventricle).[2] As afterload increases, so does ventricular contractility (within limits) as a compensatory mechanism to maintain cardiac output. Afterload is also a major influence on myocardial oxygen consumption.[1] The higher the resistance, the more the ventricle must work, thus increasing myocardial oxygen demand. Increased diastolic blood pressure can be used as an indicator of increased systemic resistance.[4]

Contractility refers to the intrinsic ability of myocardial muscle to shorten and develop tension independent of preload and afterload. Stimulation of the sympathetic nervous system increases contractility and stimulation of the parasympathetic nervous system decreases contractility.[1] Contractility is also influenced by myocardial oxygen supply and is a major influence on myocardial oxygen consumption.[2]

Oxygen

The primary functions of the pulmonary system are ventilation and respiration. Ventilation is the movement of air in and out of the lungs and is a product of the mechanical function of the pulmonary system. Respiration is the process of gas exchange by movement of oxygen from the atmosphere into the bloodstream and movement of carbon dioxide from the bloodstream into the atmosphere. Respiration is dependent on ventilation, as gas exchange cannot take place without the movement of oxygen into the lungs. Oxygen is transported to cells, where it is required for energy production via the citric acid cycle and oxidative phosphorylation. Carbon dioxide and water are metabolic byproducts.[5] Low levels of oxygen in blood is known as hypoxemia. Low level of oxygen at the tissue level is known as hypoxia.

Hemoglobin

Once respiration has taken place, the gases must be transported to the tissues for use. Oxygen in blood is carried two ways: (1) dissolved in the liquid part of the blood plasma (3%) and (2) in chemical combination with hemoglobin (97%). Most oxygen in the body is transported to the cells in combination with hemoglobin. Oxygen combines loosely and reversibly with the heme portion of hemoglobin. The average individual has about 15 grams (g) of hemoglobin in each 100 milliliters (mL) of blood. Each gram of hemoglobin has the maximum ability to combine with 1.34 mL of oxygen. Therefore, at 100% saturation, 100 mL of blood with a hemoglobin level of 15 grams would bind 20.1 mL of oxygen.[5] Low levels of hemoglobin in blood is known as *anemia.*

General Appearance

The patient's general appearance provides a wealth of information about the patient's hemodynamic status. The patient's level of consciousness and mentation provide information about perfusion of the brain. Changes in the level of consciousness, mentation, or both are indicative of inadequate perfusion of the brain and may be the result of decreased cardiac output, hypoxemia, or stroke.[6] Patient reports of fatigue, weakness, or evidence of anxiety may be indicative of decreased cardiac output or hypoxemia.[7]

TABLE 2-1	**Clarifying Chest Pain Symptoms**
DETERMINE	**TYPICAL QUESTION**
Location	Where is it?
Radiation	Does it move or stay in one place?
Quality	What is it like?
Quantity	How severe is it? How frequent?
	How long does it last?
Chronology	When did it begin?
	Have you experienced it before? How has it progressed?
	What are you doing when it occurs?
	What do you do to get rid of it?
Associated findings	Do you feel any other symptoms at the same time?
Treatment sought and effect	Have you seen a health care provider in the past for this same problem?
	What tests were done (if any), and what were the results? What was the treatment?

Modified from Urden LD, Stacy KM, Lough ME: *Critical care nursing: diagnosis and management*, ed 7, St. Louis, 2014, Mosby.

Cardiopulmonary Distress

When assessing the patient, it is important to note any signs of cardiac or pulmonary distress. Complaints of chest pain are indicative of decreased myocardial oxygen supply or increased myocardial oxygen demand, either of which may impair cardiac output. All complaints of chest pain should be followed up with clarifying questions to ascertain the source of the pain (Table 2-1). The patient may also present with pallor, palpitations, and diaphoresis. The patient with severe hypoxemia is tachypneic and may present with nasal flaring, stridor (noisy respirations), and labored breathing with use of accessory muscles and supraclavicular and intercostal retractions. In addition, the patient may complain of dyspnea and breathlessness.[8] In either event, the patient requires immediate intervention to prevent further hemodynamic compromise.

Physical Assessment

The following discussion is limited to those physical assessment findings that are suggestive of impaired tissue perfusion and altered hemodynamics.

Skin, Mucous Membranes, and Nail Beds

The color of the patient's skin and mucus membranes provides useful information on hemoglobin saturation.[8] The skin, lips, tongue, and mucous membranes should be observed for abnormal findings such as pallor and for a gray, blue, or dark purple tint or discoloration, which indicates central cyanosis. Central cyanosis is an ominous life-threatening sign of inadequate oxygenation of the blood. It occurs when the amount of unsaturated hemoglobin exceeds 5 grams per deciliter (g/dL).[9] The sublingual portion of the tongue is the most sensitive site for observation of central cyanosis given a wide variety of skin tones.

The patient's nail beds are inspected for signs of clubbing and peripheral cyanosis. *Clubbing* refers to the enlargement of the terminal phalanges of the fingers, toes, or both. The nail loses the normal angle between the finger and the nail root, and as a result, the nail becomes wide and curved (Figure 2-2). Clubbing is a rare sign of severe central cyanosis related to cardiopulmonary disease.[9] The nail beds of the fingers or toes may also have a bluish discoloration, an indication of the presence of peripheral cyanosis. Peripheral cyanosis results from decreased oxygen in the peripheral extremities caused by vascular disease or decreased cardiac output.[9]

The patient's nail beds should be assessed for capillary refill. Capillary refill is an indicator of overall perfusion as well as the adequacy of blood circulation to the extremity. Capillary refill is evaluated by compressing the nail bed to produce blanching and then releasing the pressure to observe the time it takes for the nail to regain its color. Normal capillary refill takes less than 2 seconds. Capillary refill that is greater than 2 seconds is indicative of a variety of disorders, including arterial insufficiency, decreased cardiac output, and hypovolemia.[10]

Arterial Pulses

Arterial pulses are good indicators of the adequacy of cardiac output. Alterations in the amplitude and contour of the pulse wave are reflective of the adequacy of left ventricular stroke volume.[4] Arterial pulses are palpated separately and then compared

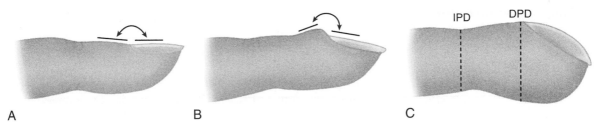

FIGURE 2-2 A, Normal digit configuration. **B,** Mild digital clubbing with increased hyponychial angle. **C,** Severe digital clubbing; the depth of the finger at the base of the nail is greater than the depth of the interphalangeal joint with clubbing. *DPD,* Distal phalangeal depth; *IPD,* interphalangeal depth. (From Kallet RH: Bedside assessment of the patient. In Kacmarek RM, Stoller JK, Heuer AJ, editors: *Egan's fundamentals of respiratory care,* ed 10, St. Louis, 2013, Mosby.)

bilaterally. When focusing on evaluating cardiac function, usually just the carotid and femoral arteries are used.[4] However, when assessing the status of perfusion to the extremities, all of the following pulses may be palpated as part of a comprehensive assessment: carotid, brachial, radial, ulnar, femoral, popliteal, posterior tibial, and dorsalis pedis arteries.

The quality of the pulse, or *pulse amplitude*, is a reflection of the strength of ventricular contraction and the elasticity of the arterial walls. Pulses may be described as absent, diminished, normal, or bounding. A number of pulse rating scales are also available. Diminished pulses are indicative of a variety of conditions, including peripheral arterial disease, hypovolemia, and decreased cardiac output. Bounding pulses are suggestive of sepsis, aortic regurgitation, and hypervolemia. The pulse contour is assessed by examination of the speed of the pulse wave upstroke, the duration of the peak, and the speed of the downstroke. It is best palpated at the carotid artery. A normal pulse wave contour may be described as smooth with rapid upstroke, rounded peak, and slightly slower downstroke. A number of different arterial pulse configuration abnormalities exist (Table 2-2), and all indicate that the patient is experiencing hemodynamic alternations.[11]

TABLE 2-2   Variations in Pulse Contour

DESCRIPTION	ASSOCIATED WITH
Weak, "Thready" Pulse—1+	
Hard to palpate, need to search for it, may fade in and out, easily obliterated by pressure.	Decreased cardiac output, peripheral arterial disease, aortic valve stenosis
Full, Bounding Pulse—3+	
Easily palpable, pounds under your fingertips.	Hyperkinetic states (exercise, anxiety, fever), anemia, hyperthyroidism

TABLE 2-2 Variations in Pulse Contour—cont'd	
DESCRIPTION	**ASSOCIATED WITH**
Water-Hammer (Corrigan) Pulse—3+	
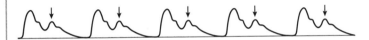	
Greater than normal force, then collapses suddenly.	Aortic valve regurgitation, patent ductus arteriosus
Pulsus Bigeminus	
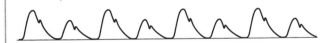	
Rhythm is coupled, every other beat comes early, or normal beat followed by premature beat, force of premature beat is decreased because of shortened cardiac filling time.	Conduction disturbance (e.g., premature ventricular contraction, premature atrial contraction)
Pulsus Alternans	
Rhythm is regular, but force varies with alternating beats of large and small amplitude.	When heart rate (HR) is normal, pulsus alternans occurs with severe left ventricular failure, which, in turn, is caused by ischemic heart disease, valvular heart disease, chronic hypertension, or cardiomyopathy

Continued

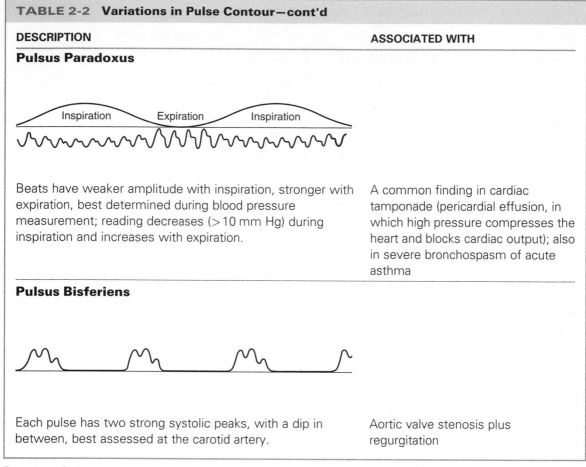

TABLE 2-2	Variations in Pulse Contour—cont'd
DESCRIPTION	**ASSOCIATED WITH**
Pulsus Paradoxus	
Beats have weaker amplitude with inspiration, stronger with expiration, best determined during blood pressure measurement; reading decreases (>10 mm Hg) during inspiration and increases with expiration.	A common finding in cardiac tamponade (pericardial effusion, in which high pressure compresses the heart and blocks cardiac output); also in severe bronchospasm of acute asthma
Pulsus Bisferiens	
Each pulse has two strong systolic peaks, with a dip in between, best assessed at the carotid artery.	Aortic valve stenosis plus regurgitation

From Jarvis C: *Physical examination and health assessment*, ed 6, St. Louis, 2012, Mosby.

Jugular Venous Pressure

Assessment of jugular vein pressure provides valuable information about right ventricular function and intravascular volume status.[4] A number of methods are available to estimate jugular vein pressure, but some of them are not practical in the clinical setting. The following method is quick and easy and does not require any extra equipment: The patient should be placed in the supine position with his or her head elevated on a pillow. The external jugular vein column (from the clavicle to the level of the jaw) can then be observed for signs of distention (Figure 2-3). If the veins collapse on inspiration, jugular vein pressure is considered normal. If the veins do not collapse on inspiration, jugular vein pressure is considered elevated. Absence of jugular venous distention (JVD) in a supine patient indicates that jugular vein pressure is low. Elevated jugular vein pressure is an indicator of right heart failure or fluid overload, and low jugular vein pressure may be an indicator of hypovolemia.[4]

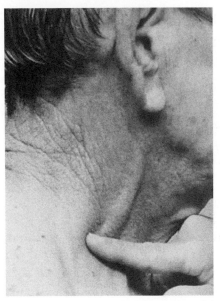

FIGURE 2-3 Elevated Jugular Venous Pressure. Note the distention of the external jugular vein. (From Urden LD, Stacy KM, Lough ME: *Critical care nursing: diagnosis and management*, ed 7, St. Louis, 2014, Mosby.)

Apical Impulse

The apical impulse, also referred to as the point of maximal impulse (PMI), is normally located at the fifth intercostal space just medial to the left midclavicular line. The PMI is about 1 to 2 centimeters (cm) in diameter, or about the size of a penny. It occurs during systole when the left ventricle contracts and rotates forward, causing the left ventricular apex to hit the chest wall. Generally only observed in thin patients, the apical impulse is the only normal pulsation visualized on the chest wall. When palpated, the apical impulse feels like a quick gentle tap. Displacement of the apical impulse either laterally or downward or a PMI greater than 2 cm in diameter is suggestive of left ventricular enlargement.[4] Feeling a double impulse may indicate the presence of an abnormal extra heart sound.

Heart Sounds

The first heart sound (S1) and the second heart sound (S2) are the normal heart sounds. These are high-pitched sounds that are heard best with the diaphragm of the stethoscope. S1 is the sound produced by closure of the atrioventricular valves during systole. It is heard most clearly at the apex of the heart, which is located at the fifth intercostal space midclavicular line (Figure 2-4). S2 is the sound produced by closure of the semilunar valves (aortic and pulmonic) during diastole. It is heard best at the base of the heart, which is located at the second intercostal space to the right of the

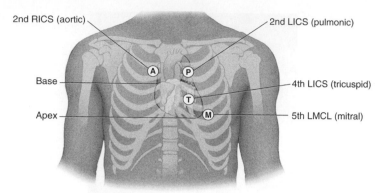

FIGURE 2-4 Auscultatory landmarks for cardiac assessment.

sternum (see Figure 2-4). Auscultation of heart sounds is performed to assess cardiac function and to identify the presence of abnormal sounds.

The third heart sound (S3) and the fourth heart sound (S4) are abnormal extra heart sounds that are sometimes present in patients. These are low-pitched sounds that are heard best with the bell of the stethoscope positioned lightly over the apical impulse. S3, also referred to as *ventricular gallop*, occurs at the beginning of diastole after S2. A third heart sound is sometimes heard in adolescents, young adults, and pregnant women, in whom it is considered benign or physiologic. However, when heard in older adults, it is indicative of acute heart failure. S4, also referred to as *atrial gallop*, occurs late in diastole just before S1. Common causes of a fourth heart sound are severe hypertension, aortic stenosis, cardiomyopathy, and such conditions as thyrotoxicosis or anemia associated with an increased cardiac output. S4 occurs with atrial contraction, and therefore, it is never heard in atrial fibrillation.

Heart Murmurs

Murmurs are abnormal extra heart sounds that are audible via auscultation during systole, diastole, or both. The most common cause of a murmur is a structural defect of the valve that results in either blood flowing backward into the chamber through an insufficient valve (regurgitation) or being forced forward through a narrowed or malformed valve (stenosis). Murmurs may also be caused by septal wall defects. The sound arises from the continuous shunting of blood back and forth between the ventricular chambers. Stenosis of the aortic or pulmonic valves increases the afterload of the left or right ventricle, and subsequently these chambers must generate higher-than-normal pressure to pump blood forward. Regurgitation of the aortic or pulmonic valves results in blood flowing back into the heart overloading the ventricle, and ultimately these chambers must pump harder to eject the additional volume. Regardless of the cause, murmurs may be indicative of problems within the heart that could lead to significant hemodynamic compromise, ventricular dysfunction, and heart failure.[12]

TABLE 2-3 Auscultation and Listening to Heart Murmurs

When you identify a heart murmur, consider the following variables for documentation:

Timing and duration	At what part of the cycle is the murmur heard? Is it associated with S1 or S2, or is it continuous?
Pitch	Is it a low or high pitch? Low pitches are best heard with the bell of the stethoscope.
Quality	Quality refers to the type of sound, including a harsh sound; a raspy, machinelike sound; or a vibratory, musical, or blowing sound.
Intensity	Murmur intensity refers to how loud the murmur is: • Grade I is barely audible in a quiet room. • Grade II is quiet but clearly audible. • Grade III is moderately loud. • Grade IV is loud and associated with a thrill. • Grade V is very loud, and a thrill is easily palpable. • Grade VI is very loud, and a thrill is palpable and visible.
Location	Where is the sound heard loudest? Most often, it is over one of the five anatomic landmarks used to auscultate heart sounds.
Example of documentation	S1, grade II, low-pitch murmur auscultated at fifth ICS, MCL. No thrill palpable.

ICS, Intercostal space; *MCL,* midclavicular line.
From Wilson SF, Giddens JF: *Health assessment for nursing practice,* ed 5, St. Louis, 2013, Mosby.

Systolic murmurs are heard between S1 and S2 and are caused by obstruction of the outflow of the semilunar valves (aortic or pulmonic stenosis) or by incompetent atrioventricular valves (mitral or tricuspid regurgitation). Diastolic murmurs are heard between S2 and the next S1 and are caused by incompetent semilunar valves (aortic or pulmonic regurgitation) or stenotic atrioventricular valves (mitral or tricuspid stenosis). The characteristics of a murmur depend on various factors, including the competence of the valve, the size of the opening, the rate of blood flow through the valve, the strength of the myocardial contraction, and the thickness of the chest wall through which the murmur must be heard. Table 2-3 outlines the different factors that should be evaluated when listening to a murmur. Figure 2-4 illustrates the location of each valve for auscultation. Table 2-4 presents the characteristics of commonly heard murmurs.

Peripheral Edema

Edema is fluid accumulation in the extravascular spaces of the tissues, and it is often an indication of fluid overload. However, in some cases, it may be caused by the loss of

TABLE 2-4 Characteristics of Some Murmurs

DEFECTS	TIMING IN THE CARDIAC CYCLE	PITCH, INTENSITY, QUALITY	LOCATION, RADIATION
Systolic Murmurs			
Mitral regurgitation	S₁ — S₂	High Harsh Blowing	Mitral area May radiate to axilla
Tricuspid regurgitation	S₁ — S₂	High Often faint, but varies Blowing	Tricuspid RLSB, apex, LLSB, epigastric areas Little radiation
Ventricular septal defect	S₁ — S₂	High Loud Blowing	Left sternal border
Aortic stenosis	S₁ ◆ S₂	"Chhhh hh" Medium Rough, harsh	Aortic area to suprasternal notch, right side of neck, apex
Pulmonary stenosis	S₁ ◆ S₂	Low to medium Loud Harsh, grinding	Pulmonic area No radiation
Diastolic Murmurs			
Mitral stenosis	Atrial kick S₂ — S₁	Low Quiet to loud with thrill Rough rumble	Mitral area Usually no radiation
Tricuspid stenosis	Atrial kick S₂ — S₁	Medium Quiet; louder with inspiration Rumble	Tricuspid area or epigastrium Little radiation
Aortic regurgitation	S₂ — S₁	High Faint to medium Blowing	Aortic area to LLSB and aorta Erb point
Pulmonic regurgitation	S₂ — S₁	Medium Faint Blowing	Pulmonic area No radiation

LLSB, Left lower sternal border; *RLSB*, right lower sternal border.
From Urden LD, Stacy KM, Lough ME: *Critical care nursing: diagnosis and management*, ed 7, St. Louis, 2014, Mosby.

TABLE 2-5	Pitting Edema Scale			
		INDENTATION DEPTH		
SCALE	**EDEMA**	**ENGLISH UNITS**	**METRIC UNITS**	**TIME TO BASELINE**
0	None	0	0	Rapid
1+	Trace	0–0.25 inch	<6.5 mm	Rapid
2+	Mild	0.25–0.5 inch	6.5–12.5 mm	10–15 sec
3+	Moderate	0.5–1 inch	12.5 mm–2.5 cm	1–2 min
4+	Severe	>1 inch	>2.5 cm	2–5 min

cm, Centimeters; *min*, minutes; *mm*, millimeters; *sec*, seconds.
From Urden LD, Stacy KM, Lough ME: *Critical care nursing: diagnosis and management*, ed 7. St. Louis, 2014, Mosby.

plasma proteins such as albumin, resulting in fluid leaking into the tissues resulting from low oncotic pressure. Edema may also be caused by poor venous return after prolonged sitting with the legs in a dependent position. When assessing the patient with edema, it is important to note if the edema is dependent, unilateral, or bilateral and whether it is pitting or nonpitting. Edema is assessed by pressing the fingertip gently into the swollen area over a bony prominence, such as the ankles, pretibial areas, or sacrum, and observing for an indentation. If the indentation does not disappear within 15 seconds, pitting edema exists. Pitting edema is rated on a scale of 0 to 4+ (Table 2-5), with 0 indicating absence of edema and 4+ indicating severe edema. Edema is often associated with heart failure.[3] A rapid weight gain of more than 2 pounds per day is also indicative of edema. A gain of 1 kilogram (kg; 2.2 pounds) is approximately equal to 1 L of fluid.

Lung Sounds

Auscultation of lung sounds is performed to assess air movement through the pulmonary system and to identify the presence of abnormal sounds. Auscultation should be done in a systematic sequence: side-to-side, top-to-bottom, posteriorly, laterally, and anteriorly. Normal lung sounds sound different according to the location and are classified as vesicular, bronchovesicular, or bronchial. Vesicular breath sounds are low in pitch, soft in intensity, and heard at the periphery of the lungs. Bronchovesicular breath sounds are moderate in pitch, moderate in intensity, and normally heard around the upper part of the sternum and between the scapulae. Bronchial breath sounds are high in pitch, loud in intensity, and heard over the trachea. It is important to be able to distinguish normal lung sounds from abnormal lung sounds.

Abnormal lung sounds are categorized as absent or diminished breath sounds, displaced bronchial breath sounds, and adventitious breath sounds. Absent or diminished breath sounds indicate that air flow to a portion of the lung(s) is inadequate or absent.

Displaced bronchial breath sounds are normal bronchial sounds that are heard in the periphery of the lungs instead of over the trachea. This condition is suggestive of fluid or exudate in the alveoli. Adventitious breath sounds are extra or added sounds heard along with other lung sounds. They are classified as crackles, wheezes, and rhonchi.

Crackles are short, discrete popping sounds produced by fluid in the small airways or alveoli or by the snapping open of collapsed airways during inspiration. They are heard on both inspiration and expiration and may clear with coughing. Crackles are further classified as fine, medium, or coarse, depending on pitch. Wheezes are high-pitched, squeaking, whistling sounds produced by air flow through narrowed small airways. They are heard mainly on expiration but may be heard throughout the inspiration–expiration cycle. Depending on their severity, wheezes are further classified as mild, moderate, or severe. Rhonchi are coarse, rumbling, low-pitched sounds produced by air flow over secretions in the larger airways or by the narrowing of the large airways. They are heard mainly on expiration and sometimes can be cleared with coughing. Rhonchi are further classified as bubbling, gurgling, or sonorous, depending on the characteristics of the sound.[9] Table 2-6 describes the various abnormal breath sounds and the conditions associated with them.

Clinical Reasoning Pearl

Although rarely assessed in clinical practice, voice sounds are particularly useful in detecting lung consolidation or lung compression, which may be the result of fluid in the alveoli or solidification of the lung tissue resulting from a tumor. The three kinds of voice sounds are described below:

- *Bronchophony* refers to a condition in which the spoken voice is heard on auscultation with higher intensity and clarity than usual. Normally, the spoken voice is muffled when heard through the stethoscope. This condition is assessed by placing the diaphragm of the stethoscope against the posterior side of the patient's chest and instructing the patient to say "ninety-nine." If bronchophony is present, the sound heard is clear, distinct, and loud.

- *Egophony* describes voice sounds increased in intensity with a nasal, bleating quality on auscultation. This condition is assessed by placing the stethoscope against the posterior side of the patient's chest and instructing the patient to say "e-e-e." If egophony is present, the "e" sound changes to an "a" sound.

- *Whispering pectoriloquy* refers to unusually clear transmission of the whispered voice on auscultation. Normally, the whispered word is unintelligible when heard through the stethoscope. This condition is assessed by placing the stethoscope against the posterior side of the patient's chest and instructing the patient to whisper "one, two, three." If whispering pectoriloquy is present, the sound heard is clear and distinct.

TABLE 2-6   Abnormal Breath Sounds and Their Associated Conditions

ABNORMAL SOUND	DESCRIPTION	CONDITION
Absent breath sounds	No air flow to particular portion of lung	Pneumothorax
		Pneumonectomy
		Emphysematous blebs
		Pleural effusion
		Lung mass
		Massive atelectasis
		Complete airway obstruction
Diminished breath sounds	Little air flow to particular portion of lung	Emphysema
		Pleural effusion
		Pleurisy
		Atelectasis
		Pulmonary fibrosis
Displaced bronchial sounds	Bronchial sounds heard in peripheral lung fields	Atelectasis with secretions
		Lung mass with exudates
		Pneumonia
		Pleural effusion
		Pulmonary edema
Crackles	Short, discrete popping or crackling sounds	Pulmonary edema
		Pneumonia
		Pulmonary fibrosis
		Atelectasis
		Bronchiectasis
Rhonchi	Coarse, rumbling, low-pitched sounds	Pneumonia
		Asthma
		Bronchitis
		Bronchospasm
Wheezes	High-pitched, squeaking, whistling sounds	Asthma
		Bronchospasm
Pleural friction rub	Creaking, leathery, loud, dry, coarse sounds	Pleural effusion
		Pleurisy

From Urden LD, Stacy KM, Lough ME: *Critical care nursing: diagnosis and management*, ed 7, St. Louis, 2014, Mosby.

Ascites

The abdomen should be assessed for signs of distention. Distention may be caused by a variety of factors, including ascites, increased bowel contents, obesity, or tumors in the abdomen. Ascites is the result of excess fluid accumulation in the abdominal cavity caused by right-sided heart failure. However, in patients with liver dysfunction, ascites may also be caused by loss of plasma proteins, which allows fluid to leak into the abdominal cavity, or increased portal pressure from cirrhosis, which forces fluid and plasma proteins into the abdominal cavity. Therefore, when assessing the patient, it is important to note if a history of liver disease exists. Patients with ascites usually present with generalized distention of the abdomen, abdominal striae, and bulging flanks. Testing for a fluid wave may help differentiate between ascites and some of the other causes of distention.

To perform a fluid wave test, the patient is placed in the supine position and instructed to gently press the edge of his or her hand along the vertical midline of the abdomen (Figure 2-5). Placement of the patient's hand on the abdomen helps stop the transmission of the vibrations generated by the tap from dissipating through the abdominal wall. If the patient is unable to participate, another staff member should assist with the test. The examiner then places his or her hands on either side of the patient's abdomen. With the fingertips of the right hand, the examiner firmly taps the abdomen and feels for the presence or absence of a fluid wave with the fingertips of the left hand. The patient's abdomen is observed at the same time for a wave or ripple moving across it. If the abdominal distention is the result of ascites, the tapping will cause a fluid wave through the abdomen.[11]

Hepatojugular Reflux

The hepatojugular reflux, also referred to as the abdominojugular reflux, is an assessment maneuver that can assist with determining the presence of systemic congestion

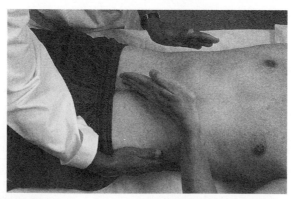

FIGURE 2-5 Testing for Fluid Wave. Strike one side of the abdomen sharply with the fingertips. Feel for the impulse of a fluid wave with the other hand. (From Wilson SF, Giddens JF: *Health assessment for nursing practice*, ed 5, St. Louis, 2013, Mosby.)

caused by right ventricular failure. This maneuver is performed by placing the patient in the supine position, with the head of the bed elevated by 30 to 45 degrees. The jugular veins are assessed with the patient in this position, and the level of JVD is noted. The patient is instructed to relax and breathe normally. Firm pressure is then applied to the patient's middle to upper abdomen for 15 to 30 seconds while the jugular veins are observed for a rise in pressure. In the patient with right ventricular failure, a sustained elevation of jugular vein pressure of greater than 3 cm will be observed for at least 15 seconds (positive hepatojugular reflux).[4]

Measurements

Pulse Rate and Rhythm

The patient's pulse rate and rhythm are assessed by palpation of the carotid or femoral artery. Alterations in rate and rhythm are reflective of issues with the patient's heart rate and rhythm.[7] The normal arterial pulse rate is 60 to 100 beats per minute (beats/min) with a regular rhythm.[11] The pulse rate may increase slightly with inspiration. Both tachycardia (rate >100 beats/min) and bradycardia (rate <60 beats/min) may adversely affect cardiac output. Tachycardia may also be a compensatory mechanism for hypovolemia or hypoxemia. Irregularities in the patient's rhythm may adversely affect cardiac output. When evaluating the rhythm of the pulse, it is important to note if it is regular, regularly irregular, or irregularly irregular.[11] A rhythm that is totally irregular is indicative of atrial fibrillation, whereas a rhythm that is basically regular with occasional irregularities is suggestive of premature beats.

If the patient has an irregularly irregular rhythm suggestive of atrial fibrillation, the patient's pulse should be assessed for a pulse deficit.[13] A *pulse deficit* is a condition in which the peripheral pulse rate is less than the apical pulse rate. This finding may indicate inadequate perfusion to the extremities and is assessed by simultaneously auscultating the apical heart rate and palpating the radial artery for 1 minute. The two numbers are then compared. If the numbers are the same, no deficit exists, and this indicates that the heart is perfusing the extremities with each beat. If a difference exists between the apical and radial heart rates, a pulse deficit is present.

Blood Pressure

The patient's blood pressure is evaluated to identify any abnormalities that would affect hemodynamic status. Blood pressure is the pressure exerted by circulating blood on the walls of blood vessels. It is determined by heart rate, the force and amount of blood pumped (stroke volume), and the size and flexibility of the arteries (systemic vascular resistance). Systemic vascular resistance is influenced by a variety of factors, including intravascular volume and the autonomic nervous system. Thus, alterations in blood pressure are reflective of hemodynamic alterations, since pressure is the product of flow and resistance.[14]

Pulse pressure describes the difference between the systolic and diastolic values and can be used as an estimate of stroke volume. Normal systolic blood pressure is 100 to 140 mm Hg (millimeters of mercury) and normal diastolic blood pressure is 60 to 90 mm Hg. The normal pulse pressure is 40 mm Hg. Pulse pressure helps with differentiating etiology. A narrow pulse pressure in may be indicative of hypovolemia. The systolic pressure may decrease as a result of a decline in cardiac output, while the diastolic pressure rises as arterial vasoconstriction occurs to compensate for the hypovolemic state. A wide pulse pressure in the patient with hypotension is indicative of sepsis. In this instance, the diastolic pressure decreases because of profound vasodilation. In both instances, alterations in pulse pressure signal that tissue perfusion is impaired.[15]

Orthostatic vital sign measurements provide information regarding the fluid status of the patient. This procedure involves taking a series of blood pressure measurements with the patient in the lying, sitting, and standing positions. The first measurement is taken with the patient placed in the supine position for at least 5 to 10 minutes. The subsequent blood pressure measurements are obtained within 1 to 3 minutes after the position change. A decrease in systolic blood pressure of 20 mm Hg or more, a decrease in diastolic blood pressure of 10 mm Hg or more, or an increase in pulse rate of more than 20 beats/min from lying to sitting or from sitting to standing indicates orthostatic hypotension. Orthostatic hypotension is the result of decreased venous return caused by hypovolemia or autonomic failure.[16]

If pericardial tamponade is suspected, assessment for pulsus paradoxus is warranted. Normally, the systolic blood pressure fluctuates with patient breaths, decreasing during inspiration and increasing during expiration. This is caused by pressure changes within the chest cavity. During inspiration, pressure in the chest cavity increases, causing a normal decrease in systolic blood pressure. Typically, less than a 10 mm Hg difference exists between inspiration and expiration. A decrease in systolic blood pressure greater than 10 mm Hg on inspiration is considered diagnostic of pulsus paradoxus.[17] Pulsus paradoxus is measured by using a manual sphygmomanometer. The patient should be placed in the supine position and instructed to breathe normally. The cuff is inflated until Korotkoff sounds are no longer heard. The cuff is then slowly deflated until the first Korotkoff sounds are heard. Sounds will be intermittent at this point and heard only during expiration.[17] The expiratory systolic blood pressure is noted. The cuff is then slowly deflated again until Korotkoff sounds are heard continuously. The inspiratory systolic blood pressure is noted. If the difference between these two systolic blood pressure values is greater than 10 mm Hg, pulsus paradoxus is present.

Respiratory Rate

Normal breathing at rest is effortless and regular and occurs at a rate of 12 to 20 breaths per minute (breaths/min) with an inspiration to expiration ratio of approximately 1:2. Alterations in the rate and rhythm of breathing are indicative of a variety of conditions, including hypoxemia. The most commonly seen pattern in patients with hypoxemia is tachypnea.[8] Tachypnea is manifested by an increase in the rate and decrease in the depth of ventilation. Tachypnea is a compensatory mechanism to increase the level of oxygen in blood. Any patient with tachypnea should be further evaluated for hypoxemia. Cheyne-Stokes respiration is an abnormal breathing pattern that may occur in patients with decompensated heart failure. It is characterized by progressively increasing depth of breathing, followed by progressively decreasing depth of breathing, followed by a period of apnea.

Oxygen Saturation

Oxygen saturation is a measure of the amount of oxygen bound to hemoglobin, compared with hemoglobin's maximal capability for binding oxygen. Oxygen saturation is measured noninvasively using a pulse oximeter, and abbreviated as SpO_2. It can be used as an indicator for hypoxemia. Normal SpO_2 values range from 95% to 99%. SpO_2 values of 91% to 94% indicate mild hypoxemia; values of 86% to 90% indicate moderate hypoxemia; and values of 85% or lower indicate severe hypoxemia, which warrants immediate medical intervention.[18]

It is important to evaluate the percent of saturated oxygen in context with the hemoglobin level. For example, SpO_2 of 95% means that 95% of the available hemoglobin is bound with oxygen. Therefore, the patient could have a hemoglobin level of 5 g/dL, 10 g/dL, or 15 g/dL and still have SpO_2 of 95%. Obviously, the patient with a hemoglobin level of 15 g/dL would have a lot more oxygen delivered to tissues compared with a patient with a hemoglobin level of 5 g/dL. Thus, the hemoglobin level must also be evaluated before a decision on oxygenation status can be made.

Case Study

Mr. C, a 65-year-old man, was admitted to the progressive care unit with a diagnosis of chest pain and respiratory insufficiency.

Patient History. Mr. C has a history of hypertension that has been controlled with medication.

Chief Complaint. Mr. C complains of chest pain on exertion that is relieved by rest, dyspnea, and fatigue. He reports a weight gain of 4.5 kg (10 pounds) over the last 5 days.

General Appearance. Mr. C appears short of breath, pale, and diaphoretic. He described the pain as a deep pressure that was unrelieved by rest, antacids, or three sublingual nitroglycerin tablets.

Physical Assessment. The following abnormal assessment findings were noted during the physical examination:
- Bluish tint of lips and tongue
- Capillary refill of 3 to 4 seconds

Continued

Case Study—cont'd

- Regular pulse, but force varies with alternating beats of large and small amplitude (pulsus alternans)
- JVD
- Apical impulse is displaced downward and 3 cm in diameter
- S_3
- Systolic murmur heard over second intercostal space right sternal border
- +3 pitting edema over the feet up to the mid-shins
- Coarse crackles in the right and left lower lobes
- Mild ascites with positive fluid wave test
- Hepatojugular reflux

MEASUREMENTS	
Heart rate	120 beats/min
Heart rhythm	Irregularly irregular
Pulse deficit	Present
Respiratory rate	28 breaths/min
Respiratory rhythm	Tachypnea
Blood pressure	150/90 mm Hg
SpO_2	89% on room air

Diagnostic Procedures. Electrocardiography shows atrial fibrillation. Echocardiography shows acute heart failure secondary to aortic stenosis. ■

Conclusion

Physical assessment yields a wealth of information regarding the hemodynamic status of the patient. Many signs and symptoms evident during the physical assessment reveal the presence of hemodynamic alterations and often suggest the source of the problem. Any evidence of cardiopulmonary dysfunction must be fully investigated and treated to ensure adequate tissue perfusion.

References

1. In Hall JE: *Guyton and Hall textbook of medical physiology,* ed 12., Philadelphia, 2011, Saunders.
2. Brashers VL, McCance KL: Structure and function of the cardiovascular and lymphatic systems. In McCance KL, Huether SE, Brashers VL, et al., editors: *Pathophysiology: the biologic basis for disease in adults and children*, 6 ed., St. Louis, 2010, Mosby, pp 1091–1141.

3. From AM, Lam SPC, Pitta SR, et al.: Bedside assessment of cardiac hemodynamics: the impact of noninvasive testing and examiner experience, *Am J Med* 124(11):1051–1057, 2011.

4. Conn RD, O'Keefe JH: Cardiac physical diagnosis in the digital age: an important but increasingly neglected skill (from stethoscopes to microchips), *Am J Cardiol* 104(4):590–595, 2009.

5. Brashers VL: Structure and function of the pulmonary system. In McCance KL, Huether SE, Brashers VL, et al., editors: *Pathophysiology: the biologic basis for disease in adults and children*, 6 ed., St. Louis, 2010, Mosby, pp 1242–1265.

6. Koita J, Riggio S, Jagoda A: The mental status examination in emergency practice, *Emerg Med Clin North Am* 28(3):439–451, 2010.

7. Thackwray J, Walton A: Clinical assessment of a patient with stable heart failure, *Br J Card Nurs* 6(3):110–117, 2011.

8. Higginson R, Jones B: Respiratory assessment in critically ill patients: airway and breathing, *Br J Nurs* 18(8):456–461, 2009.

9. Kallet RH: Bedside assessment of the patient. In Kacmarek RM, Stoller JK, Heuer AJ, editors: *Egan's fundamentals of respiratory care*, 10 ed., St. Louis, 2013, Mosby, pp 330–356.

10. Seidel HM, Ball JW, Dains JE, et al.: *Mosby's guide to physical examination*, ed 7., St. Louis, 2011, Mosby.

11. Wilson S, Giddens J: *Health assessment for nursing practice*, ed 5., St. Louis, 2013, Mosby.

12. Hanifin C: Cardiac auscultation 101: a basic science approach to heart murmurs, *JAAPA* 23 (4):44–48, 2010.

13. Khasnis A, Thakur RK: Atrial fibrillation: a historical perspective, *Cardiol Clin* 27(1):1–12, 2009.

14. Singh M, Mensah GA, Barkris G: Pathogenesis and clinical physiology of hypertension, *Cardiol Clin* 28(4):545–559, 2010.

15. Carlson B, Fitzsimmons L: Shock, sepsis, and multiple organ dysfunction syndrome. In Urden LD, Stacy KM, Lough ME, editors: *Critical care nursing: diagnosis and management*, 7 ed., St. Louis, 2014, Mosby, pp 887–925.

16. 2011 ENA Emergency Nursing Resources Development Committee: Emergency nursing resource: orthostatic vital signs, *J Emerg Nurs* 38(5):447–453, 2012.

17. Argulian E, Messerli F: Misconceptions and facts about pericardial effusion and tamponade, *Am J Med* 126(10):858–861, 2013.

18. Des Jardins T, Burton GG: *Clinical manifestation and assessment of respiratory disease*, ed 6., St. Louis, MO, 2011, Mosby.

Arterial Pressure Monitoring

Mary E. Lough

3

Arterial blood pressure is one of most frequently measured indicators of hemodynamic function in adults.[1] Blood pressure can be obtained intermittently and noninvasively using a brachial cuff and sphygmomanometer or measured continuously via an invasive arterial catheter. Blood pressure values and waveform morphology are incorporated into a range of hemodynamic equations to estimate blood flow and vascular resistance. Straightforward and ubiquitous, measurement of arterial pressure is at the heart of hemodynamic monitoring.

Historical Milestones

The pulse has been palpated since ancient times, but invasive measurement of blood pressure was not reported until 1733, when the Reverend Stephen Hales documented arterial blood pressure measured in a horse.[2] With the horse restrained on the ground, a narrow-gauge brass tube (1/6 inch diameter) was inserted into a major artery, and a tall slender glass tube was then attached. The glass tube was 9 feet long and was positioned vertical to the horse. Hales reported that the horse's blood pressure, in the glass tube, was elevated 8 feet 3 inches above the heart and pulsated 3 to 4 inches with each heartbeat.[3]

In 1828, Jean Marie L. Poisseulle made the process more manageable by using a U-shaped "hemodynamometer" to measure blood pressure in animals. It was Poisseulle who set the standard of blood pressure measurement in millimeters of mercury (mm Hg).[4] In 1905, Nikolai Korotkoff, a Russian surgeon, devised the noninvasive blood pressure auscultation method that is used today. His name is still used to identify the audible sounds that are heard as the blood pressure cuff is gently released.[4]

In 1949, Peterson and colleagues reported directly accessing the brachial artery during surgery in 100 patients—a small intra-arterial catheter was connected to a "capacitance manometer" to directly measure and record the arterial pressure waveform on an "ink-writer". In 1953, Sven-Igar Seldinger, a Swedish radiologist, pioneered percutaneous arterial cannulation over a guide wire. With the development of the critical care unit and the need for hemodynamic monitoring outside the operating room, the percutaneous *Seldinger technique* became the primary method for arterial

TABLE 3-1   Historical Technology Milestones for Blood Pressure and Intra-arterial Pressure Monitoring

YEAR	INVENTOR	TECHNOLOGY MILESTONES
1733	Stephen Hales	Measured arterial blood pressure in a horse.
1816	Rene Laennec	Invented the first stethoscope. This was a single wooden short hollow tube. The physician placed one end on the patient's chest and the other end to their ear (monoaural). Before this invention, physicians would put their ear directly on the patient's chest to listen to heart and lung sounds.
1828	Jean Poisseulle	Invented a U-shaped "hemodynamometer" to measure blood pressure in animals. Established the standard of blood pressure measurement in millimeters of mercury (mm Hg).
1829	Nicholas Commis	Invented the first stethoscope with two earpieces (binaural). His invention was described in the *London Gazette*. In the decades following Laennec's discovery, many physicians worked independently to improve stethoscope designs. Most devices were fragile, constructed with hollow tubes and hinges.
1851	George Cammann	Development and production of the first commercially available binaural stethoscope.
1896	Scipione Riva-Rocci	Invented the first mercury sphygmomanometer. This was a glass manometer filled with mercury attached to an inflatable arm cuff. It was used to quantify human systolic blood pressure.
1905	Nikolai Korotkoff	Identified the audible sounds auscultated as the blood pressure cuff is released. Discovered how to identify diastolic blood pressure. The auscultated sounds are still referred to as Korotkoff sounds.
1929	Edgar Van Nuys Allen	The Allen test was described in patients with thromboangiitis obliterans. A modified Allen test remains in use today for insertion of radial arterial catheters.
1949	Lyle H. Peterson	Arterial waveform and arterial pressures recorded from the brachial artery during surgery.
1953	Sven-Igar Seldinger	Percutaneous vascular access described.

vascular access. About the same time, the radial artery became the principal site for arterial pressure monitoring.[2] Additional historical technology milestones are listed in Table 3-1.

Currently, in the United States, 56% of surgical patients are admitted to the critical care unit with an arterial catheter in situ.[1] Arterial catheters are placed in 22% of medical critical care patients and are usually inserted in the unit.[1] This pattern of arterial catheter use has remained very similar for over a decade.[1]

Key Physiologic Concepts

The arterial waveform represents the upper part of the left ventricular (LV) pressure curve as described in Chapter 1 and shown in Figure 3-1. The opening of the aortic valve marks the beginning of systole as blood is rapidly ejected into the aorta from the left ventricle. Figure 3-1 shows the drop in systolic LV volume that mirrors the rise in systolic arterial pressure.

The arterial pressure is a result of the force exerted on the distensible arterial walls by the circulating blood and represents the sum of hemodynamic, hydrostatic, and kinetic pressures.[5] When LV volume is ejected during systole, the aorta expands to accommodate the LV stroke volume (Figure 3-2, *A*), and then recoils to propel the blood toward the periphery (Figure 3-2, *B*). Arteries and arterioles modulate blood pressure through control of the arterial vessel diameter. Innervation of the vasculature by

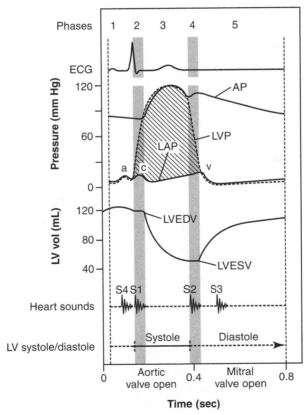

FIGURE 3-1 Cardiac cycle shows the left ventricular pressure (LVP) waveform (dashed line). The area shaded below this waveform represents the pressure changes in the left ventricle during systole. The top of the LVP waveform during systole is synonymous with the systemic arterial pressure (AP) waveform. The left atrial waveform (LAP) is also shown. The volume in the left ventricle is ejected during systole, as shown by the the change in left ventricular end-diastolic volume (LVEDV) compared with left ventricular end-systolic volume (LVESV).

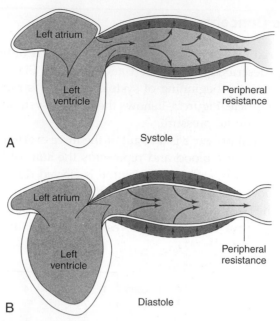

FIGURE 3-2 A, The healthy aorta is distensible and the aortic wall expands in response to the ejected stroke volume. **B,** The aortic wall recoils to propel blood toward the peripheral vessels (Modified from Koeppen BM, Stanton BA: *Berne & Levy Physiology*, ed 6, St. Louis, 2010, Elsevier.)

the sympathetic nervous system results in vasoconstriction, while innervation by the parasympathetic nervous system results in vasodilation (see Chapter 1).

Arterial Pressure Waveform

The upstroke of the arterial pressure wave is known as the anacrotic limb and reflects LV ejection pressure. The downslope of the arterial waveform is called the *dicrotic limb*. The end of systole occurs with closure of the aortic valve, which causes an abrupt change in blood flow that creates a visible notch on the arterial waveform. This is usually known as the *dicrotic notch* and less commonly labeled as the *incisura*. As the distance from the aortic root to the site of measurement increases, the notch appears farther down the dicrotic limb as shown in Figure 3-3. The remainder of the waveform represents diastolic run-off throughout the arterial vasculature. Systolic blood pressure (SBP) is measured at the peak of ejection. Diastolic blood pressure (DBP) is measured at the lowest point (Figure 3-4). Mean arterial pressure (MAP) represents the average (mean) pressure across a single cardiac cycle in systole and diastole. Because in normal sinus rhythm approximately one third of the cardiac cycle is spent in systole and two thirds in diastole, MAP calculation takes into account the longer diastolic period. Manual formulas can be used to calculate MAP (listed below), but these have some limitations, especially with faster heart rates.[5]

$$\text{MAP} = \text{SBP} \, (\times 1) \, + \, \text{DBP} \, (\times 2) \, \div \, 3$$

$$\text{MAP} = \text{DBP} \, + \, (\text{SBP} - \text{DBP}) \, \div \, 3$$

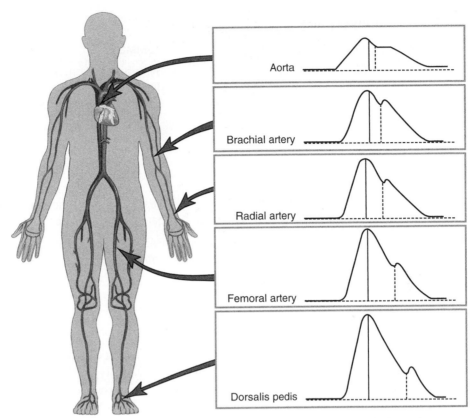

FIGURE 3-3 The shape of the arterial pressure wave changes as it travels from the aorta to the periphery. The peak becomes taller, the base becomes wider and the dicrotic notch appears lower on the waveform descent.

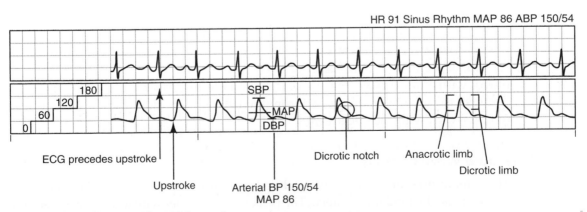

FIGURE 3-4 The normal arterial waveform.

TABLE 3-2   Normal Values

PARAMETER	VALUES	COMMENTS
Systolic blood pressure	90–140 mm Hg	Systolic blood pressure target may vary by diagnosis and clinical management. Considerable physiologic variation exists.
Diastolic blood pressure	<80 mm Hg	
Mean arterial pressure (MAP)	70–100 mm Hg	MAP target may vary by diagnosis and clinical management.
Pulse pressure variation (PPV)	PPV >13% predicts positive responsive to a fluid challenge	Research studies support this value for patients on controlled mechanical ventilation.
Stroke volume variation (SVV)	SVV >13% predicts positive responsive to a fluid bolus SVV <13% signifies patient will NOT be fluid responsive	Research studies support this value for patients on controlled mechanical ventilation.

> Indicates greater than; < indicates less than.

With tachycardia, diastolic filling time is shortened, whereas systolic ejection time remains relatively constant. This affects the validity of the manual formulas listed above. The bedside computer calculates MAP using the area under the arterial pressure curve, with adjustments for a shorter diastolic filling time, as needed. Decreased diastole filling time reduces output from the left ventricle and consequently lowers arterial pressure in critically ill patients who lack physiologic reserve. Normal arterial pressure values are listed in Table 3-2.

Pulse Wave Velocity

The arterial vascular tree is dynamic and distensible. A healthy aorta is compliant and readily expands to accommodate the ejected LV stroke volume (see Figure 3-2, *A*). The systolic ejection of blood produces a pulsatile pressure wave that traverses the arterial vasculature from the aorta to the periphery. It is this pressure pulse, rather than a volume pulse, that a clinician detects when palpating a patient's pulse at the radial, carotid, or femoral site.[5] The arterial pulse wave travels much faster than the flowing blood, with a pulse wave velocity of 0.3 second from aortic root to the periphery.[6] In contrast, the blood volume ejected from the left ventricle moves about 20 centimeters (cm) forward with each heartbeat.[6]

Arterial Pressure Wave Contour

The arterial pressure wave changes shape as it encounters smaller peripheral arteries and increased vascular resistance. The peak becomes taller with a wider base as shown

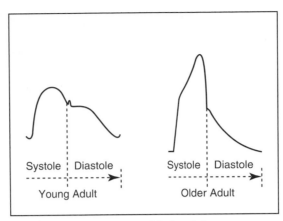

FIGURE 3-5 Arterial waveform: young versus elderly adult.

in Figure 3-3.[6] As arteries bifurcate and become smaller, this leads to backflow of arterial blood in a process known as *wave reflection*. A common analogy used to describe this process is to visualize waves on a beach, where waves coming onto the beach collide with waves that are receding. The receding waves are additive to the height of the oncoming waves. It is for this same reason that the arterial upstroke becomes more upright, the systolic peak becomes taller, and, as described previously, the dicrotic notch occurs later in the waveform (see Figure 3-3).[5] Consequently, systolic blood pressure is higher, with a wider pulse pressure, when measured at the radial arterial site, than at the aorta. In contrast the MAP changes very little as the pulse wave moves from aorta to periphery. This is the reason many clinical protocols and formulae rely on MAP rather than systolic blood pressure.

The amplitude (height) of the arterial waveform is determined by three factors, LV stroke volume, velocity of ejection, and aortic stiffness.[6] The rapid upstroke of the arterial waveform is generated by the ejection and velocity of the LV stroke volume. A higher peak is generated when the left ventricle ejects blood into a noncompliant "stiff" aorta.[6] Aortic stiffness results from atherosclerotic changes and from the normal aging process.[7] Older adults have less compliant vascular systems and are more likely to have elevated systolic pressures,[8] as illustrated in Figure 3-5. In one study of adults over 65 years of age, the intra-arterial systolic blood pressure was 5 millimeters of Mercury (mm Hg) higher than the cuff blood pressure and the intra-arterial diastolic blood pressure was 8 mm Hg lower than the cuff blood pressure.[8]

Clinical Procedure and Technical Considerations

Arterial lines are inserted to facilitate clinical management when continuous blood pressure monitoring is required or frequent arterial blood gas assessments are required. Clinical reasons to insert an arterial catheter are for hemodynamic management when continuous monitoring of arterial pressure may help treat a patient in any form of shock (cardiogenic, hemorrhagic, distributive, neurogenic) or in severe sepsis, with a goal of maintaining the systolic blood pressure above 65 mm Hg. Other reasons include titration of vasoactive medications to a specified target MAP or systolic blood pressure (see Chapter 9), or use of arterial waveform-based cardiac output monitoring as described in Chapter 12. Arterial catheters are most often inserted into the radial artery and less frequently into the femoral artery. Although, when emergency arterial access is required because of bleeding, or shock with severe hypotension, the femoral artery is often the most easily accessible vessel. Other sites such as the axillary or brachial arteries in the arm or the dorsalis-pedis in the foot may be used when other arterial access is unavailable.

Arterial Catheter Site and Insertion

The choice of site for insertion of an arterial catheter is not trivial. The radial artery is the most frequently accessed site for insertion of an arterial catheter. This artery is preferred because the hand has a second arterial supply in the ulnar artery, and the radial artery runs over a bone, which provides a compressible site in the case of bleeding. Prior to radial catheter insertion, an Allen test is performed to ensure that arterial circulation to the hand via the palmer arch is adequate (Figure 3-6). The palmer arch consists of four interconnected arterial "arches."[2] Three of the arches occur on the palm side of the hand and include the palmar carpal arch, the deep palmar arch, and the superficial palmar arch. The arch on the back (dorsal) side of the hand is the dorsal palmar rete.[2] The superficial and deep palmer arches provide blood flow to all the fingers in the hand. This rich anastomotic network ensures that blood supply to the hand is adequate during radial arterial cannulation.[9]

The Allen Test

Before a radial catheter is inserted, collateral circulation is assessed using Doppler flow or by the modified Allen test.[10] In the Allen test, the radial and ulnar arteries are compressed simultaneously. The patient is asked to clench and unclench the hand until it blanches. One of the arteries is then released, and the hand should immediately flush from that side. The same procedure is repeated for the remaining artery (Figure 3-6). If the patient is not sufficiently alert to perform the hand movements, Doppler assessment for return of blood flow can be used instead.

Arterial catheters are inserted percutaneously by one of two methods: an "over the needle" approach or for larger arteries, an "over the wire" approach, also known as the *Seldinger technique*[10] (Figure 3-7). To improve insertion accuracy, reduce vascular complications, and reduce the number of unsuccessful insertion attempts, ultrasound guidance is increasingly used. Research studies have demonstrated that successful cannulation is achieved with fewer attempts using ultrasound.[11,12] Portable ultrasound devices designed for use at the bedside are now considered a standard of care. Ultrasound guidance for arterial cannulation is recommended by ultrasonography and echocardiography professional societies.[13-15]

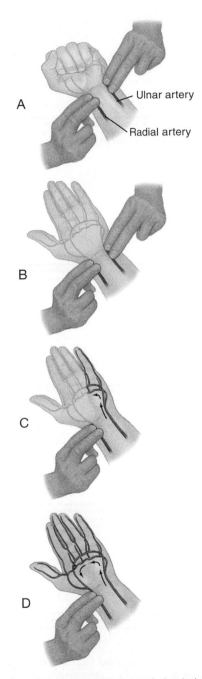

FIGURE 3-6 The Allen test is used to assess collateral circulation in the hand before insertion of an arterial catheter in the radial artery. The steps are: **A,** both arteries are simultaneously compressed to occlude blood flow and the patient is asked to clench and unclench the fist. **B,** Fingers are extended and the patient's hand should have blanched, as pressure on both arteries is maintained. **C,** The examiner removes pressure from the ulnar artery and blood flow should return from that side. **D,** If the normal hand color does not return with 5–10 seconds, this suggests that the arterial arch arteries are not intact and an arterial catheter should not be inserted. The process is then repeated for the radial artery.

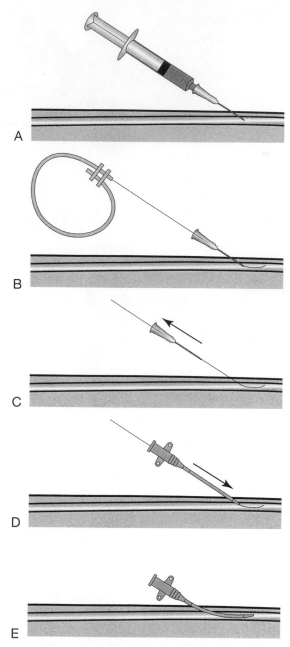

FIGURE 3-7 Insertion of an arterial catheter using an over-the-wire Seldinger technique. **A,** A beveled needle is inserted into the artery, and access is established by blood return in the syringe. **B,** A flexible guide wire is advanced through the needle. **C,** The needle is removed while maintaining the guide wire in position. **D,** The catheter is inserted over the wire until the hub is in contact with the skin. The guide wire is then removed. **E,** The catheter is in position with the artery, ready to be connected to the arterial pressure monitoring system.

Arterial Pressure Monitoring

Arterial Pressure Transducer and Tubing

The hemodynamic monitoring system is assembled before the artery is cannulated. As soon as the arterial catheter is inserted, it is connected to the pressure-monitoring setup as described below.

1. High-pressure tubing (noncompressible) connects the arterial catheter to the disposable transducer.
2. The transducer receives the pressure wave signal via the fluid-filled tubing and converts it into electrical energy.
3. The bedside monitor contains the amplifier with recorder, which increases the volume of the electrical signal and displays it on an oscilloscope and digital scale in mm Hg.
4. A bag of saline (0.9%) with all air removed, is used to prime the system, which incorporates a manual flush to maintain patency. The saline bag is compressed inside an opaque high-pressure cuff at 300 mm Hg to maintain a pressure higher than the patient's own blood pressure. (See Chapter 5, Figure 5-5.)
5. Arterial tubing pressure systems contain an access port for blood sampling for laboratory analysis. Most systems are configured to permit needleless access.

Arterial Pressure Fundamentals

Zeroing the Transducer

To ensure accuracy of hemodynamic pressure readings, the system is calibrated to local atmospheric pressure. This is termed *zeroing the transducer* as the three-way zero-reference stopcock is turned to be open to air (closed off to the monitor and off to the patient) for this calibration. The zero shown on the monitor represents an atmospheric pressure of 760 mm Hg at sea level. If a patient's blood pressure is 120/80 mm Hg, this is additive to the local atmospheric pressure; that is, the measurement is actually an unwieldy 880/840 mm Hg.[16] Additionally, atmospheric pressure fluctuates with weather conditions.[16] Thus, the purpose of zeroing the transducer is to standardize the baseline to achieve accurate arterial pressure measurements.

Leveling the Transducer

If the transducer is situated on the same holder as a central venous pressure catheter, it is likely that transducer height placement will be leveled to the phlebostatic axis which is measured on the side of the chest, at the intersection of the fourth intercostal space and midway between the anterior – posterior chest. The position of the phlebostatic axis is preferably marked on the patient's lateral chest wall with a small x to ensure that all clinicians are using the same reference point. A carpenter's level can be used to ensure the phlebostatic axis and the air reference transducer are at the same height. This is called *leveling the transducer* and is described in Chapter 4 (see Figures 4-3 and

4-4) and Chapter 5 (see Figure 5-5). This is a reasonable location for leveling of the arterial pressure transducer as it approximates both the atria and the aortic root. The purpose of leveling is to eliminate the effects of hydrostatic pressure.

Baseline Blood Pressure

A baseline arterial pressure is also established with the patient's cuff blood pressure, although in hypotensive states, the arterial pressure is considered more accurate. In many critical care units, it is standard practice to check the cuff blood pressure once a shift to correlate the cuff and arterial pressure.

Square Wave Test

Another mechanism for verifying accuracy of blood pressure measurement is to perform a square wave test, also called a dynamic frequency response test.[5] The test makes use of the manual flush system to deliver a small bolus of fluid into the high-pressure tubing and catheter. With the normal waveform displayed, the fast-flush will generate a rapid increase in pressure that is seen on the monitor as a "square wave." An optimal waveform with few oscillations determines that the hemodynamic system is sufficiently dynamic and will accurately reflect the patient's arterial pressure.

All hemodynamic systems have some damping applied to them. If they were not damped, the vibrations of the arterial fluid column would vibrate indefinitely and accurate measurements could not be obtained.[5] When the system is overdamped (usually called a damped waveform), the pressure tracing is unusually smooth and rounded, the systolic pressure is falsely low, the diastolic pressure is falsely high and the dicrotic notch is not visible.[5] In the presence of air bubbles, clots, or kinked tubing, the patient's arterial pressure waveform will appear damped and produce an overdamped square waveform result. One frequent cause of a damped radial arterial waveform is the patient bending the wrist and inadvertently obstructing the arterial catheter. In this situation, the arterial pressure is not accurate. A small wrist support may be needed to maintain optimal wrist position. See Chapter 4 (Figure 4-5) for more information on how to interpret and use this test.

Catheter Patency

A patent catheter is essential for accurate arterial pressure measurements. Heparin has traditionally, if controversially, been added to the arterial pressure bag flush-system at 1 to 2 unit per milliliter (mL) to prevent clots forming in the arterial catheter.[17,18] The 1993 landmark multi-site randomized controlled trial by the American Association of Critical Care Nurses (AACN) compared continuous 0.9% saline (sodium chloride) flush with continuous heparinized flush in 5139 adult patients with arterial catheters (88% radial; 9% femoral; 4% brachial; pedal <1%) at 198 sites. The study showed that catheters maintained with a heparinized flush were statistically more likely to remain patent over time, although the clinical differences were small as displayed in Table 3-3.[17] Catheter patency was determined from visible blood backflow into the arterial line and by a normal square wave test (see Figure 4-5). Clinically, if a radial arterial catheter will be in use for less than 72 hours, the likelihood of the catheter

TABLE 3-3   Arterial Catheter Patency and Continuous Flush Solution

	PROBABILITY OF ARTERIAL CATHETER PATENCY		
	24 HOURS	48 HOURS	72 HOURS
0.9% saline flush	(0.93) 93%	(0.86) 86%	(0.79) 79%
Heparinized saline flush	(0.97) 97%	(0.94) 94%	(0.90) 90%

Probability (decimal) and probability of remaining patent (%) at 24 hours, 48 hours, and 72 hours duration depending on type of continuous flush solution; 88% of the catheters were in the radial artery, 9% were in the femoral artery.
Data from Evaluation of the effects of heparinized and nonheparinized flush solutions on the patency of arterial pressure monitoring lines: AACN Thunder Project. By the American Association of Critical-Care Nurses, *Am J Crit Care* 2(1);3–15, 1993.

remaining patent is very high, irrespective of the flush solution (see Table 3-3). Femoral arterial catheters remain open at equal rates with both types of flush solution (98% patency at 24 hours and over 90% patency at 72 hours).[17] Patency is enhanced by the administration of other anticoagulants or thrombolytics, a catheter longer than 2 inches, femoral catheter placement, and use in male patients.[17] A deflated pressure cuff was one of the factors noted when a nonfunctional catheter was identified.[17]

A recent Cochrane systematic review of seven randomized controlled trials of 0.9% saline flush versus heparinized flush in 606 patients confirmed that 0.9% saline flush is as effective as a heparinized flush in maintaining arterial catheter patency.[18] Clinical guidelines in Britain recommend the use of sodium chloride 0.9% for maintenance of arterial lines.[19] Given the risk of heparin induced thrombocytopenia, it is prudent to eliminate heparin exposure whenever possible, and as illustrated in Table 3-3, the risk of catheter occlusion is small.

Arterial Catheter Blood Conservation Devices

One of the challenges with frequent blood withdrawal is managing the diluted dead space intraluminal volume that is in the arterial tubing. In many critical care units, the traditional three-way stopcock has been replaced by a blood conservation system that is connected to the arterial setup (Figure 3-8). Blood conservation devices permit withdrawal of the diluted tubing "dead space" volume into a reservoir within the closed system attached to the arterial line tubing. The dead space intraluminal volume will vary (5 to 10 mL), depending on the length of tubing between the catheter and the reservoir. The blood sample is withdrawn from a sampling port near the insertion point of the catheter (see Figure 3-8). The dead space intraluminal volume is then gently returned to the patient, and the line is flushed until clear, by using the flush-mechanism from the in-line flush mechanism. The advantage of blood conservation devices is minimal blood loss that reduces the need for blood transfusions[20] and potentially a lower arterial catheter infection rate compared with the traditional three-way stopcock access method.[21]

Errors to Avoid

An uncommon, but significant error, is the use of a 5% dextrose solution, instead of 0.9% saline as the flush solution. The dead space withdrawal volume required to clear

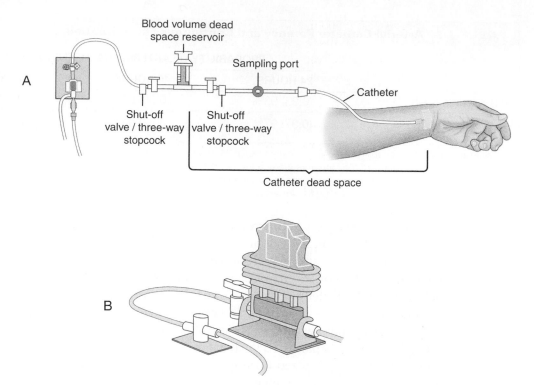

FIGURE 3-8 Blood conservation device on an arterial catheter (**B,** Courtesy Edwards LifeSciences Product).

glucose is much larger than that needed to clear saline. Blood withdrawn from an arterial catheter with an erroneous dextrose solution may produce artificially high blood glucose values.[19] Inappropriate insulin treatment based on these elevated values may result in harm to the patient.[19]

Mobility with Arterial Catheters

Early mobility is an important goal for critically ill patients. Lines and tubes are often perceived as barriers to early mobilization. Femoral arterial catheters are of particular concern. Two observational studies have demonstrated that patients can safely mobilize with femoral arterial catheters in situ.[22,23] Important safety measures when mobilizing a patient with an arterial catheter include having adequate staff members available to help the patient and manage all the lines.

Maintenance and Troubleshooting

Hemodynamic pressure lines require constant vigilance to maintain accuracy of the arterial waveform. The arterial waveform can become damped for a number of reasons: (1) a decrease in catheter lumen size from any cause such as a kink, air bubbles, biofilm "tail" or clot at the end of the catheter, or (2) a loss of pressure in the system (check pressure bag is at 300 mm Hg). If the length of noncompliant pressure tubing from the arterial catheter to the transducer is longer than 48 inches (122 cm), this can increase the dynamic resonance and the systolic peak may be amplified above the true value.[5] Other potential problems include inaccurate transducer zero or leveling. If the transducer is placed too high above the phlebostatic axis the arterial pressure reading will be erroneously low. Conversely, if the transducer is incorrectly placed below the phlebostatic axis the reading will be inaccurately high. Common problems along with suggested solutions are listed in Table 3-4.

> **Clinical Reasoning Pearl**
>
> Hypotension is an important but late sign of hemodynamic compromise.[24]

Complications of Arterial Catheters

The major complications associated with continuous arterial pressure monitoring, infection, distal ischemia, and bleeding, are discussed below.

Infection in Arterial Catheters

Similar to other intravascular devices, arterial catheters may become a portal for bacterial or other infections. Historically, arterial catheters were considered to carry a lower infection risk compared with central venous catheters (CVC), but this belief has now been discredited.[25,26] Lucet et al. (2010) examined 3532 catheters (arterial and venous) for 27,541 days, in 2095 patients, in a multi-center trial.[25] Colonization rates were similar for both catheters (7.9% arterial; 9.6% CVC). Infection rates were also similar: 0.68% (1.0/1000 catheter-days) for arterial, and 0.94% (1.09/1000 catheter-days) for CVCs. These small differences were not statistically significant. The risk of infection from an arterial line increased over time, especially after 7 days in situ. A higher infection rate existed for the femoral artery location compared with the radial artery.[25] Higher infection rates for femoral arterial catheters were confirmed in a recent meta-analysis of 49 arterial catheter randomized controlled trials.[26]

Although the hemodynamic monitoring setup is a closed system, the arterial line is frequently accessed to withdraw blood. Often, patients who are critically ill require not only hemodynamic monitoring but also frequent arterial blood gases, hourly blood glucose checks,[27] or other laboratory studies. Blood conservation devices are often used to limit blood loss associated with these tests. Oto et al. (2012) examined the infection risk of an arterial line blood conservation device compared with the traditional three-way stopcock access method in a randomized controlled trial of 216 arterial catheters. The study results showed an intraluminal volume contamination rate of 52% for three-way stopcocks and 18% for blood conservation devices ($p = 0.03$). In this study, intraluminal contamination was not associated with contamination at the catheter tip. Arterial catheter tip contamination was linked to a longer number of days in situ. Other studies have reported that most bacterial contamination (intraluminal or catheter tip)

TABLE 3-4   Troubleshooting Hemodynamic Pressure Monitoring Systems

PROBLEM	CAUSES	INTERVENTIONS	MAINTENANCE AND PREVENTION
• No waveform on monitor • Straight line on monitor • Sudden loss of waveform	**Monitor Causes** • Transducer cable has a loose connection. • Wrong scale: scale selected is too small for an arterial waveform. **Tubing/Transducer Causes** • Stopcock turned to the "off to patient" position meaning, no communication between patient and transducer/monitor. • Faulty transducer (rare). **Clinical Causes** • Catheter kinked. • Catheter clotted.	**Monitor interventions** • Check electrical connections between transducer and monitor module. • Change monitor module: the module can be sent to the hospital clinical engineering department. • Recalibrate monitor. • Check appropriate scale is selected on monitor. **Tubing/Transducer Interventions** • Check that stopcocks are open as intended. • Replace faulty transducer. **Clinical Interventions** • Reposition patient's limb (hand, leg) to unkink catheter. For example, provide a radial hand splint. • If the waveform has been sub-par, prior to loss, assess if the arterial line should be removed. It may be at the end of clinical usefulness. • Also see clinical interventions for damped waveform.	• Always visually monitor the hemodynamic waveform so that sudden loss can be detected. • Verify monitor settings are as expected. • Perform a "square wave" test every 8 to 12 hours to verify that the system has adequate dynamic resonance Maintain a working continuous flush system. Some hospitals use heparin 1unit/mL for patency, others do not because of concerns of heparin-induced thrombocytopenia (HIT). Follow hospital protocol. • Daily assessment of the need for an arterial catheter.

- Damped waveform with inaccurate digital numbers

Tubing/Transducer Causes

- System is over damped.
- Air bubbles in tubing
- Pressure bag not inflated to 300 mm Hg, low pressure allows blood to backflow into tubing.
- Loose Luer connections open system to atmospheric pressure, and to leaks; blood will backflow into tubing.

Clinical Causes

- Fibrin-clot-biofilm tail at end of catheter.
- Catheter tip up against vessel wall, or enmeshed in a biofilm tail that extends from the tip of the catheter.
- Positional catheter, may be kinked.

Tubing/Transducer Interventions

- Test the dynamic response by doing a fast flush test. The system is over-damped if the fast-flush maneuver produces damped or no oscillations.
- Eliminate all air from the system during set-up.
- If air bubbles are in a system connected to a patient, carefully back-flush all air bubbles out of the system and away from the patient.
- Check pressure bag is at 300 mm Hg.
- Tighten all Luer connections.

Clinical Interventions

- Verify with a cuff blood pressure that the digital numbers are in fact inaccurate, rule out hypotension.
- If a clot is suspected as the cause of a damped arterial line, do not irrigate the catheter with a syringe, this will only force fibrin-clot-biofilm into the blood stream and increase risk of infection.
- Reposition limb if catheter is positional, may be kinked (see above) or it may be due to a biofilm tail or flap that partially occludes the catheter tip.

- Check cuff blood pressure once a shift. Use the opposite arm if a radial arterial catheter is in situ.
- During hemodynamic system setup, remove all air bubbles from the system. Remove all air from the 0.9% saline bag that will be inside the pressure cuff.
- Use needleless blood access systems, and blood conservation systems, whenever possible, to reduce risk of air-entry into system.
- Use fast-flush system to clear line after blood withdrawal to maintain patency.

Continued

TABLE 3-4 Troubleshooting Hemodynamic Pressure Monitoring Systems—cont'd

PROBLEM	CAUSES	INTERVENTIONS	MAINTENANCE AND PREVENTION
• Inaccurate low pressure values with normal waveform	**Monitor Causes** • Inaccurate calibration (not zeroed correctly) where the stopcock was not opened to atmospheric pressure, i.e., solid cap was on. **Clinical causes** • Transducer air-fluid stopcock is positioned higher than the zero reference (phlebostatic axis). • For every 1 inch (2.5 cm) the transducer level is ABOVE the phlebostatic axis, the pressure value is reduced by about 2 mm Hg.	**Monitor Interventions** • Calibrate to "zero" (local atmospheric pressure) when system is setup. Modern disposable transducers are so reliable that repeated calibration is not required unless the transducer is disconnected from the monitor. However, many hospitals have policies that require recalibration on a regular basis such as every 8 to 12 hours. • Re-zero after transport off the unit, when connected to a transport monitor, or whenever the transducer has been disconnected from the monitor. **Clinical Interventions** • Re-level to the phlebostatic axis with any position change. • False low readings often occur when the bed height is raised and the transducer is not re-leveled at the same time. • It is not necessary to continually re-zero the monitor with bed height changes (as long as cables remain connected) because atmospheric pressure differences are minimal.	• Use a standardized method to verify the transducer air-fluid reference stopcock is correctly aligned (carpenters level or similar). • When the height of the transducer is changed this will alter the digital pressure numbers and also the position of the waveform within the monitor scale. • Because many bedside monitors automatically upload hemodynamic pressure information to an electronic health record (EHR), it is important to make sure accurate information is recorded.
• Inaccurate high pressure values with normal waveform	**Monitor Causes** • Inaccurate calibration (not zeroed correctly) where the stopcock was not opened to atmospheric pressure.	**Monitor Interventions** • Calibrate to "zero" (local atmospheric pressure) when system is set up. Rationale is described in prior section. • Re-zero after transport off the unit, when connected to a transport monitor, or whenever the transducer is disconnected from the transducer-monitor cable.	• Prevention and maintenance interventions are the same as in prior section.

	Clinical Causes	Clinical Interventions
	• Transducer air-fluid stopcock is positioned higher than the zero reference level (phlebostatic axis). • For every 1 inch (2.5 cm) that the transducer level is BELOW the phlebostatic axis, the pressure value is increased by about 2 mm Hg.	• Re-level to the phlebostatic axis with any position change. • Falsely high readings may occur when the bed is lowered and the transducer is not re-leveled at the same time. • It is not necessary to continually re-zero the monitor with bed height changes (as long as cables remain connected) because atmospheric pressure differences are minimal.
• Underdamped waveform • Catheter "fling" in waveform	• Underdamping of the system. • Addition of longer extension lengths of high-pressure non-compressible tubing. • Additions of multiple stopcocks.	• The system is "underdamped" if use of the fast-flush mechanism produces a square wave with undulations and many dynamic oscillations. • Use short lengths of high-pressure noncompressible tubing (under 48 inches length). • Perform a "square wave" test every 8 to 12 hours to verify that the system has normal dynamic resonance.

comes from the skin surface.[28] This affords the opportunity to use the same infection prevention methods that have been so successful in lowering the rate of CVC infections as discussed in Chapter 4. In fact, the growing consensus is that the same infection control principles should be applied to arterial catheter placement and maintenance.[28]

Standard infection prevention measures include antimicrobial site preparation and sterile technique for insertion. Chlorhexidine-impregnated dressings over the insertion site have been shown to reduce arterial catheter colonization and infection rates.[29] Prevention of contamination during blood access includes the use of clean gloves and thorough disinfection of the access port before blood is withdrawn. The arterial flush system is used to flush the line after blood draws to maintain catheter patency. Arterial pressure-transducer tubing sets are changed every 96 hours[30] or per hospital policy. Daily assessment of the clinical need for an arterial catheter is essential. One center reduced arterial catheter infections by using a scheduled replacement every 5 days.[31] Alternatively, if the patient is sufficiently stable, a transition to cuff blood pressure can be considered.

Published survey and quality improvement data suggest that some clinicians may be complacent about the infection risk associated with arterial catheters and arterial pressure-monitoring transducer-tubing systems.[19,32] Compliance with central line infection prevention bundles is closely monitored in most hospitals, but arterial catheter practices are not closely scrutinized.[28] However, as more published reports highlight the arterial catheter as a source of bloodstream infection, this may be re-evaluated. The 2011 Centers for Disease Control (CDC) recommendations for infection prevention in arterial pressure-monitoring systems are listed in Box 3-1.[33]

Vascular Complications with Arterial Catheters

The most serious complication of continuous arterial blood pressure monitoring is ischemia of the tissues distal to the arterial catheter insertion site. Hand ischemia that is severe enough to require a surgical repair is rare, it occurs in fewer than 1 in 500 to 1000 cases.[34] Nevertheless, because this complication can be so devastating, it is standard practice is to assess circulation beyond the artery, including skin color, temperature, and perfusion (capillary refill). Acute interruption of arterial circulation results in ischemic injury identified by the five Ps—pain, pallor, pulselessness, parathesia, polar (cold skin temperature). Unfortunately, in critical illness, a cascade of other confounding factors may impact peripheral perfusion in addition to obstruction from the arterial catheter. These include clinical conditions such as hypovolemia and shock; iatrogenic sequela such as vasoconstriction from vasoactive infusions; thrombosis as a result of heparin-induced thrombocytopenia from heparin in the arterial flush[35]; inadequate collateral arterial perfusion; and in some cases, patients who are unable to report their symptoms because of intubation or because of sedative or opiate infusions. Some clinicians use Doppler or pulse oximetry to quantify clinical assessment when any suspicion of ischemia exists.[35] The radial artery and dorsalis pedis artery are considered to be at greater risk of thrombosis than the femoral artery, mainly because of the smaller size of these peripheral arteries.[36] Because arterial obstruction could result in tissue death, when ischemia is suspected, the catheter must be removed immediately.

BOX 3-1 CDC Guidelines for Prevention of infection for Peripheral Arterial Catheters and Pressure Monitoring Devices in Adult Patients, with Level of Evidence

- In adults, use of the radial, brachial, or dorsalis pedis sites is preferred over the femoral or axillary sites of insertion to reduce the risk of infection. *Category IB*
- A minimum of a cap, mask, sterile gloves and a small sterile fenestrated drape should be used during peripheral arterial catheter insertion. *Category IB*
- During axillary or femoral artery catheter insertion, maximal sterile barriers precautions should be used. *Category II*
- Replace arterial catheters only when a clinical indication exists. *Category II*
- Remove the arterial catheter as soon as it is no longer needed. *Category II*
- Use disposable, rather than reusable, transducer assemblies when possible. *Category IB*
- Do not routinely replace arterial catheters to prevent catheter-related infections. *Category II*
- Replace disposable or reusable transducers at 96-hour intervals. Replace other components of the system (including the tubing, continuous-flush device, and flush solution) at the time the transducer is replaced. *Category IB*
- Keep all components of the pressure monitoring system (including calibration devices and flush solution) sterile. *Category IA*
- Minimize the number of manipulations of and entries into the pressure monitoring system. Use a closed flush system (i.e., continuous flush), rather than an open system (i.e., one

that requires a syringe and stopcock), to maintain the patency of the pressure monitoring catheters. *Category II*
- When the pressure monitoring system is accessed through a diaphragm, rather than a stopcock, scrub the diaphragm with an appropriate antiseptic before accessing the system. *Category IA*
- Do not administer dextrose-containing solutions or parenteral nutrition fluids through the pressure monitoring circuit. *Category IA*
- Sterilize reusable transducers according to the manufacturers' instructions if the use of disposable transducers is not feasible. *Category IA*

Level of Evidence

Category IA: Strongly recommended for implementation, strongly supported by well-designed experimental, clinical, or epidemiologic studies.

Category IB: Strongly recommended for implementation and supported by some experimental, clinical, or epidemiologic studies, a strong theoretical rationale; or an accepted practice (e.g., aseptic technique) supported by limited evidence.

Category IC: Required by state or federal regulations, rules, or standards.

Category II: Suggested for implementation and supported by suggestive clinical or epidemiologic studies or a theoretical rationale.

Data from O'Grady NP, et al.: Guidelines for the prevention of intravascular catheter-related infections, *Am J Infection Control* 39(4 Suppl 1):S1–S34, 2011.

Removal of any arterial catheter may be associated with complications. Hematoma is the most commonly seen complication and is normally managed by local compression at the site. Pseudoaneurysm is a less frequent complication that occurs when the artery insertion hole does not close normally and is instead covered by a clot, posing a risk of hemorrhage. Pseudoaneurysm is initially treated with compression at the site. If this is unsuccessful, surgical repair may be required.[35]

Bleeding

The arterial monitoring setup is a closed system from the pressure bag to the arterial catheter. Arterial blood does not flow into the tubing because the system is pressurized to be higher than the systolic blood pressure by the inflated pressure bag (300 mm Hg). However, if a loose connector, vented cap on a stopcock, or an open stopcock exists, arterial blood will flow along the path of least resistance, and a large blood loss may occur. It is imperative that all hemodynamic monitoring tubing connections have a Luer (screw) lock system and are tightly screwed shut. Loose or open connectors can be life threatening. For this reason, it is prudent to keep arterial pressure line tubing in view, on top of bed coverings whenever possible. To increase patient safety, monitor alarms must be turned on to detect any loss in arterial pressure from tubing disconnection or other causes.

Targeted Arterial Pressures in Critical Illness

Arterial catheters and continuous blood pressure monitoring are used to guide clinical management. Blood pressure guidelines are frequently incorporated into clinical practice guidelines and will vary, depending on the intervention.

Sepsis

In the Surviving Sepsis guidelines,[37] arterial hypotension in adults is defined as systolic blood pressure less than 90 mm Hg, MAP less than 70 mm Hg, or a decrease in systolic blood pressure of 40 mm Hg or more (or less than two standard deviations below age-normal). In the initial sepsis resuscitation period (first 6 hours), the goal is to increase blood pressure to a MAP 65 mm Hg or greater by crystalloid volume resuscitation.[37] Sepsis resuscitation targets also include a central venous pressure (CVP) of 8 to 12 mm Hg, urine output 0.5 mL/kg/hr or greater, normalization of serum lactate levels, and superior vena cava oxygenation levels above 70%.[37] With adequate volume resuscitation, vasopressor support may be added to achieve the target of MAP 65 mm Hg. The target MAP is not a goal in itself; the intent is to increase blood supply to tissues, preserve organ perfusion, and prevent tissue hypoxia.

Because it was not known whether a higher MAP range would be beneficial in treatment outcomes for sepsis, Asfar and associates (2014) studied two different MAP targets in septic shock.[38] No difference was found between 28-day and 90-day mortality rates for the 776 patients randomized to either a MAP of 65-70 mm Hg (low-MAP target), or to 80-85 mm Hg (high-MAP target) for the initial 5 days of treatment.[38] As a secondary aim, this study used stratified randomization to assign patients with a history of chronic hypertension to both the high-MAP-target and low-MAP-target groups.

The premise was that patients with chronic hypertension would have better physiologic outcomes if they were in the higher MAP group. Interestingly, there was no difference in mortality based on history of hypertension.[38] Patients in the higher MAP target group experienced more atrial fibrillation, which the authors surmised was caused by the increased doses of vasopressor catecholamines used to maintain the MAP in the 80 to 85 mm Hg range.[38]

Permissive Hypotension in Trauma

Traditional management of trauma patients has been to provide large amounts of volume to raise blood pressure. Results of a recent surgical research study suggests that permissive hypotension, with a low target MAP, might benefit trauma patients without head injury. Morrison et al. (2011)[39] examined permissive hypotension in a randomized controlled trial of 81 trauma patients undergoing laparotomy or thoracotomy for blunt and penetrating trauma. To be enrolled in the study, patients had to have at least one hypotensive episode (systolic blood pressure ≤90 mm Hg), which had usually occurred in the emergency department. Trauma patients were randomized on arrival at the operating room door to either (1) a target minimum MAP of 50 mm Hg or (2) to a target minimum MAP of 65 mm Hg (standard care). The target minimum MAP of 50 mm Hg group received less intraoperative fluids and had a lower risk of coagulopathy and early postoperative death, compared with the 65 mm Hg group.[39] This study has excited considerable controversy and will undoubtedly encourage more researchers to examine the role of perioperative arterial pressure monitoring targets.

Arterial Waveform Derived Variables and Volume Responsiveness

Indicators of volume responsiveness can be mathematically calculated from the arterial pressure waveform. Two indicators are: pulse pressure variation (PPV), and stroke volume variation (SVV).[40] Advanced hemodynamic monitors display these values on the screen as aids to assess patient volume responsiveness. These two values (PPV and SVV) are not direct surrogates for preload. Instead, the variation in these values over one respiratory cycle may indicate preload responsiveness, that is, determine whether the patient is likely to benefit hemodynamically from a fluid volume challenge.

Clinical Reasoning Pearl

Dynamic Versus Static Parameters: Volume Responsiveness

The arterial pressure waveform, in combination with advanced hemodynamic monitoring systems, is now used to derive dynamic parameters that can predict volume responsiveness in selected patients. Dynamic parameters (PPV and SVV percentages) are calculated over a full respiratory cycle. Dynamic parameters more accurately predict which critically ill mechanically ventilated patients will positively respond to a volume challenge.[40,41]

Pulse Pressure Variation

Pulse pressure is the difference between the maximum (systolic) and minimum (diastolic) values on the arterial pressure waveform. Numerically, this is calculated as: SBP – DBP = pulse pressure. PPV is calculated as a percentage and is available on many advanced hemodynamic monitoring systems to assist with fluid volume responsiveness.

The normal systolic pressure difference between inspiration and expiration is 5 to 10 mm Hg, with spontaneous breaths. A respiratory-associated decrease in systolic pressure of greater than 10 mm Hg during inspiration is known as *pulsus paradoxus* and may indicate volume depletion or cardiac tamponade. With mechanical ventilation the difference in the systolic arterial pressure between inspiration and expiration is accentuated, especially with larger tidal volumes. Ventricular stroke volume is potentially reduced during positive pressure ventilation when elevated intrathoracic pressures impede venous return to the heart, resulting in lower stroke volumes. Conversely, lower intrathoracic pressures during exhalation will facilitate venous return from the periphery to the thorax, and produce larger stroke volumes. See Chapter 14 for additional information on the impact of mechanical ventilation on hemodynamic function.

PPV is measured over the course of the respiratory cycle and reflects the variation in arterial pulse pressure between inspiration and expiration calculated as a percentage (see Figure 3-9 for PPV waveform). In a now classic study, Michard et al. (2000)[42]

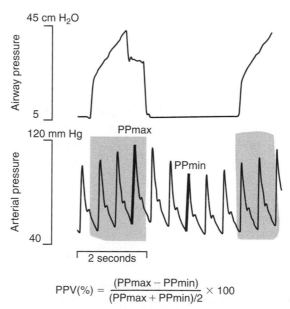

$$PPV(\%) = \frac{(PPmax - PPmin)}{(PPmax + PPmin)/2} \times 100$$

FIGURE 3-9 Systolic pulse pressure variation Note that the inspiratory phase of mechanical ventilation, shown by the airway pressure waveform, precedes the decline in arterial pressure. Higher pressure during the inspiratory phase of positive pressure ventilation decreases blood flow into the thorax and right heart, which leads to a lower stroke volume from the left ventricle and a lower arterial pressure. (Adapted from Michard, F, Boussat S, Chemla D, et al.: Relation between respiratory changes in arterial pulse pressure and fluid responsiveness in septic patients with acute circulatory failure, *Am J Respir Crit Care Med* 162(1):134–138, 2000.)

examined the impact of volume expansion on cardiac index and PPV in 40 patients on controlled mechanical ventilation (no spontaneous breaths) with acute circulatory failure caused by sepsis. In this study, a patient with a baseline PPV at or above 13% was likely to respond positively to a fluid challenge and to an increase in their cardiac index by 15% or more (positive predictive value 94%). In contrast, if the PPV was lower than 13%, the patient was unlikely to respond to a fluid challenge (negative predictive value 96%).[42] The same researchers also showed that a similar PPV percentage was predictive of fluid volume responsiveness in a small study of patients with acute lung injury who were mechanically ventilated with high levels of positive end expiratory pressure (PEEP).[43] Clinician–researchers continue to investigate the predictive role of PPV percentage in ventilated patients with spontaneous breaths. One small single-center study recently reported that PPV can be used to predict fluid volume requirements based on changes in arterial pressure in mechanically ventilated patients taking spontaneous breaths.[44]

Although still a relatively new parameter, PPV percentage has the potential to be very helpful for fluid volume management in critical illness. This is important because it is known that only about 50% of hemodynamically unstable critically ill patients respond to a fluid challenge.[41] This means that the other half receive excess volume that does not confer hemodynamic benefit and may be harmful. As with all derived parameters the baseline data must be accurate to avoid a "garbage in, garbage out" situation, meaning the arterial pressure waveform, from which these parameters are derived, must be accurate.

Stroke Volume Variation

SVV is a proprietary algorithm that predicts fluid volume responsiveness. SVV value is displayed on monitors that support this technology. Normal SVV values range from 10% to 15% for patients on controlled mechanical ventilation (no spontaneous breaths).[45] A clinical value of 13% is often used to determine fluid responsiveness.[45] SVV is calculated over one respiratory cycle, by the bedside computer, using the following equation and then converted to a percent value. Some advanced hemodynamic monitoring systems calculate and display the SVV percentage to assist with fluid volume management.

Stroke Volume Variation Calculation

$$\% \, SVV \; = \; \frac{SVmax - SVmin}{SVmean}$$

When SVV is high ($\geq$13%) the patient is predicted to be volume responsive; that is, a fluid challenge will potentially increase stroke volume and increase cardiac output. When there is less SVV variability (<13%) the patient is considered non–volume responsive, suggesting that fluid volume is already optimized and that further fluid boluses will not increase cardiac output.[45] This is graphically illustrated in Figure 3-10. It is important to emphasize that no single variable should be used to manage fluid volume status and patient care in critically ill patients. The SVV is additive to other hemodynamic, respiratory, and patient assessment data.

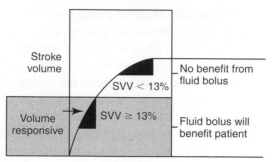

FIGURE 3-10 Stroke volume variation in response to a volume challenge.

The movement away from the use of static pressure values (blood pressure, CVP, pulmonary artery occlusion pressure) toward dynamic arterial indices (PPV, SVV) to determine patients' preload responsiveness has been research based. Marik et al. (2009)[40] conducted a meta-analysis of 29 randomized controlled studies that compared dynamic arterial waveform derived variables with conventional static measures during volume controlled mechanical ventilation.[40] The analysis demonstrated that dynamic variables (PPV, SVV) identified fluid volume responsiveness in mechanically ventilated critically ill patients, with better predictive capability than the traditional static measures.[40] See Chapter 12, Arterial Waveform and Pressure-Based Hemodynamic Monitoring, for more information on the application of these parameters.

Passive Leg Raise

Passive leg raise is a method to provide an endogenous fluid bolus by raising the patient's legs and observing the effect on hemodynamic parameters. To obtain the largest fluid volume effect from a passive leg raise, the patient is initially positioned on the back with the head of bed elevated to 45 degrees, then the bed position is changed so that the patient is lying supine, and both legs are raised off the bed at a 45 degree angle.[41] This offers the equivalent of a small fluid volume bolus as blood flows from the legs into the large veins of the abdomen and thorax (Figure 3-11). If the patient is flat in bed to begin with, the passive leg raise volume challenge may not be sufficient to demonstrate fluid responsiveness.[41] A response to passive leg raise will be evident within 1 minute if the patient is volume responsive. The patient's legs can also be supported by raising the foot of the bed or using a wedge or pillows.[41]

Monnet et al. (2006) demonstrated that an increase in aortic blood flow of ≥10% in response to a passive leg raise accurately predicted fluid responsiveness (sensitivity 97%, specificity 94%).[46] To accurately measure aortic blood flow the researchers used an esophageal Doppler probe. The arterial waveform was monitored to evaluate change in arterial pulse pressure over a respiratory cycle. This change is known as pulse pressure variation, or PPV. In response to a passive leg raise, a PPV change of

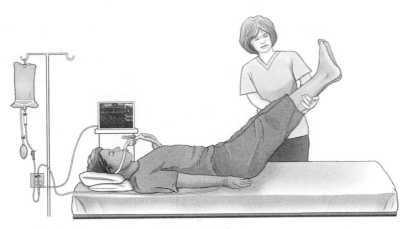

FIGURE 3-11 Passive leg raise in an intubated patient.

12% or greater, across the mechanical ventilator cycle indicated volume responsiveness (sensitivity 88%, specificity 93%), in patients who were fully mechanically ventilated (no spontaneous breaths) and without arrhythmias.[46]

However, in the same study, when ventilated patients had spontaneous breaths or arrhythmias, the predictive value of a change in PPV ($\geq$12%) was weaker (sensitivity 88%, specificity 46%).[46] In this study, the researchers used a gold standard to measure the impact of passive leg raise, namely, blood flow in the aorta. The dynamic arterial waveform parameter (PPV) was only predictive when the circumstances were tightly controlled (mechanical ventilation, no spontaneous breathing, no arrhythmias).[46] Other factors may also influence PPV. In mechanically ventilated patients change in PPV over the respiratory cycle may also be affected by large tidal volumes.[41]

Other researchers have examined the impact of a passive leg raise in spontaneously breathing patients, using measures such as echocardiography,[47,48] Doppler,[49] or stroke volume using advanced monitoring systems.[48] However, evidence that changes in PPV or SVV alone are sufficient to predict fluid responsiveness in spontaneously breathing patients is lacking.

Arterial Waveform Monitoring for Other Devices

The arterial pressure waveform is integral to several noninvasive or minimally invasive hemodynamic monitoring systems that use sophisticated technology and proprietary algorithms to formulate advanced hemodynamic variables as listed in Table 3-5 and discussed in Chapter 12. The arterial blood pressure waveform is also vital to assessment of intra-aortic balloon pump (IABP) efficacy (see Chapter 15). In all situations, these advanced hemodynamic technologies can only produce precise and reliable data if the arterial waveform is accurate and of good quality.

TABLE 3-5   Hemodynamic Devices That Use the Arterial Pressure Waveform

DEVICE	PURPOSE	ARTERIAL WAVEFORM	DESCRIPTION
IABP	Arterial diastolic augmentation to lower systemic vascular resistance and increase cardiac output	IABP can be timed from the dicrotic notch of the arterial waveform	Augments the arterial waveform and pressure during diastole. See Chapter 15.
PiCCO	Hemodynamic monitoring and minimally invasive cardiac output	Pulse contour analysis	Continuous arterial waveform analysis using a proprietary algorithm provides information on the cardiac output, stroke volume, SVV% and PPV%. See Chapter 12.
LiDCO	Hemodynamic monitoring and minimally invasive cardiac output	Pulse power analysis	Continuous arterial waveform analysis using a proprietary algorithm provides information on the cardiac output, stroke volume, SVV% and PPV%. See Chapter 12.
FlowTrac	Hemodynamic monitoring and minimally invasive cardiac output	Arterial pressure	Continuous arterial waveform analysis using a proprietary algorithm that incorporates age, BSA, and whether male or female, to calculate stroke volume, cardiac output, and SVV%. See Chapter 12.

BSA, Body surface area; *IABP*, intra-aortic balloon pump; *PPV*, pulse pressure variation; *SVV*, stroke volume variation.

Conclusion

Arterial pressure monitoring remains an important vital sign, but that is not its only function. A target MAP is incorporated into the sepsis clinical guidelines. The pressure waveform is used as a component of sophisticated hemodynamic algorithms, and dynamic arterial waveform derived variables are being investigated to identify their role in assessment of fluid responsiveness. Yet it all comes back to the basics, as these advanced hemodynamic technologies can only produce precise and reliable data if the arterial waveform is accurate and of good quality. This requires careful clinical assessment and knowledge of the fundamentals of arterial pressure monitoring.

Case Study

Mrs. P is a 66-year-old female with a diagnosis of long-standing interstitial lung disease. She uses oxygen via nasal cannula at home and takes steroids. Her warfarin dose was recently reduced because of a prolonged international normalized ratio (INR). Over the last week, she has been feeling increasingly short of breath and tired, and her family doctor had increased her dose of steroids. Today, she started feeling more tired and "light-headed" at home, and called 9-1-1 for help to go to the emergency department.

Syncopal Event: In the emergency department, she experienced a brief syncopal event as she attempted to walk to the bathroom. She regained consciousness quickly, and vital signs at that time were heart rate 124 beats/min; cuff blood pressure 62/palpation mm Hg; respiratory rate 38 breaths/min; and pulse oximetry (SpO_2) 64% on 2 liters nasal cannula. An arterial blood gas (ABG) showed:

pH 7.44

$PaCO_2$ 41.3

PaO_2 28

SaO_2 54%

HCO_3^- 27

One Minute Later: Mrs. P was placed on a 100% non-rebreather mask with a 15-liter oxygen flow, achieving a SpO_2 of 98%, HR 89 beats/min, BP 126/73 mm Hg.

Computed tomographic angiography (CTA) of the thorax showed a submassive pulmonary embolism in the right pulmonary artery. A Doppler ultrasound scan revealed a large clot in the right peroneal and right tibial leg veins.

Critical Care Unit Admission: Mrs. P. was admitted to the critical care unit, where a radial arterial line was placed and an intravenous (IV) heparin infusion was started. The heparin will stop new clots from developing but does not reduce existing thrombus.[50] She was alert and orientated, although very short of breath with any small movement. Vital signs on admission to the critical care unit were stable.

Hypotensive Episode on Heparin Infusion: Mrs. P remained alert and communicative but short of breath on 80% high-flow oxygen. She was only comfortable sitting upright in bed and desaturated to SpO_2 85% with mild exertion such as repositioning. Six hours later, she developed acute chest pain with a sustained period of hypotension (BP 77/46 mm Hg). Her blood pressure increased with an IV crystalloid bolus and vasopressor support. This change in hemodynamics, with a hypotensive episode of longer than 15 minutes was instrumental in the decision to use fibrinolysis to decrease the size of the pulmonary embolism.[51]

Stable after tPA: The heparin was stopped for an hour and an IV infusion of Alteplase (tissue plasminogen activator) 100 mg was administered over 2 hours.[51] Mrs. P tolerated the treatment well, with no untoward side effects. Vital signs were taken every 15 minutes during the infusion and for an hour afterward. Follow-up vital signs were stable and the heparin infusion was restarted. One day later, her oxygen requirement was reduced to 4 L

Continued

Case Study—cont'd

nasal cannula with non-labored respirations and SpO$_2$ 96%. After another 48 hours she transferred to the progressive critical care unit (telemetry) in stable condition. The plan is to transition to low-molecular-weight heparin (LMWH) and then to warfarin for long-term INR management. ◾

PARAMETERS	SYNCOPAL EVENT	1 MINUTE LATER	ADMIT TO CRITICAL CARE UNIT	HYPOTENSIVE EPISODE ON HEPARIN	POST-TPA
Temp °C		37.1	36.8	38.3	37.2
Heart rate	124	89	96	180	95
Blood pressure (mm Hg)	62/palp cuff	126/73 cuff	137/85 A-line	77/46 A-line	118/74
MAP (mm Hg)			100		
Respiratory rate	38	22	24	36 with mild exertion	24
SpO$_2$	64%	98%	98%	85% with mild exertion	96%
Oxygen	2 liters (L) per nasal cannula (NC)	15 L non-rebreather mask	15 L non-rebreather mask	80% high flow oxygen mask	4-L NC
pH	7.44		7.43	7.44	
PaCO$_2$	41.3		43.4	45.7	
PaO$_2$	28		113	65	
Oxygen saturation	54%		99%	94%	
HCO$_3^-$	27		29	29	
INR	1.3			1.3	
aPTT	28.6			134.5	

aPTT, Activated partial thromboplastin time; *TPA*, tissue plasminogen activator.

Patient Education

- Explain the reason for insertion of the arterial catheter.

- If the catheter is to be inserted into the radial artery, describe the procedure for the Allen test (see Figure 3-6) and explain why it is performed.

- Explain that insertion of the needle may be painful. A local anesthetic will be given to numb the pain. Once inserted, the catheter is not painful.

- Describe that all invasive catheters have a risk of infection and describe the precautions that are taken to avoid infection both during insertion and during catheter maintenance.

- The patient is asked not to move or bend the wrist (radial artery) or hip (femoral artery and to avoid flexion that may dislodge the arterial catheter.

- Show the arterial waveform on the bedside monitor and explain why this waveform is important to monitor.

- The major complications from an arterial catheter are bleeding, catheter clotting, and infection.

- When the catheter is removed, the clinician will firmly hold pressure on the pulse or insertion site until a stable clot has formed.[52,53]

Patient Safety

Prevention of Bleeding

- Use Luer (screw) locks on all tubing connections.

- If the catheter is not sutured (this varies by hospital), tape the catheter securely in place.

- Tape a U-loop of tubing to the skin near the insertion site so that a direct pull on the tubing (from any cause) will not dislodge the catheter.

Prevention of Infection

- Insertion of the arterial catheter is a sterile procedure (see Box 3-1).

- Apply chlorhexidene on the skin before insertion.

- "Scrub the hub" to thoroughly disinfect the hub of all needleless access ports, before and after drawing a blood sample.

- Ask the patient to tell you if the catheter site becomes painful.

Safe Use of Monitor Alarms

- Arterial pressure monitor alarms must be on.

- Adjust arterial pressure alarms 10 mm Hg above or below the target mean arterial pressure or systolic blood pressure.

Patient Comfort

Explain the purpose of the arterial catheter and that blood samples may also be withdrawn from the catheter. This is an alternative to a venipuncture or finger stick and is more comfortable for the patient.

References

1. Gershengorn HB, Garland A, Kramer A, et al.: Variation of arterial and central venous catheter use in United States intensive care units, *Anesthesiology* 120(3):650–664, 2014.
2. Brzezinski M, Luisetti T, London MJ: Radial artery cannulation: a comprehensive review of recent anatomic and physiologic investigations, *Anesth Analg* 109(6):1763–1781, 2009.
3. Booth J: A short history of blood pressure measurement, *Proc Royal Soc Med* 70(11):793–799, 1977.
4. Paskalev D, Kircheva A, Krivoshiev S: A centenary of auscultatory blood pressure measurement: a tribute to Nikolai Korotkoff, *Kidney Blood Pressure Res* 28(4):259–263, 2005.
5. McGhee BH, Bridges EJ: Monitoring arterial blood pressure: what you may not know, *Crit Care Nurse* 2:60–64, 2002, 66–70, 73 passim.
6. London GM, Pannier B: Arterial functions: how to interpret the complex physiology, *Nephrol Dial Transplant* 25(12):3815–3823, 2010.
7. Devos DGH, Rietzschel E, Heyse C, et al.: MR pulse wave velocity increases with age faster in the thoracic aorta than in the abdominal aorta, *J Magn Reson Imag*, http://dx.doi.org/10.1002/jmri.24592, 2014.
8. Reddy AK, Jogendra MR, Rosendorff C: Blood pressure measurement in the geriatric population, *Blood Press Monit* 19(2):59–63, 2014.
9. Habib J, Baetz L, Satiani B: Assessment of collateral circulation to the hand prior to radial artery harvest, *Vasc Med* 17(5):352–361, 2012.
10. Tegtmeyer K, Brady G, Lai S, et al.: Videos in clinical medicine. Placement of an arterial line, *N Engl J Med* 354(15):e13, 2006.
11. Shiloh AL, Savel RH, Paulin LM, Eisen LA: Ultrasound-guided catheterization of the radial artery: a systematic review and meta-analysis of randomized controlled trials, *Chest* 139 (3):524–529, 2011.
12. Seto AH, Abu-Fadel MS, Sparling JM, et al.: Real-time ultrasound guidance facilitates femoral arterial access and reduces vascular complications: FAUST (Femoral Arterial Access With Ultrasound Trial), *JACC Cardiovasc Interv* 3(7):751–758, 2010.
13. Troianos CA, Hartman GS, Glas KE, et al.: Guidelines for performing ultrasound guided vascular cannulation: recommendations of the American Society of Echocardiography and the Society of Cardiovascular Anesthesiologists, *J Am Soc Echocardiogr* 24(12):1291–1318, 2011.
14. Lamperti M, Bodenham AR, Pittiruti M, et al.: International evidence-based recommendations on ultrasound-guided vascular access, *Intensive Care Med* 38(7):1105–1117, 2012.
15. American Institute of Ultrasound in Medicine: AIUM practice guideline for the use of ultrasound to guide vascular access procedures, *J Ultrasound Med* 32(1):191–215, 2013.

16. Magder SA: The highs and lows of blood pressure: toward meaningful clinical targets in patients with shock, *Crit Care Med* 42(5):1241–1251, 2014.

17. American Association of Critical-Care Nurses: Evaluation of the effects of heparinized and nonheparinized flush solutions on the patency of arterial pressure monitoring lines, *Am J Crit Care* 2(1):3–15, 1993.

18. Robertson-Malt S, Malt GN, Farquhar V, Greer W: Heparin versus normal saline for patency of arterial lines, *Cochrane Database Syst Rev* 5;2014, CD007364.

19. Leslie RA, Gouldson S, Habib N, et al.: Management of arterial lines and blood sampling in intensive care: a threat to patient safety, *Anaesthesia* 68(11):1114–1119, 2013.

20. Mukhopadhyay A, Yip HS, Prabhuswamy D, et al.: The use of a blood conservation device to reduce red blood cell transfusion requirements: a before and after study, *Crit Care* 14(1):R7, 2010.

21. Oto J, Nakataki E, Hata M, et al.: Comparison of bacterial contamination of blood conservation system and stopcock system arterial sampling lines used in critically ill patients, *Am J Infect Contr* 40(6):530–534, 2012.

22. Damluji A, Zanni JM, Mantheiy E, et al.: Safety and feasibility of femoral catheters during physical rehabilitation in the intensive care unit, *J Crit Care* 28(4):535, e9–15, 2013.

23. Perme C, et al.: Safety and efficacy of mobility interventions in patients with femoral catheters in the ICU: a prospective observational study, *Cardiopulm Phys Ther J* 24(2):12–17, 2013.

24. Cove ME, Pinsky MR: Perioperative hemodynamic monitoring, *Best Pract Res Clin Anaesthesiol* 26(4):453–462, 2012.

25. Lucet JC, Bouadma L, Zahar JR, et al.: Infectious risk associated with arterial catheters compared with central venous catheters, *Crit Care Med* 38(4):1030–1035, 2010.

26. O'Horo JC, Maki DG, Krupp AE, Safdar N: Arterial catheters as a source of bloodstream infection: a systematic review and meta-analysis, *Crit Care Med* 42(6):1334–1339, 2014.

27. Raurell-Torredà M, Del Llano-Serrano C, Almirall-Solsona D, Nicolás-Arfelis JM, Dulhunty J, Tower M: Arterial catheter setup for glucose control in critically ill patients: a randomized controlled trial, *Am J Crit Care* 23(2):150–159, 2014.

28. Safdar N, O'Horo JC, Maki DG: Arterial catheter-related bloodstream infection: incidence, pathogenesis, risk factors and prevention, *J Hosp Infect* 85(3):189–195, 2013.

29. Safdar N, O'Horo JC, Ghufran A, et al.: Chlorhexidine-impregnated dressing for prevention of catheter-related bloodstream infection: a meta-analysis, *Crit Care Med* 42(7):1703–1713, 2014.

30. Ullman AJ, Cooke ML, Gillies D, et al.: Optimal timing for intravascular administration set replacement, *Cochrane Database Syst Rev* 9:2013, CD003588.

31. Pirracchio R, Legrand M, Rigon MR, et al.: Arterial catheter-related bloodstream infections: results of an 8-year survey in a surgical intensive care unit, *Crit Care Med* 39 (6):1372–1376, 2011.

32. Reynolds H, Dulhunty J, Tower M, et al.: A snapshot of guideline compliance reveals room for improvement: a survey of peripheral arterial catheter practices in Australian operating theatres, *J Adv Nurs* 69(7):1584–1594, 2013.

33. O'Grady NP, Alexander M, Burns LA, et al.: Guidelines for the prevention of intravascular catheter-related infections, *Am J Infect Contr* 39(4 Suppl 1):S1–S34, 2011.

34. Valentine RJ, Modrall JG, Clagett GP: Hand ischemia after radial artery cannulation, *J Am Coll Surg* 201(1):18–22, 2005.

35. Garg K, Howell BW, Saltzberg SS, et al.: Open surgical management of complications from indwelling radial artery catheters, *J Vasc Surgery* 58(5):1325–1330, 2013.

36. Cousins TR, O'Donnell JM: Arterial cannulation: a critical review, *AANA J* 72(4):267–271, 2004.

37. Dellinger RP, Levy MM, Rhodes A, et al.: Surviving sepsis campaign: international guidelines for management of severe sepsis and septic shock: 2012, *Crit Care Med* 41 (2):580–637, 2013.

38. Asfar P, Meziani F, Hamel JF, et al.: High versus low blood-pressure target in patients with septic shock, *N Engl J Med* 370(17):1583–1593, 2014.
39. Morrison CA, Carrick MM, Norman MA, et al.: Hypotensive resuscitation strategy reduces transfusion requirements and severe postoperative coagulopathy in trauma patients with hemorrhagic shock: preliminary results of a randomized controlled trial, *J Trauma* 70 (3):652–663, 2011.
40. Marik PE, Cavallazzi R, Vasu T, Hirani A: Dynamic changes in arterial waveform derived variables and fluid responsiveness in mechanically ventilated patients: a systematic review of the literature, *Crit Care Med* 37(9):2642–2647, 2009.
41. Marik PE, Monnet X, Teboul JL: Hemodynamic parameters to guide fluid therapy, *Ann Intensive Care* 1(1):1, 2011.
42. Michard F, Boussat S, Chemla D, et al.: Relation between respiratory changes in arterial pulse pressure and fluid responsiveness in septic patients with acute circulatory failure, *Am J Respir Crit Care Med* 162(1):134–138, 2000.
43. Michard F, Chemla D, Richard C, et al.: Clinical use of respiratory changes in arterial pulse pressure to monitor the hemodynamic effects of PEEP, *Am J Respir Crit Care Med* 159 (3):935–939, 1999.
44. Grassi P, Lo Nigro L, Battaglia K, et al.: Pulse pressure variation as a predictor of fluid responsiveness in mechanically ventilated patients with spontaneous breathing activity: a pragmatic observational study, *HSR Proc Intensive Cardiovasc Anesth* 5(2):98–109.
45. McGee WT: A simple physiologic algorithm for managing hemodynamics using stroke volume and stroke volume variation: physiologic optimization program, *J Intensive Care Med* 24 (6):352–360, 2009.
46. Monnet X, Rienzo M, Osman D, et al.: Passive leg raising predicts fluid responsiveness in the critically ill, *Crit Care Med* 34(5):1402–1407, 2006.
47. Préau S, Saulnier F, Dewavrin F, et al.: Passive leg raising is predictive of fluid responsiveness in spontaneously breathing patients with severe sepsis or acute pancreatitis, *Crit Care Med* 38 (3):819–825, 2010.
48. Biais M, Vidil L, Sarrabay P, et al.: Changes in stroke volume induced by passive leg raising in spontaneously breathing patients: comparison between echocardiography and Vigileo/FloTrac device, *Crit Care* 13(6):R195, 2009.
49. Chan CP, Cheung PL, Man Tse M, et al.: Influence of different positions on hemodynamics derived from noninvasive transcutaneous Doppler ultrasound, *Physiol Rep* 1(4):e00062, 2013.
50. Smithburger PL, Campbell S, Kane-Gill SL: Alteplase treatment of acute pulmonary embolism in the intensive care unit, *Crit Care Nurse* 33(2):17–27, 2013.
51. Jaff MR, McMurtry MS, Archer SL, et al.: Management of massive and submassive pulmonary embolism, iliofemoral deep vein thrombosis, and chronic thromboembolic pulmonary hypertension: a scientific statement from the American Heart Association, *Circulation* 123 (16):1788–1830, 2011.
52. American Thoracic Society (ATS): Patient information series: arterial catheterization, *Am J Respir Crit Care Med* 170:P1–P2, 2004.
53. Balaji NR, Shah PB: Cardiology patient page. Radial artery catheterization, *Circulation* 124(16): e407–e408, 2011.

Central Venous Pressure Monitoring

Deborah Tuggle

4

Central venous pressure (CVP) is the pressure inside the thoracic vena cava near the right atrium. It is considered equal to the right atrial pressure and right ventricular (RV) pressure at the end of diastole when the tricuspid valve is open. Measurement of the CVP has a long history (Box 4-1).[1] The pressures from the central veins have been used extensively as an indirect reflection of intravascular volume (preload) and RV function. However, recent evidence has provided new knowledge that is projected to change practice in the future. At this time, many institutions lack newer equipment for evaluating volume status, so this chapter will review both past and current thinking on CVP monitoring.

Key Physiologic Concepts

Central pressure in the venous system is of clinical interest as a determinant of the filling pressure or preload of the right heart and thus a regulator of stroke volume. Starling's law of the heart describes this physiologic relationship: the greater the muscle fiber stretch (preload) the greater the reflexive force of the muscle (contractility). Changes in CVP (ΔCVP) are a result of changes in blood volume (ΔV) within the thoracic veins divided by the compliance in the veins (Cv). This relationship is depicted by the following equation:

$$\Delta CVP = \Delta V \div Cv$$

Thus, CVP will be increased by either an increase in venous return volume or by a decrease in venous compliance. Compliance changes result from changes in vascular tone. Decreased compliance is most commonly caused by contraction of smooth muscle and by narrowing of smaller veins outside the thorax in response to sympathetic stimulation. Venous constriction results in increased pressure transmitted back to the vena cava. Central venous pressures will be decreased by either a decrease in venous volume or by an increase in vein compliance. Increased compliance is generally caused by relaxation of smooth muscle, followed by a widening of the veins mediated by the parasympathetic nervous system in the resting state.

BOX 4-1　Historic Milestones in Central Venous Cannulation and Pressure Monitoring

1616　William Harvey announced his discovery that blood flow is continuous and in one direction.

1656　Sir Christopher Wren used a goose quill connected to a pig's bladder to infuse a mixture of fluids into dogs' veins.

1733　Stephen Hales inserted a glass tube into a major vein in a horse to measure vascular pressure.

1844　Claude Bernard cannulated a horse's jugular vein to measure intracardiac pressures and temperatures; he also recorded the first central venous insertion complication: right ventricular perforation in a dog.

1912　Frizt Bleichroeder and associates inserted the first central venous pressure (CVP) catheter in a human being.

1941　André Cournand, Hilmert Ranges, and Dickinson Richards used right heart catheterization to assess heart function.

1956　Cournand, Richards, and Forssmann shared the Nobel Prize in Physiology and Medicine for their contributions to the advancement of right heart catheterization.

1959　Hughes and Magovern published a nonstatistically tested study drawing a relationship between right atrial pressure and blood volume.

1962　Wilson and Grow further popularized the use of CVP as a measure of blood volume in thoracic surgery patients.

Venous volume and pressure are dynamic properties of the vascular system, and many factors influence them. For example, a deep breath (inspiration) increases venous return to the heart through the development of negative intrathoracic pressure generating a "sucking" action on blood flow. Mechanically delivered breaths, in contrast, employ positive pressure that can decrease venous return to the thorax. Hydrostatic forces related to gravity impact CVP. Standing may pool blood away from the chest and thus decrease CVP, whereas lying supine, especially with legs elevated, may pool blood in the thorax and increase CVP.

Medications that manipulate venous tone may alter CVP. Nitroglycerin, a venodilator, may decrease CVP by pooling blood in the venous circulation. Norepinephrine, a vasopressor, may raise CVP by increasing venous tone. Inotropes may decrease CVP by moving blood forward in the cardiopulmonary circuit and out of the thorax. These factors influence CVP by either changing thoracic venous blood volume or changing venous compliance.

Measurement of Central Venous Pressure

Central venous pressures were originally estimated noninvasively by inspecting neck veins as part of the physical examination (Figure 4-1). With the advent of vessel cannulation, readings could be obtained directly using intravenous catheters placed via the jugular, subclavian, or femoral vein and threaded into the superior or inferior vena cava in proximity to the right atrium. With advances in cannulation, CVP readings

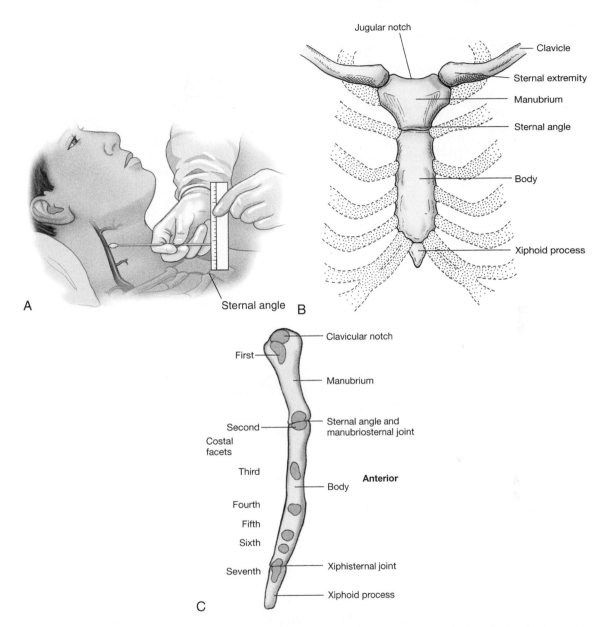

FIGURE 4-1 A, Position the patient supine and at 45 degrees elevation. Locate the level of pulsation of the internal jugular vein (or the visible top of the external jugular if pulsations are not apparent). Measure the horizontal distance in centimeters from this point to the sternal angle. **B** and **C,** Anterior views showing the protruding segment of the sternum at the manubrium junction. The sternal angle is estimated to lie 5 centimeters (cm) above the atrium. Thus, the sum of the distance above the angle plus 5 cm provides a bedside estimate of central venous pressure. (Parts **B** and **C** from Ballinger PW, Frank ED: *Merrill's atlas of radiographic positions and radiologic procedures,* ed 11, vol 1, St. Louis, 2012, Mosby.)

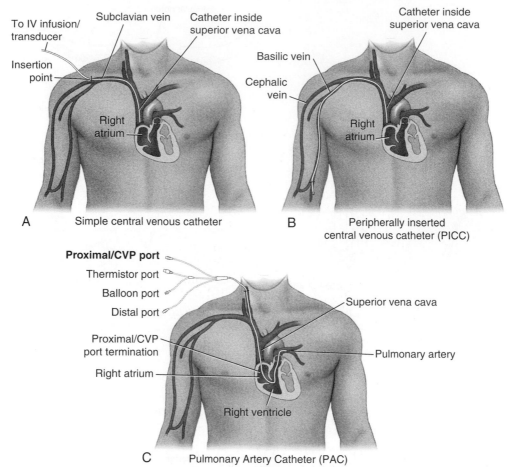

FIGURE 4-2 A, Simple central venous catheter: normally inserted via the subclavian (*shown*) or jugular approach; may be a single (*shown*), double- or triple-lumen device to better accommodate fluid and medication administration. **B,** Peripherally inserted central catheter (PICC): may be inserted via the basilic vein (*shown*), cephalic vein or brachial vein. **C,** Pulmonary artery catheter (PAC): generally inserted via the subclavian vein or internal jugular vein (*shown*); the PAC is threaded into position with the proximal port terminating in the right atrium, and the distal port terminating in the pulmonary artery.

were measured from the central venous port (right atrial port) of pulmonary artery catheters and from peripherally inserted central catheters, often abbreviated as a PICC (Figure 4-2).[2]

Originally, CVP readings were recorded manually in centimeters of water (cm H_2O) utilizing an in-line manometer device (Figure 4-3). However, they are now almost exclusively obtained digitally as millimeters of mercury (mm Hg) using a saline-filled pressure tubing and transducer set-up (Figure 4-4). Currently, a central venous catheter is typically a multi-lumen catheter and is employed for fluid infusions, intravenous medications, parenteral nutrition, hemodialysis, temporary pacemaker insertion, blood specimen collection, and the measurement of venous oxygen saturation (see Chapter 7) far more than for pressure monitoring.

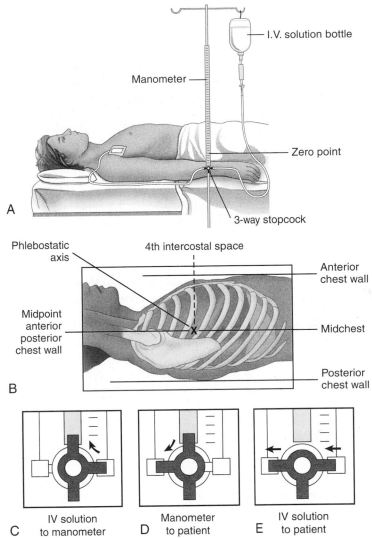

FIGURE 4-3 Water Manometer Technique for Central Venous Pressure Monitoring. A, The system attached to the central line consists of an intravenous (IV) solution with tubing, a manometer with centimeter markings, and a special, three-way stopcock. To measure central venous pressure (CVP), the manometer must first be "zeroed" by placing the zero point denoted on the manometer at the level of the patient's phlebostatic axis, the external landmark for the right atrium. **B,** The phlebostatic axis is located at the fourth intercostal space at the mid anteroposterior diameter of the chest. **C,** Next, the stopcock is turned to fill the manometer with IV fluid. **D,** After that, the stopcock is positioned to connect the manometer to the patient. Fluid in the manometer will be seen to oscillate and gradually fall until the pressure of the column of fluid in the manometer equilibrates with the pressure in the central vein. Once the fluid column stabilizes, the CVP is read in centimeters of water (cm H_2O) by comparing the fluid height in the manometer to its centimeter scale. **E,** After reading is taken, the stopcock is placed in position to deliver fluid to the patient.

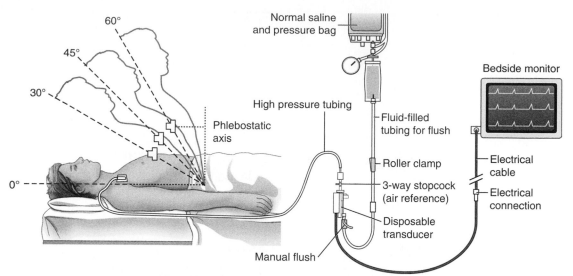

FIGURE 4-4 Pressure-Transducer Technique for Central Venous Pressure Monitoring.
Pre-primed, fluid-filled pressure tubing with an inline transducer transforms pulsatile intravascular pressures into an electronic signal for display on the bedside monitor. The transducer-stopcock must be leveled to the phlebostatic axis for accuracy, but the head of the bed may be positioned up to 60 degrees. A pressure bag is inflated over the normal saline bag to maintain continuous, minimal infusion for catheter patency.

Central venous cannulation is a procedure carried out by a trained health care provider with the assistance of the bedside nurse. Patients are placed in the supine position, with the head of the bed flat, or in a slight Trendelenburg position to augment vascular flow to the neck and upper chest vessels to increase ease of insertion. A procedural timeout is allowed for patient safety, and the catheter is inserted under strict sterile technique (see the Troubleshooting Primary Complications of CVP Lines section). Once the catheter is positioned, the pre-primed, fluid-filled pressure tubing and hemodynamic transducer are attached. The transducer device will transform the patient's pulsatile blood pressure into an electronic signal that can be displayed on the bedside monitor. The tubing is connected to a bag of normal saline inserted into a pressure bag inflated to approximately 300 mm Hg. The pressure on the system ensures a continuous flow of saline, at a rate of 3 milliliters per hour (mL/hr), to maintain catheter patency. The system also contains a manual flush device for intermittently clearing the line following blood sampling and as needed. After the catheter and the system are in place, a sterile dressing is applied, the catheter and line are secured, and chest radiography is performed to detect any inadvertent vessel injury or lung complication such as a pneumothorax.

Patient Comfort

- Insertion of a central venous catheter to obtain the CVP is not without risk and may be a painful procedure for the patient, especially if multiple insertion attempts are required.

- Preferentially, central venous catheters are inserted into the larger thoracic veins, primarily the subclavian vein. One challenge with cannulation of these large veins is the existence of many vascular anatomic variations between individuals.

- Mechanical complications after more than three central venous insertion attempts are six times higher when compared with the complication rate following a single attempt.[3]

- The use of real-time ultrasonography at the bedside reduces the number of insertion attempts. This results in a more comfortable and safer experience for the patient. Static ultrasound is used for pre-puncture vein localization. Dynamic ultrasound is used to guide the needle to an optimal location inside the vein.[4]

When measuring CVP, it is important to compare all readings with the patient's clinical picture. Serial readings and trends in pressure are more clinically meaningful compared with single measures. In addition, certain steps must be taken to ensure accuracy. Most importantly, all CVP readings must be referenced to the anatomic position of the atrium regardless of the method measurement used. A landmark on the chest, known as the *phlebostatic axis*, is the point of reference for the atrium.[5] At the phlebostatic axis, the mid-chest line (half the anteroposterior diameter) intersects the fourth intracostal space. Locating this axis and marking the chest may aid in uniformity of readings among practitioners. For accuracy, the pressure transducer is leveled to the phlebostatic axis when measures are being recorded. Patients are generally placed in the supine position for CVP readings, with the head of the bed elevated no more than 60 degrees. It is important to consider individual variations and compare readings with the head of the bed elevated with those taken at 0 degrees to ensure that they are consistent.[6] Measures may also be taken in the side-lying position, but research has only confirmed lateral rotations of 20, 30, or 90 degrees, and each has a different, rotation-specific reference point. Many find this to be overly cumbersome, so the recumbent position is the most frequently used.[7]

As with all pressure transducer systems, dynamic response should be assessed by using the square wave test,[8,9] as shown in Figure 4-5. Dynamic response is the ability of the system to reproduce pressure waves created in a patient's bloodstream. The square wave test analyzes the fluctuations that result from flush device activation. If the system accurately records this standard configuration, it is believed to be capable of accurately recording patient pressure waveforms as well. Abnormal square wave configurations require interventions to eliminate air bubbles, tighten loose connections,

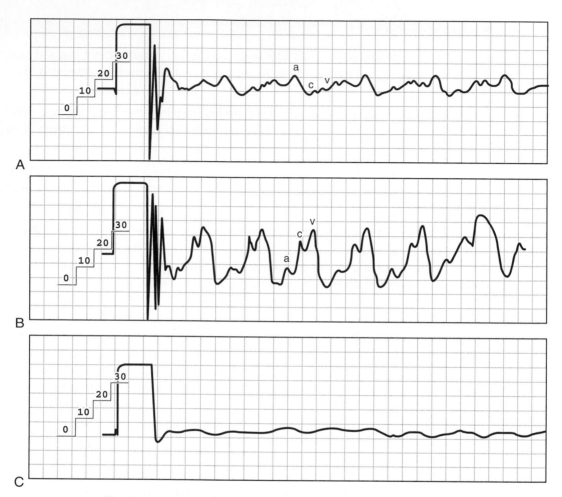

FIGURE 4-5 The Square Wave Test for Dynamic Response. Dynamic response can be evaluated clinically using the fast-flush device on the system and noting the square wave that is produced. Systems with appropriate dynamic response will return to baseline pressure waveforms within one to two oscillations following the flush. If dynamic response is deemed inadequate, clinicians should troubleshoot the system as stated below until acceptable system response is achieved. **A,** Normal square wave test: Note the second peak following the flush is less than a third the height of the first and less than 1 millimeter (mm) in distance from the first; this represents normal dissipation of the pressure created with the flush and an accurate system. **B,** Underdamped square wave: Note the multiple oscillations following the square wave; this may result in overestimation of central venous pressure (CVP); ensure that no tubing extensions are added and replace the transducer. **C,** Overdampened square wave: Note that no downward movement follows the square wave; this may result in underestimation of CVP; ensure correct scale, correct reference point, adequate air in the pressure bag, tight connections, no air bubbles, no micro-clots, and no kinks.

and unclog catheter tips and mitigating other sources of error until the configuration improves.[10] Improvements in monitor software and built-in pressure acquisition algorithms have improved the accuracy of digitally displayed pressures.[11] However, manual measurement via waveform inspection is a helpful skill to acquire.[12,13]

Central Venous Pressure Waveforms

Normal CVP waveforms consist of *a, c,* and *v* waves and *x* and *y* descents (Figure 4-6). These are low-pressure waves consistent with the low pressures of the venous system.

- The *a* wave reflects an increase in pressure created by atrial contraction. It is the first hemodynamic wave that follows the electrocardiographic *P* wave and generally falls at the beginning of the QRS complex.
- The *c* wave is a small wave created by the upward movement of the tricuspid leaflets during valve closure. It falls on the downslope of the *a* wave, within the *x* descent.
- The *v* wave is created by ventricular contraction and the resultant bulging of the tricuspid valve into the atrium. It falls after the *T* wave on electrocardiography (ECG).[14]

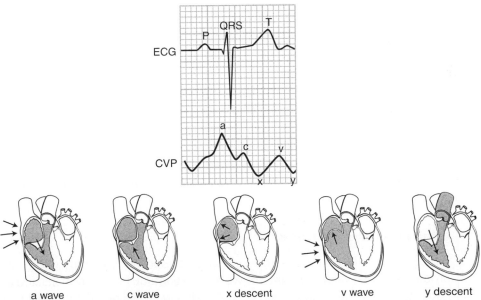

FIGURE 4-6 Normal Central Venous Pressure (CVP) Waveforms. *a* wave: **a**trial contraction (follows the *p* wave of the ECG). *c* wave: **c**losure of the tricuspid valve (generally at the end of the QRS). *v* wave: **v**entricular contraction (tricuspid bulging into the atrium, follows the *T* wave of the ECG). *x* descent: atrial relaxation. *y* descent: passive atrial emptying.

Clinical Reasoning Pearl

For a variety of reasons, it may be difficult to identify the individual *a*, *c*, and *v* waves from the moving waveforms on a bedside monitor. The CVP scale may be too large, or the monitor may be positioned above eye-range of the clinician.

To accurately identify individual waves in sinus rhythm:

- Print out a dual channel (ECG and CVP) tracing on ECG paper. If this is not possible, briefly freeze the monitor frame.

- Draw a straight line from the *p* wave downward through the CVP waveform.

- The wave to the immediate right will be the *a* wave (response to atrial contraction).

- Draw a straight line downward from the middle of the *T* wave.

- The vertical line may pass through the beginning of the *v* wave, or the wave will be to the immediate right (response to ventricular contraction).

Once the waves are identified, manual pressure readings can be noted. The mean of the *a* wave has traditionally been considered the best reflection of right ventricular preload.[15] Although it has little clinical relevance overall, the *c* wave is generally positioned at the mean of the *a* wave and serves as a convenient point for measurement. The leading edge of the *c* wave is called the Z *point* and signals the end of diastole.[16] Using the Z point for pinpointing measures is particularly useful when no *a* waves are present, as in atrial fibrillation. Pressure readings are also impacted by changes in intrathoracic pressure related to breathing, adding further complexity to obtaining useful measures. It is recommended that reading of CVP be done at the end of expiration when breathing "artifact" is less.[17] End expiration varies, depending on whether the patient is spontaneously breathing (negative pressure inspiration) or receiving mechanical ventilator breaths (positive pressure inspiration) (Figure 4-7). Once the Z point at end expiration is located, it is referenced to a scale that is displayed at the beginning of any printed strip or to the left of the wave sweep on the monitor screen (Figure 4-8). Stop cursors are available on many monitor systems to "freeze" visual display image to assist with manual CVP readings. Although it is a little more labor intensive, manual readings are more accurate than digital readings when obtained by a trained practitioner.[18]

Clinical Reasoning Pearl

Research has shown that using the monitor cursor-line to identify end expiration produces similar values to a graphic waveform printout. In a study of 25 cardiac surgery patients, no statistical differences in CVP value were observed with the two methods (cursor line or printout) when patients were mechanically ventilated or were breathing spontaneously. If a graphic printout is not available, the monitor cursor is a helpful alternative to identify end expiration.[19]

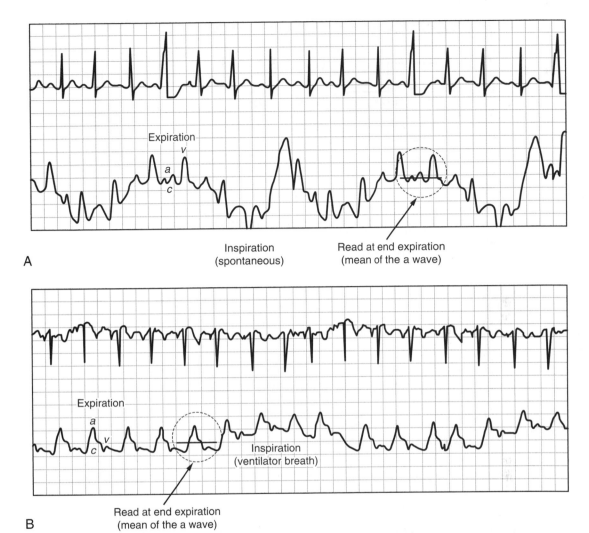

FIGURE 4-7 Effects of Breathing on Central Venous Pressure (CVP) Waveforms. Because of its placement within the chest, the CVP tracing is subject to the pressure variations of breathing. To avoid measuring respiratory artifact, end expiration readings are recommended. The digital reading on the monitor pressure averages CVP across the entire respiratory cycle. Therefore, manual measures are recommended. The appearance of end expiration differs between spontaneous breathing and mechanical ventilation. **A,** Spontaneous breaths: Inspiration creates a negative pressure to "suck" air into the chest, and the decrease in pressure pulls CVP waveform downward; readings are taken just before the waves dip down into a breath. **B,** Ventilator breaths: Inspiration is by positive pressure delivered by the machine. This moves the CVP waveform upward; readings are taken just before the waves move upward with a mechanical breath.

In addition to assessing pressure readings, CVP waveforms may be analyzed to obtain other clinical information. For example, enlarged *a* waves may indicate right atrial contraction against a closed tricuspid valve, as seen in third-degree heart block and other atrioventricular dissociated rhythms. Enlarged *a* waves may also be seen in

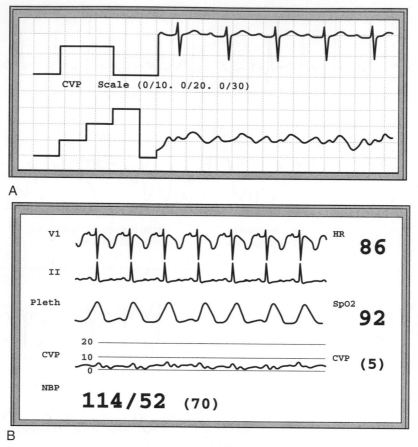

FIGURE 4-8 Central Venous Pressure (CVP) Monitoring Scales. A, Scale on Monitor Waveform: Each level of the "staircase" at the beginning of the waveform represents one of the numbers in the parenthesis, 0–30 mm Hg in this case. **B,** Scale on Monitor Screen: Monitor screens may be placed in "freeze" to stop wave sweep and allow waves to be lined up for manual reading. *CVP,* Central venous pressure; *HR,* heart rate (Lead V1 and Lead II); *NBP,* noninvasive blood pressure; *Pleth,* pulse oximetry waveform; *SpO₂,* pulse oximetry oxygenation saturation.

atrial hypertrophy. In certain dysrhythmias, *a* waves will be absent because true atrial contraction is lacking (i.e., atrial fibrillation) or because atrial contraction occurs simultaneously with ventricular contraction (i.e., re-entry supraventricular tachycardia). Enlarged *v* waves may be seen when ventricular contraction occurs with an open tricuspid valve, as with premature ventricular beats. The cause of *v* wave increase in this situation is blood moving backward into the atrium. Enlarged *v* waves may also occur with tricuspid valve regurgitation (Figure 4-9). With these pathologies, if CVP pressure readings are elevated because of structural changes in the right atrium or the tricuspid valve, the CVP value will not accurately reflect right heart filling pressures.

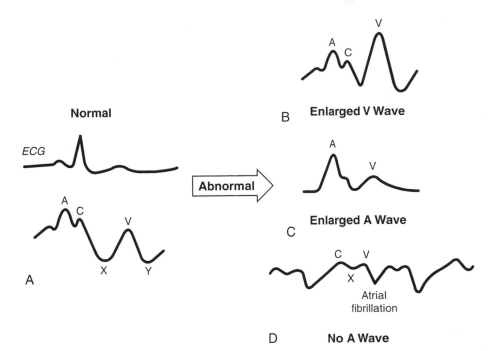

FIGURE 4-9 **Waveforms Are Analyzed to Establish Cardiovascular Pathology. A,** The normal central venous pressure (CVP) waveform. **B,** Enlarged *v* wave: This abnormality is seen with tricuspid regurgitation and intermittently with dissociated rhythms when the ventricular contracts against an open tricuspid valve. **C,** Enlarged *a* wave: This abnormality is seen in situations causing increased atrial pressure during contraction; examples include tricuspid stenosis or dissociated rhythms that cause the atrium to intermittently contract against a closed tricuspid valve (i.e., third degree heart block, ventricular ectopic beats); with dysrhythmias, the enlarged *a* wave is called a *cannon wave*. **D,** No *a* wave: This abnormality is seen in atrial fibrillation when no coordinated atrial contraction exists and therefore no *P* waves.

Establishing Baseline—Normal Pressure Ranges

The normal range for CVP in healthy adults varies, depending on the source quoted, but is generally listed as 2 to 6 mm Hg. Because of the effects of aging and disease on heart muscle compliance, textbook normal ranges for CVP are not especially applicable to the critically ill. An adjusted and more realistic range for CVP has been promoted as 8 to 12 mm Hg. Research by Rivers et al. (2001) on severe sepsis resuscitation and early goal-directed therapy, established this range and advocated for fluid infusion to achieve a CVP of greater than 8 mm Hg.[20] Originally, because of the effects of mechanical ventilation on right ventricular compliance, a CVP of 12 to 15 mm Hg was thought to be most reflective of an adequate vascular volume in the ventilated population. This recommendation has since gone out of favor because of concerns about abdominal compartment syndrome following excessive fluid resuscitation.[21] Many clinicians have adopted a target CVP of greater than or equal to 8 mm Hg as the goal for fluid optimization in all hemodynamically compromised patients, not only in those with sepsis.

Assessment of Central Venous Pressure Readings

Changes in CVP are usually attributed to changes in vascular volume, with lower than "normal" readings interpreted as hypovolemia, and higher readings interpreted as hypervolemia. However, many other factors may impact CVP readings. The CVP is a direct measure of pressure in the right heart and only an indirect reflection of pressure in the entire vascular compartment.

A fall in CVP may indicate a problem with blood inflow to the right heart. Obstructions to flow may occur with venous dilation, upper arm deep vein thrombosis, superior vena cava syndrome, abdominal tumor compression, or, rarely, vena cava filter blockage (Box 4-2).

Mechanical ventilation alters CVP. Positive pressure ventilation with large tidal volumes may decrease venous return and inflow to the right heart. Conversely, adjunctive positive airway pressure such as positive end-expiratory pressure (PEEP) transmitted to the cardiovascular system may increase the CVP value.

A pathophysiologic state that could falsely elevate CVP, despite low vascular volume, is intra-abdominal hypertension (IAH), also known as abdominal compartment syndrome. In this situation, abdominal trauma or surgical procedures result in inflammation and fluid shifts out of the vascular compartment and into the abdominal tissues. This may result in a relative hypovolemia, as the aorta and vena cava are compressed by increased pressure in the abdomen. The increase in abdominal pressure is transmitted directly to the thorax and erroneously raises CVP (i.e., the increased CVP is not reflective of intravascular volume status). The enlarged abdomen pushes upward on the diaphragm, decreasing lung volumes, increasing thoracic pressures, and causing an increase in CVP that may mask hypovolemia.[22]

Elevations in CVP are generally an indication of either hypervolemia or right-sided heart failure with congestion of the right atrium and ventricle. Causes of hypervolemia are excessive volume resuscitation and sodium and water retention, as seen in kidney, heart, or liver failure. Causes for right heart failure include direct muscle dysfunction, valvular or structural abnormalities, and increased resistance to forward blood flow. Direct muscle dysfunction encompasses pathologies such as right ventricular infarction and right-sided heart failure. Because of the anatomic position of the heart, traumatic injury to the chest typically results in damage to the right heart chambers. Cardiac contusion, may, therefore, involve the right atrium and ventricle and lead to muscle failure.

Abnormal heart valve function may also decrease the productivity and output of the heart. Tricuspid stenosis impedes forward movement of blood into the right heart and tricuspid regurgitation sends blood backward to the atrium. Either way, blood accumulates on the right side, leading to high CVP. Lastly, increased pulmonary vascular

---

BOX 4-2 Causes of Changes in Central Venous Pressure (CVP) Measurements

HIGH CVP (GREATER THAN 12 mm Hg)

Muscle Dysfunction
Ischemia or infarction
Chronic heart failure
Cardiac contusion
Cardiomyopathy
Electrolyte or acid–base imbalances
Decreased cardiac compliance

Valvular or Structural Abnormalities
Tricuspid stenosis or regurgitation
Pulmonic stenosis or regurgitation
Atrial septal defect
Ventricular septal defect

Increased Resistance to Forward Blood Flow
Left heart failure with increased intracardiac
    pressures
Pulmonary hypertension (cor pulmonale)
Pulmonary pathologies (chronic obstructive lung
    disease, pulmonary emboli, acute respiratory
    distress syndrome)
Excessive vasopressor use
Coarctation of the aorta

Hypervolemia
Excessive fluid resuscitation
Sodium and water retention related to kidney,
    heart, or liver dysfunction
Cushing syndrome
Hyperaldosteronism
Postoperative stress
Pregnancy or eclampsia

Other
Elevated intrathoracic pressure
Intra-abdominal hypertension (IAH) or abdominal
    compartment syndrome

LOW CVP (LESS THAN 8 mm Hg)

Hypovolemia
Inadequate fluid intake
Excessive diuresis or diaphoresis
Vomiting and diarrhea
Uncontrolled diabetes mellitus
Diabetes insipidus

Vascular Dilation
Severe sepsis
Excessive vasodilator therapy

---

resistance (PVR) or increased afterload, may raise resistance to blood flow beyond what the heart can overcome, causing blood to remain in the right heart and elevating the CVP. Causes of high pulmonary afterload include pulmonary hypertension, pulmonary emboli, pneumothorax, and other lung-related pathologies that strain the right heart.

Controversies Regarding Central Venous Pressure

At the time of this writing, increasing evidence suggests that CVP has little, if any, correlation to static volume status. One of the more provocative papers was a systematic review of the literature published in 2008 by Marik and colleagues.[23] In 29 studies involving 685 patients with signs of hypoperfusion, only 56% responded to a fluid bolus despite low cardiac filling pressures documented by CVP and pulmonary artery occlusion pressure (PAOP). Thus, static measures of volume status such as CVP may be poor indicators of preload and inaccurate in predicting fluid responsiveness. Fluid responsiveness is a more contemporary term used to describe intravascular volume status.[24] A patient is said to be fluid responsive with a 10% to 15% increase in stroke volume after a 500-milliliter (mL) crystalloid bolus is administered over 10 to 15 minutes.[25] The controversy surrounding CVP was brought into further focus after the Surviving Sepsis Campaign opted to continue recommending a CVP of 8 to 12 mm Hg as a guide for fluid resuscitation in its updated 2012 guidelines.[26] Arguably the best explanation for this stance is the lack of a widely accepted better option and the prevalent use of CVP in critical care units around the world. In 2013, Marik and Cavallazzi published an updated meta-analysis and a "plea for some common sense."[27] The authors expressed concern that CVP values could misguide clinicians, lead to inappropriate therapy, and result in harm to the patient. They suggested that routine use of CVP monitoring be abandoned until supporting data are published.

Since the reason for fluid resuscitation is improved cardiac function, fluid loading to achieve a target CVP is of no value if cardiac output does not increase. The strategy of fluid loading to improve cardiac contractility may be taken to the extreme, resulting in excessive fluid administration, widespread fluid "third spacing," pulmonary edema, abdominal hypertension, and other complications. Excessive fluid therapy is also known to increase critical care unit length of stay, hospital stay, and mortality.[28] Perhaps the best use of CVP readings is to make it part of a thorough hemodynamic and clinical assessment of the patient, which includes more conservative reflections of fluid status such as weight, urinary output, blood pressure, heart rate, level of consciousness, and breath sounds.

Troubleshooting Primary Complications of CVP Lines

Although viewed as a convenient tool for accessing the cardiovascular system, CVP lines may cause harm to the patient. Safety during the insertion, maintenance, and removal phases of use is an ongoing concern. Prior to insertion, an assessment of patient risk for complications should be completed. High-risk patients are those with coagulopathies, overt delirium or combative behavior, skin or vascular disease at the site, immunosuppression, severe lung disease, and inability to survive possible pneumothorax. Complications of CVP catheters may include line disconnection with hemorrhage, vascular injury, thrombus formation, clot embolization, and dysrhythmias (with catheter migration). The following sections review the top three concerns associated with central vein cannulation.[29]

A formal assessment to determine whether the patient really needs a central line for hemodynamic management or another clinical indication should be a daily procedure. The risk of catheter-associated bloodstream infection increases with the duration of days in situ for both central venous catheters and peripherally inserted central catheters.[30,31] Double-lumen and triple-lumen catheters have slightly higher rates of infection compared with single-lumen catheters.[30,31] Prompt removal of central lines decreases risk of infection. Without formal assessment, it is easy to lose track of the number of days a central venous catheter has been in place.[32]

Infection

In 2004, the Institute of Healthcare Improvement (IHI) launched the 100 K Lives Campaign and selected central line–associated bloodstream infections (CLABSI) as one of their key targets for improvement. Besides a reported 18% mortality rate, CLABSI was shown to significantly increase health care costs. Following a thorough literature review by the IHI, a set of preventive interventions known as the *central line bundle* were adopted (Box 4-3).[33]

Aseptic maintenance of central lines on a daily basis is vitally important. Strict hand hygiene, antiseptic scrubbing of access ports and hubs prior to use, and timely replacement of wet or loose dressings are basic strategies for the prevention of infection. Administrative support empowers staff to stop procedures if proper techniques are breached. Making needed supplies, educational materials, and surveillance data readily available is mandatory for a successful CLABSI reduction program.[34] Some facilities

---

BOX 4-3 Institute of Healthcare Improvement: Central Line Bundle

- Hand hygiene before and after the procedure
- Maximum barrier precautions during insertion:
  - Provider and assistants—cap, mask, sterile gown and gloves
  - Patient—full sterile drape covering head to toe with only a small opening over the insertion site
- Chlorhexidine skin antisepsis—2% solution in 70% isopropyl alcohol, applied with a back and forth friction scrub for at least 30 seconds, and allowed to dry completely without wiping or blotting
- Optimal site selection—avoid femoral vein due to higher infection potential; consider subclavian vein for most patients
- Review of line—necessity daily; promptly remove all unnecessary lines

Data from Institute of Healthcare Improvement. *How-to guide: prevent central line-associated bloodstream infections (CLABSI),* <www.ihi.org>. 2012 (Accessed January 10, 2014.).

have also instituted the use of chlorhexidine bathing, chlorhexidine impregnated dressings, and antimicrobial catheters to drive their CLABSI rates to zero.[35] The reduction in infection rates that followed the widespread implementation of the central line bundle launched by the IHI resulted in the selection of CLABSI prevention as a National Patient Safety Goal (NPSG 7.04).

Patient Education

- Explain the rationale for placement of a central line, including hemodynamic monitoring, intravenous medication administration, and fluid therapy to the patient and to the family.

- Depending on the location of the central venous catheter, the patient may have movement restrictions such as not turning the head toward the catheter (internal jugular vein placement), or not bending at the hip (femoral vein placement).

- Review the procedures associated with central lines (insertion, daily maintenance, and removal) with the patient and with the family.

- Explain monitor waveforms, numerical displays, and alarms in straightforward language to the patient and to the family.

Pneumothorax

Lung trauma from central venous catheter insertions into the chest, particularly at the subclavian site, may lead to lung collapse. Many patients in the critical care unit setting have underlying pulmonary pathologies that may be rapidly exacerbated by the development of pneumothorax, threatening overall oxygenation. In some cases, a one-way valve is created by damaged tissue, leading to a *tension pneumothorax* with a dramatic increase in intrathoracic pressure. This is a life-threatening emergency, as a tension pneumothorax could obstruct blood flow through the chest and result in profound shock or cardiac standstill. It is important to perform chest radiography after central line insertions. This procedure is just as important after unsuccessful attempts so that any inadvertent damage to the lung may be identified. Even if the x-ray film is cleared, patients should be monitored closely over the next hour for any changes in vital signs that might indicate delayed lung collapse. Most pneumothoraces require chest tube insertion to reinflate the lung. A tension pneumothorax generally requires an emergency needle insertion to release pressure and re-establish blood flow with insertion of a chest tube.[36]

Air Emboli

Air embolism is a preventable, hospital-acquired condition that may result in serious patient harm, including death. It is also a serious reportable event, which may result in nonpayment to hospitals by the Centers for Medicare and Medicaid Services (CMS).[37] Central lines placed directly in the chest (jugular or subclavian) have the highest risk for air insufflation because of their proximity to the thorax and the pressure changes involved in breathing. With all central lines, it is vital to remove air from infusion bags and tubes, secure all ports and connections, utilize air-eliminating filters and air-in-line sensors, and maintain a closed system at all times. When central lines are removed, utmost care should be employed. The patient should always be in bed (never in a chair), either lying flat or with the head down to increase intrathoracic pressure and discourage air entry. In spontaneously breathing patients, the greatest risk is during the negative-pressure inspiratory phase. If the patient is able to cooperate reliably, he or she should be asked to take a deep breath and hold it while the line is removed. If the patient is not able to cooperate reliably, the bed is placed in the Trendelenburg position and the catheter withdrawn during exhalation.[38] For mechanically ventilated patients, the safest time to withdraw the catheter is during inspiration because of the positive pressure of a ventilator breath.

Catheters should be pulled in one continuous motion with the dominant hand. Immediately after withdrawal, pressure must be applied over the site with the nondominant hand to reduce the chance of air entry and to stop bleeding. Pressure should be maintained for 5 minutes or until hemostasis is achieved. Then an *air-occlusive* dressing such as Vaseline-gauze or a bacteriostatic ointment–infused gauze is applied. The dressing is to be left in place for 24 hours to allow the catheter track to close.[39]

Following line discontinuation, it is important to monitor the vital signs, pulse oximetry, and level of consciousness. Tachycardia, tachypnea, hypotension, oxygen desaturation, and changes in level of consciousness may indicate air emboli. If an embolus is suspected, the patient should be placed on the left side in the Trendelenburg position. This maneuver will help limit how much air passes through the right heart and into the lungs, thus reducing the risk of impaired gas exchange and right ventricular outflow obstruction (airlock). Additional treatments include fluid infusion to increase CVP, 100% oxygen or hyperbaric oxygen therapy, and Advanced Cardiac Life Support (ACLS) measures.[40]

Case Study

Mrs. G is a 77-year-old female with a history of hypertension, obesity, arthritis, and congestive heart failure. She presents to the emergency department with shortness of breath that had started earlier in the day and worsened over the course of the morning.

Physical Examination

General: Female, awake, alert and in no obvious distress

Lungs: Crackles in the right base

Cardiovascular: Regular rate and rhythm; no gallops or murmurs; mild jugular venous distention

Continued

Case Study—cont'd

Abdomen: Mildly distended and tympanic
Rectal: Waived

Vital Signs

Temperature: 34.5° C
Pulse: 97 beats/min
Blood pressure: 150/88 mm Hg
Respiratory rate: 27 breaths/min
Sepsis screen: positive

Testing

Arterial blood gas (ABG): partial pressure of arterial oxygen (PaO_2) 78; saturation 89%; partial pressure of carbon dioxide (PCO_2) 32; bicarbonate (HCO_3^-) 19; pH 7.31
Chest radiography: right-lower-lobe infiltrate; increased vascular markings
Electrocardiography (ECG): within normal limits; no signs of ischemia
Urine output (UO): cloudy; positive for white blood cells (WBCs)
Laboratory: lactate: 4.8 millimoles per liter (mmol/L); WBC 14.5/microliter (µL); platelet 40/µL. Blood, sputum, and urinary culture specimens collected.

Diagnoses

1. Urinary tract infection
2. Right lower lobe pneumonia
3. Mild coagulopathy
4. Mildly decompensated heart failure (sepsis exacerbated)

Management. Mrs. G was started on empiric antibiotics to address her two potential sources of sepsis. Because of her mild heart failure and adequate blood pressure, she was given only 500 milliliters (mL) of normal saline as her initial fluid bolus and transferred to the critical care unit for hemodynamic assessment and therapy for lactic acidosis and apparent hypoperfusion.

In the critical care unit, a central venous catheter was inserted and her CVP was measured as 4 mm Hg. She was given a liter of normal saline and monitored for signs of worsening heart function. CVP increased to 6 mm Hg. Two hours after arrival and following a total of 1.5 L of normal saline, the lactate level remained elevated at 4.7 mmol/L, and the CVP was 5 mm Hg. The passive leg raise maneuver was performed to assess fluid responsiveness. Findings of this test corroborated the low CVP reading and indicated a continued need for additional fluid therapy. Another liter of saline was cautiously administered. In addition, dobutamine at 2.5 micrograms per kilogram per minute (mcg/kg/min) was initiated to address her unresolved hypoperfusion (without hypotension) and to reduce the need for additional fluid therapy that could possibly aggravate the underlying heart failure.

Case Study—cont'd

Two hours later, the lactate level had decreased to 2.8 mmol/L, and the CVP was at 8 mm Hg. She had no signs of increased shortness of breath, had stable oxygen saturation with pulse oximeter oxygen saturation (SpO_2) of 95% on 4 L of oxygen by nasal cannula. The next morning, she was weaned off her dobutamine and transferred to a medical-surgical unit. The following day, she was discharged home. ∎

PARAMETERS	ED ADMISSION	CVP LINE INSERTED	AFTER VOLUME RESUSCITATION	AFTER DOBUTAMINE INFUSION
Temperature (° C)	34.5		36.0	
Heart rate (beats/min)	97	108	102	98
Blood pressure (mm Hg)	150/88	138/80	142/78	148/82
Respiratory rate (breaths/min)	27	28	22	20
Sepsis screen	+			
pH	7.31			
PaO_2	78			
SaO_2 / SpO_2	89% (SaO_2)	90%	91%	95% (SpO_2)
$PaCO_2$	32			
HCO_3^-	19			
Chest radiography	Right-lower-lobe infiltrate; increased vascular markings			
ECG	Within normal limits; no signs of ischemia			
CVP (mm Hg)		4	5	8
Urine	Cloudy; positive for WBC			
Lactate (mmol/L)	4.8		4.7	2.8
WBC (µL)	14.5			
Platelet (µL)	40			

Conclusion

With the move away from static measures of preload such as CVP and PAOP (wedge pressure), newer concepts in hemodynamics have been proposed.[41] Dynamic or "functional" hemodynamics are gaining popularity in determining whether fluid therapy will improve cardiac output, blood pressure, and ideally, overall perfusion. An early example of a functional hemodynamic assessment is postural blood pressure checks. Patients have been shown to maintain supine blood pressure despite significant losses of vascular volume. However, when outside forces are applied, in this case gravity, compensation can fail resulting in a fall in blood pressure. Most consider a systolic blood pressure drop of 10 to 15 mm Hg to be a sign of hypovolemia.[42] Another example of a functional hemodynamic evaluation is measuring the effect of a different outside force, a positive pressure ventilator breath.[43-45] Pulse paradox may be noted in fluid responsive patients being mechanically ventilated. Patients on low volume ventilation to reduce lung injury may temporarily require larger tidal volumes of 8 mL/kg or greater to increase accuracy of this maneuver. A systolic blood pressure variation of greater than 10 to 15 mm Hg could imply that fluid loading may improve cardiac function. To perform ventilator breath assessment, patients need to be sedated and ventilated on control mode ventilation with no negative pressure triggering. Sustained dysrhythmias have also been shown to alter the accuracy of ventilator-based assessments of fluid responsiveness.

A more recently appreciated bedside test for fluid responsiveness is the passive leg raise maneuver.[41,46] This test involves placing a semirecumbent patient in a supine position with legs elevated to 45 degrees (see Chapter 3, Figure 3-11). Lakhal et al. (2010) explored the response of CVP to passive leg raise and found that a CVP increase of 2 mm Hg or more was significant for fluid responsiveness.[47]

Clinical Reasoning Pearl

The static CVP value is not used to assess volume in isolation. It is one component of a comprehensive hemodynamic fluid volume assessment that includes heart rate, blood pressure, and urine output and may include passive leg raise to assess the effect of dynamic fluid volume on CVP, stroke volume variation (SVV), or pulse pressure variation (PPV). Bedside echocardiography may also be used to assess the collapsibility of the inferior vena cava.

Over the last 15 years, demands for safer and more accurate hemodynamic monitoring have led to the development of less invasive and even noninvasive devices. These emerging technologies measure stroke volume, cardiac output, and other parameters by a variety of methods including arterial waveform analysis and bioreactance.[48,49] Bioreactance is the analysis of the variation in frequency of an oscillating current traversing the thoracic cavity. For fluid assessment, use of passive leg raise and ventilator-induced changes to pulse pressure and stroke volume.[50] Both PPV and SVV are considered to be indicative of fluid responsiveness when more than a 13% variation is seen with passive leg raise, with a positive pressure ventilator breath, or in response to a fluid challenge. In addition, application of bedside ultrasonography has also been promoted. Echocardiography-derived dimensions of the inferior vena cava, right atrium, and systemic and hepatic veins have allowed noninvasive reflections of central venous volume and overall fluid status.[51-54]

In summary, the era of CVP monitoring for hemodynamic volume assessment may be coming to an end. Historically, changes in health care are slow, and giving up such a longstanding staple of critical care practice will be even slower. With new concepts and technologies in hemodynamic monitoring, future practitioners may become more successful in guiding fluid resuscitation and medication titration. Accurate monitoring and more effective therapy will improve patient outcomes and potentially decrease costs.

References

1. Nossaman BD, Scruggs BA, Nossaman VE, et al.: History of right heart catheterization: 100 years of experimentation and methodology development, *Cardiol Rev* 18(2):94–101, 2010.
2. Latham HE, Rawson ST, Dwyer TT, et al.: Peripherally inserted central catheters are equivalent to centrally inserted catheters in intensive care unit patients for central venous pressure monitoring, *J Clin Monit Comput* 26(2):85–90, 2012.
3. McGee DC, Gould MK: Preventing complications of central venous catheterization, *N Engl J Med* 348:1123–1133, 2003.
4. American Society of Anesthesiologists Task Force on Central Venous Access: Practice guidelines for central venous access, *Anesthesiology* 116:539–573, 2012.
5. Paolella LP, Dorfman GS, Cronan JJ, Hasan FM: Topographic location of the left atrium by computed tomography: reducing pulmonary artery catheter calibration error, *Crit Care Med* 16(11):1154–1156, 1988.
6. Courtois M, Fattal PG, Kovács SJ, et al.: Anatomically and physiologically based reference level for measurement of intracardiac pressures, *Circulation* 92(7):1994–2000, 1995.
7. Tuggle D: Obtaining pulmonary artery catheter data is too labor intense to be reliable, *Crit Care Med* 37(5):1833, 2009.
8. Gardner RM: Direct blood pressure measurement—dynamic response requirements, *Anesthesiology* 54(3):227–236, 1981.
9. Bridges ME, Middleton R: Direct arterial vs oscillometric monitoring of blood pressure: stop comparing and pick one (a decision-making algorithm), *Crit Care Nurse* 17(3):96–97, 1997, 101–102.
10. Bridges EJ: Pulmonary artery pressure monitoring: when, how, and what else to use, *AACN Adv Crit Care* 17(3):286–303, 2006.
11. Tyler L, Greco S, Bridges E, et al.: Accuracy of stop-cursor method for determining systolic and pulse pressure variation, *Am J Crit Care* 22(4):298–305, 2013.
12. Jain RK, Antonio BL, Bowton DL, et al.: Variability in central venous pressure measurements and the potential impact on fluid management, *Shock* 33(3):253–257, 2010.
13. Bridges E: Pulmonary artery/central venous pressure measurement. AACN Practice Alert. <aacn.org> 2013 (Accessed September 29, 2013.).
14. Rhodes A, Grounds E, Bennett D: Hemodynamic monitoring. In Vincent JL, editor: *Textbook of critical care*, 6 ed., St. Louis, MO, 2011, Saunders, pp 523–546.

15. Magder S: Invasive intravascular hemodynamic monitoring: technical issues, *Crit Care Clin* 23(3):401–414, 2007.

16. Magder S: How to use central venous pressure measurements, *Curr Opin Crit Care* 11(3):264–270, 2005.

17. Berryhill RE, Benumof JL, Rauscher LA: Pulmonary vascular pressure reading at the end of exhalation, *Anesthesiology* 49(5):365–368, 1978.

18. Ahrens TS, Schallom L: Comparison of pulmonary artery and central venous pressure waveform measurements via digital and graphic measurement methods, *Heart Lung* 30(1):26–38, 2001.

19. Paison E: Good, Tizon J, et al.: Evaluation of the monitor cursor line method for measuring pulmonary artery and central venous pressures, *Am J Crit Care* 19(6):511–521, 2012.

20. Rivers E, Nguyen B, Havstad S, et al.: Early goal-directed therapy in the treatment of severe sepsis and septic shock, *N Engl J Med* 345(19):1368–1377, 2001.

21. Regueira T, Bruhn A, Hasbun P, et al.: Intra-abdominal hypertension: incidence and association with organ dysfunction during early septic shock, *J Crit Care* 23(4):461–467, 2008.

22. Papavramidis TS, Marinis AD, Pliakos I, et al.: Abdominal compartment syndrome–intra-abdominal hypertension: defining, diagnosing, and managing, *J Emerg Trauma Shock* 4:279–291, 2011.

23. Marik PE, Baram M, Vahid B: Does central venous pressure predict fluid responsiveness? A systematic review of the literature and the tale of seven mares, *Chest* 134(1):172–178, 2008.

24. Kupchik N, Bridges E: Critical analysis, critical care: central venous pressure monitoring: what's the evidence? *Am J Nurs* 112(1):58–61, 2012.

25. Cecconi M, Parsons AK, Rhodes A: What is a fluid challenge? *Curr Opin Crit Care* 17(3):290–295, 2011.

26. Dellinger RP, Levy MM, Rhodes A, et al.: Surviving Sepsis Campaign: international guidelines for management of severe sepsis and septic shock, 2012, *Intensive Care Med* 39(2):165–228, 2013.

27. Marik PE, Cavallazzi R: Does the central venous pressure predict fluid responsiveness? An updated meta-analysis and a plea for some common sense*, *Crit Care Med* 41(7):1774–1781, 2013.

28. Magee G, Zbrozek A: Fluid overload is associated with increases in length of stay and hospital costs: pooled analysis of data from more than 600 US hospitals, *Clinicoecon Outcomes Res* 5:289–296, 2013.

29. Kusminsky RE: Complications of central venous catheterization, *J Am Coll Surg* 204(4):681–696, 2007.

30. Dezfulian C, Lavelle J, Nallamothu BK, et al.: Rates of infection for single-lumen versus multilumen central venous catheters: a meta-analysis, *Crit Care Med* 31:2385–2890, 2003.

31. Chopra V, Ratz D, Kuhn L, et al.: PICC-associated bloodstream infections: prevalence, patterns, and predictors, *Am J Med* 127:319–328, 2014.

32. Burdeu G, Currey J, Pilcher D: Idle central venous catheter-days pose infection risk for patients after discharge from intensive care, *Am J Infect Control* 42(4):453–455, 2014.

33. Institute of Healthcare Improvement. How-to guide: prevent central line-associated bloodstream infections (CLABSI), <www.ihi.org>. 2012 (Accessed January 10, 2014.).

34. Han Z, Liang SY, Marschall J: Current strategies for the prevention and management of central line-associated bloodstream infections, *Infect Drug Resist* 3:147–163, 2010.

35. Scheithauer S, Lewalter K, Schröder J, et al.: Reduction of central venous line-associated bloodstream infection rates by using a chlorhexidine-containing dressing, *Infection* 42:155–159, 2014.

36. Ayas NT, Norena M, Wong H, et al.: Pneumothorax after insertion of central venous catheters in the intensive care unit: association with month of year and week of month, *Qual Saf Health Care* 16(4):252–255, 2007.

37. Centers for Medicare and Medicaid Services: listening session on hospital-acquired conditions in inpatient settings and hospital outpatient healthcare-associated conditions in outpatient settings, *Fed Regist* 73(211):64618–64619, 2008.

38. Ingram P, Sinclair L, Edwards T: The safe removal of central venous catheters, *Nurs Stand* 20(49):42–46, 2006.

39. Preuss T, Wiegand DJ: Central venous catheter removal. In Wiegand DJ, editor: *Procedure manual for critical care*, ed 6, St. Louis, MO, 2011, Saunders, pp 595–599.

40. Gordy S, Rowell S: Vascular air embolism, *Int J Crit Illn Inj Sci* 3(1):73–76, 2013.

41. Marik PE, Monnet X, Teboul JL: Hemodynamic parameters to guide fluid therapy, *Ann Intensive Care* 1(1):1, 2011.

42. Truijen J: Van lieshout JJ, Wesselink WA, Westerhof BE: Noninvasive continuous hemodynamic monitoring, *J Clin Monit Comput* 26(4):267–278, 2012.

43. Michard F, Teboul JL: Predicting fluid responsiveness in ICU patients: a critical analysis of the evidence, *Chest* 121(6):2000–2008, 2002.

44. Monnet X, Teboul JL: Assessment of volume responsiveness during mechanical ventilation: recent advances, *Crit Care* 17(2):217, 2013.

45. Freitas FG, Bafi AT, Nascente AP, et al.: Predictive value of pulse pressure variation for fluid responsiveness in septic patients using lung-protective ventilation strategies, *Br J Anaesth* 110(3):402–408, 2013.

46. Monnet X, Rienzo M, Osman D, et al.: Passive leg raising predicts fluid responsiveness in the critically ill, *Crit Care Med* 34(5):1402–1407, 2006.

47. Lakhal K, Ehrmann S, Runge I, et al.: Central venous pressure measurements improve the accuracy of leg raising-induced change in pulse pressure to predict fluid responsiveness, *Intensive Care Med* 36(6):940–948, 2010.

48. Marik PE, Levitov A, Young A, Andrews L: The use of bioreactance and carotid Doppler to determine volume responsiveness and blood flow redistribution following passive leg raising in hemodynamically unstable patients, *Chest* 143(2):364–370, 2013.

49. Benomar B, Ouattara A, Estagnasie P, et al.: Fluid responsiveness predicted by noninvasive bioreactance-based passive leg raise test, *Intensive Care Med* 36(11):1875–1881, 2010.

50. Michard F, Lopes MR, Auler JO: Pulse pressure variation: beyond the fluid management of patients with shock, *Crit Care* 11(3):131, 2007.

51. Michard F, Teboul JL: Using heart-lung interactions to assess fluid responsiveness during mechanical ventilation, *Crit Care* 4(5):282–289, 2000.

52. Berkenstadt H, Margalit N, Hadani M, et al.: Stroke volume variation as a predictor of fluid responsiveness in patients undergoing brain surgery, *Anesth Analg* 92(4):984–989, 2001.

53. Reuter DA, Kirchner A, Felbinger TW, et al.: Usefulness of left ventricular stroke volume variation to assess fluid responsiveness in patients with reduced cardiac function, *Crit Care Med* 31(5):1399–1404, 2003.

54. Beigel R, Cercek B, Luo H, Siegel RJ: Noninvasive evaluation of right atrial pressure, *J Am Soc Echocardiogr* 26(9):1033–1042, 2013.

Pulmonary Artery Pressure and Thermodilution Cardiac Output Monitoring

Jonathan Judy-del Rosario and Amy Salgado

A pulmonary artery catheter (PAC) is a flow-directed central venous catheter inserted into the right side of the heart to obtain both direct and indirect hemodynamic measurements (Box 5-1). During insertion, when the catheter tip reaches the right atrium, a small balloon near the tip of the distal end of the catheter is inflated. The catheter is floated through the right ventricle and advanced into the pulmonary artery until the tip reaches one of the smaller pulmonary blood vessels where, because of the inflated balloon, it is too large to advance further—this is termed the "wedge" position. These intracardiac catheters are inserted and used in operating rooms, cardiac catheterization suites, and critical care units, to diagnose heart conditions and guide therapeutic interventions.

This chapter will provide a historical overview of PACs; physiologic review, including cardiac function, indications for use, insertion procedure, measurement methods and waveform interpretation.

Historical Milestones

The first human heart catheterization was performed in 1929 by Warner Forssmann, a German physician who inserted a catheter into the right atrium of his own heart.[1,2] In 1941, André Frédéric Cournand and Hilmert Ranges performed eight heart catheterizations in four patients and measured cardiac output using the Fick method. The catheters were left in place for several days.[2] In 1956 Cournand, Forssmann, and Dickinson W. Richards were awarded the Nobel Prize in Physiology and Medicine for their work on heart catheterization and intracardiac catheter development.

The PAC with a balloon flotation device and temperature measurement for thermodilution cardiac output was introduced in 1970 by William Ganz and HJC Swan.[2,3] These catheters have since been developed to not only measure right atrial pressure (RAP), pulmonary artery pressure PAP, pulmonary artery occlusion pressure (PAOP) also known as the 'wedge' pressure but also measure cardiac output, and some catheters measure venous oxygen saturation and provide intracardiac pacing. Table 5-1 provides a summary of historical milestones in the development of diagnostic right heart catheterization.

BOX 5-1   Data Obtained from Pulmonary Artery Catheters

Direct Measurement	Indirect Measurement for Calculated Values*
RAP or CVP	SV
PAOP	CI
PAP	PVR
CO	SVR
SvO$_2$#	O$_2$ delivery#
RVEDP	LVEDP

*See Box 5-2 and Table 5-4 for calculation of values using data obtained from a pulmonary artery catheter
*See Box 5-3 for calculation of the cardiac index
#See Chapter 6 for calculations related to venous oxygen saturation and oxygen delivery
CI, Cardiac index; *CO*, cardiac output; *CVP*, central venous pressure; *LVEDP*, left ventricular end-diastolic pressure; *O$_2$*, oxygen; *PAOP*, pulmonary artery occlusion pressure; *PAP*, pulmonary artery pressure; *PVR*, pulmonary vascular resistance; *RAP*, right atrial pressure; *SV*, stroke volume; *SVO$_2$*, mixed venous oxygen saturation in the pulmonary artery; *SVR*, systemic vascular resistance.

Table 5-1   Pulmonary Artery Catheter Historical Milestones

DATE		PULMONARY ARTERY CATHETER
1844	Claude Bernard	Physiologist credited with inventing the term cardiac catheterization. Inserted a glass tube into the internal jugular vein to reach the right ventricle, and into the left carotid artery to reach the left ventricle in a horse.
1870	Adolf Fick	Published the formula for calculating cardiac output
1929	Warner Forssmann	Performed a right heart catheterization on himself by inserting a ureteral catheter into his right atrium and taking a chest radiograph as proof.
1941	Cournand and Ranges	Described right atrial catheterization and calculation of cardiac output in 4 patients
1945	Cournand et al.	Right heart catheterization (right atrium or ventricle) with calculation of Fick Cardiac Output in 260 catheterizations published in the *Journal of Clinical Investigation*
1949	HK Hellems et al.	Right heart catheterization with a venous catheter advanced into a pulmonary artery capillary in 13 patients, both wedge pressures and waveforms were obtained, published in the *Journal of Applied Physiology*.
1956	Cournand, Forssmann and Richards	Nobel prize awarded for advancements in heart catheterization
1970	HJC Swan and William Ganz	Right heart catheterization with the "Swan-Ganz" pulmonary artery catheter (PAC) in 70 patients. Case series published in *The New England Journal of Medicine*. The "Swan-Ganz" PAC was novel because it could be inserted at the bedside using waveform analysis and did not require fluoroscopy in the cardiac catheterization laboratory

Although pulmonary artery catheters are used to guide various therapies, their use has not come without controversy. In the 1980s, several early observational studies reported an increase in mortality in patients with PACs, although it was hypothesized that these patients were often the most critically ill and had a poor prognosis.[4,5] Following the observational studies, several randomized controlled trials (RCTs) have been completed.[6–8] Many report little evidence of efficacy and possible complications and costs.[5–8] More recent reviews of these studies showed no significant changes in morbidity or mortality and possible increase in complications and costs.[9,10] A review by Koo et al. (2011) concluded that there was a lack of significant evidence to support the use of PACs in patients with acute coronary syndrome, high-risk noncardiac surgery, congestive heart failure, shock, acute respiratory distress syndrome (ARDS), and critical illness. In addition, Koo reported a decline in PAC use by greater than 50% between 2002 and 2006.[11] Criticisms of these studies cite poor patient selection, misinterpretation of hemodynamic data, inappropriate therapy in response to the data obtained, and complications occurring because of less experienced clinicians.[1]

In 2013, the Cochrane Collaboration published a review on 13 randomized controlled trials that evaluated the use of the PAC.[12] Nine of these studies had adequate randomization and consequently a decreased risk for bias. In all randomized controlled trials combined, 5686 patients were included. There was no significant difference in overall mortality rate between the PAC group and the central venous catheter (CVC) group. Also, no significant difference was observed in hospital length of stay in the 9 randomized controlled trials that reported hospital length of stay; nor was a significant difference seen in critical care unit length of stay in the 11 randomized controlled trials that reported critical care unit length of stay. Of the 13 studies, 4 of the trials based in the United States reported an increased cost in the PAC group versus the CVC group. However, because of lack of data, only 2 of the trials were statistically analyzed, and no significant difference existed in overall hospital cost.

To date, no randomized controlled trial has conclusively proven that any form of monitoring will improve outcomes.[2] Ultimately, the decision to insert a PAC should be based on clinical judgment, preferably by an experienced operator who can accurately interpret data and guide treatments using the PAC as a diagnostic tool as one component of a comprehensive clinical assessment.

Key Physiologic Concepts

Cardiac Function

Cardiac output or the volume of blood pumped by the heart, delivers oxygen and nutrients to the body to meet metabolic demands. As physiologic demands increase, cardiac output must also increase. Cardiac output is determined by two factors: heart rate and stroke volume. Heart rate multiplied by stroke volume produces cardiac output, expressed in liters per minute (L/min) (see Chapter 1, Figure 1-7).

Heart rate is regulated by both the parasympathetic and sympathetic nervous systems. As metabolic demands increase, heart rate should also increase to provide adequate cardiac output. Careful consideration should be paid to this rising heart rate, as excessively rapid heart rates are associated with decreased diastolic filling time, which contributes to cardiac ischemia, decreased contractility, and reduced cardiac output.

Stroke volume is the amount of blood pumped from the ventricle with each cardiac contraction, usually measured in milliliters (mL). It is calculated in the cardiac catheterization laboratory by subtracting the end-systolic volume from the end-diastolic volume within the ventricle (see Chapter 1, Figure 1-8). Stroke volume is determined by three factors: preload, afterload, and contractility. When using the PAC it is calculated by dividing the cardiac output by the heart rate.

Preload is a measure of force, but conceptually, it relates to the end-diastolic volume of the ventricle. The stretch of the cardiac muscle fibers at the end of diastole is directly related to ventricular compliance. For example, a heart with a thick ventricular wall and decreased compliance will require increased preload, or volume, compared with a heart of normal size with normal compliance. Decreased preload in an injured heart greatly decreases stroke volume, ultimately decreasing cardiac output. Measurement of pressure in the right atrium (RAP) is used as a proxy for preload volume in the right heart, and PAOP is used to estimate preload volume in the left heart.

Afterload is the tension against which the ventricular muscle fibers must eject during systole. Afterload is affected by ventricular size, ventricular wall thickness, and blood pressure. A quantitative assessment of afterload can be calculated using hemodynamic pressure and flow data obtained from the PAC. The calculations for pulmonary vascular resistance (PVR), and systemic vascular resistance (SVR) are listed in Box 5-2.

PVR represents the afterload on the right ventricle. When pressures in the pulmonary vasculature rise, as is seen with volume overload or left heart failure, PVR increases, which results in an increased afterload for the right ventricle. Any increase in PVR increases the workload of the right ventricle.

BOX 5-2   Equations for Calculated Values Obtained via the Pulmonary Artery Catheter

$$CO = SV \times HR$$
$$SV = (CO \times 1000) / HR$$
$$SVI = (CI \times 1000) / HR$$

$$PVR = \frac{(\text{mean PA} - \text{mean PAOP})}{CO} \times 80$$

$$SVR = \frac{(MAP - CVP)}{CO} \times 80$$

CI, Cardiac index; *CO*, cardiac output; *HR*, heart rate; *MAP*, mean arterial pressure; *mean PA*, pulmonary artery mean pressure; *PAOP*, pulmonary artery occlusion pressure; *PVR*, pulmonary vascular resistance; *SV*, stroke volume; *SVI*, stroke volume index; *SVR*, systemic vascular resistance.

SVR represents the afterload on the left ventricle. Increased afterload may be seen with conditions that cause vasoconstriction, for example, systemic hypertension or hypothermia induced vasoconstriction. Afterload reduction can be accomplished with peripheral vasodilators such as nitroprusside or nitroglycerin. Decreased afterload is seen in conditions that cause vasodilation, for example, hyperthermia and sepsis-induced vasodilation. Afterload or SVR may be increased by using vasopressors such as phenylephrine or norepinephrine. Although increasing SVR may improve blood pressure initially, the increased afterload may ultimately decrease cardiac output if there is a fall in the ejected stoke volume in a poorly contractile heart. The physiologic effects of vasopressors, vasodilators, and inotrope medications are discussed in detail in Chapter 9.

Contractility is the ability of the heart muscle to forcibly contract and, thus, to eject blood. Independent of preload and afterload, many forces may affect contractility. Sympathetic activity and circulating catecholamines may increase contractility. In addition, various medication infusions such as epinephrine, dobutamine, and milrinone are used to improve contractility. Contractility may decrease with acidosis, electrolyte abnormalities, hypoxia, ischemia, or medications that slow the heart rate such as beta-blockers. Sepsis may decrease cardiac output and contractility because of the effects of circulating cytokines. Myocardial infarction also decreases contractility due to lack of myocardial blood flow and poor oxygenation to the area of damaged heart muscle.

Clinical Procedures and Technical Considerations

Indications

The PAC is used to assess volume status, for regulating fluid management, monitoring cardiac output, and titration of vasoactive and inotropic medications. Pulmonary artery catheterization is necessary for the diagnosis of pulmonary hypertension. These catheters are often used in patients undergoing major cardiac or vascular surgery and refractory shock states. The decision to use a PAC should be based on a clinical need. It is important to understand that the catheter is a diagnostic tool and not a therapeutic intervention.

In a 2012 review on the role of the PAC, Jean-Louis Vincent suggested the following indications for use in critically ill patients:

- Severe circulatory shock (not straightforward hypovolemia or clearly hyperkinetic states)
- Right ventricular failure
- Acute respiratory failure caused by pulmonary edema (not pulmonary edema responsive to therapy)
- Complex fluid management, with impending acute kidney injury

For patients with acute heart failure, the American College of Cardiology (ACC) and the American Heart Association (AHA) have published guidelines for PAC use.[13] See Table 5-2.

TABLE 5-2   Recommendations for Invasive Hemodynamic Monitoring

CLASS OF RECOMMENDATION	NO BENEFIT	BENEFICIAL	LEVEL OF EVIDENCE
I		Invasive hemodynamic monitoring with a pulmonary artery catheter should be used to guide therapy in patients who have respiratory distress or clinical evidence of impaired perfusion in whom the adequacy or excess of intracardiac filling pressures cannot be determined from clinical assessment	C
IIa		Invasive hemodynamic monitoring can be useful for patients with acute heart failure and persistent symptoms despite standard therapies, and: • When fluid status, perfusion, SVR or PVR status is uncertain • When systolic blood pressure remains low • When systolic blood pressure is associated with symptoms, despite initial therapy • When kidney function is worsening with therapy • Need intravenous vasoactive medications • When consideration for mechanical circulatory support (MCS) or transplantation	C
III No Benefit	Routine use of invasive hemodynamic monitoring is not recommended in normotensive patients with acute decompensated heart failure and congestion with symptomatic response to diuretics and vasodilators		B

Data from Yancy CW, Jessup M, Bozkurt B. et al.: ACCF/AHA 2013 Guideline for the management of heart failure: A report of the American College of Cardiology Foundation /American Heart Association Task Force on Practice Guidelines. *Circulation*, 128:e240-e327, 2013.

A major benefit of using a PAC is its ability to guide therapy when the patient's clinical trajectory does not follow an expected pattern, as described in the case study at the end of this chapter. The PAC monitors intracardiac pressures from the right heart, the pulmonary vasculature, and end-diastolic pressures in the left heart (Figure 5-1). The PAC also provides real-time data on volume status, cardiac output, and venous oxygen saturation. In addition, PVR and SVR may be calculated, along with other calculated data to give estimates of left-sided heart function (see Box 5-2). The immediate availability of information is useful in providing ongoing assessment of a patient's clinical picture to assist a clinician with therapeutic interventions.

Equipment

Introducer

Typically, an 8-French (Fr) introducer catheter is used for insertion of a PAC (Figure 5-2). This catheter has a port with a one-way valve through which the PAC can be inserted (Figure 5-3). In addition, the introducer usually has a side port that can be used to infuse medications or large volumes of fluid.

Pulmonary Artery Catheter

Most current PACs have multiple lumens. The different lumens are identified by a terminal "port" with a distinctive color or shape for easy identification. The basic PAC includes a proximal right atrial lumen, a distal pulmonary artery lumen, a thermistor,

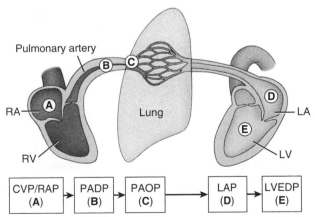

FIGURE 5-1 Sources of hemodynamic monitoring data from within the cardiopulmonary vascular system, measured in millimeters of mercury (mm Hg): **A,** Right atrium for measurement of right atrial pressure (RAP)/ central venous pressure (CVP); **B,** Pulmonary artery for measurement of pulmonary artery diastolic pressure (PADP), systolic pressure and mean pressure; **C,** Small pulmonary arteriole for measurement of pulmonary artery occlusion pressure (PAOP) also described as a "wedge" pressure or pulmonary capillary pressure; **D,** Left atrium is the source for left atrial pressure (LAP), which is indirectly measured by the PAOP, which displays a left atrial waveform when the pulmonary artery catheter (PAC) balloon is inflated and accurately positioned; **E,** Left ventricle is the source for left ventricular end-diastolic pressure (LVEDP). The LVEDP represents the pressure created by the volume in the left ventricle at the end of diastolic when the mitral valve is open. LVEDP is estimated from the PAOP mean value and the left atrial waveform at end-diastole.

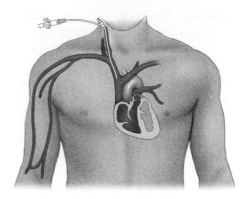

FIGURE 5-2 Introducer.

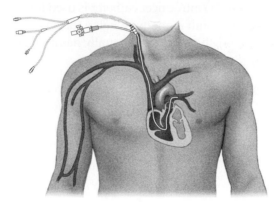

FIGURE 5-3 Pulmonary artery catheter placement through the right heart chambers.

and an inflation balloon (Figure 5-4, *A*). The proximal injectate lumen rests in the right atrium and measures the RAP or central venous pressure (CVP). This lumen is also used to obtain a bolus thermodilution cardiac output. The distal lumen rests in the pulmonary artery and is used for measuring PAP and PAOP. Some PAC catheters have an additional right atrial proximal infusion lumen for infusion of medications (Figure 5-4, *B*). Some multilumen PACs have a specialized electrical wire that connects to a filament on the catheter to obtain continuous cardiac output waveform on the bedside monitor (Figure 5-4, *C*). Some PACs have yet another lumen that allows for transvenous pacing in patients who require invasive hemodynamic monitoring and temporary pacing. Other PACs provide continuous measurement of SVO_2 (see Chapter 7).

Transducer

Two transducer setups are needed to measure the waveforms of both the right atrium and the pulmonary artery from the catheter. The transducers are connected separately to the catheter proximal port (RA) and distal port (PA) using saline-flushed, noncompliant tubing. The tubing maintains patency via a 500 mL bag of normal saline, enclosed by a pressure bag inflated to 250 to 300 millimeters of mercury (mm Hg).

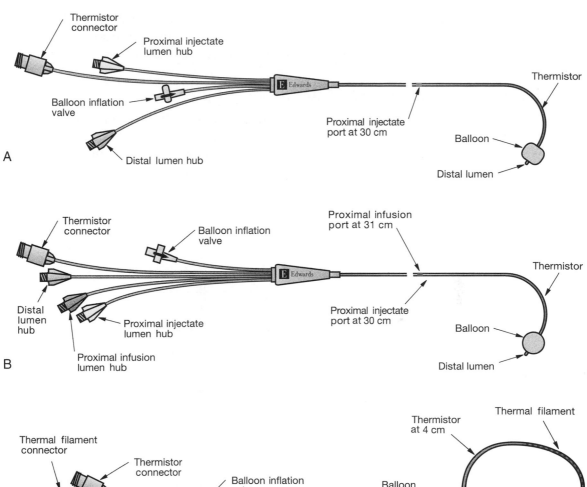

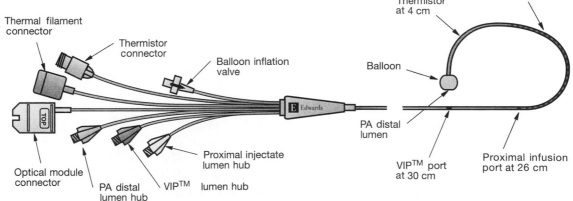

FIGURE 5-4 Pulmonary artery catheters with various features. **A,** Basic PAC with four lumen hubs—proximal right atrial, distal pulmonary artery, thermistor and balloon inflation; **B,** PAC with additional venous infusion lumen hub; **C,** PAC with additional venous infusion port (VIP), thermal filament and connector for continuous cardiac output monitoring, and fiberoptic lumen and connector for mixed venous oxygen (SVO$_2$) monitoring. (Courtesy Edwards LifeSciences, LLC.)

Approximately 3 mL per hour of saline is delivered to the patient. The tubing is connected to the transducer and an electrical cable connects the transducer to the monitor to display the hemodynamic waveforms and pressure measurements (Figure 5-5).

Insertion of a Pulmonary Artery Catheter

Intravenous access is obtained by placement of an introducer into a central vein. The PAC is inserted through the introducer. To promote ease of insertion, the preferred site is the right internal jugular (IJ) vein, but other options include the left IJ vein the subclavian vein or the femoral vein. The PAC comes packaged with a natural preformed

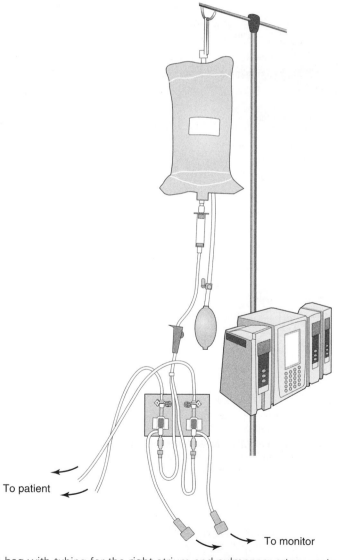

To patient

To monitor

FIGURE 5-5 Pressure bag with tubing for the right atrium and pulmonary artery ports.

curve that facilitates placement of the catheter. Given the curve of the catheter, the right IJ vein provides the easiest and most direct access to the right heart. The second best access point is the left subclavian vein. Femoral vein sites are the most challenging and may require placement via fluoroscopy. Black marks on the catheter, at 10 centimeter (cm) intervals, assist with placement.

Once the access for the introducer has been obtained, the PAC is inserted under continued sterile conditions. The balloon at the catheter tip must be tested first by using the syringe provided in the packaging. This syringe has a maximum volume of 1.5 mL and is the only syringe that should be used on the catheter to prevent over inflation of the balloon. The balloon is first inflated and then deflated to ensure integrity. The proximal (RA) and distal (PA) ports are then connected to a transducer setup, and the lines are thoroughly flushed with saline. Finally, if an extra port is available, the line is flushed with saline and a screw cap should be placed on the extra port to exclude all air. A sleeve for the PA catheter must be placed prior to insertion. Once the catheter is inserted into the introducer, the tip is advanced to the right atrium (approximately 15 cm) and a right atrial waveform should be visualized on the monitor (Figure 5-6). At this point, the balloon is inflated. The catheter is then carefully advanced to the right ventricle (see Figure 5-7) and then into the pulmonary artery (see Figure 5-8). The catheter is advanced, or "floated," using the balloon on the catheter tip, until the tip of the catheter wedges into a small pulmonary blood vessel (see Figure 5-9). Once the catheter is in the wedge position, the PAOP pressure should be noted, and then the air in the balloon is released. Once the balloon is deflated, the PAOP waveform should return back to the PA waveform, with corresponding PA digital pressure values (see Figure 5-7) on the monitor. At this time, the black mark at the insertion site of the PAC should be documented (in cm) to note the distance of the catheter from the insertion site into the heart. If any difficulty arises during the process of advancing the catheter, the balloon should be deflated, and the catheter withdrawn back into the RA to re-attempt insertion. During insertion, the bedside nurse assists the physician or the advanced practice provider with the setup and flushing of the catheter. The nurse will also assist in monitoring the catheter waveforms and

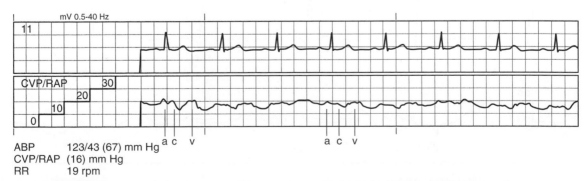

FIGURE 5-6 Right atrial pressure (RAP) waveform. Simultaneous ECG and RAP waveforms illustrate that the p wave occurs prior to the a wave; that the QRS initiates ventricular systole and results in the c wave and the v wave.

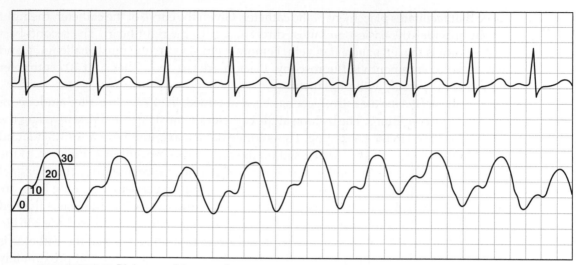

FIGURE 5-7 Right ventricle waveform.

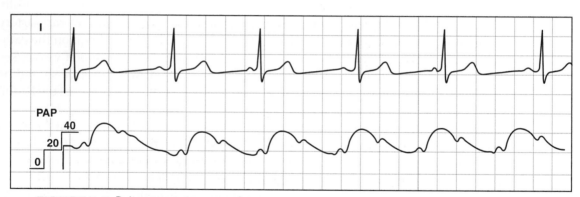

FIGURE 5-8 Pulmonary artery waveform.

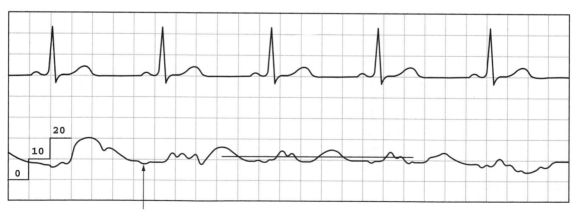

PAC balloon inflated

FIGURE 5-9 Pulmonary artery occlusion pressure (PAOP) waveform. The PAOP is read as a mean pressure as indicated by the line.

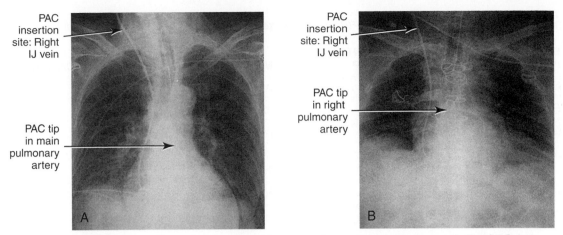

FIGURE 5-10 Chest radiography showing pulmonary artery catheter placement. **A,** The PAC tip is in the main pulmonary artery and the catheter balloon will not wedge from this location. **B,** The PAC tip is in the right pulmonary artery in optimal position to wedge to obtain a PAOP waveform.

electrocardiography (ECG) reading during insertion. Portable anteroposterior chest radiography is performed to confirm placement (Figure 5-10). Once the catheter is correctly placed, waveform analysis may begin.

Risks

The use of invasive catheters does not come without risk. Clinicians are not uniformly trained or competent at catheter insertion or data interpretation.[13] However, when performed by an experienced clinician complications associated with a PAC are rare.[2] Of the 13 randomized controlled trials reviewed by the Cochrane Collaboration in 2013, 11 listed specific complications of PAC use.[12] However, because there is no clinical consensus as to which PAC complications should be reported, the complication rates vary widely between the studies, as listed in Table 5-3. Transient arrhythmia was the most commonly reported complication, and none of the incidents required further intervention.[6,7,14–20] Some studies reported complications such as hematoma, arterial puncture, hemothorax, or pneumothorax, which were related to central line insertion but were not unique to the PAC.[21] Other complications of central line insertion include pain, bleeding, and air embolus. Thrombosis and line infection were rarely reported in the studies, and since these complications may occur with any indwelling catheter, they were not included in Table 5-3.

Arrhythmias are typically associated with movement of the PAC through the right side of the heart, especially as the catheter tip is advanced through the right ventricle. Premature ventricular contractions (PVCs) are the most common, are mostly transient, and typically resolve once the catheter is passed into the pulmonary artery. Right bundle branch block may also occur during insertion but is rare. Additional complications related to PAC insertion include cardiac tamponade, balloon rupture, and knotting or coiling of the catheter. A knotted or coiled catheter may be removed under fluoroscopic

TABLE 5-3 **Complications of Pulmonary Artery Catheter Insertion**

STUDY & YEAR PUBLISHED	TOTAL PATIENTS IN PAC GROUP	COMPLICATIONS REPORTED	TOTAL COMPLICATION RATE
Shoemaker 1988[19]	310	Arrhythmia = 37	11.9%
Pearson 1989[22]	33	No complications reported	0
Isaacson 1990[15]	49	Arrhythmia = 5	10.2%
Joyce 1990[16]	32	Arrhythmia = 9 Catheter looping = 4	40.6%
Berlauk 1991[21]	66	Pneumothorax = 1	1.5%
Guyatt 1991[23]	16	No complications reported	0
Bender 1997[14]	51	Arrhythmia = 3	5.9%
Valentine 1998[20]	60	Arrhythmia = 5 Pneumothorax = 1	10.0%
Rhodes 2002[18]	95	Arrhythmia = 3	3.2%
Richard 2003[7]	335	Arrhythmia = 60 Arterial puncture = 17 Catheter looping = 6 Hemothorax = 1	25.1%
Sandham 2003[8]	941	Arterial puncture = 3 Hemothorax = 2 Pneumothorax = 8 Pulmonary hemorrhage = 3 Pulmonary infarction = 1	1.8%
Harvey 2005[6]	506	Arrhythmia = 16 Arterial Puncture = 16 Hematoma = 17 Hemothorax = 1 Pneumothorax = 2 Retrieval of lost guidewire = 2	10.7%
NHLBI 2006[17]	513	Arrhythmia = 34 Air embolism = 1 Pneumothorax = 2 Hemothorax = 1 Hematoma = 1	7.6%

visualization, but sometimes surgery is required to remedy the situation. Meticulous care must be taken in managing the catheter to prevent infection, including the use of the catheter sleeve and adherence to aseptic technique when administering medications. As with any indwelling catheter, thrombus formation on the catheter itself and at the insertion site is a risk. Pulmonary infarction is not commonly seen but may be caused by a thrombus or embolus or by a malpositioned catheter resulting in prolonged wedging into a smaller vessel. Arteriovenous fistula formation is a rare complication that can occur.

A rare, and usually fatal, complication that may occur is pulmonary artery rupture. Risk factors for pulmonary artery rupture include age (>60 years), anticoagulation therapy, cardiopulmonary bypass surgery, pulmonary hypertension, and operator error, either during insertion of the catheter, or failure to recognize a malpositioned catheter after insertion. The balloon on the catheter should only be inflated with the prescribed amount of air and should not be forcefully inflated or inflated with liquid. If pulmonary artery rupture is suspected, as evidenced by hemoptysis, hypoxia, shortness of breath, or chest pain, the patient should be placed in the lateral recumbent position with the affected side down. The physician or advanced practice provider should be immediately notified. Diagnostics include immediate chest radiography. A double lumen endotracheal tube may be inserted to provide ventilation to the unaffected lung. Immediate surgical evaluation should be obtained, and the patient should be prepared for a potential lung lobectomy.

Measurement Method

Leveling the Transducer

After placement of the PAC, the transducer should be placed at the level of the phlebostatic axis. The phlebostatic axis is located at the fourth intercostal space, midaxillary line (Figure 5-11). The transducer should always be at the level of the phlebostatic axis to ensure accurate measurement, and this is best accomplished with the head of the bed at 0 to 45 degrees.

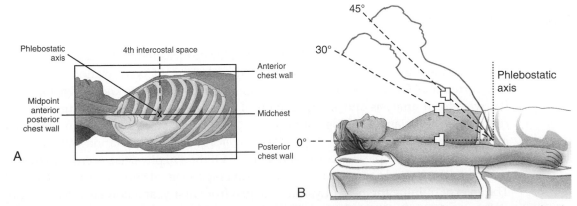

FIGURE 5-11 A, Location of the phlebostatic axis. **B,** Level of the phlebostatic axis according to patient's head of the bed 0 to 45 degrees.

Head of Bed Elevation

Multiple studies have confirmed the accuracy of measurements with the head of bed 0 to 45 degrees.[24–29] For consistency, all measurements are preferably obtained with the patient in the same body position each time. If the transducer is at the level of the phlebostatic axis and the head of bed is 0 to 45 degrees, the readings should be accurate.

Zeroing the Transducer

The next step is to zero the transducer to ambient air pressure for calibration. The three-way stopcock is turned off toward the patient, opening the port that is closest to the transducer to air. Once the transducer is calibrated (zeroed) using the monitor, the cap is placed back on the transducer and the stopcock opened from patient to transducer.

Square Wave Test

To assess the dynamic response accuracy of the monitoring system, the line is flushed, using the flushing mechanism on the pressure tubing. On the waveform, this should produce a distinct sharp rise with a plateau, followed by a distinct drop, or the formation of a square wave. Information about the use of the square wave test is found in Chapter 4 (Figure 4-5). After flushing, and the pulmonary arterial waveform should be present on the monitor

Scale

Once the waveforms are present, the appropriate scale is selected to ensure accurate measurements. The scale is usually located on the left of the waveform and measured in mm Hg. Using a scale that is too large will result in less accurate readings, as it will be difficult to see the subtle changes in the waveform necessary for accurate measurement and waveform analysis. Bedside monitors also have an option for "optimal waveform," which will automatically adjust the scale to the ideal size, if preferred.

Waveform Interpretation

Several principles must be followed to ensure accurate measurement of data with a PAC. These include transducer leveling, waveform morphology, ECG correlation, and respiratory correlation. Clinicians who do not routinely use PACs are less knowledgeable about PA waveform analysis and interpretation of data. A few studies have surveyed and reported on clinician knowledge of the PAC.[1,2,13,30–32] In a study by Iberti and associates in 1990, physician knowledge about PAC waveform and interpretation was measured using a 31-item multiple-choice questionnaire.[31] Of the 496 physicians across 13 medical centers in the United States and Canada, the average score of correct answers was 67%. The level of training for these physicians ranged from first-year fellows to attending physicians. In 1996, Burns et al. used 29 of the same 31 questions to poll 168 critical care nurses.[30] The average correct score was 56.8%, and 39% were unable to accurately measure the PAOP. In 2006, Parviainen et al. tested 47 physicians and 22 critical care unit nurses in a critical care unit training program about accurate leveling of a transducer and PAOP measurement.[32] Although the study was conducted unannounced, review materials had been passed out weeks in advance. The nurses were able to level the transducer more accurately compared with physicians, but both groups demonstrated major variations in accurate reading of PAOP. It is important to understand how to read PAC waveforms and to gather accurate data to make appropriate treatment decisions.

Measuring Right Atrial Pressure or Central Venous Pressure

To obtain intrathoracic RAP pressure readings, the patient is placed on the back with head of bed at 0 to 45 degrees, ensuring that the transducer is at the level of the phlebostatic axis. A printed strip of both the ECG reading and the RA tracing is obtained. ECG correlation is important when analyzing waveforms. It may be difficult at times to identify subtleties in some of the waveforms such as the RAP and the PAOP. Correlation with the ECG tracing will help ensure precise identification of the waves to provide an accurate assessment of values. The reading is measured at end expiration.

First, the P wave is located on the ECG and a vertical line drawn from the P wave to the *a* wave of the RA tracing. The *a* wave reflects atrial contraction. The next positive deflection is the *c* wave (sometimes not seen), followed by the *v* wave. The *c* wave represents closure of the tricuspid valve, and the *v* wave represents filling of the atrium. Second, returning to the *a* wave, the mean of the wave is taken to determine the pressure in the right atrium (see Figure 5-6). This information is also discussed in Chapter 4 under CVP monitoring (see Figure 4-6).

Measuring the Pulmonary Artery Pressure

To obtain the PA, a dual waveform strip of both the ECG and PA tracing is printed. A vertical line is drawn from the end of the QRS complex to the PA tracing. The lowest portion of the waveform runoff is the PA diastolic (PAD) pressure. The peak of the positive deflection following the QRS is the PA systolic (PAS) pressure (see Figure 5-8). When measuring PA pressures, distinct systolic and diastolic phases should be present. The rise of the systolic phase should be sharp. As the blood is ejected out of the pulmonary artery, a decline in pressure occurs, resulting in a downward waveform, often with a notch seen during the fall. This notch, called the *dicrotic notch*, is caused by the closure of the pulmonic valve (see Figure 5-8). Again, using the appropriate scale on the monitor will ensure accurate assessment of pressures.

Measuring the Pulmonary Artery Occlusion Pressure

The PAOP, also known as the *pulmonary artery wedge pressure*, is obtained by carefully inflating the balloon of the PA catheter, and allowing the tip of the catheter to passively float, or "wedge," into the capillary bed. To obtain the PAOP, the gate valve or stopcock on the balloon port is unlocked and air, up to 1.5 mL, is inserted until the waveform dampens as evidence of the wedge position. A strip of the ECG and PAOP waveforms is printed. The balloon should not be left inflated for more than 10 seconds. The balloon is released and the valve closed when the wedge pressure reading is complete. Next, the *a* and *v* waves are identified. A vertical line is drawn from the QRS to the PAOP tracing (see Figure 5-9). The wave following the line is the *a* wave. Measure the mean of the *a* wave, at end expiration, as this represents the PAOP. Often, the *c* wave is not seen on the PAOP tracing. The *v* wave represents ventricular systole.

The PAOP is a reflection of the left ventricular end-diastolic pressure, which is an estimate of preload volume in the heart. In a healthy heart and in LV failure, the PAOP usually correlates with the PAD pressure, and both may be considered an indirect measurement of left ventricular end-diastolic pressure.

However, in some pathophysiologic circumstances, the PAOP and the PAD pressure will not correlate. These conditions are well known and include:

1. Conditions that impact the pulmonary vasculature and lungs but spare the left ventricle, such as chronic obstructive pulmonary disease (COPD), acute respiratory distress syndrome (ARDS), and pulmonary hypertension, or pulmonary embolus that leads to right heart failure. In these conditions the left ventricle is unaffected so that the PAOP value will be within normal limits while PAD will be abnormally elevated.
2. Mitral stenosis will increase the pressure in the left atrium, which will raise the wedge pressure although the left ventricle is protected.
3. Mitral regurgitation may cause giant *v* waves on the PAOP tracing. The *v* waves reflect the increased pressure from the blood ejected retrograde into the left atrium. The rise in left atrial pressure caused by systolic regurgitation distorts the normal PAOP wedge tracing, and makes waveform interpretation difficult.

Pulmonary Artery Waveform Analysis

It is important to recognize conditions that alter normal pressure readings, for example, variation associated with breathing, arrhythmias, and issues with the catheter itself. Although these scenarios may not always be present, an experienced clinician should be able to recognize the following situations and understand their effects on accurate pressure monitoring.

Respiratory Variation

Breathing causes cyclic fluctuations in pressure within the thoracic cavity that are recorded by hemodynamic pressure measurements. With spontaneous breathing, intrathoracic pressures decrease at the beginning of inspiration (inhalation) and intrathoracic pressures rise during expiration (exhalation). When examining the waveform, in a spontaneously breathing patient, a negative deflection occurs during inspiration, so the measurement should be taken just before this point (Figure 5-12). One can also estimate end expiration by observing the respiratory rise and fall of the patient's chest. Or, find end expiration by correlating the respiratory tracing that is derived from movement of the electrocardiogram (ECG) leads with the pulmonary arterial waveform on the bedside monitor.

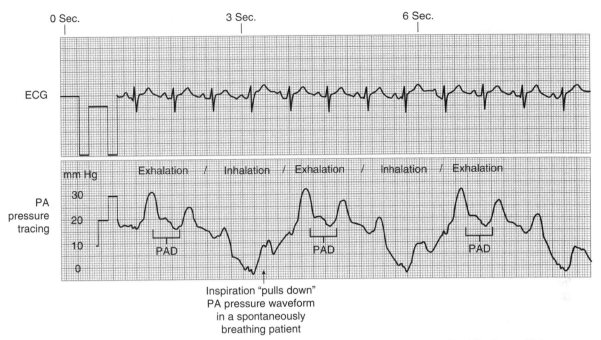

FIGURE 5-12 End expiration reading for spontaneous breathing. (From Urden LD, Stacy KM, Lough ME: *Critical care nursing: diagnosis and management*, ed 7, St. Louis, 2014, Mosby.)

With mechanical ventilation the opposite effect occurs: Intrathoracic pressure increases with inspiration due to the effects of positive pressure ventilation (air being forced in) and decreases with passive expiration (exhalation). That being known, waveforms are analyzed at the point where intrathoracic pressures are least affected by air movement, which is at end expiration. During positive pressure mechanical ventilation, a positive deflection occurs during inspiration, so the measurement should be taken just before the waveform rises (Figure 5-13). Other options are to correlate the PA waveform with another respiratory waveform such as the respiratory tracing derived from the ECG leads, the capnography ($ETCO_2$) waveform, or continuous airway pressure monitoring, if available.

Respiratory variation in the waveforms cannot always be seen, although when variation exists, it is important to record the measurement at end expiration to record the most accurate hemodynamic values.

Clinical Reasoning Pearl

To accurately assess respiratory variation, it is important to understand that the inspiration to expiration ratio is usually about 1:2. Look for the longest portion of the waveform that occurs without deflection (up or down). In volume cycled ventilation, the end of that longest portion will be the end of expiration, especially with slower respiratory rates of less than 16 breaths per minute.

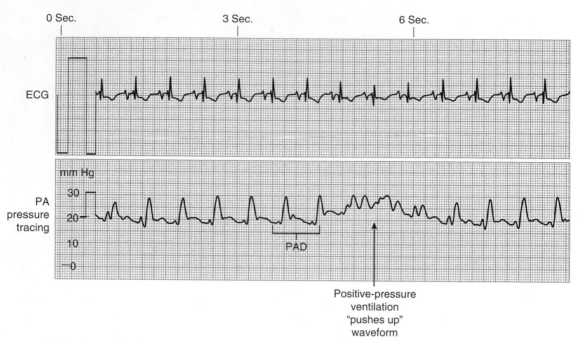

FIGURE 5-13 End expiration reading for mechanical ventilation. (From Urden LD, Stacy KM, Lough ME: *Critical care nursing: diagnosis and management*, ed 7, St. Louis, 2014, Mosby.)

Atrial Fibrillation

With atrial fibrillation, the ventricular filling will vary with each beat, resulting in fluctuating stroke volumes and pressures. Tachycardia may decrease filling time, which, in turn, decreases stroke volume. The decreased time spent in diastole may result in PAD values that are higher or lower than those if the heart rate were within normal limits.

Damping

Over-damping of the pressure waveform may occur for various reasons, including air in the line; improper flushing of the catheter, fibrinous clot at the end of the catheter, or the catheter tip migrated up against the vessel wall. When this occurs, the waveforms become rounded out (damped), resulting in inaccurate measurements.

Underdamping

Underdamping of the pressure waveform may cause the waveform to look jagged or erratic. When underdamping occurs, waveforms will be distorted and pressures will be inaccurate.

Spontaneous Wedge

This complication may occur when the PAC has floated an excessive distance forward into the pulmonary vascular bed usually without the balloon being inflated.

A spontaneous wedge tracing is identified by the left atrial waveform but also by the position of the tip of the PAC on chest radiography. When spontaneous wedge position is identified, the catheter must be repositioned by withdrawing it back by several centimeters.

Overwedging

This complication may occur when inflating the balloon to obtain a PAOP waveform and measurement. The danger of over-inflation of the balloon is that it may precipitate a balloon leak, or worse, rupture of a pulmonary blood vessel. For this reason PAC insertion kits include a specific syringe designed to instill a limited amount of air into the balloon. In addition, the clinician must observe the shape of the waveform and stop inflation once the expected PAOP waveform is observed on the monitor.

Inability to Wedge

If an attempt is made to inflate the balloon and the PA waveform does not dampen or change to a wedged waveform, the air should be passively released from the balloon. The PAC may have been slightly pulled back, have migrated back into the PA, or may not be advanced far enough to obtain a wedge pressure. The physician or provider trained to advance PACs may attempt to refloat the tip into a small pulmonary vessel to obtain the wedge pressure. Then again, the attempt to obtain a wedge pressure should not be continued if it has already failed.

Right Ventricular Waveform

If the tip of the PAC slips back into the right ventricle, the classic RV waveform will be displayed (see Figure 5-7). It is important that clinicians recognize the distinctive RV waveform shape. The first clue may be a decrease in the diastolic pressure recorded from the catheter tip. The RV tracing is identified by the waveform but can also be confirmed by the position of the tip of the PAC on chest radiography. When the tip of the catheter is in the right ventricle, a high risk of irritation of the ventricular endocardium exists, especially when ventricular dysrhythmias are present. The physician or advanced care provider must be notified immediately if a RV waveform is noted during routine monitoring so that the catheter can be repositioned.

Measuring Thermodilution Cardiac Output

Another useful function of the PAC is the ability to measure or calculate cardiac output. A more precise measurement of cardiac performance is the cardiac index, which adjusts the cardiac output to the body surface area (BSA) of the individual (Box 5-3). Using the PAC, cardiac output can be obtained by any of three methods: continuous cardiac output measurement; bolus thermodilution cardiac output measurement; or the Fick principle.

BOX 5-3   Body Surface Area (BSA) and Cardiac Index (CI)

CI = CO / BSA

Body surface area (m^2) = Square root of: height (cm) × weight (kg)

BSA, Body surface area; *CI*, cardiac index; *CO*, cardiac output.

Continuous Cardiac Output

The most commonly used method for cardiac output measurement is the continuous cardiac output. The PAC is equipped with a thermal filament between the proximal port and distal end of the catheter (Figure 5-4, *C*). With proper placement, the filament sits in the right ventricle. Heat impulses are transmitted every 30 to 60 seconds, in an on–off fashion, and blood temperature changes are measured throughout the filament. The data are transferred to the monitor, which displays the average cardiac output obtained over the previous 3 to 6 minutes, on a continuous basis. In addition to providing continuous readings, these catheters are usually equipped with fiberoptic capability to continuously measure the saturation of oxygen (SvO$_2$) in the pulmonary artery (Figure 5-4, *C*) (see Chapter 7 for more information).

A major benefit of using continuous cardiac output catheters is the availability of up-to-date data on which to base clinical decisions and interventions. Several studies have shown that continuous cardiac output is an accurate and reliable method of measuring cardiac output.[33–35] In addition, compared with intermittent bolus thermodilution cardiac outputs, this method does not use extra volume and has a decreased risk of infection, as frequent injections of crystalloid are not needed. It is important to note that continuous cardiac output readings may be less accurate with large volume infusions through the proximal port, as this will affect the blood temperature around the filament, resulting in falsely low cardiac output readings.[36]

Intermittent-Bolus Thermodilution Cardiac Output

Intermittent-bolus thermodilution cardiac output is another method of measuring cardiac output. It was the primary method of obtaining data prior to the availability of continuous cardiac output catheters. The bolus thermodilution cardiac output method requires multiple injections (3–5) of an injectate, usually 10-mL of sterile normal saline, at room temperature, to obtain the measurements. The clinician injects the 10-mL bolus into the proximal port of the PAC, at end expiration, while simultaneously pressing a foot pedal/soft key on the monitor, to indicate the timing of the injectate. As the bolus of saline travels from the proximal port past the thermistor near the tip of the PAC, a thermodilution curve is generated and viewed on the bedside computer-monitor (Figure 5-14, *A*).

The bolus thermodilution method not only delivers large amounts of additional volume over a 24-hour period, but if not in a closed delivery system, may increase the risk of infection to the patient. In addition, the injection must be performed in a consistent manner so that each waveform is consistent, and the average measurement will be accurate (see Figure 5-14, *A*). Consistency of injections can vary by clinician or a single user may not inject fluid at a consistent rate, which would cause inconsistent waveforms and reduced accuracy (Figure 5-14, *B*).

Fick Method

The Fick principle determines flow, or cardiac output, by assessing the relationship of arterial blood and mixed venous blood samples to tissue oxygen consumption. In other words, blood will absorb the quantity of oxygen from the lungs that will be used by tissues. Three variables must be measured to calculate a Fick cardiac output: VO_2 (oxygen consumption), CaO_2 (arterial oxygen content), and CvO_2 (venous oxygen content). In clinical practice this formula is typically modified to use a standardized VO_2 value, and to use the arterial oxygen saturation (SaO_2) and mixed venous oxygen saturation (SvO_2) values. The substitution of oxygen saturation for oxygen content is reasonable since saturated hemoglobin makes up 97% of the oxygen content of blood. The dissolved oxygen (partial pressure) makes up only 3% of the total.

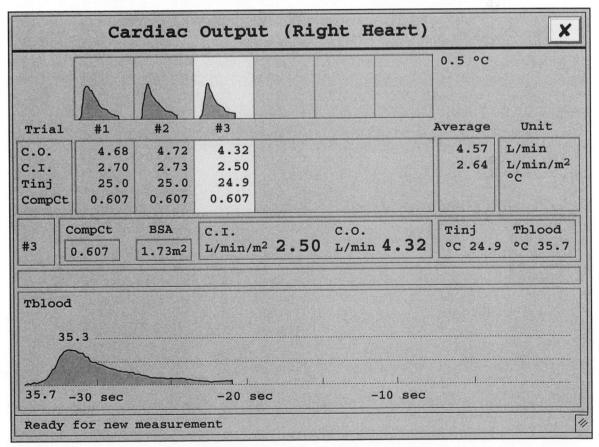

A

FIGURE 5-14 A, Accurate thermodilution cardiac output waveforms.

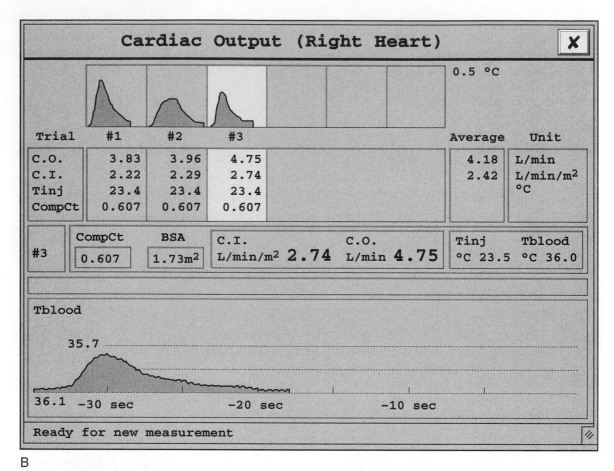

B

FIGURE 5-14, cont'd B, Inaccurate thermodilution cardiac output waveforms. *BSA*, Body surface area; *°C*, centigrade; *C.I.*, cardiac index; *C.O.*, cardiac output; *CompCt*, computation constant; *L/min*, liters per minute; *L/min/m²*, liters per minute per meter squared; *sec*, seconds; *Tblood*, patient's blood temperature; *Tinj*, injectate temperature.

Oxygen Consumption

VO_2 can be measured by collection of exhaled gases, or by indirect calorimetry. Because this may be time consuming or simply not feasible, oxygen consumption is usually estimated. The most commonly used formula for resting oxygen consumption is $125 \text{ mL} \times BSA$.

Next, two blood samples representing arterial oxygen saturation (SaO_2) and mixed venous oxygen saturation (SvO_2) are obtained in a blood gas syringe for each analysis. The CaO_2 sample is drawn from an arterial line, while the CvO_2 is simultaneously drawn from the distal port of the PAC. A current hemoglobin level (drawn within 6–12 hours) should also be available at the time the blood samples are obtained.

Using the modified Fick method, the cardiac output is calculated with the given data. In this formula, 1.34 mL represents the amount of oxygen carried by each gram of hemoglobin. In addition, 10 is a conversion factor to convert milliliters per deciliter (mL/dL) to liters per minute (L/min). To calculate the cardiac index, divide the cardiac output by BSA (see Box 5-3).

$$\text{Step 1: Oxygen consumption (VO}_2) = 125 \text{ mL} \times \text{BSA}$$
$$\text{Step 2: CO} = \text{VO}_2 \div \text{(Arteriovenous O}_2 \text{ saturation difference)}$$
$$\times \text{ hemoglobin} \times 1.34 \times 10$$

Result = cardiac output
For example:

Patient data:
BSA $= 2.0 \text{ m}^2$
Hb $= 11$ g
$SaO_2 = 98\%$
$SvO_2 = 63\%$

$$\text{Step 1: Oxygen consumption (VO}_2) = 125 \times 2 = 250 \text{ mL}$$
$$\text{Step 2: } 250 \div (0.98 - 0.63) \times 11 \times 1.34 \times 10$$

Result = 4.26

The Fick method is often considered the "gold standard" for determining cardiac output. Unlike the other two methods, Fick is not affected by tricuspid regurgitation. In addition, the Fick method may be more accurate in conditions with a lower cardiac output. While the calculation may be more accurate than using continuous cardiac output or bolus thermodilution cardiac output, the Fick method only provides a "snapshot" in time. When drawing the SvO_2 sample from the distal PA port, it is important not only to remove an adequate deadspace volume (waste) but also to draw back slowly to avoid drawing oxygenated blood from the pulmonary capillaries into the syringe.

Clinical Reasoning Pearl

- Patients with severe tricuspid regurgitation have an alteration in blood flow across the tricuspid valve, and may not have accurate cardiac output measurements using the thermodilution method. It is important to use either continuous cardiac output if available, or the Fick method to calculate cardiac output.

- A mixed venous oxygen saturation (SvO_2) is obtained only from the distal port of a PAC. The term "mixed" refers to the mixing of venous blood from the lower body (via the inferior vena cava) and the blood returning from the upper portion of the body (via the superior vena cava) including blood returned from the brain. Since brain cells consume a higher oxygen level, blood returning from the superior vena cava may have a lower oxygen concentration than blood returning from the inferior vena cava at rest.

Interpretation of Data

Normal or Expected Values

Although it is important to obtain accurate data from PAC waveforms and cardiac output, it is equally important to interpret and analyze the data accurately with knowledge of the normal values. See Table 5-4 for normal values.

TABLE 5-4 Normal Values

PARAMETER	EQUATION	NORMAL VALUE RANGES
HR		60-100 beats/min
BSA*	kilogram × centimeter × 0.007184	0.6-2.9 m^2
SV	CO × 1000 ÷ HR	60-100 mL/beat
SVI	SV ÷ BSA	30-65 mL/beat/m^2
CO	HR × SV	4-8 L/min
CI*	CO ÷ BSA	2.5-4.0 L/min/m^2
RAP		2-6 mm Hg
PAS		15-30 mm Hg
PAD		8-15 mm Hg
PA mean	PAD + ⅓ (PAS − PAD)	9-18 mm Hg
PAOP		4-12 mm Hg
MAP	DBP + ⅓ (SBP − DBP)	70-100 mm Hg
PVR	[(PA mean − PAOP) × 80] ÷ CO	100-250 dynes·sec/cm^5
PVRI	[(PA mean − PAOP) × 80] ÷ CI	255-315 dynes·sec/cm^5/m^2
SVR	[(MAP − CVP) × 80] ÷ CO	800-1200 dynes·sec/cm^5
SVRI	[(MAP − CVP) × 80] ÷ CI	2000-2400 dynes·sec/cm^5/m^2

*See Box 5-3 for the calculation of cardiac index using body surface area
BSA, Body surface area; *CI*, cardiac index; *CO*, cardiac output; *DBP*, diastolic blood pressure; *HR*, heart rate; *MAP*, mean arterial pressure; *PA mean*, pulmonary artery mean pressure; *PAD*, pulmonary artery diastolic pressure; *PAOP*, pulmonary artery occlusion pressure; *PAP*, pulmonary artery pressure; *PAS*, pulmonary artery systolic pressure; *PVR*, pulmonary vascular resistance; *PVRI*, pulmonary vascular resistance index; *RAP*, right atrial pressure; *SBP*, systolic blood pressure; *SV*, stroke volume; *SVI*, stroke volume index; *SVR*, systemic vascular resistance; *SVRI*, systemic vascular resistance index.

Patient Safety

- Prior to placement of a PAC, review the patient's history for possible venous access issues or history of deep vein thrombosis. Also, review the patient's laboratory values such as bleeding time or platelet count, which may need to be corrected prior to PAC insertion.

- Chest radiography should be performed after insertion to check placement and rule out complications such as pneumothorax.

- Note the position of the 10-cm increment black marks on the PAC at the insertion site. If the PAC tip is pulled back into the right ventricle it may cause cardiac dysrhythmias. If the PAC tip is advanced too far, it could spontaneously wedge in the pulmonary vascular bed and result in a pulmonary infarction.

- All hemodynamic tubing should be thoroughly flushed before initial setup. Zero the transducer on initial setup and again if a disconnection occurs in the system. All vented caps on the three-way stopcocks should be changed to nonvented caps to decrease risk of air-entry and infection. A pressure bag with saline should be maintained at 300 mm Hg at all times, with the date and time noted.

- The distal port of the PAC should never be used to infuse medications. Avoid albumin or blood products through the PAC. Dressings to the insertion site should remain intact at all times and be changed per hospital policy to decrease risk of infection.

- Prior to removing a PAC, the patient should be placed flat or in the Trendelenburg position (head downwards) to decrease risk of air embolism. All flushes, medications, or infusions should be discontinued or placed in another venous access line prior to PAC removal. Remove the catheter with a steady motion while the patient exhales or holds their breath. If the patient is mechanically ventilated, the catheter pull is timed during exhalation. The introducer may be left in place or removed using the same technique.

Patient Education

- Prior to insertion of the PAC, ensure that the patient understands the procedure and informed consent has been obtained. Assess the patient's ability to participate in the procedure—the patient must be able to lie flat for an extended period.

- Prior to repositioning the patient to obtain PAC readings, explain the process. Although readings may be obtained anywhere between 0 and 45 degrees, using the same position with each reading allows for more accurate comparison of results, and patients need to understand the need for repositioning.

Case Study

Mrs. J, a 73-year-old female with a history of coronary artery disease, myocardial infarction with multiple stent placements, and ischemic cardiomyopathy presented to the emergency department with severe shortness of breath and worsening bilateral lower extremity edema. She was unable to finish an entire sentence without having to stop to catch her breath.

PARAMETERS	INITIAL ASSESSMENT	AFTER FUROSEMIDE	AFTER PAC PLACEMENT	AFTER DOBUTAMINE
Temperature (°C)	37.6	38.0	37.9	37.8
HR (beats/min)	102	113	94	87
RR (breaths/min)	32	40	24	22
BP (cuff) / A-line (MAP)	88/47	83/palp	92/50 (64)	98/52 (67)
SpO_2	90% on a 0.5 (50%) Venturi mask	89% on 100% non-rebreather mask	98% on 0.8 FiO_2 mechanically ventilated	97% on 0.6 FiO_2 mechanically ventilated
RAP (mm Hg)			16	14
CI (L/min/m²)			1.7	2.1
SVR (dynes·sec/cm⁵)			1250	850
PAP S/D (mean) mm Hg			48/30 (36)	36/25 (28)
PAOP (mm Hg)			32	25

Initial Assessment and Interventions: On physical examination, Mrs. J's temperature was elevated; she was tachycardic, hypotensive and short of breath with a SpO_2 90% on 50% FiO_2 ventimask. On auscultation she had crackles throughout her posterior lung fields bilaterally. On exam she had 3+ pitting bilateral lower extremity edema and her legs were pale and cool. A 12-lead electrocardiogram revealed sinus rhythm with a left bundle branch block, which was her baseline. Laboratory studies were: Na^+ 133 mmol/L, K^+ 4.0 mmol/L, Cl^- 101 mmol/L, HCO_3^- 20 mmol/L, BUN 45 mg/dL, creatinine 1.8 mg/dL (her baseline was 1.2 mg/dL), glucose 96 mg/dL, Ca^{2+} 8.5 mg/dL.

Case Study—cont'd

Furosemide (Lasix) 40 mg intravenous (IV) was administered and she was placed on a non-rebreather mask with 100% FiO$_2$. The cardiology team was called stat to evaluate her cardiac status.

After Furosemide: There was no urine output response to the IV furosemide. The cardiology team arrived quickly, to find her condition had worsened with an increased temperature, increased respiratory rate to 40 breaths/min, tachycardia, and hypotension with a barely audible cuff blood pressure, palpated at systolic 83 mm Hg, with SpO$_2$ 89% on 100% FiO$_2$ non-rebreather mask. Mrs. J was intubated in the emergency department before transferring to the critical care unit. Due to her lack of response to diuretics, borderline kidney function and hypotension, a PAC was inserted and a radial arterial line was placed.

After PAC Placement: After intubation and insertion of the PAC and arterial line, her respiratory rate was controlled at 24 breaths/min. Her blood pressure remained low with elevated cardiac filling pressures: RAP 16 mm Hg, PAP 48/30 (36) mm Hg, and PAOP 32 mm Hg. Her cardiac index was low (1.7) with an elevated SVR (1250) consistent with a diagnosis of acute heart failure and progression to cardiogenic shock. To treat her high SVR and low cardiac output, a dobutamine infusion was initiated at 5 mcg/kg/min.

After Dobutamine: Two hours after initiation of dobutamine her intracardiac filling pressures were trending downward in a favorable direction to RAP 14 mm Hg, PAP 36/25 (28) and PAOP 25 mm Hg. Her cardiac index increased (2.1) with vasodilation decreasing the SVR (850) in response to dobutamine. Her urine output remained less than 30 milliliters per hour.

The dobutamine dose was increased to 8 mcg/kg/min and a combination of bumetanide (Bumex) and furosemide were administered. Mrs. J responded to diuresis, resulting in further improvement of her condition. The PAC was utilized to guide the initiation and up-titration of dobutamine therapy in the setting of acute heart failure and volume overload. ∎

Conclusion

Despite evidence that PACs do not improve morbidity or mortality, they continue to be used today in many cardiothoracic surgical critical care units, to diagnose pulmonary hypertension and to guide therapeutic interventions. It is important to weigh the risk versus benefits before deciding to use a PAC and to discuss these with the patient. Success in using these catheters depends on the experience of the person inserting the catheter, as well as those monitoring the patient and interpreting the data.[1,2,13,30-32] Careful attention should be paid to the subtleties of interpreting the waveforms, proper positioning of the patient, selection of optimal scales, identifying end expiration, and recognizing appropriate waveforms to ensure accurate data comparison. Taking these steps will provide the best opportunity for positive outcomes when using the PAC and cardiac output measurements to guide therapy.

References

1. Chatterjee K: The Swan-Ganz catheters: past, present, and future. A viewpoint, *Circulation* 119 (1):147–152, 2009.
2. Vincent JL: The pulmonary artery catheter, *J Clin Monit Comput* 26(5):341–345, 2012.
3. Swan HJ, Ganz W, Forrester J, et al.: Catheterization of the heart in man with use of a flow-directed balloon-tipped catheter, *N Engl J Med* 283(9):447–451, 1970.
4. Connors AF Jr, Speroff T, Dawson NV, et al.: The effectiveness of right heart catheterization in the initial care of critically ill patients. SUPPORT Investigators, *JAMA* 276(11):889–897, 1996.
5. Zion MM, Balkin J, Rosenmann D, et al.: Use of pulmonary artery catheters in patients with acute myocardial infarction. Analysis of experience in 5,841 patients in the SPRINT Registry, *Chest* 98(6):1331–1335, 1990, SPRINT Study Group.
6. Harvey S, Harrison DA, Singer M, et al.: Assessment of the clinical effectiveness of pulmonary artery catheters in management of patients in intensive care (PAC-Man): a randomised controlled trial, *Lancet* 366(9484):472–477, 2005.
7. Richard C, Warszawski J, Anguel N, et al.: Early use of the pulmonary artery catheter and outcomes in patients with shock and acute respiratory distress syndrome: a randomized controlled trial, *JAMA* 290(20):2713–2720, 2003.
8. Sandham JD, Hull RD, Brant RF, et al.: A randomized, controlled trial of the use of pulmonary-artery catheters in high-risk surgical patients, *N Engl J Med* 348(1):5–14, 2003.
9. Binanay C, Califf RM, Hasselblad V, et al.: Evaluation study of congestive heart failure and pulmonary artery catheterization effectiveness: the ESCAPE trial, *JAMA* 294(13):1625–1633, 2005.
10. Shah MR, Hasselblad V, Stevenson LW, et al.: Impact of the pulmonary artery catheter in critically ill patients: meta-analysis of randomized clinical trials, *JAMA* 294(13):1664–1670, 2005.
11. Koo KK, Sun JC, Zhou Q, et al.: Pulmonary artery catheters: evolving rates and reasons for use, *Crit Care Med* 39(7):1613–1618, 2011.
12. Rajaram SS, Desai NK, Kalra A, et al.: Pulmonary artery catheters for adult patients in intensive care, *Cochrane Database Syst Rev* (Issue 2), 2013, CD003408.
13. Yancy CW, Jessup M, Bozkurt B, et al.: ACCF/AHA 2013 Guideline for the management of heart failure: A report of the American College of Cardiology Foundation /American Heart Association Task Force on Practice Guidelines, *Circulation* 128:e240–e327, 2013.
14. Bender JS, Smith-Meek MA, Jones CE: Routine pulmonary artery catheterization does not reduce morbidity and mortality of elective vascular surgery: results of a prospective, randomized trial, *Ann Surg* 226(3):229–236, 1997, discussion 236-237,.
15. Isaacson IJ, Lowdon JD, Berry AJ, et al.: The value of pulmonary artery and central venous monitoring in patients undergoing abdominal aortic reconstructive surgery: a comparative study of two selected, randomized groups, *J Vasc Surg* 12(6):754–760, 1990.
16. Joyce W, Provan JL, Ameli FM, et al.: The role of central haemodynamic monitoring in abdominal aortic surgery. A prospective randomised study, *Eur J Vasc Surg* 4(6):633–636, 1990.
17. National Heart and Lung Institute: Pulmonary-artery versus central venous catheter to guide treatment of acute lung injury, *N Engl J Med* 354(21):2213–2224, 2006.
18. Rhodes A, Cusack RJ, Newman PJ, et al.: A randomized, controlled trial of the pulmonary artery catheter in critically ill patients, *Intensive Care Med* 28(3):256–264, 2002.
19. Shoemaker WC, Appel PL, Kram HB, et al.: Prospective trial of supranormal values of survivors as therapeutic goals in high-risk surgical patients, *Chest* 94(6):1176–1186, 1988.
20. Valentine RJ, Duke ML, Inman MH, et al.: Effectiveness of pulmonary artery catheters in aortic surgery: a randomized trial, *J Vasc Surg* 27(2):203–211, 1998, discussion 211-212.
21. Berlauk J, Abrams JH, Gilmour IJ, et al.: Preoperative optimization of cardiovascular hemodynamics improves outcome in peripheral vascular surgery. A prospective, randomized clinical trial, *Ann Surg* 214(3):289–297, 1991, discussion 298-299.

22. Pearson KS, Gomez MN, Moyers JR, et al.: A cost/benefit analysis of randomized invasive monitoring for patients undergoing cardiac surgery, *Anesth Analg* 69(3):336–341, 1989.

23. Guyatt G: A randomized control trial of right-heart catheterization in critically ill patients. Ontario Intensive Care Study Group, *J Intensive Care Med* 6(2):91–95, 1991.

24. Cason CL, Holland CL, Lambert CW, et al.: Effects of backrest elevation and position on pulmonary artery pressures, *Cardiovasc Nurs* 26(1):1–6, 1990.

25. Chulay M, Miller T: The effect of backrest elevation on pulmonary artery and pulmonary capillary wedge pressures in patients after cardiac surgery, *Heart Lung* 13(2):138–140, 1984.

26. Dobbin K, Wallace S, Ahlberg J, et al.: Pulmonary artery pressure measurement in patients with elevated pressures: effect of backrest elevation and method of measurement, *Am J Crit Care* 1(2):61–69, 1992.

27. Keating D, Bolyard K, Eichler E, et al.: Effect of sidelying positions on pulmonary artery pressures, *Heart Lung* 15(6):605–610, 1986.

28. Lambert CW, Cason CL: Backrest elevation and pulmonary artery pressures: research analysis, *Dimens Crit Care Nurs* 9(6):327–335, 1990.

29. Wilson AE, Bermingham-Mitchell K, Wells N, et al.: Effect of backrest position on hemodynamic and right ventricular measurements in critically ill adults, *Am J Crit Care* 5 (4):264–270, 1996.

30. Burns D, Burns D, Shively M: Critical care nurses' knowledge of pulmonary artery catheters, *Am J Crit Care* 5(1):49–54, 1996.

31. Iberti TJ, Fischer EP, Leibowitz AB, et al.: A multicenter study of physicians' knowledge of the pulmonary artery catheter. Pulmonary Artery Catheter Study Group, *JAMA* 264 (22):2928–2932, 1990.

32. Parviainen I, Jakob SM, Suistomaa M, et al.: Practical sources of error in measuring pulmonary artery occlusion pressure: a study in participants of a special intensivist training program of The Scandinavian Society of Anaesthesiology and Intensive Care Medicine (SSAI), *Acta Anaesthesiol Scand* 50(5):600–603, 2006.

33. Albert NM, Spear BT, Hammel J: Agreement and clinical utility of 2 techniques for measuring cardiac output in patients with low cardiac output, *Am J Crit Care* 8(1):464–474, 1999.

34. Della Rocca G, Costa MG, Pompei L, et al.: Continuous and intermittent cardiac: pulmonary artery catheter versus aortic transpulmonary technique, *Br J Anaesth* 88(3):350–356, 2002.

35. Medin DL, Brown DT, Wesley R, et al.: Validation of continuous thermodilution cardiac output in critically ill patients with analysis of systematic errors, *J Crit Care* 13(4):184–189, 1998.

36. Wetzel RC, Latson TW: Major errors in thermodilution cardiac output measurement during rapid volume infusion, *Anesthesiology* 62(5):684–687, 1985.

Oxygenation and Acid–Base Balance Monitoring

6

Barbara McLean

The assessment of hemodynamic status, in combination with evaluation of oxygenation and ventilation is essential for achievement of best practice in the care of critically ill patients. The endpoints of hemodynamic monitoring provide practitioners with the data that allow assessment of the fluid status, vascular tonal changes, and the cardiovascular response to delivery of adequate oxygen to meet the demands of tissues.[1]

The arterial blood gas (ABG), in combination with selected chemistry variables, provides direct information about ventilation and oxygenation, as well as indirect information about internal respiration (tissue metabolism, tissue perfusion, tissue oxygenation). The ABG adds to the primary hemodynamic indicators that are usually measured, namely, heart rate, blood pressure, central venous pressure (CVP), stroke volume, cardiac output, and corresponding derived, calculated values. However, changes in these parameters may be late indicators of tissue hypoperfusion.

The ultimate goal of hemodynamic evaluation is the assessment of tissue perfusion. To support this goal, assessment of the indicators of oxygen availability and metabolic derangements are important for directed management. In most environments, perfusion and metabolic derangements are evaluated by correlating the ABG, parameters that represent the availability of oxygen with either a mixed venous blood gas (SvO_2) or a central venous blood gas ($ScvO_2$), representing the oxygen delivery–to–consumption ratio. That comparative analysis provides answers to the most important daily question for the clinician to ask: "Are the tissues adequately oxygenated?"

This chapter is designed to answer that question. The chapter initially focuses on assessment of oxygenation and ventilation, followed by the evaluation of metabolism at the cellular level, as assessed by the acid–base balance.

Historical Milestones

As stated by Dr. Barry Shapiro, it is difficult to "appreciate the rapid evolution of technology relevant to pH and blood gas measurements. Discovery of the scientific foundations took three centuries, whereas development of practical methods for clinical application took only three decades from the realization of their potential clinical importance."[2]

The pH concept was introduced in 1909 but was later stalled by controversy over the labeling and the significance of acid and base. Danish scientists in 1923 defined *acid* as a substance able to give off a proton at a given pH, and *base* as a substance that could bind a proton; in 1948, the North American Singer-Hasting school defined acids as strong nonbuffer anions and bases as nonbuffer cations. The consequence of this last definition, was that electrolyte disturbances were mixed up with acid–base disorders, and the variable "strong ion difference" (SID) was introduced as a measure of non-respiratory acid–base disturbances.[3,4] Since that time, blood gas analysis has been established as a powerful diagnostic tool in critical care and an essential component of hemodynamic evaluation.

One groundbreaking invention was development of carbon dioxide and oxygen electrodes in the 1950s, which led to construction of the blood gas analyzer by Severinghaus and Bradley in 1959.[5]

ABG analysis supports the diagnosis and management of the patient's pulmonary oxygenation and ventilation capabilities as well as an understanding of tissue respiration and metabolism. The analysis may be complex and it is completely dependent on the clinician's ability to correctly identify and interpret the results. Accurate interpretation of the ABG provides essential keys for ventilator management and to metabolic monitoring and enriches the evaluation of oxygen demand and delivery.

Basics in Pulmonary Gas Exchange: External Respiration

Gas exchange in the lungs takes place between the blood circulating in the capillary network surrounding the alveoli and the gas in the alveoli. In the optimal lung, oxygen is driven into blood, and carbon dioxide is driven into the alveolus. The relationship between alveoli and capillaries is shown in Figure 6-1.

Blood Flow

All of the blood ejected from the right ventricle flows through the pulmonary artery, which then rapidly divides into the capillary network that surrounds the alveoli.

Alveolar Gas Exchange Physiology

The capillary and alveolar walls are both very thin, which facilitates a rapid exchange of gases by passive diffusion along concentration gradients. This gas exchange between the alveoli and blood in the pulmonary capillaries occurs by passive diffusion; that is, oxygen moves from a region of high partial pressure in the alveolus to a region of low partial pressure in the pulmonary capillaries down a pressure gradient. Carbon dioxide moves in the opposite direction, from a region of high partial pressure in the pulmonary capillaries to low partial pressure within the alveolus (Figure 6-2).

In pulmonary physiology, the alveolus is abbreviated with an upper case "A," whereas pulmonary capillary arterial blood is abbreviated as a lowercase "a."

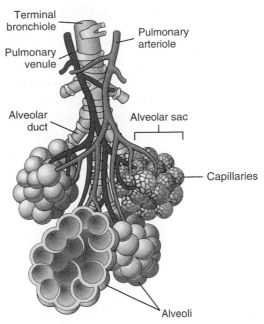

FIGURE 6-1 Relationship of alveoli and pulmonary capillaries. (From Patton KT, Thibodeau GA: *Anatomy & physiology,* ed 7, St. Louis, 2010, Mosby.)

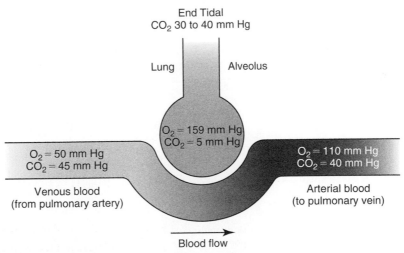

FIGURE 6-2 Partial pressures of oxygen (O_2) and carbon dioxide (CO_2).

Pulmonary venous blood is abbreviated with a lowercase "v." The *partial pressure* is abbreviated as "P" and describes the dissolved state of the gas that exerts pressure to cross membranes. The normal partial pressure values of oxygen (O_2) and carbon dioxide (CO_2) in the pulmonary capillaries and the alveolus are shown in Figure 6-2.

Dissolved venous carbon dioxide ($PvCO_2$) moves from the capillaries into the alveolus ($PACO_2$) because the concentration of carbon dioxide is higher in venous blood than in the alveolus (see Figure 6-2). Alveolar oxygen (PAO_2) moves out of the alveolus into the pulmonary capillaries (PaO_2) because the concentration of oxygen is higher in the alveolus than in the capillary and then onto the hemoglobin, thus saturating the hemoglobin with oxygen (see Figure 6-2). PaO_2 represents the oxygen dissolved in arterial blood plasma. SaO_2 represents the saturation of hemoglobin with oxygen when measured in arterial blood.

The distance between the alveolus and the capillary is approximately 0.7 micrometers. This tiny distance allows for extremely fast and efficient gas diffusion driven by the gas pressure gradients (see Figure 6-3). Once oxygen has passed through the alveolar and capillary walls, the oxygen primarily binds with hemoglobin to form oxyhemoglobin (SaO_2) for transport throughout the circulatory system. The bound oxygen is the major component of *oxygen content* or availability as described in Box 6-1.

Alveolar Gas Exchange in Disease States

With alveolar disorders the amount of alveolar ventilation may be reduced. The alveolar wall may be thickened by fibrosis, the functional alveolar surface area may be diminished by collapse of the alveoli, or the diffusion distance may be widened by pulmonary edema. These conditions limit the mobilization of gas across the membrane.

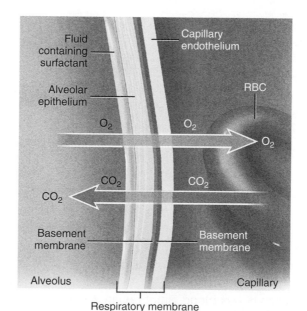

FIGURE 6-3 Dissolved venous carbon dioxide (CO_2) moves from the capillaries to the alveolus. Oxygen (O_2) moves from the alveolus to the pulmonary capillaries, where dissolved oxygen will saturate the red blood cell (RBC). (From Patton KT, Thibodeau GA: *Structure and function of the body*, ed 14, St. Louis, 2012, Mosby.)

BOX 6-1   Content of Oxygen: CaO₂ or CvO₂

Oxygen Content (CaO₂ or CvO₂): The total amount of oxygen carried by the hemoglobin is known as the content of oxygen and is measured in milliliters per deciliter (mL/dL) sometimes referred to (in the past) as *volume percent*. A deciliter equals 10 milliliters.

The content calculation represents the oxygen saturation % (SO_2) multiplied by the total hemoglobin multiplied again by the amount of oxygen per milliliter carried per saturated hemoglobin (1.38).

Calculation example: If the hemoglobin is 10 mg/dL, with an arterial oxygen saturation of 1.0 (100%), and every molecule of hemoglobin carries 1.38 mL of oxygen (standard factor) this is written as: $10(1.0) \times 1.38 = 13.8$ mL/dL of oxygen.

Alternatively, blood supply (perfusion) may be impaired by a reduced cardiac output, in which case insufficient gas exchange occurs despite sufficient ventilation. It is imperative to remember that the only purpose of the pulmonary blood flow, which is powered by the right ventricle, is to provide a blood flow and gradient for gas exchange, which occurs between the thin membranes of the capillaries and the alveoli (see Figure 6-3).

Oxygen Transport and the Oxyhemoglobin Curve

Because oxygen is transported around the circulatory system attached to hemoglobin in blood, the saturation of hemoglobin with oxygen predicts the total content of oxygen (CaO_2). The saturation mechanism is designed so that in circumstances where cellular demand is increased, hemoglobin will release oxygen to a dissolved state much more readily.

After leaving the alveolar capillary interface and the left ventricle, red blood cells flow and deform (change shape) as they move through systemic capillaries, continuously dissociating oxygen to maintain a relatively constant capillary partial pressure of oxygen in arterialized blood (PaO_2). The PaO_2 exerts an arterialized capillary partial pressure creating a diffusion gradient between two concentrations (capillary to cell) that will drive oxygen from high-pressure areas to low-pressure areas and from hemoglobin to dissolved state in the arterial vasculature (see Figure 6-4).

The rate of release of reservoir oxygen (SaO_2) to the dissolved state (PaO_2) and ultimately to the tissues depends on both cell demand and blood flow through the capillaries.[6] This means that at all times, hemoglobin should release its bound oxygen reservoir (SaO_2 or oxyhemoglobin), to the dissolved state (usable PaO_2) when the cell "demands" more. This unique relationship is graphically represented by the oxyhemoglobin dissociation curve as shown in Figure 6-5. In other words, when cells consume more oxygen, the reserve or bound oxygen is released from hemoglobin, dissolves in blood, exerts a partial pressure, and is then available to be taken up by the cells. In order

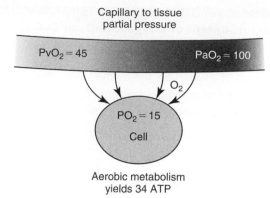

FIGURE 6-4 Dissolved oxygen moves from the capillary to the cell.

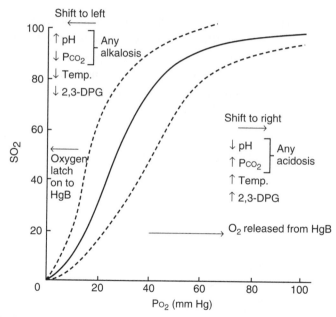

FIGURE 6-5 Oxyhemoglobin dissociation curve. *Hgb,* Hemoglobin; *O$_2$,* oxygen; *PCO$_2$,* partial pressure of carbon dioxide; *PO$_2$,* partial pressure of oxygen; *SO$_2$,* oxygen saturation; *Temp,* temperature. (From Weinberger S, Cockrill B, Mandel J: *Principles of pulmonary medicine,* ed 6, St. Louis, 2014, Elsevier.)

to meet the cell demand, which may be increased due to increased work of breathing, poor perfusion or hyper-inflammation, or because the delivery of oxygen is inadequate, hemoglobin releases oxygen more rapidly, shifting to the dissolved state. This is described as a shift to right of the oxyhemoglobin curve as indicated in Figure 6-5.

In the oxyhemoglobin curve, a *shift to the right* represents increased oxygen release and indicates that the proportional relationship between delivery and demand is increased on the demand side. Because the role of the hemoglobin is to transport and release oxygen where more dissolved oxygen is needed, higher tissue demand will result in a lower venous saturation in most clinical situations. Consequently, the evaluation of mixed venous (SvO_2) and central venous ($ScvO_2$) saturations, which represent the desaturation of hemoglobin, have become commonplace measurements in the critical care unit.[7]

When the oxyhemoglobin curve is said to *shift to the left*, this represents a decrease in the release of oxygen and may indicate that demand is low. Or failure of release of oxygen may be due to pathophysiologic conditions (shunt, sepsis, hemoglobin deformability) (see Figure 6-5).

Clinical Reasoning Pearl

The Importance of Saturated Hemoglobin

The percentage of saturated hemoglobin, both in the arterial and the central venous compartments, reflects the potential for the dissociation of oxygen—a function that uniquely occurs in an environment where the cells are using oxygen and perfusion is optimized.

Cellular operations are accomplished through the biochemical reactions that take place within the cell. Reactions are turned on and off, sped up, and slowed down according to immediate cellular needs and functions. Each process consumes cellular energy to produce energy, predominantly adenosine triphosphate (ATP). That energy (ATP) is best stored and created in the presence of oxygen (aerobically). Therefore, when tissues are more metabolically active, more oxygen is needed, and oxygen is released from circulating hemoglobin from reserve saturation of hemoglobin or SvO_2, promoting a shift to the right in the dissociation curve (see Figure 6-5).

Basics in Cellular Gas Exchange and Metabolism: Internal Respiration

Energy metabolism is the general process by which living cells acquire and use the energy needed to stay alive, grow, heal, and reproduce. The production of acid associated with energy metabolism is a continuous process.

Under normal physiologic conditions, the human body generates 50 to 100 milliequivalents per day (mEq/day) of acid from metabolism of carbohydrates, proteins, and fats. To maintain acid–base homeostasis, the cellular acid production must be balanced by neutralization or excretion of acid. The lungs and kidneys are the main regulators of acid–base homeostasis. The lungs regulate carbon dioxide, an end product of carbonic acid (H_2CO_3), and the kidneys regulate the hydrogen ion (H^+), also an end product of H_2CO_3.

Carbon dioxide is generated during the complete oxidation of carbohydrates and fatty acids. Most carbon dioxide is transported as H_2CO_3 in the bloodstream, as a combination of carbon dioxide (CO_2) and water (H_2O). The transformation of carbon dioxide and water ultimately yields H_2CO_3. When H_2CO_3 is presented to the alveoli by the pulmonary circulation, rapid dissociation takes place, yielding carbon dioxide and water, both of which are eliminated via the alveoli.

Acid Classification

Acids are primarily classified by the method utilized for excretion. Volatile acids require respiratory excretion, and fixed acids are cleared metabolically. Additionally, acids are named in accordance with their donation molecules (i.e., lactate, acetoacetate, beta-hydroxybutyrate, or carbon dioxide). For every one donator produced, one H^+ is donated so the quantity of donator measured generally reflects the number of H^+ ions that have been produced and donated into the blood in the original dissociation. The terms *lactic acidosis* or *ketoacidosis* indicate a dysfunctional metabolic process that results in a higher level of H^+ released into the bloodstream. This is termed *metabolic acidosis*.

Lactate Production and Clearance

Cells balance catabolic and anabolic pathways to control levels of critical metabolites and ensure that sufficient energy is always available. During critical illness, lactate levels can be increased by a number of mechanisms. Originally, increased lactate was considered to only reflect tissue hypoxia. Hyperlactemia in critical illness is now considered to also result from, among other causes, reduced lactate clearance in the liver, relative to production or accelerated aerobic glycolysis that exceeds the oxidative capacity of mitochondria. This may be cytokine driven or catecholamine driven.[8] Lactate measurement in critical illness may reflect the degree of global tissue anoxia and is one of the better predictors of potential organ damage.[9]

Evaluation of Pulmonary Blood Flow and Gas Exchange

Although lung oxygenation and ventilation are intimately related, each should be evaluated separately.

Ventilation–Perfusion Ratio and the Zones of the Lung

Pulmonary gas exchange represents the communication between recruited alveoli (V: ventilation) and pulmonary blood flow (Q: perfusion). The adequacy of pulmonary gas exchange is called the *V/Q ratio*. When alveoli receive optimal amounts of blood flow, at about 5 liters per minute (L/min) and optimal alveolar ventilation, at about 4 L/min, this will optimize gas exchange. In normal physiology, the match between ventilation and perfusion is about 80%. This is described as a normal V/Q ratio: 4 L alveolar ventilation divided by 5 L pulmonary perfusion = 0.8 (Box 6-2).

BOX 6-2 Pulmonary Gas Exchange

Pulmonary gas exchange can be divided into four functional components:

- **Ventilation** is the movement of air out of the lungs, measured primarily by the $PaCO_2$ and end-tidal carbon dioxide ($ETCO_2$).
- **Perfusion** is the movement and distribution of blood through pulmonary circulation, measured by PaO_2, relationship of alveolar to arterial oxygen differences and the $PaCO_2$ to $ETCO_2$ gradient.

- **Diffusion** is the movement of oxygen and carbon dioxide across the alveolar–blood barrier known as the *alveolar–capillary membrane*, primarily measured by PaO_2, relationship of alveolar to arterial oxygen differences, $PaCO_2$ and the $ETCO_2$.
- **Control of breathing** is a process of regulating gas exchange to meet metabolic needs of the moment, measured by tidal volume (V_T), respiratory rate (F) or the minute ventilation (V_E).

An important contributor to the V/Q ratio is the anatomical position of the lung and the pressurized distribution of gas. The zones of the lung divide each lung into three regions, based on the relationship between the pressure in the alveoli (PA), pressure in the arteries (Pa), and pressure in the veins (Pv) (Figure 6-6):

- Zone 1: PA > Pa > Pv
- Zone 2: Pa > PA > Pv
- Zone 3: Pa > Pv > PA

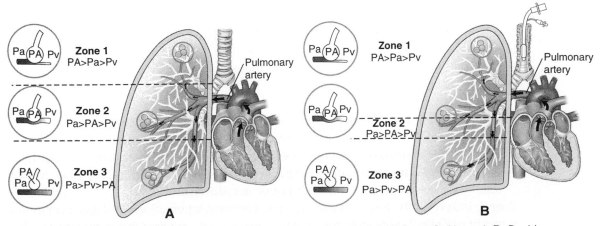

FIGURE 6-6 West's lung zone relationship of ventilation to blood flow. **A,** Normal. **B,** Positive pressure ventilation. (Modified from Wukitsch MW, Petterson MT, Tobler DR, Pologe JA: Pulse oximetry: Analysis of theory, technology, and practice, *J Clin Monit* 4(4):290–301, 1988.)

TABLE 6-1   Characteristics of Lung Zones: Normal and Positive Pressure Ventilation

DESCRIPTION	NORMAL LUNG*	POSITIVE PRESSURE VENTILATION (INSPIRATION)** + INCREASED IMPACT IF PEEP ADDED (EXPIRATION)
Relationship of alveolar ventilation (V) to blood flow and perfusion (Q) in the three lung zones.	Zone 1: blood flow < alveolar pressure	Zone 1: gas without blood flow significant alveolar deadspace
	Zone 2: blood flow = alveolar pressure: OPTIMAL	Zone 2: small blood flow = alveolar pressure: OPTIMAL
	Zone 3: blood flow > alveolar pressure	Zone 3: blood flow without gas significant (shunt)
Amount of lung affected by regional changes in pulmonary blood flow (Q) and alveolar ventilation (V) by lung zone.	Zone 1: PA>Pa>Pv: ⅛ lung	Zone 1: PA>Pa>Pv: ¼ or more lung
	Zone 2: Pa>PA>Pv: majority of lung	Zone 2: Pa>PA>Pv: ½ or smaller
	Zone 3: Pa>Pv>PA: ⅛ lung	Zone 3: Pa>Pv>PA: ¼ or more

< Less than; > greater than; = equals; *PA*, pulmonary alveolar pressure; *Pa*, pulmonary arterial pressure; *PEEP*, positive and expiratory pressure; *Pv*, pulmonary venous pressure; *Q*, perfusion; *V*, ventilation.
*See Figure 6-6, *A.*
**See Figure 6-6, *B.*

This model of the lung was developed by John B. West as shown in Figure 6-6.[10] Other researchers also noted that vascular pressures in the pulmonary arteries and veins were lower at the top of the lung compared with the bottom of the upright lung; that is, pulmonary arterial pressures were lower than alveolar pressures in the upper lung regions when a person was upright. The characteristics of the three lung zones are listed in Table 6-1. The lung zones are altered by positive pressure ventilation as described next.

Zone 1: The zone 1 effect is usually exacerbated when a person is ventilated with positive pressure. In these circumstances, blood vessels may become completely collapsed by the increased alveolar pressure, and blood does not flow through these regions. That lung surface does not participate in gas exchange and is termed *alveolar dead space* (gas is present, blood is not or is reduced).

Zone 2: In zone 2, the gas exchange surface is optimal where blood and gas meet in proportion. Zone 2 represents the alveolar surface that clinicians try to maximize when utilizing ventilation techniques, for example, positive end-expiration pressure (PEEP) and strategies to enhance mean airway pressure, or to optimize vascular perfusion with volume, inotropes, or position therapies (optimal gas and optimal blood flow). *Zone 3*: In zone 3, alveolar pressure is lower, and blood flow is continuous throughout the cardiac cycle. The most dependent surface receives more of the blood flow, creating a higher blood to collapsible alveolar pressure (blood is present, gas is not or is reduced).

In the unhealthy lung, the V/Q ratio reflects a much slower gas mix resulting from altered distribution of gas to blood, often caused by atelectasis, acute respiratory distress syndrome (ARDS), or pulmonary embolism. When ventilation and perfusion do not match (V is higher than Q, or V is lower than Q) gas exchange will be significantly affected. When describing ventilation and perfusion matching, the surface areas of the lung are also dependent on lung positioning. Evaluation of the V/Q ratio and pulmonary gas exchange can be performed at any bedside by an array of parameters.

Oxygenation Monitoring

Continuous Oxygenation Monitoring—Pulse Oximetry

Oxygenation measured from the pulse oximeter assesses the amount of oxygen that is bound to hemoglobin (SpO_2), measured by noninvasive plethysmography via a finger probe, ear sensor, or similar oximetry device. The value of pulse oximetry readings lies in its ability to noninvasively monitor oxygen exchange.

Pulse oximetry technology utilizes the light absorptive characteristics of hemoglobin in the arterial blood flow. The calculation of the percentage of arterial oxyhemoglobin is based on the distinct characteristics of light absorption (the red and near infrared light spectra) by oxygenated hemoglobin (O_2Hb) versus deoxygenated hemoglobin (HHb). The light is absorbed differently by completely saturated hemoglobin versus deoxygenated hemoglobin and absorption varies by the monitoring wavelength used as shown in Figure 6-7.[11]

To obtain the SpO_2 reading two light emitting diodes project a light through skin and tissues to detect visible red light at the 660 nanometer (nm) wavelength and near infrared light at the 940 nm wavelength. The pulse oximeter uses information from both wavelengths to measure the oxygen saturation. When hemoglobin is deoxygenated, near infrared light passes through easily and more red light is absorbed. In contrast, with highly oxygenated hemoglobin, red light passes more easily through the hemoglobin and more infrared light is absorbed.[11] The normal SpO_2 range is from 0.90 to 1.00 (90% to 100%) saturation of hemoglobin.

SpO_2 is defined as the fraction of oxygenated hemoglobin relative to the total amount of hemoglobin. The pulse oximeter is a noninvasive measure of the saturation of hemoglobin using light wavelengths transmitted through a well-perfused area of the body such as the finger. The pulse oximeter measures the saturation of hemoglobin but one caveat is that it is not able to identify when the gas attached to the hemoglobin is

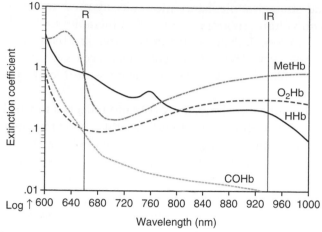

FIGURE 6-7 Light absorption of oxyhemoglobin (O_2Hb), which represents the saturation of hemoglobin with oxygen (SO_2). Other dyshemoglobins are identified by wavelength reading. The vertical lines indicate the monitoring wavelengths used in many pulse oximeters: Red (R) at 660 nanometers (nm) and near infrared (IR) at 940 nm. *COHb*, Carboxyhemoglobin; *HHb*, deoxyhemoglobin; *MetHb*, methemoglobin. (Modified from Wukitsch MW et al.: Pulse oximetry: analysis of theory, technology, and practice. *J Clin Monit* 4(4), 1988, Springer.)

not oxygen but is carbon monoxide, termed *carboxyhemoglobin* (COHb). Also, the pulse oximeter cannot identify other hemoglobin variants with altered oxygen binding. These are known as dyshemoglobinemias. Only co-oximetry using a blood sample in the clinical laboratory can accurately detect dyshemoglobins.[11]

Co-oximetry, technically called spectrophotometry is generally used in the clinical laboratory as part of the ABGs analysis, although some portable co-oximeter devices are now available. Co-oximetry uses a light emission and absorption methodology to directly measure non-oxygen carrying dyshemoglobins, each one having an individual wavelength signature. The dyshemoglobins include carboxyhemoglobin (COHb), methemoglobin (MetHb) and sulfhemoglobin (SulfHb)[11] (see Figure 6-7). Normal blood oxygen saturation, abbreviated as O_2Hb or SO_2, has its own individual wavelength pattern as shown in Figure 6-7. See Table 6-2 for a comparison of the different methods of oxygen measurement and the capability of different technologies to detect dyshemoglobins.[11]

SaO_2 is measured from a blood sample by a laboratory or a point-of-care co-oximeter. Laboratory co-oximeters use multiple wavelengths to distinguish additional types of hemoglobin such as carboxyhemoglobin (carbon monoxide+hemoglobin). In healthy persons, SaO_2 and the SpO_2 will be almost identical. However, in the setting of carbon monoxide poisoning, only the SaO_2 blood gas value measured by co-oximetry will be accurate.

Because oxygen is transported around the vascular system primarily attached to hemoglobin in blood, SpO_2 can provide an approximation of the total amount of oxygen available, if needed. Saturated hemoglobin (oxyhemoglobin) provides the

TABLE 6-2 Comparison of Devices Used to Measure Oxygen

DEVICE	SAMPLE	ANALYSIS	REPORTED RESULTS	CLINICAL ISSUES
Arterial blood gas analyzer	Blood	Arterial blood gas analyzers have three electrodes: pH – glass electrode PO_2 – Clark electrode PCO_2 – Severinghaus electrode	Measured Values • PO_2 • SO_2 • PCO_2 • pH Calculated values • HCO_3^- • TCO_2 • Base excess or base deficit	• Requires a blood sample. • Analyzers are usually in the clinical laboratory • When ABG and pulse oximetry values are dissimilar, the presence of a dyshemoglobin that does not bind oxygen should be considered
Co-oximeter	Blood	• In the clinical laboratory the co-oximeter measures the oxygen saturation of hemoglobin and dyshemoglobins using up to 100 different wavelengths. • Portable co-oximeters that use up to 8 wavelengths are now available.	There are co-oximetry wavelengths to measure dyshemoglobins: • O_2Hb • $COHb$ • $MetHb$ • SHb • $SulfHb$	• Co-oximetry may be requested for arterial (SaO_2) or venous (SvO_2 and $ScvO_2$) blood gas measurements. • Blood sample must be drawn slowly from the catheter to not introduce air bubbles into the syringe. • Labeled syringe must be immediately transported to the clinical laboratory, if a portable co-oximeter is not available. • Sometimes transported on ice; because, when the blood sample remains at room temperature for more than 10 minutes the PO_2 will be falsely low as white blood cells and platelets continue to consume oxygen during this time.

Continued

TABLE 6-2 Comparison of Devices Used to Measure Oxygen—cont'd

DEVICE	SAMPLE	ANALYSIS	REPORTED RESULTS	CLINICAL ISSUES
Point of Care Test	Blood	Point of care cartridge sensors measure: pH –potentiometry* PO_2 –amperometry** PCO_2 –potentiometry*	Measured Values • PO_2 • SO_2 • PCO_2 • pH Calculated values • HCO_3^- • TCO_2 • Base excess or base deficit	• Blood sample volume is small • Convenient for rapid interpretation of arterial blood gases at the bedside • Anemia and hemodilution may make results less accurate
Pulse oximeter	Transcutaneous	Measures oxygen saturation of hemoglobin by pulsed light with absorption at 2 different wavelengths: Red spectrum 660 nm Near infrared 940 nm	SpO_2	• Noninvasive, continuous used for clinical bedside monitoring. Verify perfusion by a pulsatile plethsmography waveform. • SpO_2 may not be accurate with poor peripheral perfusion. • SpO_2 is unreliable in hypoxemia when values are below 80%. • SpO_2 is inaccurate in carbon monoxide poisoning. • SpO_2 is inaccurate with MetHb in amounts greater than 30%.

COHb, Carboxyhemoglobin; *HCO_3^-*, bicarbonate; *HHb*, deoxygenated hemoglobin; *MetHb*, methemoglobin; *O_2Hb*, oxyhemoglobin; *PCO_2*, partial pressure of carbon dioxide in blood; *PO_2*, partial pressure of oxygen in blood; *SaO_2*, oxygen saturation in arterial blood; *$ScvO_2$*, mixed venous oxygen saturation; *SHb*, sickle cell hemoglobin; *SO_2*, oxygen saturation in blood; *SpO_2*, oxygen saturation from a pulse oximeter; *SulfHb*, sulfhemoglobin; *TCO_2*, total carbon dioxide.

*Potentiometry uses two electrodes; one is the reference electrode with a known electrode potential. The other electrode is the test electrode. The Nernst Equation is used to calculate the result.

**Amperometry is the measurement of current flow produced by an oxidation-reduction reaction.

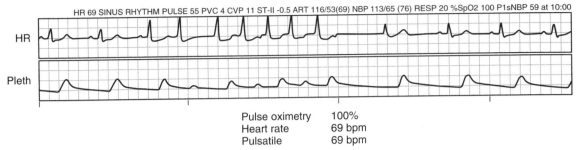

HR 69 SINUS RHYTHM PULSE 55 PVC 4 CVP 11 ST-II -0.5 ART 116/53(69) NBP 113/65 (76) RESP 20 %SpO2 100 P1sNBP 59 at 10:00

Pulse oximetry	100%
Heart rate	69 bpm
Pulsatile	69 bpm

FIGURE 6-8 Pulse plethysmography waveform variability with an irregular heart rate.

reservoir for available oxygen to be used at the cellular level. The oximetry sensor does not measure or predict cellular use of oxygen.

The pulse oximeter waveform, known as *plethysmography*, may also be used to monitor perfusion and variability of perfusion, as seen with an irregular heart rate that results in variable stroke volumes as shown in Figure 6-8. Pulse oximetry may inaccurately reflect saturation of hemoglobin in low-perfusion states. This often occurs when patients are critically ill, and lung gas exchange is negatively affected by alveolar dysfunction, pulmonary blood flow, poor perfusion, cardiac dynamics, and amount of hemoglobin. It is not uncommon to accept a lower SpO_2 (88%)[10] in the absence of tissue hypoxia indicators, such as lactic acid, unexpected hyperkalemia, wide anion gap, decreasing bicarbonate, base deficit, and decreasing serum carbon dioxide, on a venous blood sample.

SpO_2 and SaO_2 are often used to successfully guide oxygen therapy administration. However, there are clinical circumstances where the SpO_2 may not be accurate, as listed in Box 6-3.

SpO_2 monitoring does not provide information about level of carbon dioxide in the bloodstream. In the setting of hypoventilation where supplemental oxygen is administered, the high flow of oxygen into the alveoli and bloodstream produces a normal SpO_2, which may provide a false sense of security in the setting of hypoventilation and rising $PaCO_2$, as described in Box 6-4.

Pulse oximetry does not provide any information about ventilation. That information is obtained by clinical assessment of respiratory rate, chest movement, level of consciousness, ABG analysis and capnography monitoring of end-tidal carbon dioxide ($ETCO_2$). Capnography monitoring is discussed in detail in Chapter 8.

BOX 6-3 SpO_2 Caveats

SpO_2 is unreliable in low perfusion states.
SpO_2 is unreliable when saturation drops below 80%.
SpO_2 is falsely elevated in high carboxyhemoglobin environments.

SpO_2 is falsely elevated in a high-methemoglobin environment.
Sickle cells may create a false high or low SpO_2.

BOX 6-4   Pulse Oximetry and Hypercapnia Case Example

In the post-anesthesia recovery unit (PACU) a 54-year-old male with a history of chronic obstructive pulmonary disease (COPD) is recovering from anesthesia and extubation. Two hours after an orthopedic procedure, he remains minimally responsive to verbal and physical stimuli.

Vital signs are within normal limits: heart rate 98; blood pressure 107/68 mm Hg; respiratory rate 8 breaths per minute (shallow); and SpO_2 98% on high-flow oxygen. As part of the assessment to determine the reasons for his lack of responsiveness, an arterial blood gas is obtained by arterial puncture: pH 7.28;

PaO_2 439 mm Hg; $PaCO_2$ 124 mm Hg; SaO_2 100%.

Extreme hypercapnia was the cause of his failure to regain full consciousness after anesthesia. At this point, he was reintubated, ventilated, and transferred to the critical care unit.

Patients on high-flow oxygen with an inadequate respiratory drive may have a pulse oximeter reading close to 100%. Without effective ventilation (movement of air in and out of the lungs), carbon dioxide levels can rise to extremely high levels in blood (hypercapnia).

Arterial Blood Gas

The most common reasons for obtaining an ABG are summarized in Box 6-5. Other less obvious reasons include assessment of metabolic derangements and the need to provide evidence that tissues are functioning aerobically (using oxygen) or anaerobically (without oxygen, thus producing lactic acid). One of the most important considerations when drawing an ABG is to minimize the time delay that may occur between obtaining the sample, analysis, and notification. The increased use of bedside point-of-care measurement has significantly improved data retrieval.[13]

BOX 6-5   Most Common Reasons for Obtaining Arterial Blood Gases[12]

Changes in ventilator settings (27.6%)
Respiratory events (26.4%)
   Respiratory compromise
   Hypoxemia by pulse oximeter
   Diminished ventilation
Peri- or post-cardiopulmonary arrest or
   collapse
Routine (25.7%)

Metabolic reasons
   Sepsis
   Diabetic ketoacidosis
   Kidney failure
   Heart failure
   Liver failure
   Toxic substance ingestion
   Drug overdose
   Trauma
   Burns

Bound Oxygen in Arterial Blood

Hemoglobin is the second most important component contributing to oxygen delivery. In an acute short-term crisis, the saturation–desaturation ratios are rapidly responsive to changes in ventilation, cardiac output, hemoglobin oxygen affinity, and the cellular environment. The oxygen saturation of hemoglobin is defined as the amount of oxygen combined with hemoglobin in proportion to the amount of oxygen the hemoglobin is capable of carrying. It is expressed as a percentage of a ratio of content to capacity. When measured by co-oximetry in arterial blood, this is referred to as saturation of the arterial blood (SaO_2), and in the venous blood as saturation of the venous blood (SvO_2).

SaO_2 should be directly reflective of the oxygen administered written as the fraction of inspired oxygen (FiO_2) and the gas in the alveoli (PAO_2) as shown:

$$FiO_2 \Rightarrow PAO_2 \Rightarrow SaO_2.$$

Dissolved Oxygen in Arterial Blood

PaO_2 is a measure of the dissolved gas in the bloodstream that creates a pressure and is immediately usable. The PaO_2 is normally about 70 to 100 millimeters of mercury (mm Hg) and is an important measure for the assessment of the V/Q ratio. In healthy lungs, the higher the alveolar oxygen (PAO_2) relating to oxygen administration and alveolar recruitment, the higher the arterial oxygen (PaO_2) should become. In a normal healthy lung, PaO_2 should equal about five times the oxygen administered or FiO_2; that is, if the FiO_2 is 1.0 (100%) the PaO_2 should be close to 500 mm Hg. This may be described as:

$$FiO_2 \Rightarrow PAO_2 \Rightarrow SaO_2 \Rightarrow PaO_2$$

When breathing at sea level, the normal oxygen concentration of room air is 0.21, or 21%. The normal PaO_2 is between 70 and 100 mm Hg, and an SaO_2 of greater than 94% is considered acceptable. Age and disease process may affect what would be considered normal.

The adequacy of the V/Q ratio depends on the oxygen concentration gradient on either side of the pulmonary surface area, alveolar recruitment, the permeability and width of the alveolar–capillary membrane, and the contact time of hemoglobin with this gas exchange membrane based on heart rate and cardiac output (refer to Figures 6-1 through 6-3). Pathologies affecting the functional diffusion layer or the gas exchange surface area, such as pulmonary edema or pulmonary fibrosis, will lower the PaO_2, particularly when measured in proportional ratio to the FiO_2. Disturbances of the V/Q ratio in asthma, pulmonary embolism, ARDS, and circulatory failure also lower the PaO_2.

PaO_2 directly affects the amount of oxygen available to the mitochondria within the cell, as cells voraciously consume oxygen. In other words, PaO_2 may be considered as an indirect measure of the oxygen available for tissue metabolism.

$$FiO_2 \Rightarrow PAO_2 \Rightarrow SaO_2 \Rightarrow PaO_2 \Rightarrow Cellular\ O_2\ (Cellular\ Demand)$$

When the level of oxygen dissolved in plasma is inadequate for tissue consumption, ideally the cardiac output will increase by increasing heart rate and/or stroke volume. Additionally the oxyhemoglobin curve may shift to the right representing a release of oxygen more rapidly. This is often evaluated with continuous or intermittent SvO_2 monitoring. If these adaptations are unsuccessful, ultimately cells may shift to anaerobic metabolism (without oxygen), consuming more adenosine triphosphate (ATP) than can be produced and yielding higher levels of lactate, while donating H^+ into the plasma.

$$FiO_2 \Rightarrow PAO_2 \Rightarrow SaO_2 \Rightarrow PaO_2 \Rightarrow Cellular\, O_2\, (Cellular\, Demand) \Rightarrow PvO_2 \Rightarrow SvO_2$$

Methods for Evaluating the Relationship of Ventilation to Perfusion

To evaluate the relationship of ventilation to perfusion more thoroughly, PaO_2 must always be correlated with the ventilation therapy applied to the patient. The PaO_2 level that prompts many clinicians to make a diagnosis of hypoxemia and failure of lung gas exchange is generally in the range of 60 to 75 mm Hg. Hypoxemia increases the likelihood of tissue deficits,[14] Table 6-3 lists the terms of hypoxemia classification.

Acute Respiratory Distress Syndrome

The ARDSnet trial was a landmark study that demonstrated that mechanical ventilation with smaller tidal volumes and standardized levels of positive end expiratory pressure (PEEP) reduced mortality in patients with acute respiratory distress syndrome

---

TABLE 6-3 Categorization of Hypoxemia Based on Physiologic Responses and Duration of Onset

HYPOXEMIA TERM	DESCRIPTION AND ONSET
Acute hypoxemia	A rapid decline in arterial oxygenation developing over <6 hours (e.g., acute upper airway obstruction)
Subacute hypoxemia	Reduced arterial oxygenation occurring in 6 hours to 7 days (e.g., pneumonia)
Sustained hypoxemia	Reduced arterial oxygenation for 7 to 90 days (e.g., prolonged acute respiratory distress syndrome, high-altitude climbing expeditions)
Chronic hypoxemia	Prolonged reduction of arterial oxygenation for over 90 days (e.g., chronic obstructive pulmonary disease)
Generational hypoxemia	Cross-generational reduced arterial oxygenation (e.g., Tibetan highland residents)

Note: In the absence of any universally accepted terminology describing the time-related differences in responses to hypoxemia, the proposed criteria are based on human physiologic adaptations to hypoxemia.

TABLE 6-4 Comparison of ARDSnet and Berlin Criteria for Acute Respiratory Distress Syndrome (ARDS)

CRITERIA	ARDSnet[15]	BERLIN[16]
Onset	Acute	Acute within 1 week of clinical insult
PEEP	Not included in definition	Incorporated into categories
Chest radiograph CT (Berlin only)	Diffuse or homogenous Patchy infiltrates	Bilateral opacities not explained by effusions, lung collapse or nodules
CLASSIFICATION WITH P/F RATIO		
P/F < 300 on 0.4 FiO$_2$	ALI (Acute Lung Injury)	Mild ARDS: PEEP or CPAP $\geq$ 5 cm H$_2$O
P/F $\leq$ 200 on 0.4 FiO$_2$	ARDS regardless of PEEP	Moderate ARDS: PEEP or CPAP $\geq$ 5 cm H$_2$O
P/F < 100	– – – – – – – – – – – –	Severe ARDS: PEEP or CPAP $\geq$ 5 cm H$_2$O
Left heart dysfunction	PAOP < 18 mm Hg	Respiratory failure not explained by heart failure, overload or history. Echocardiography for objective assessment

cm H$_2$O, Centimeters of water; *CPAP*, continuous positive airway pressure; *CT*, computed tomography; *FiO$_2$*, fraction of inspired oxygen; *mm Hg*, millimeters of mercury; *P/F*, PaO$_2$/FiO$_2$ ratio; *PAOP*, pulmonary artery occlusion pressure; *PEEP*, positive end expiratory pressure.

(ARDS) (see Table 6-4).[15] The American-European Consensus Conference on ARDS (2012) defined ARDS predominantly by degree of hypoxemia using the PaO$_2$/FiO$_2$ ratio (P/F ratio) as the major oxygenation criterion (The Berlin Definition).[16]

The previous ARDS definition (1992) did not take into consideration the level of PEEP required to maintain acceptable levels of oxygenation.[17] The issue of hypoxemia is typically addressed first by increasing the FiO$_2$. Clinicians evaluate the proportional gas exchange and response to therapy in a number of ways, typically beginning with the P/F ratio. The P/F ratio is based on the gold standard alveolar (A) to arterial (a) difference or gradient (A-a gradient). Therapeutic considerations for managing PaO$_2$ are listed in Box 6-6.

PaO$_2$/FiO$_2$ Ratio

The most frequently used pulmonary oxygenation assessment method is the P/F ratio. Normal ratio values are greater than 250 on 0.4 (40%) FiO$_2$. A P/F ratio less than 300 indicates severe respiratory failure usually ARDS. See Box 6-7 for a case example demonstrating P/F ratio assessment.

Alveolar–Arterial Gradient

The gold standard to evaluate the relationship of ventilation to perfusion is the comparison of FiO$_2$ delivered into the alveoli (PAO$_2$) and the responding measure of gas

---

BOX 6-6 PaO$_2$ Therapeutic Considerations[13]

The safest limit of PaO$_2$ in critically ill patients is unknown. However, the following concerns must be discussed at the bedside:

- High fractional inspired concentrations of oxygen (FiO$_2$) cause pulmonary damage, possibly more so in patients with injured lungs, but this damage is difficult to identify clinically, and information on safety thresholds for oxygen administration is unclear.
- Precise control of arterial oxygenation in critically ill patients may improve outcomes by reducing the harm associated with unnecessary extremes of oxygen administration.
- For selected critically ill patients, permissive hypoxemia (the tolerance of lower arterial oxygenation levels) may better balance the harms and benefits of oxygen therapy.
- Clinical evidence supporting permissive hypoxemia is not currently available, and robust studies are required to evaluate safety and efficacy before implementation can be advocated.

BOX 6-7 P/F Ratio: Case Example

Ms. A. is a 65-year-old female, who presents to the emergency department with rapid shallow breathing, hypotension, and acute prodrome. She suffers a respiratory arrest before an arterial blood gas (ABG) or any laboratory studies are performed. Following resuscitation and intubation, she is placed on assist control with a tidal volume of 375 mL (7 mL/kg), ventilator frequency of 20. ABG oxygenation values are as follows:

- FiO$_2$ 1.0 (100%) and PEEP 5 cm H$_2$O
- PaO$_2$ 90
- P/F ratio: 90/1.0 = 90

This patient has severe respiratory failure.

Case example continues in Box 6-11.

dissolved in the arterial blood (PaO$_2$). Since oxygen enters the pulmonary capillary blood by passive diffusion (see Figure 6-1), it follows that in a steady state the alveolar pressure (PAO$_2$) must always be higher than the arterial pressure of oxygen (PaO$_2$). The difference between alveolar oxygen (calculated PAO$_2$) and arterial oxygen (measured PaO$_2$) on room air (0.21) is usually less than 20 mm Hg. When FiO$_2$ is 1.00 (100%) the difference should be less than 95 mm Hg.[18]

This evaluation, known as the alveolar–arterial difference in oxygen (A-a DO_2 or A-a gradient) requires some calculations to assure that the ventilation support and oxygen support provided to the patient is appropriate especially when making changes in ventilatory and oxygen therapies. The A-a difference is helpful primarily when a patient retains carbon dioxide, as in chronic obstructive pulmonary disease (COPD) or severe asthma. See Box 6-8 for a calculation using this formula and Box 6-9 for a clinical example.

Arterial/Alveolar Ratio

Another method of oxygen assessment is the arterial/alveolar ratio (a/A ratio or the PaO_2 measured/PAO_2 calculated). The ratio is a more appropriate method for evaluation of patients who are receiving increased FiO_2 as the division corrects for FiO_2. Whenever the ratio is less than 85%, concern should be focused on alveolar recruitment. Refer to Box 6-10 for a case example demonstrating calculation of the a-A ratio assessment method.[13]

In critical care, alveolar opening (recruitment) strategies to optimize mean airway pressures are frequently employed in patients with hypoxemia. Causes of hypoxemia

---

BOX 6-8 Calculation of the Alveolar–Arterial (A-a) Gradient

The alveolar gas equation makes it simple to calculate PAO_2. This simplified formula incorporates the following steps:

Step 1: Alveolar partial pressure calculation
  a. Barometric pressure (PB) fixed at 760 mm Hg at sea level
  b. % of that pressure that is oxygenated (FiO_2)
  c. Subtract partial pressure that is lost as a result of humidification (Pw): Fixed at 47 mm Hg
  d. Example: FiO_2 (PB − Pw)
Step 2: Reduce for the presence of carbon dioxide in the alveoli
  a. Measured $PaCO_2$, which is relatively the same in both blood and alveoli (except with perfusion deficits).

  b. Multiply by 1.2: standard respiratory quotient or divide by 0.8, standard respiratory quotient
  c. Example: $1.2 \times PaCO_2$
Step 3: Step one minus step two: yields the calculated alveolar partial pressure of oxygen
  a. Example:
   $PAO_2 = [FiO_2 − (PB − Pw)] − [1.2 \times PaCO_2]$
Step 4: Subtract the PaO_2 (measured from the arterial blood gas) from the calculated PAO_2
  a. Normal A-a difference (also known as: A-a gradient $= <20$ mm Hg)
  b. A-a difference: evaluated primarily when patients are carbon dioxide retainers.

BOX 6-9   **Alveolar–Arterial (A-a) Gradient: Case Example**

Ms. H. is a 27-year-old woman, who comes to the emergency room complaining of pleuritic chest pain of at least 4-hour duration. Chest radiography and physical examination were normal, although she was splinting during deep inspirations. Her PaO_2 was 81 mm Hg, and $PaCO_2$ was 31 mm Hg (room air FiO_2 0.21). Local barometric pressure is 747 mm Hg.

Example:

Step 1: $0.21(760 - 47) = 157$ (rounded up)
Step 2: $1.2 \times 31 = 32$

Step 3: $157 - 32 = 125$ (this is the estimated alveolar partial pressure of oxygen)
Step 4: PAO_2 (calculated) 125 mm Hg $- PaO_2$ (measured) 81 mm Hg $= 44$
A-a difference $= 44$.

Interpretation: The normal A-a gradient in a healthy person on room air is less than 20. This patient's A-a gradient is higher because oxygen is not distributing into the bloodstream. This patient is hypoxemic, likely a problem caused by shunting or poor alveolar recruitment.

Case example continues in Box 6-10.

BOX 6-10   **Arterial–Alveolar (a-A) Oxygen Ratio: Case Example***

Ms. H. has a calculated PAO_2 of 125 mm Hg and a measured PaO_2 of 81 mm Hg.
   $81/125 = 0.648$, or 65%.
   PaO_2 measured / PAO_2 calculated (refer to Box 6-8 for PAO_2 calculation)
   Interpretation: A normal arterial–alveolar oxygen ratio is greater than 0.85

(85%). This test evaluates the ability of oxygen to diffuse from the alveoli to the pulmonary capillaries. The a-A ratio is most helpful to assess a patient on higher levels of FiO_2 with PEEP of less than 10 cm H_2O. This patient's a-A ratio is low, consistent with hypoxemia.

*Case example continues from Box 6-9.

---

are listed in Table 6-5. Mean airway pressure, which can be measured or read from the ventilator, is affected by tidal volume, loss of compliance, alveolar collapse, increased resistance, or by a combination of these. The result may elevate peak and/or plateau pressure. Optimally, a transition to pressure control ventilation occurs, which eliminates tidal volume as a contributing factor. If the patient is profoundly hypoxemic when placed on pressure control or if the patient does not tolerate a lower FiO_2, other strategies must be employed to open the alveoli and improve lung compliance.

TABLE 6-5	Causes of Hypoxemia and Effect on the Alveolar–Arterial (A-a) Oxygen Difference			
CAUSE OF HYPOXEMIA	**EFFECT ON P/F RATIO**	**EFFECT ON P(A-a) OXYGEN GRADIENT**	**COMMENT**
Reduced FiO_2	Normal >225	Unchanged or reduced	Resolved by increasing FiO_2
Hypoventilation	Normal >225	Unchanged	Causes included pharmacologic, neurologic, and muscular weakness. Alleviated by increasing FiO_2
Ventilation–perfusion mismatch	Low <225	Increased	Most frequent cause of hypoxemia in the critically ill
Right-to-left shunt	<225	Increased	Anatomic or physiologic. Cannot be alleviated by increasing FiO_2
Diffusion limitation	<225	Increased	Rare cause of hypoxemia that can be alleviated by increasing FiO_2

FiO_2, Fraction of inspired oxygen.

The strategy for opening collapsed alveoli is to provide an opening (recruitment) pressure to the alveoli. These strategies include PEEP greater than 10 centimeters of water (cm H_2O), high-frequency oscillation ventilation (HFOV), high-frequency percussive ventilation (HFPV) and airway pressure release ventilation (APRV). The recently published Berlin definitions for ARDS[16] places considerable value on mean airway pressure ventilator strategies[19] and incorporated these measures into the evaluation of gas exchange (see Table 6-4).

Because the previously described tools to evaluate efficacy of therapy do not take mean airway pressure into account, they may offer a false sense of security and lead to inappropriate early weaning attempts. In this case, one may consider the use of the oxygenation index to evaluate the acuity of ARDS or the degree of alveolar derecruitment.

Oxygenation Index

The oxygenation index (OI) incorporates the severity of oxygenation impairment (PaO_2/FiO_2 ratio) and mean airway pressure (MawP) into a single measure.

$$OI = (FiO_2 \times MawP) \div PaO_2$$

The normal oxygenation index value is less than 6, and those patients with ratios greater than 25 typically have severe acute respiratory failure or ARDS. A case example demonstrates use of the oxygenation index in Box 6-11.[20]

BOX 6-11   Oxygenation Index: Case Example*

Ms. A. has noncompliant lungs and is placed on pressure control with a PEEP of 15 cm H_2O, and an FiO_2 0.80 (80%).

Her ABG reflects an improvement in oxygenation.

PaO_2 is now 110. The goal is to decrease her FiO_2.

The P/F ratio is $110/0.8 = 137$, indicating that she remains profoundly hypoxemic.

Calculation of the Oxygenation Index

Her mean peak airway pressure (read from the ventilator) is 21 cm H_2O.

Oxygenation index $= (FiO_2 \times$ mean airway pressure)$/PaO_2$ or $(0.8 \times 21)/110 = 15$

Interpretation: The oxygenation index of 15 is relatively poor ($2 \times$ normal). A normal oxygenation index value is less than 6.

---

*Case example continues from Box 6-7.

Summary of Oxygenation Measures

Oxygenation measures from the ABG and the pulse oximeter are used to evaluate the amount of oxygen that is bound to hemoglobin (SaO_2, SpO_2) and is dissolved in arterial blood, exerting pressure for cellular use (PaO_2). See Box 6-12 for the full list of oxygenation measures.

Without adequate dissolved oxygen in plasma, patients rapidly progress to metabolic dysfunction, producing lethal amounts of lactic acid as a byproduct of anaerobic metabolism. The notion that oxygenation is only an indicator of appropriate alveolar–blood interchange and a stable V/Q match is problematic. To protect patients and improve outcomes, the clinician must evaluate the oxygenation component of the ABG as a reflection of the amount and the appropriateness of support needed to generate optimal gas exchange (see Table 6-5).

BOX 6-12   Oxygenation Measures

- PAO_2—Partial pressure of oxygen in the alveoli
- PaO_2—Partial pressure of oxygen in arterial blood (hypoxemia)
- SpO_2—Saturation of arterial blood (pulse oximeter) as a percentage
- SaO_2—Percentage of arterial hemoglobin saturated with oxygen
- PvO_2—Partial pressure of oxygen in venous blood

- $ScvO_2$—Percentage of hemoglobin saturated with oxygen in the central venous circulation in the superior vena cava; measured from a fiberoptic-tipped central venous catheter
- SvO_2—Percentage of hemoglobin saturated with oxygen in the pulmonary arterial circulation; measured from a fiberoptic-tipped pulmonary artery catheter

---

Clinical Reasoning Pearl

Clinical situations that require oxygenation analyses:

1. P/F or the a-A ratio is used for alveolar–arterial gas assessment when evaluating an increase in FiO_2 and PEEP of less than 10 cm H_2O.

2. A-a difference is the best tool when patients are retaining carbon dioxide at levels higher than 50 mm Hg.

3. The oxygenation index is used when PEEP is greater than 10 cm H_2O, inspiratory time is prolonged, or strategies for alveolar recruitment such as APRV (airway pressure release ventilation) or HFOV (high-frequency oscillation ventilation) are employed.

Ventilation Measures and Assessment of Partial Pressure of Arterial Carbon Dioxide and End-Tidal Carbon Dioxide

Carbon dioxide is the end-product of complete oxidation of carbohydrates and fatty acids. The arterial partial pressure of carbon dioxide is termed the $PaCO_2$. Of necessity, considering the amounts involved in continuous oxidation, there needs to be a very efficient and functional physiologic system to rapidly excrete carbon dioxide. Even though carbon dioxide is produced as an end product of metabolism, it is excreted as gas via the lungs and is therefore known as the *respiratory acid*.

The $PaCO_2$ is regulated by the minute ventilation (V_E). The lungs are the sole regulator of carbon dioxide (the respiratory acid), and a huge amount of carbon dioxide needs to be excreted every 24 hours—at least 12,000 to 13,000 millimoles per day (mmol/day).[6] Even minor changes in ventilation affect the arterial $PaCO_2$ level and the intracellular pH, which profoundly affects ion transport and stability.

$PaCO_2$ measures the partial pressure of dissolved carbon dioxide in arterial blood. Carbon dioxide is released during aerobic and anaerobic tissue metabolism and is the main contributor of acid in the bloodstream. Because carbon dioxide diffuses rapidly across all membranes, including the alveolar capillary surface, as long as ventilation is adequate, carbon dioxide is always moving from pulmonary arterioles to alveoli. The PCO_2 in the capillaries is higher than that in the alveoli; thus, carbon dioxide diffuses into alveoli and is then a major component of exhaled gas. Capnography is the measurement and graphical display of carbon dioxide concentration within the expired gas, as described in Chapter 8. In healthy lungs, the normal $PaCO_2$ is about 40 mm Hg (range 35–45 mm Hg). The exhaled $ETCO_2$ is usually only slightly lower than the corresponding arterial $PaCO_2$. In contrast, with hypoperfusion the difference (gradient) between arterial and exhaled carbon dioxide can be large.

> **BOX 6-13   PaCO$_2$ Proportional to [VCO$_2$/V$_A$]**
>
> Where:
> - PaCO$_2$ = Arterial partial pressure of carbon dioxide
> - VCO$_2$ = Carbon dioxide production by the body
> - V$_A$ = Alveolar ventilation

Regulation of arterial carbon dioxide is very precise.

$$FiO_2 \Rightarrow PAO_2 \Rightarrow SaO_2 \Rightarrow PaO_2 \Rightarrow Cellular\,O_2\,(Cellular\,Demand)$$
$$\Rightarrow PaCO_2 \Rightarrow PACO_2 \Rightarrow ETCO_2$$

The way to truly measure the ventilation capacity (ability to regulate carbon dioxide) is via the minute ventilation or measurement of exhaled ventilation gases (V_E). The minute ventilation measures the amount of volume exhaled per minute (V_E), calculated as respiratory rate (RR) $\times V_T$ (Box 6-13). Normal V_E is about 8 to 10 L/min. Another way to measure effective V_E is to evaluate alveolar ventilation V_A. Some of the current generations of "smart" ventilators estimate the alveolar ventilation (V_A). For most clinical decision-making purposes, V_A and V_E are considered the same measure, although that is true in healthy lungs only. In the unhealthy lung, a large number of alveoli do not participate in gas exchange, and V_E will not equal V_A. When alveoli are not recruited, gas exchange is affected. PaO$_2$ will go down first, and PaCO$_2$ will eventually go up as the functional alveolar surface is decreased.

PaCO$_2$ is directly measured (not calculated) and is a reliable indicator of respiratory regulation of acid. The correlation between acute changes in PaCO$_2$ and pH is direct, consistent, and linear. This changed PaCO$_2$ will affect intracellular pH, and this effect is rapid.

> **Clinical Reasoning Pearl**
>
> A fall in pH signals a significant change in intracellular metabolism.
>   A 0.1 unit fall in pH from 7.40 to 7.30 represents a 25% increase in H$^+$ ions. To put this into perspective, a similar percentage change in serum sodium would increase the sodium value from a normal 140 mEq/L to 175 mEq/L.

Carbon dioxide (CO$_2$) is not technically an acid because it does not contain a hydrogen (H$^+$), so it cannot be a proton donor. However, in order to be transported in the bloodstream, carbon dioxide chemically combines with water to form H$_2$CO$_3$ (carbonic acid) directly affecting pH.

The Acid–Base Balance

In the clinical environment, the primary variable that requires significant attention is the unmeasured proton H$^+$ and its acid effects, including loss of vascular tone and ionic cellular exchange with potassium (K$^+$). When the bloodstream is in an acidic range, the

TABLE 6-6 Correlation of Acute Changes in pH and $PaCO_2$	
$PaCO_2$	**pH**
40	7.4
50	7.3
60	7.2

extracellular potassium level rises as cells exchange K^+ with H^+, moving potassium out of the cell, as H^+ enters the cell. This occurs with acute changes in pH and $PaCO_2$, as listed in Table 6-6.

In 1987, 7% of surveyed physicians at a large University Hospital stated that they had a clear understanding of ABG evaluation and acid–base balance, but when those same physicians were tested, only 40% diagnosed the clinical scenarios correctly.[21] In the critical care unit, where 9 of 10 patients have acid–base imbalance, hypoxemia, or both, these misinterpretations may lead to serious deficiencies in therapeutic management.[22]

The Physiology of pH

Arterial pH is an indirect measurement of carbon dioxide and H^+ acid concentration in blood, which reflects the overall acid production, regulation and buffering capabilities of the cells, lungs, and kidneys, as defined in Box 6-14.

$$CO_2 + H_2O \leftrightarrow H_2CO_3 \leftrightarrow H^+ + HCO_3^-$$

The acid–base balance depends primarily on the concentration of carbonic acid (H_2CO_3) in the bloodstream, which is a product of the respiratory acid carbon dioxide bound to water, as well as H^+ plus any bicarbonate buffer. It is essential to understand that unless the patient has ingested acid, all acid in the bloodstream has been produced at the cellular level (see Box 6-13).

The normalization of the pH of the blood is dependent only on the ratio of the amount of carbon dioxide to the amount of HCO_3^- (bicarbonate ion) present in blood. This ratio remains relatively constant because the concentrations of both buffering components (HCO_3^- and carbon dioxide) are very large compared with the amount of H^+ produced by metabolism. Blood pH, partial pressure of oxygen (pO_2), partial pressure of carbon dioxide (pCO_2), and HCO_3^- are carefully regulated. The cells,

---

BOX 6-14   Evaluation of Acid–Base Balance

An *acid* is a chemical compound that can give up a free hydrogen ion (H^+) in aqueous solution.

A *base* is a compound that can accept a free H^+.

BOX 6-15   Regulating Acid–Base Balance

Cells: Regulate pH

Acidosis: acid (H^+) uptake in exchange for potassium release provides buffer effect and promotes intracellular hypokalemia

Alkalosis: acid (H^+) release in exchange for potassium uptake provides buffer effect and promotes intracellular hyperkalemia

Kidney: Acid–Base Regulator

Major volume and electrolyte regulator
Acid regulator
Base regulator

Lung: Acid Regulator

Rate and depth of breaths depends on the carbonic acid and therefore the pH

kidneys, and lungs work together to maintain a blood pH of 7.4 primarily via acid excretion through ventilation and kidney excretion of acidotic waste (Box 6-15).

The normal arterial blood pH is 7.4 (range 7.35 to 7.45). A pH less than 7.35 indicates acidosis, and a pH greater than 7.45 indicates alkalosis. Because pH is an inverse reflection of H^+ concentration, an increase in H^+ concentration decreases pH, and vice versa (see Table 6-7). H^+ is formed as an end product of cellular metabolism. Any alteration of this balance causes derangements in pH. Acidosis is diagnosed when extra acids are present or base is lost, with a pH below 7.40.

Carbon dioxide enters the red blood cell as a waste product as shown in Figure 6-9. In the red blood cell, it reacts with water to form carbonic acid (H_2CO_3) as shown in Figure 6-10. In the kidney, the H_2CO_3 dissociates into HCO_3^- and H^+ (see Figure 6-11).

TABLE 6-7   pH and Hydrogen Ion Concentration

BLOOD pH	[H^+] (nmol/L)	% CHANGE FROM NORMAL
Acidemia		
7.00	100	+150
7.10	80	+100
7.30	50	+25
Normal		
7.40	40	
Alkalemia		
7.52	30	−25
7.70	20	−50
8.00	10	−75

nmol/L, Nanomoles per liter.

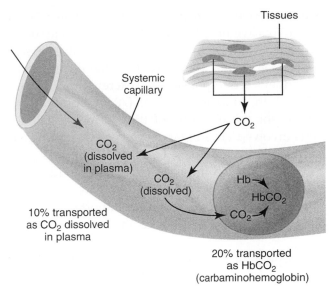

FIGURE 6-9 Carbon dioxide enters the red blood cell as a waste product from the tissues. (From Patton KT, Thibodeau GA, Douglas M: *Essentials of anatomy and physiology*, St. Louis, 2012, Mosby.)

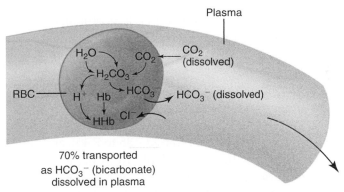

FIGURE 6-10 Transport of CO_2 in the blood. *Cl*, Chloride; *CO_2*, carbon dioxide; *H^+*, hydrogen ion; *Hb*, hemoglobin; *HCO_3^-*, bicarbonate; *HHb*, deoxygenated hemoglobin; *H_2O*, water; *RBC*, red blood cell (From Patton KT, Thibodeau GA, Douglas M: *Essentials of anatomy and physiology*, St. Louis, 2012, Mosby.)

These products diffuse into plasma, where H^+ is buffered by hemoglobin. Approximately 10% of the total body carbon dioxide dissolves in the plasma, 20% of the total body carbon dioxide is carried as carboxyhemoglobin (COHb) on proteins, and the remaining 70% is carried as HCO_3^- in plasma (see Figure 6-10). Whenever carbon dioxide is dissolved in arterial blood, $PaCO_2$ rises. H^+ also rises, and the pH goes down because the pH is inversely related to the H^+ concentration in the blood.

Whenever $PaCO_2$ rises and the pH is acidotic, consideration must be focused on the most important reason: decreased alveolar ventilation. Improving alveolar ventilation may require the control of ventilator tidal volume and frequency to increase the minute ventilation (V_E), as well as time and ability to exhale, as exhalation is when carbon dioxide is removed from the bloodstream. This will require mechanical ventilation, either noninvasive or invasive. In addition, it may become vital to decrease the work of breathing and metabolic rate, utilizing analgesia, sedation, and, possibly, pharmacologic neuromuscular paralysis, although this is a controversial decision.

The kidneys are responsible for excretion of the fixed acids. This is a critical role, even though the amounts involved (70–100 mmol/day) are relatively small. No other way exists for the excretion of these acids, and it should be appreciated that the amounts involved are still large compared with the total plasma H^+ of only 40 nanomoles per liter (nmol/L) (see Figure 6-11).

The other extremely important role that the kidneys play in acid–base balance is the reabsorption of filtered bicarbonate. Bicarbonate is the predominant extracellular buffer against the fixed acids, and it important that its plasma concentration always be defended. In acid–base balance, the kidney is responsible for two major activities:

1. Reabsorption of filtered bicarbonate: 4000 to 5000 mmol/day
2. Excretion of the fixed acids (acid anion and associated H^+) is about 1 mmol/kg/day.

In order for cells to efficiently transport ions and metabolites, the cellular milieu must have an optimal acid-base balance. The intracellular environment is complex and has a considerable capability to provide buffer via electrolytes and proteins, and therefore maintain a fairly stable pH. Unfortunately, that environment can only be measured by the blood pH, and the blood pH must be chemically close to normal (pH 7.40) for the system to function appropriately.

State of the pH

Theoretically, values of pH could range from (−) infinity to (+) infinity, but human arterial pH is normally about 7.40 (range 7.35 to 7.45), and the limits of survival cover a 10-fold range of H^+ within a blood pH from 6.8 to 7.8. The pH is regarded as a "dimensionless" representation of the H^+ and is not measured as a concentration; nor does it have any units. The pH reference is a mere reflection of the presence or absence of H^+. Considering the importance of the H^+, it may be problematic that it is not measured but assumed by the indicators of $PaCO_2$ and bicarbonate—base or serum carbon dioxide measured in the chemistry profile (see Table 6-8).

Clinicians must instinctively understand and assign the H^+ when evaluating the three primary acid effectors of the acid–base balance: ventilation, metabolism, and clearance by the kidney. The reversible relationship of H^+ and HCO_3^- in the kidney is shown below:

$$H_2CO_3 \leftrightarrow HCO_3^- + H^+$$

Carbonic Acid $\leftrightarrow$ Bicarbonate Ions + Hydrogen Ions

Blood $\leftrightarrow$ Kidney

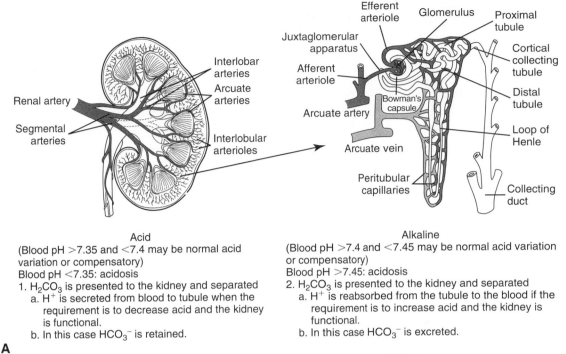

Acid
(Blood pH >7.35 and <7.4 may be normal acid variation or compensatory)
Blood pH <7.35: acidosis
1. H_2CO_3 is presented to the kidney and separated
   a. H^+ is secreted from blood to tubule when the requirement is to decrease acid and the kidney is functional.
   b. In this case HCO_3^- is retained.

Alkaline
(Blood pH >7.4 and <7.45 may be normal acid variation or compensatory)
Blood pH >7.45: acidosis
2. H_2CO_3 is presented to the kidney and separated
   a. H^+ is reabsorbed from the tubule to the blood if the requirement is to increase acid and the kidney is functional.
   b. In this case HCO_3^- is excreted.

A

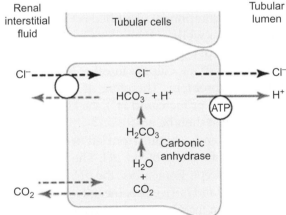

B

FIGURE 6-11 Kidney handling of acid and base H_2CO_3 is presented to kidney where it slowly dissociates into 2 H^+ and CO_2. (**A,** Modified from Kacmarek R, Dimas S, Mack C: *Essentials of respiratory care*, ed 4, St. Louis, 2006, Mosby; **B,** from Hall JE: *Guyton and Hall textbook of medical physiology*, ed 12, Philadelphia, 2011, Saunders.)

When evaluating patients, it is essential to have a basic understanding of the acid–base balancing system. The processing of both carbon dioxide and H^+ requires binding of the acid (H^+) and transfer to carbonic acid (H_2CO_3) in the bloodstream as well as reversible dissociation.

TABLE 6-8	**Acid–Base Definitions**
Acidosis	An abnormal process or condition that would lower arterial pH if no secondary changes occur in response to the primary etiologic factor
Alkalosis	An abnormal process or condition that would raise arterial pH if no secondary changes occur in response to the primary etiologic factor
Simple (acid–base) disorders	Those in which a single primary etiologic acid–base disorder is present
Mixed (acid–base) disorders	Those in which two or more primary etiologic disorders are present simultaneously
Acidemia	Arterial pH <7.35 (i.e., $[H^+] > 44$ nmol/L)
Alkalemia	Arterial pH >7.45 (i.e., $[H^+] < 36$ nmol/L)

nmol/L, Nanomoles per liter.

$$CO_2 + H_2O \leftrightarrow H_2CO_3 \leftrightarrow HCO_3^- + H^+$$

$$\text{Lung Alveoli} \leftrightarrow \text{Blood} \leftrightarrow \text{Kidney}$$

The most important component identified is H_2CO_3, which is an intermediary of carbon dioxide and water as well as H^+ and HCO_3^-. As the amount of H_2CO_3 in the bloodstream goes up, the pH goes down. Whatever causes the change of H_2CO_3 concentration is the primary culprit; in other words, identifying the directional pH change identifies the problem. Therefore, if the problem is too much acid (either increased carbon dioxide or increased H^+), the H_2CO_3 goes up, and the pH goes down. The primary cause must then be acidosis.

The equation is constantly shifting from left to right and right to left to maintain a normal H_2CO_3 and, thus, a normal blood pH. The bi-directional arrows in the equations above illustrate this concept. Remember, the pH is a measure of the acidity or alkalinity of the extracellular fluid and is inversely (negative logarithm) proportional to the number of H^+ in the blood. When the plasma contains either too many hydrogen ions (acidemia: pH <7.35) or too few hydrogen ions (alkalemia: pH >7.45), the pH will change.

A pH change reflects a change in the absence or presence of H^+. For example, if metabolic acids have accumulated H^+ increases, binding to bicarbonate or HCO_3^-, which is calculated and presented as a decreasing Bicarbonate. If able, the hyperventilation response will begin, and the lungs should respond effectively, which means that more carbon dioxide than normal will be exhaled (Table 6-9).

If either the kidneys or the lungs do not respond to a pH change or if they provide an ineffective response, the patient will remain in acid–base imbalance and will be considered to have a mixed acid–base problem with both a primary cause driving the pH change, and a secondary problem of failure to compensate.

TABLE 6-9 Normal Values for Arterial Blood Gas and Central or Mixed Venous Blood Gas on Room Air (0.21) at 760 mm Hg Sea Level	
ARTERIAL VALUES (ABG)	**VENOUS VALUES (VBG)**
pH: 7.40 (range) 7.35–7.45	pH: 7.32–7.38
$PaCO_2$: 40 (range 35–45) mm Hg	$PvCO_2$: 42–50 mm Hg
PaO_2: 80–100 mm Hg	PvO_2: 40 mm Hg
Saturation: 95%–100%	Saturation: 60%–80%
Base excess/deficit: −2 to +2	
Serum HCO_3^-: 22–26 mEq/L	Serum CO_2: 23–27 mEq/L
Serum lactate, less than 2 mmol/L in critically ill patients with normal liver function	
Mixed venous saturation values should always be correlated with other tissue indicators of hypoxia, base deficit, wide anion gap, serum bicarbonate, and lactate level.	

The Metabolic Acid Hydrogen Ion Correlated to the Inverse Buffer Bicarbonate Ion

The essence is that whether volatile or fixed, all measured acids are about the presence or absence of H^+. Although H^+ does not truly exist by itself in plasma, because it must always be bound to any H^+ acceptor, this is the commonly utilized terminology. H^+ is very small in size and easily moves across the cell wall seeking a bond to proteins and all other negatively charged ions. This may create a profound cellular dysfunction and is the main reason the pH of the extracellular environment (blood) is physiologically tightly regulated.

The presence or absence of H^+ is what affects the simplest measure of acid–base balance, which is the pH. H^+ concentration in the extracellular fluid that is either too high (H^+ high, low pH: acidemia) or too low (low H^+, high pH: alkalemia) will cause potentially fatal cardiovascular disturbances, including decreased myocardial contractility, vasomotor instability, and cardiac arrhythmias. The acid, which affects the blood pH, is always related to the presence of H^+. The relationship of carbon dioxide and water to carbonic acid is expressed below, where there is a reversible association between the two components.

$$CO_2 + H_2O \leftrightarrow H_2CO_3^-$$

Lung Alveoli $\leftrightarrow$ Blood

Respiratory carbon dioxide and metabolic acids (H^+) are generated from cell metabolism and excess H^+ must be buffered or eliminated to maintain a neutral chemical environment. For acid–base balance, the daily amount of acid excreted must equal the amount produced per day. Common acid–base disorders are listed in Table 6-10.

TABLE 6-10   **Primary Acid–Base Disorders with Compensation**

ACID–BASE DISORDER	PRIMARY CHANGE	COMPENSATION
Respiratory acidosis	$PaCO_2$ ↑	HCO_3^- ↑, H^+ ↓
Respiratory alkalosis	$PaCO_2$ ↓	HCO_3^- ↓, H^+ ↑
Metabolic acidosis	HCO_3^- ↓, H^+ ↑	$PaCO_2$ ↓
Metabolic alkalosis	HCO_3^- ↑, H^+ ↓	$PaCO_2$ ↑

Bases

All bases collect acids (H^+) but do so with a varying affinity. Buffers (bases) are present in all body fluids. In acid cells, bases act within 1 second after acid accumulation begins. They combine with excess acid to form substances that may not greatly affect pH. Some buffers have a strong affinity with acid; others are weak. The three primary plasma buffers are HCO_3^-, intracellular proteins, and chloride (Cl^-). All are negatively charged to facilitate attraction to H^+. Combining positively charged ions with negatively charged ions yields a chemically neutral substance.

Base Excess or Base Deficit (Normal Range −2 to +2, Ideal 0)

Base excess or base deficit is a calculated indicator of circulating buffer, or the quantity of available base in the bloodstream. This indirectly reflects the tissue and kidney tubular presence (or absence) of acid. As the proportion of acid rises, the relative amount of base decreases, and vice versa. Abnormally high values ($>+2$) reflect alkalosis; low values (<-2) reflect acidosis. Base excess or base deficit is a calculated value that estimates the metabolic component of the blood pH. Base excess and anion gap reflect lactate levels only in pure lactic acidosis. Acute kidney injury, pre-existing acid–base disorders, decreased albumin levels, and intraoperative administration of bicarbonate or any other base may alter the base excess or deficit values.

   Serum Bicarbonate (Normal Range 22 to 26 mEq/L, Ideal 24). Serum HCO_3^- is one of the major components of acid–base regulation contributed by the kidney. It is generated or excreted by the functional kidneys to maintain a normal acid–base environment in direct proportion to the amount of circulating acid. Because bicarbonate is affected by both the respiratory and metabolic components of the acid–base system, the relationship between metabolic acidosis and bicarbonate is not particularly linear or predictable. When the bicarbonate level changes, acid level changes in the opposite direction. To determine the cause of bicarbonate changes (problem versus compensation), the relationship to pH must be evaluated. The pH will respond to the presence or absence of acid, and the directional relationship reflects how the pH alteration was caused. The kidney is responsible for the regeneration of HCO_3^-, as well as excretion of the H^+.

   Although bicarbonate is a buffer, it is usually reported in the venous blood sample as "carbon dioxide content" or "total carbon dioxide" or "carbon dioxide" and not as HCO_3^-. The serum bicarbonate concentration is usually calculated and reported separately with an ABG analysis. Either total carbon dioxide or HCO_3^- must be considered when determining the acid–base status.

Note that serum is a term used in the clinical laboratory to describe the pale yellow fluid that remains after all the red cells, white cells, and clotting factor proteins have been removed by centrifuge from the blood sample. When the sample contains white cells and clotting factors, it is described as plasma.

Proteins. Extracellular and intracellular proteins offer a significant contribution to buffering acids. Hemoglobin is not only used for oxygen transport, but it also provides a very strong buffer for H^+. Albumin is also a significant buffer, and hypoalbuminemia must be considered when performing anion gap calculations.[23]

Chloride (Cl^-). The number of positive and negative ions in the plasma must remain balanced at all times. Besides plasma proteins, bicarbonate and chloride are the two most abundant negative ions (anions) in the plasma. To maintain electrical neutrality, any change in chloride must be accompanied by an opposite change in bicarbonate concentration. If chloride increases, bicarbonate decreases, a situation described as *hyperchloremic acidosis*. Thus, the serum chloride concentration may influence the acid–base balance.[24]

Cellular Electrolytes. The cells also offer protection in the metabolic acid environment. H^+ may exchange across the cell wall, attracted by negatively charged intracellular proteins. When this happens, K^+ shifts out of the cell, causing an excess of K^+ in the bloodstream.[25]

Other Buffers. Other buffers, including phosphate and ammonium, are present in very limited quantities and have a lesser impact on the regulation of acid. The body's response to a change in the acid–base status has three components, as described in Box 6-16.

Lactic Acidosis

Acidosis arises from increased production of acids by the cells, or loss of alkali, or decreased excretion of acids by the lung or kidney. Lactic acidosis reflects an increased cellular production of acid and is identified by a state of metabolic acidosis as well as an elevated serum lactate. This presents as one type of anion gap metabolic acidosis and may result from a variety of conditions.[26,27]

In addition, arterial lactate concentration is dependent on the balance between its production and consumption. In the critically ill patient, increased glucose metabolism, increased energy expenditures, and profound catabolism are the norm. The

---

BOX 6-16 Three Buffering Methods to Regulate Acid

1. **Buffering**: Decrease in bicarbonate (HCO_3^-) as excess hydrogen ions (H^+) are bound to HCO_3^-. This will reduce the serum carbon dioxide level.

2. **Respiratory**: Alteration in arterial carbon dioxide ($PaCO_2$).

3. **Kidney**: Alteration in HCO_3^- excretion or retention.

corresponding lactic acidosis signals physiologic stress but may not necessarily be evidence of tissue hypoxia. The concomitant energy expenditures, along with metabolic dysfunction, will increase lactate production. Frequently, higher levels of lactate clearance will mask this disturbing trend.

Lactate Production

Tissues involved in active glycolysis produce excess lactate from glucose under normal aerobic conditions (with oxygen) within the cell cytoplasm. Major lactate producing tissues are the brain, red blood cells, the gut, skeletal muscle, and skin. The body produces about 20 mmol/kg/day of excess lactate that "spills over" into blood and is metabolized predominantly in the liver and to a lesser extent in the kidney. The excess lactate is converted to glucose by a process known as gluconeogenesis, or metabolized to carbon dioxide and water. Only the liver and the kidney have the necessary enzymatic pathways to convert lactate to glucose. This normal physiologic process does not produce H^+ and does not alter the pH. See Figure 6-12 for an illustration of aerobic and anaerobic metabolism and lactate production within the cell cytosol and mitochondria.

All tissues can produce lactate under anaerobic conditions (without oxygen). The combination of hypoxemia and inadequate blood flow is a significant threat to tissue viability and will shift metabolism from an aerobic to an anaerobic (without oxygen) mechanism. The end product of anaerobic metabolism is lactic acid. H^+ is released from the dissociation lactate which then lowers the pH and causes metabolic acidosis.

Clinical Reasoning Pearl

Lactic acidosis is the most common cause of metabolic acidosis in hospitalized patients without diabetes. Lactate concentrations greater than 5 mmol/L with severe metabolic acidosis (pH <7.35) are indicative of conditions with high mortality rates.

Blood Lactate Levels

Blood lactate concentrations reflect the balance between lactate production and clearance. The normal blood lactate concentration in physiologically unstressed patients is 0.5 to 1 mmol/L. In critical illness, lactate concentrations of less than 2 mmol/L are considered acceptable. Hyperlactatemia is defined as a mild to moderate persistent increase in blood lactate concentration (2–4 mmol/L) without metabolic acidosis. Depending on the hospital or clinical laboratory protocol, lactic acidosis is diagnosed when increased blood lactate levels rise above 3 mmol/L.

When patients are at risk of cellular hypoxia a blood sample to measure the lactate level should be drawn. This may be a patient with suspected sepsis, but also patients with sustained tachycardia, tachypnea, hyperventilation, and persistent hypotension.

An arterial lactate sample should be placed on ice and taken as soon as possible to the clinical laboratory. Any serum lactate value above 2.0 mmol/L needs to be investigated for tissue hypoxia and hypoperfusion. Lactate levels will provide more information when correlated with an arterial or central venous blood gas. The serum lactate level is used as an index of the severity of the lactic acidosis, as each lactate generally means that one H^+ has been produced. Serial serum lactate levels are obtained to

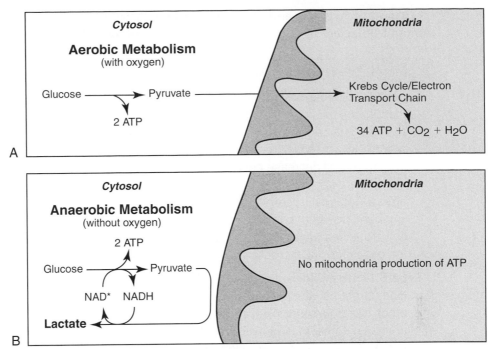

FIGURE 6-12 Human cells convert carbohydrates into energy. This process optimally occurs in aerobic conditions (with oxygen), but can also occur in anaerobic conditions (without oxygen), although much less efficiently and for a limited period of time. The first step is anaerobic and occurs in the cell cytosol where one molecule of glucose is converted into two molecules of pyruvate. At this point the metabolic pathways diverge depending on whether oxygen is present or not. **A,** In **aerobic metabolism** (oxygen present) pyruvate will diffuse from the cytosol into the mitochondria, where it enters the Krebs cycle to generate 34 adenosine triphosphate (ATP) as energy for the cell. Carbon dioxide (CO_2) and water (H_2O) are byproducts of this process. **B,** In **anaerobic metabolism** (no oxygen), pyruvate is unable to diffuse into the mitochondria. The anaerobic alternative is the conversion of pyruvate to lactate. Consequently lactate levels increase in the blood. **Note:** The liver and kidney can convert lactate to pyruvate in anaerobic conditions: 2 molecules of pyruvate are converted into 2 molecules of glucose. This is a metabolically expensive process as it uses more energy than it produces, but it does allow cells to have access to glucose in the absence of oxygen (anaerobic conditions).

evaluate therapy effectiveness or progressive dysfunction. A clearance level greater than 10% in 24 hours is a measure of successful therapeutic intervention.

Clinical Reasoning Pearl

Serial lactate measurements are helpful when patients have a persistent clinical profile of tissue hypoxia: tachycardia, hyperventilation, and a high index of suspicion regarding infection or inflammation.

Conditions Associated with Increased Lactate

High circulating levels of lactate can be divided into two groups according to etiology: (1) type A acidosis, in which lactate is increased secondary to reduced cellular perfusion or hypoxia; and (2) type B acidosis, in which clinical conditions affect the amount of lactate in blood unrelated to decreased availability of oxygen.

Clinical Reasoning Pearl

Type A lactic acidosis: Lactic acidosis (>2 mmol/L) *with* clinical evidence of inadequate tissue oxygen delivery is described as type A lactic acidosis. Hypoxemia that is sustained will result in lactic acidosis, as cellular metabolism shifts from an aerobic to anaerobic metabolism. Prolonged hypotension with low perfusion pressures will decrease cellular oxygen delivery. This is often related to a systemic shock state such as septic shock, cardiogenic shock, hypovolemic shock, or cardiac arrest. Regional ischemia that reduces perfusion to large areas of tissue such as ischemic bowel or compartment syndrome in a limb or the abdomen, will cause a shift to anaerobic metabolism in the affected tissues. Seizures will dramatically increase lactic acid production as a result of extreme muscle activity.

Type B lactic acidosis: Lactic acidosis (>2 mmol/L) *without* clinical evidence of inadequate oxygen delivery to the tissues is described as type B lactic acidosis. In other words, other clinical conditions increase the amount of lactate in blood unrelated to decreased availability of oxygen. The classic example is diabetic ketoacidosis, where lactic acidosis and hypovolemic shock may coexist. Leukemia and multiple myeloma have all been associated with type B acidosis. Drug toxicities associated with type B lactic acidosis include salicylate toxicity, nitroprusside toxicity, cyanide poisoning, and ethylene glycol poisoning. Any significant liver dysfunction may also affect the clearance of lactate.

It is important to recognize that considerable clinical overlap may exist between these two forms of acidosis (type A and type B). A patient admitted to the critical care unit with combined diabetic ketoacidosis and severe sepsis or with underlying leukemia with septic shock may have both type A and type B lactic acidosis. For this reason, the lactate level is never assessed in isolation but is combined with the ABG assessment and, if possible, central or mixed venous oxygen saturation and the clinical history. Figure 6-13 shows a format that can be used to differentiate the cause of the lactic acidosis, especially in patients with complex conditions.

Clinical Reasoning Pearl

When looking only at an abnormal pH, it is impossible to detect the source of the acid–base problem. Evaluation of both the respiratory ($PaCO_2$) and metabolic (HCO_3^-) contribution is necessary.

Identify the Cause of the pH Change

H^+ is clinically evaluated by the shift in pH. If one concentrates on the shifting pH, it becomes extraordinarily clear what the problem is. If the pH is not within range, not only

Type A Acidosis		Type B Acidosis	
Problem Regional hypoperfusion	Hypoxic (ischemic) lactic acidosis	Non-hypoxic lactic acidosis	Problem Metabolic dysfunction
☐	Cardiogenic shock	Liver dysfunction	☐
☐	Hypovolemic shock	Renal dysfunction	☐
☐	Hemorrhagic shock	Malignancies	☐
☐	Hyperglycemic hyperosmolar syndrome	Accelerated aerobic glycolysis DKA	☐
☐	Severe pulmonary dysfunction	Methanol, ethanol	☐
☐	Carbon monoxide poisoning	Anti-retrovirals, INH	☐
☐	Cardiac arrest	Cyanide poisoning	☐
☐	Any condition where oxygen delivery is inadequate	Valproic acid	☐
☐	Severe sepsis Profound tissue hypoxia	Early sepsis Pyruvate Dehydrogenase deficiency	☐

FIGURE 6-13 Type A and B lactic acidosis: discovering the source of the infection.

does an acid–base disequilibrium exist, but the opposing system has failed to respond and regulate. The organs involved in regulation of external acid–base balance are the lungs and the kidneys. An ideal pH is only achievable when the production of acid is normal and the regulation mechanisms of both the lung and the kidney are functioning optimally. Any pH that is out of range is a serious and acute problem because the acid load is extraordinarily high or low and compensation by the opposing system is inadequate.

The pH should always be as close to ideal as possible (7.40), but a small variation is acceptable (range 7.35–7.45). When a perfect balance of acid and buffer exists, the pH is deemed ideal or optimal. A normal pH occurs when the system preserves chemical neutrality inside the cells, and maintains the serum pH in the range. When the system contains too many acid ions (in the form of $\uparrow CO_2$ or $\uparrow H^+$) this causes acidemia. When the system contains too few acid ions (in the form of $\downarrow CO_2$ or $\downarrow H^+$) this causes alkalemia, and the pH will reflect the change. The clinician should investigate any variation in the pH relative to ideal (pH 7.40).

If the pH is within range, and both carbon dioxide, base or bicarbonate are within range, this may be considered a normal variant. See Table 6-9 for normal ABG ranges. If the pH is within range, but carbon dioxide or bicarbonate are not, this represents an abnormality with compensation. If production is too high or one regulator (lung or kidney) is failing or overloaded, the other will attempt to compensate, if capable. The pH goes outside of range of normal when one or both systems are failing or unable to compensate (Box 6-17). See the table below for an example:

Acid–Base Evaluation: Compensated Respiratory Acidosis

ABG Values

pH 7.36
$PaCO_2$ 50
HCO_3 48

ABG	INTERPRETATION
pH	The pH is on the acid side of ideal, but within the normal range.
$PaCO_2$	The patient's respiratory rate is 35 to 45 breaths per minute (rapid and shallow). Despite the rapid respiratory rate, the patient is failing to regulate the carbon dioxide as the $PaCO_2$ is out of range. The excess respiratory acid caused a significant increase in circulating carbonic acid (H_2CO_3) but the pH is in range, which suggests that this is not an acute (sudden) event. If excess acid is present, why is the pH not outside of range as well?
HCO_3^-	Bicarbonate is elevated and outside of range. The kidney accepted the H_2CO_3, broke it down into H^+ and HCO_3^-, and then excreted the extra H^+ ions to achieve a pH that is on the acidotic side (pH 7.35–7.39) of ideal. As always, HCO_3^- is directly inverted from H^+.

Summary: The patient has a respiratory acidosis (cannot exhale enough carbon dioxide), but the pH is in range, although on the acid side of ideal, because of metabolic compensation. This indicates that this is longstanding or chronic respiratory acidosis, with compensation, because the pH is within the normal range.

BOX 6-17   pH as a Symptom

An altered pH is often a symptom of a problem.
    Examine the pH to identify the presence or absence of acid.
    Is the pH 7.40? Unlikely any problems are present.
    If the pH is not at 7.40, even if the alteration is small, an increase or decrease in acid is present.

Arterial Blood Gas—Knowledge Application

The following five questions are applied to interpretation of an ABG.

1. What is the PaO_2? What is the P/F?
2. What is the pH? Is it ideal (pH 7.40)?

Is the pH within the normal range (pH 7.35–7.45) or out of range (pH <7.35 [acidosis], or pH >7.45 [alkalosis]).

3. If not at pH 7.40, what caused a variation?
4. What is the ventilation status? What is the $PaCO_2$?
5. What is the metabolic status? What is the bicarbonate?

Step 1: *Assess the PaO₂ and P/F ratio*

Firstly, the oxygenation status, the relationship to FiO_2, and any interventions to improve ventilation are identified. This means that an evaluation is not complete without one of the oxygen calculations mentioned earlier. When evaluating an ABG, the first step is to evaluate the A-a gradient. It is important to:

- Determine if the PaO_2 is within the range of normal.
- Compare the PaO_2 to the FiO_2. The P/F ratio is the standard method with the following exceptions: as long as the patient is not retaining carbon dioxide as a consequence of low tidal volumes with lung-protective ventilation (permissive hypercapnia) or being ventilated with alveolar recruitment strategies (high PEEP, inverse ratio ventilation: APRV, HFOV) or the patient is retaining carbon dioxide because of alveolar hypoventilation caused by lung disease.

Steps 2, 3: *Assess the pH*

The second and third steps are to evaluate the acid–base balance: An acid–base problem is named on the basis of the direction of the pH with respect to an optimal acid–base balance (pH 7.40).

- The pH has to be evaluated for the presence or absence of H^+. Any problem is always named on the basis of the direction of the pH. The pH range used in critical care is 7.35 to 7.45. If the pH is out of range (<7.35 or >7.45) the acid–base problem is acute and uncompensated. Any pH <7.40 indicates that more acid is present in blood. In contrast, any pH >7.40 indicates that less acid is present in blood.
- When looking only at the pH, it is impossible to detect whether the condition is respiratory or metabolic in origin.

Step 4: *Assess PaCO₂ and ventilation status*

The fourth step is to evaluate the ventilatory system or carbon dioxide management: The functional respiratory system quickly responds to pH changes, generally within 1 to 2 minutes. Whenever the minute ventilation is affected, the pH should be evaluated to discover if lung injury is the source of the problem, or if the increase in minute ventilation is a physiologic response to compensate for a metabolic problem.

Step 5: *Assess bicarbonate and metabolic status*

The fifth step is to evaluate the metabolic system. An increase in metabolism yields an increase in H^+. In terms of H^+ production the primary reasons are ketoacidosis, lactic acidosis, in terms of H^+ clearance kidney failure or liver failure. Any acute increase in acid (H+) will result in an acute decrease in serum bicarbonate (HCO_3^-).

Oxygenation Analysis

ABG and Oxygenation Values

FiO_2 (100% oxygen) 1.0
PaO_2 110 mm Hg
P/F ratio 110 mm Hg
FiO_2 1.0 (100% oxygen) 110/ 1.0 = 110 mm Hg

ABG & FiO_2	INTERPRETATION
FiO_2	Maximal oxygen administration. A healthy lung with an FiO_2 of 1.0 (100% oxygen) would be close to a PaO_2 of 500 mm Hg on this amount of supplemental oxygen.
PaO_2	The patient is relatively hypoxemic and is not responding as expected, meaning there is no rise in PaO_2 in response to the increased oxygen delivery (FiO_2).
P/F ratio	Low P/F ratio of 110 on 1.0 FiO_2

Summary: This patient has refractory hypoxemia.

Acid–Base Evaluation: Acute Metabolic Acidosis

ABG Values

pH	7.25
$PaCO_2$	20
HCO_3^-	16

ABG	INTERPRETATION
pH: 7.25	The pH is on the acid side and outside normal range
$PaCO_2$ 20 mm Hg	The respiratory rate is 22 to 26 breaths per minute. This patient is hyperventilating and is excessively "blowing off" carbon dioxide, thus lowering the $PaCO_2$ in the bloodstream. This is a hyperexcretion of acid on the respiratory regulation side, a situation that would normally raise the pH. Thus, hyperventilation and removal of $PaCO_2$ to 20 mm Hg cannot be the cause of the shift in the pH, as this pH (7.25) reflects the presence of too much acid. This is a ventilatory attempt to compensate, but it is inadequate.
HCO_3^- 16	A low serum bicarbonate level that is outside of range, indicates that H^+ has significantly increased.

Summary: The acid–base imbalance is acute and caused by a metabolic acidosis (uncompensated) because the pH is not within the normal range.

Respiratory Acidosis

Chronic respiratory acidosis disorder occurs in pulmonary diseases in which effective alveolar ventilation is decreased. For carbon dioxide to be removed from blood, alveolar carbon dioxide ($PACO_2$) must be lower than the arterial blood ($PaCO_2$) as shown with normal carbon dioxide values in Figure 6-2. In air-trapping syndromes, where loss of alveolar elasticity, airway obstructive disease, or profound hypoventilation occurs, the alveolar concentration of carbon dioxide will rise because it cannot be effectively exhaled. The increase in $PACO_2$ limits the removal of carbon dioxide from blood ($PaCO_2$) because of the alteration in the pressure gradient. Over time, the amount of carbon dioxide eliminated is less than the amount generated, and $PaCO_2$ levels increase in the bloodstream.

Respiratory acidosis (hypercapnia) is always a ventilation problem, which may be the result of therapeutic failure or may be pathophysiologic in origin, resulting in carbon dioxide retention. $PaCO_2$ derangements are direct reflections of the degree of ventilatory dysfunction. The degree to which the increased $PaCO_2$ alters the pH depends on the rapidity of onset and compensation via the blood buffer and regulation systems in the kidney. The pH may be profoundly affected because of the time required (hours to days) for compensation as the kidney retains bicarbonate.

The most common cause of inadequate carbon dioxide excretion, which leads to carbon dioxide retention, is inadequate alveolar ventilation, or alveolar hypoventilation. Alveolar hypoventilation may occur as a result of airway obstruction, loss of alveolar recoil, or inadequate time for exhalation affecting the ability to express carbon gas into the environment.

Acidosis Compensation

Acute rises in $PaCO_2$ precipitate a rise in extracellular buffering systems, primarily from hemoglobin and proteins, even before compensation via the kidney occurs. However, the rise in extracellular buffers is not sufficient to maintain a normal pH in the presence of an elevated $PaCO_2$. Once buffering takes place, which requires adequate kidney function, the shift will be to retain HCO_3^- and to excrete H^+ as described in Box 6-18.

The increase in carbon dioxide has resulted in a primary respiratory acidosis. For every 10 mm Hg increase in carbon dioxide ($PaCO_2$), the pH will acutely decrease 0.08 (on the acid side). This will also result in more circulating carbonic acid (H_2CO_3). If respiratory acids accumulate because of respiratory dysfunction, where carbon dioxide is retained or increased, the kidneys should respond by processing the increased H_2CO_3, breaking down the chemical bonds of the H_2CO_3, excreting H^+ and retaining HCO_3^- in the bloodstream.

When excess acid is out of range but the pH is not (7.35–7.40), compensation must be present. Once the problem is named, it becomes easier to evaluate the compensation (see Box 6-18).

Acid–Base Evaluation: Acute Respiratory Acidosis

ABG Values

pH 7.28
$PaCO_2$ 54
HCO_3^- 24

ABG	INTERPRETATION
pH	Acidosis
$PaCO_2$	The patient's respiratory rate is >32 breaths per minute and is rapid and shallow. The problem is hypercapnia ($PaCO_2$ > 45 mm Hg), which signals alveolar hypoventilation, resulting in respiratory acidosis.
HCO_3^-	The bicarbonate is within normal range and is not the cause of the acidotic pH. However, a failure to compensate is evident. It may take some hours for compensatory regulation by the kidney to start to occur.

Summary: The problem is acute respiratory acidosis.

BOX 6-18   Acidosis Compensation

- Increased H^+ caused by:
  - Respiratory failure with inability to regulate carbon dioxide
  - Kidney failure, with inability to regulate acid (hydrogen ions [H^+]) and bicarbonate (HCO_3^-) balance
  - Tissue hypermetabolism in a hypoxic state
- Buffering of acid occurs in three primary ways:
  - Rapid buffering using bicarbonate, proteins, intracellular electrolytes, and chloride.
  - If not the problem or cause of the acidosis, the respiratory center immediately stimulates hyperventilation to blow off the byproducts of carbonic acid when metabolic acidosis is the cause of the acidosis.
  - If not the cause of the acidosis, the kidney responds by conjugating and retaining more bicarbonate and excreting more acid (H^+).

COMPENSATION FOR RESPIRATORY ACIDOSIS

ABG Values	
pH	7.35
$PaCO_2$	58
HCO_3^-	36

BOX 6-18 Acidosis Compensation—cont'd

$$\uparrow CO_2 + H_2O \rightarrow H_2CO_3 \rightarrow \uparrow\uparrow HCO_3^- + H^+\downarrow\downarrow$$

$$\text{Lung Alveoli} \rightarrow \text{Bloodstream} \rightarrow \text{Kidney}$$

Problem: Increased carbon dioxide ($\uparrow CO_2$; alveolar hypoventilation)

Retained carbon dioxide adds more acid to the bloodstream and therefore more HCO_3^- is needed to achieve a neutral pH balance. The HCO_3^- value needs to be higher. Compensation will require that the kidney produce more bicarbonate ($\uparrow\uparrow HCO_3^-$).

Compensation

Excess carbon dioxide in the bloodstream lowers the pH.

Kidney produces bicarbonate ($\uparrow\uparrow HCO_3^-$) to compensate.

Kidney excretes excess acid ($H^+\downarrow$).

Result: pH is less than 7.40, on the border at 7.35.

COMPENSATION FOR METABOLIC ACIDOSIS

ABG Values	
pH	7.35
PaCO$_2$	26
HCO$_3^-$	15

$$\downarrow CO_2 + H_2O \leftarrow H_2CO_3 \leftarrow \downarrow HCO_3^- + H^+ \uparrow$$

$$\text{Lung Alveoli} \leftarrow \text{Bloodstream} \leftarrow \text{Kidney}$$

Problem: Increased H^+ acid measured by $\downarrow$pH with $\downarrow HCO_3^-$

Less acid (identified by the low pH and the low bicarbonate) requires less volatile acid (CO_2) to achieve a neutral pH. Therefore, compensation will require elimination of bicarbonate ($\downarrow\downarrow HCO_3^-$).

Compensation: The decreased $\downarrow PaCO_2$ (hyperventilation) is a response to the metabolic acidosis to "blow off" excess acid (CO_2).

The rapid respiratory rate may ultimately lead to a fall in oxygen.

In this example, the kidney has not yet adapted to produce additional bicarbonate (HCO_3^-).

Result: pH is greater than 7.35 but less than 7.40.

Alkalosis Compensation

Ongoing alkalosis will also generate a compensatory response to achieve a pH within the normal range, as described in Box 6-19.

BOX 6-19   Alkalosis Compensation

Decreased H^+ caused by:
- Uncontrolled hyperventilation,
- Kidney losses with aggressive diuresis, and/or
- Tissue hypometabolism.
  Extra base is present or loss of acid is present, with a pH >7.45.
  Compensating for an alkaline state occurs in two ways:
- First, if the respiratory system is NOT the cause of the alkalosis, the respiratory system responds by slowing ventilation and retaining carbon dioxide (acid).
- Second, if the kidney is NOT the problem or cause of the alkalosis, the kidney will excrete bicarbonate and retain H^+.

COMPENSATION FOR RESPIRATORY ALKALOSIS

ABG Values	
pH	7.44
PaCO$_2$	22
HCO$_3^-$	18

$$\downarrow CO_2 + H_2O \leftarrow H_2CO_3 \leftarrow HCO_3^- \downarrow + H^+ \uparrow\uparrow$$

Lung Alveoli ⬅ Bloodstream ← Kidney

Problem: Decreased CO_2 (hyperventilation) results in less acid in the bloodstream ($\downarrow\downarrow CO_2$). Less volatile acid requires less bicarbonate (HCO_3^-) to achieve a neutral pH balance. Therefore, the bicarbonate value needs to be lower. Compensation will require elimination of bicarbonate ($\downarrow\downarrow HCO_3^-$) by the kidney.

Compensation:
Excess bicarbonate (HCO_3^-) is excreted by the kidney.
H^+ retained by the kidney.
Result: pH is greater than 7.40, although less than 7.45.

BOX 6-19   Alkalosis Compensation—cont'd

COMPENSATION FOR METABOLIC ALKALOSIS

ABG Values	
pH	7.44
PaCO$_2$	52
HCO$_3^-$	33

$$\downarrow CO_2 + H_2O \rightarrow H_2CO_3 \leftarrow \uparrow HCO_3^- + H^+\downarrow$$

Lung Alveoli ← Bloodstream → Kidney

Problem: ↓ H$^+$ acid measured by increased ↑bicarbonate. More alkali (identified by the high bicarbonate) requires a lot more volatile acid (↑CO$_2$) to achieve a neutral pH. Therefore compensation will require retention of carbon dioxide.

Compensation: The elevated ↑PaCO$_2$ (hypoventilation) is in response to excess bicarbonate (alkali or base) in the bloodstream. The elevated carbon dioxide retains H$^+$ in the bloodstream.

Result: pH is less than 7.45 but greater than 7.40.

Anion Gap

The bicarbonate or total carbon dioxide should also be examined in relation to the other measured electrolytes, specifically to calculate the anion gap (Figure 6-14). The anion gap estimates the differences between unmeasured and measured cations (positively charged particles) and measured and unmeasured anions (negatively charged particles). Particles that possess charges tend to have high affinity to bind to other particles that are opposite their own, perhaps the origin of the saying "opposites attract." The anion gap is the Na$^+$ concentration minus total carbon dioxide plus Cl$^-$ as shown in the equation later in this section.

The normal anion gap range is 12 plus or minus 4 mEq/L. This is an artifact of measurement, since these three electrolytes are only the ones most commonly measured. Because the value of K$^+$ is small and relatively constant, it is not usually used to calculate the anion gap; if K$^+$ is used then the normal anion gap is about 16 plus or minus 4 mEq/L. If all the plasma anions and cations were measured, anions would equal cations and there would be no anion gap. Table 6-11 provides guidance for interpreting the anion gap and other acid–base disorders.[28]

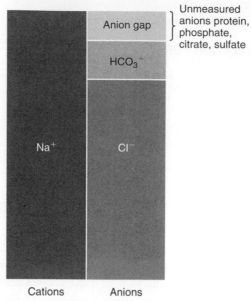

FIGURE 6-14 Anion gap.

Hyperchloremic Acidosis

The importance of the anion gap is that it can help both to diagnose the presence of a metabolic acidosis and characterize its cause. Thus, regardless of pH, an elevated anion gap suggests a metabolic acidosis from unmeasured organic anions, caused by lactic acidosis or ketoacidosis; the higher the anion gap, the more likely it reflects an organic acidosis.

TABLE 6-11	Interpretation of Acid–Base Disorders
LABORATORY VALUE	**CLINICAL CONDITION**
Wide anion gap	*Always* strongly suggests a *true* metabolic acidosis
Hyperglycemia	If ketones present, suggests diabetic ketoacidosis
Hypokalemia and/or hypochloremia	Suggests metabolic alkalosis
Hyperchloremia	Common with normal anion gap acidosis
Elevated creatinine and urea	Suggests uremic acidosis, hypovolemia (pre-renal failure), or acute kidney injury
Elevated creatinine	Consider ketoacidosis: ketones interfere in the laboratory method used for creatinine measurement and give a falsely elevated result; typically urea will be normal
Elevated glucose	Consider diabetic ketoacidosis (DKA), or hyperglycemic hyperosmolar syndrome (HHS)

In contrast, a normal anion gap in a patient with metabolic acidosis indicates a hyperchloremic acidosis, most commonly from excessive fluid resuscitation with 0.9% sodium chloride, or bicarbonate loss via the kidneys as renal tubular acidosis or via the gastrointestinal system as diarrhea. The anion gap is used to determine if a metabolic acidosis is caused by an accumulation of nonvolatile acids, such as lactic acid or ketoacid. Both lactic and ketoacids carry a positive charge resulting from excess H^+, or from net loss of bicarbonate, as in diarrhea. The anion gap is not used when a patient has metabolic acidosis purely from kidney failure.[29]

$$Na^+ - (Cl^- + HCO_3^-)$$

$$Cations - Anions$$

$$Positively\ Charged\ Ions - Negatively\ Charged\ Ions$$

Unmeasured cations, including calcium, magnesium, gamma-globulins, potassium, and hydrogen, bind negatively charged particles. Unmeasured anions, including albumin, phosphate, sulfate, and lactate, bind positively charged particles.[30] Calculation of the anion gap is shown in Box 6-20.

Clinical Reasoning Pearl

In metabolic acidosis, the anion gap is evaluated to differentiate the cause of the acidosis.

If anion gap is >20, consider lactic acidosis or ketoacidosis until proven otherwise.

If anion gap is <20, evaluate chloride levels (hyperchloremic, non-gap acidosis), and assess kidney function by measuring blood urea nitrogen (BUN) and creatinine.

BOX 6-20 Calculating the Anion Gap

In metabolic acidosis, calculate an anion gap.

Hyperventilation brings the pH back to normal range (7.35–7.39) but not to ideal (7.40).

Anion gap: Na^+ subtract the following total (HCO_3^- is less the Cl^-): in this case:

$$Na^+ 140 - (HCO_3^- [17] + Cl^- [100])$$

$$140 - 117 = 23$$

A wide anion gap often indicates lactic acidosis or ketoacidosis.

Check serum lactate and blood glucose.

Stewart Acid–Base Classification

In some clinical situations, hyperlactemia and tissue hypoperfusion occur in the absence of acidosis. In such cases, the levels of lactate may under predict the seriousness of the clinical situation. This weak correlation between hyperlactemia and metabolic acidosis may be better understood when using the Stewart acid–base classification. Stewart showed that three independent variables affect the pH:

1. Strong ion difference, defined as >3 mEq/L[31]
2. Partial pressure of carbon dioxide in blood ($PaCO_2$)
3. The sum of the weak acids and proteins in the plasma[32,33]

The Role of the Liver and Other Organs

The liver is also important in acid–base physiology, and this is often overlooked. It is important because it is a metabolically active organ that may be either a significant net producer or consumer of hydrogen ions. The amounts of acid involved may be very large. The acid–base roles of the liver may be considered under the following headings:

- Carbon dioxide production from complete oxidation of substrates
- Metabolism of organic acid anions such as lactate, ketones, and amino acids
- Metabolism of ammonium
- Production of plasma proteins, especially albumin

If the glucose is elevated a serum ketone level should also be drawn. Ketoacidosis presents with a wide anion gap metabolic acidosis resulting from the production of ketone bodies, also known as keto-anions. Ketone bodies (acetoacetate, beta-hydroxybutyrate, acetone) are released into the blood from the liver when hepatic lipid metabolism has changed to a state of increased ketogenesis. A relative or absolute insulin deficiency is present in all cases. An associated lactic acidosis may co-exist with ketoacidosis.

Applying the Methods

The above acid–base information is applied to the interpretation of the ABG adding three additional questions to the earlier questions listed here.

1. What is the PaO_2? What is the P/F?
2. What is the pH? Is it ideal (pH 7.40)?
3. If not at pH 7.40, what caused a variation?
4. What is the ventilation status? What is the $PaCO_2$?

5. What is the metabolic status? What is the bicarbonate?
6. If the problem is metabolic acidosis, what is the anion gap?
7. Is the problem compensated?
8. What interventions can be used to correct the original problem?

Table 6-12 lists acid–base disorders and possible causes.

TABLE 6-12   Acid–Base Disorders and Possible Causes

DISORDER	pH	PRIMARY PROBLEM	COMPENSATION
Metabolic acidosis	↓	↓ in HCO_3^-	↓ in $PaCO_2$
Metabolic alkalosis	↑	↑ in HCO_3^-	↑ in $PaCO_2$
Respiratory acidosis	↓	↑ in $PaCO_2$	↑ in $[HCO_3^-]$
Respiratory alkalosis	↑	↓ in $PaCO_2$	↓ in $[HCO_3^-]$

Special Situations—Mixed Acid–Base Disorders

DISORDER	CHARACTERISTICS	CLINICAL CONDITION
Respiratory acidosis with metabolic acidosis	↓ in pH ↓ in HCO_3^- ↑ in $PaCO_2$	Cardiac arrest Intoxications Multi-organ failure
Respiratory alkalosis with metabolic alkalosis	↑ in pH ↑ in HCO_3^- ↓ in $PaCO_2$	Cirrhosis with diuretics Pregnancy with vomiting Overventilation with chronic obstructive pulmonary disease (COPD)
Respiratory acidosis with metabolic alkalosis	pH in normal range ↑ in $PaCO_2$ ↑ in HCO_3^-	COPD with diuretics, vomiting, gastric suction Severe hypokalemia
Respiratory alkalosis with metabolic acidosis	pH in normal range ↓ in $PaCO_2$ ↓ in HCO_3^-	Sepsis Salicylate toxicity Kidney failure with acute heart failure or pneumonia Advanced liver disease
Metabolic acidosis with metabolic alkalosis	pH in normal range HCO_3^- normal	Uremia or ketoacidosis with vomiting, gastric suction, diuretics.

Case Study #1

A 58-year-old male is admitted to the emergency department (ED) with a change in level of consciousness. He has a known history of type 1 diabetes and COPD and uses supplementary oxygen at home. He went out with friends for lunch and might have missed his morning insulin dose. He ate fries, a burger, and a milkshake. His blood glucose was 469 mg/dL on his home glucometer, and he was feeling lethargic. His wife increased his nasal flow from 1 L/min to 6 L/min. He became more lethargic, so she called for the emergency medical services (EMS). Upon arrival in the ED his vital signs are heart rate 121 bpm; respiratory rate 5 breaths/min; and blood pressure 84/45 mm Hg. The following are his ABG values prior to intubation and at ICU admission:

PARAMETERS	AT ED (PRIOR TO INTUBATION)	AT ICU ADMISSION
SpO_2	91%	100%
SaO_2	92%	100%
PaO_2	67.2	190
$PaCO_2$	52.4	40
pH	7.19	7.36
Bicarbonate/base deficit	15/−9	20/−5
Oxygen	6 L/min (add 3% to room air FiO_2 for every 1-L flow) 21% +18% =39% oxygen	Assist-control (AC) mechanical ventilation (MV), F 18, T_V 375, PEEP +5, FiO_2 (0.6) 60%
P/F ratio	171: 67/ 0.39	316: 190/0.6
A-a: CO_2 retainer	356.9	Not applicable
Blood glucose (mg/dL)	421	150
Diagnosis	Respiratory AND metabolic acidosis	
Plan	Intubate, carbon dioxide removal; insulin, control blood glucose, and volume replacement	

Case Study #1—cont'd

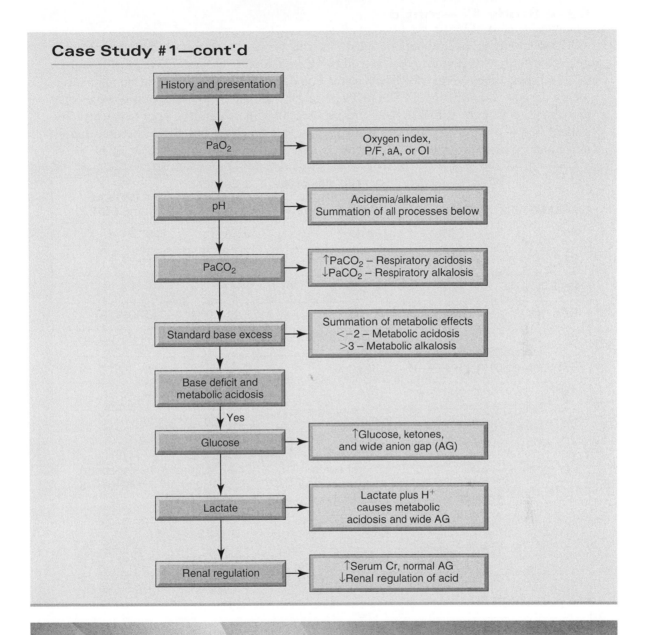

Case Study #2

A 25-year-old male with unknown medical history presented to the ED after a 52-foot fall, which had resulted in significant facial trauma, irregular respirations, and altered level of consciousness, requiring bag-mask ventilation. On admission, he was in sinus tachycardia at 120 beats per minute, but within 5 minutes of arrival, his heart rate dropped to 35 beats per minute.

Continued

Case Study #2—cont'd

Three attempts at intubation failed, as the airway was full of blood. Emergent cricothyrotomy was performed, which allowed ventilation with symmetrical breath sounds. Bilateral chest tubes were placed, with a small blood return on the right. Additional findings were Glasgow Coma Scale (GCS) 6 (eye opening: 1, verbal: 1, motor: 4); pupils were equal and reactive to light (PERRL) 4–2 mm; moving all four extremities spontaneously. The patient had a positive history for illicit drug use; his family reported that he used heroin and other opiates. Toxicology screen was positive for opiates and benzodiazepines.

PARAMETERS	1. ED	2. POST-OPERATIVE ADMITTED TO CRITICAL CARE	3. CRITICAL CARE UNIT	4. CRITICAL CARE UNIT
SpO_2	72%	96%	95%	97%
SaO_2	87%	98%	97%	100%
PaO_2	56	135	161	113
FiO_2	(100%)	0.70 (70%)	0.60 (60%)	0.40(40%)
P/F	56/1.0=56	135/0.7=192	161/0.6=268	113/0.4=282
PEEP (cm H_2O)	————	10	6	6
$PaCO_2$	51	36	57	36
TV RR V_E MV mode	RR 6 Bag-mask ventilation	350 25 8.7 L/min Assist control MV rate 20	220–260 26 6.2 L/min SIMV (without a mandatory rate) and +10 cm H_2O PS	380 20 7.6 L/min Assist control MV rate 15
pH	7.29	7.43	7.35	7.51
Base deficit / excess (HCO_3^-)	−3 (22)	−0.3 (24)	+ 5 (31)	+ 4.6 (30)
Cl^-	112	110	103	102
Na^+	142	140	140	141
Anion gap	7	5	6	9
Chest radiograph			Chest radiograph A	Chest radiograph B

cm H_2O, Centimeters of water; *MV*, mechanical ventilation; *PS*, pressure support; *SIMV*, synchronized intermittent mandatory ventilation.

Case Study #2—cont'd

1. *Initial ED Assessment and Interventions:* On physical examination, the patient was found to be severely hypoxic, and despite effective bag-mask ventilation, the SpO_2 could not be increased above 90%.

   On first intubation attempt, cords were easily and quickly visualized, but the endotracheal tube could not be passed. Because of severe hypoxia, the trauma surgeon performed emergent cricothyrotomy. Shortly after placement, the patient became bradycardic and hypotensive, requiring emergent bilateral chest tube placement. He continued to have intermittent hypotension and significant blood loss, which necessitated administration of 5 units of packed red blood cells, 3 units of fresh frozen plasma, and norepinephrine at 8 mcg/min. The patient was transported for computed tomography (CT) and then to the operating room for stabilization.

   Initial ABG: Significant hypoxemia, acute (uncompensated) respiratory acidosis, very small base deficit, and normal anion gap. Emergent cricothyrotomy performed.

2. *Post-Operative:* Admitted to critical care: After surgery, blood replacement, and stabilization, cricothyrotomy was converted to a tracheostomy and the patient was admitted to the critical care unit.

   Second ABG: Continued hypoxemia, signified by P/F ratio of 192, acid–base balance maintained at normal; relative hypoxemia was accepted, as vital signs were stable and no evidence of lactic acidosis was seen. Low-normal $PaCO_2$ resulted in normal range pH. Base and bicarbonate were within normal limits. No gap analysis was required, as no evidence of metabolic acidosis was seen.

3. *Critical Care Unit:* In the critical care unit, the patient received a total of 8 units packed red blood cells, 6 L balanced fluids (lactated Ringers), fentanyl at 2 mcg/kg/hr, and dexmedetomidine at 0.7 mcg/kg/hr. He was weaned to SIMV with no mandatory rate. As the effects of anesthesia wore off, he became more agitated. The team planned to extubate him as soon as possible. See chest radiograph A.

   Third ABG: Hypoxemia was resolving, as evidenced by P/F ratio of 268 and decrease in PEEP. The patient had a chronic (compensated) respiratory acidosis: $PaCO_2$ 57 mm Hg, and pH was on the acid side of normal 7.35. Base excess was +5.

4. *Critical Care Unit:* The patient may be oversedated, although he opens his eyes to voice (RASS -2). At this time, because he still requires a ventilator rate and volume to maintain normal $PaCO_2$ regulation, he was returned to assist control mechanical ventilation. Discontinuation of fentanyl, and reduction of dexmedetomidine were considered, with the intent to prepare for a spontaneous breathing trial.

   Fourth ABG: Hypoxemia was resolving, as evidenced by P/F ratio of 282 and low PEEP. Overcompensation for respiratory acidosis (excess exhalation of $PaCO_2$) results

Continued

Case Study #2—cont'd

in metabolic alkalosis, and it will take some time for the kidney to adjust the acid–base balance as required.

Plan: The plan is to return the patient to SIMV with a mandatory rate so that spontaneous efforts could be maintained, with his own spontaneous breaths supported by pressure support (PS). See chest radiograph B. The plan is to let the metabolic alkalosis resolve, and resume spontaneous breathing trials.

Chest radiograph A:

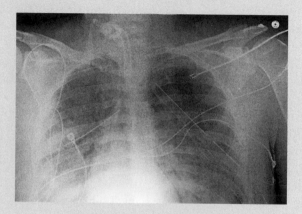

Chest radiograph B:

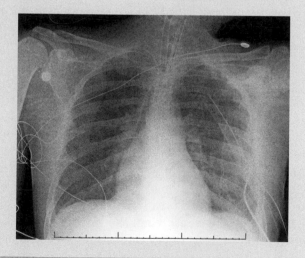

Conclusion

A careful clinician knows that understanding the data in a blood gas panel requires an appreciation for not only oxygenation, acids, and bases but also ventilation, gas exchange, dynamics of electrolyte and water movement, plasma composition, respiratory control, and kidney regulation of hydrogen ion, electrolyte, and water excretion. No single value ever gives the complete picture, and complexity in critical care is part of daily practice. Hemodynamics can only be optimized in the presence of adequate tissue oxygenation and an acid–base balance within the normal range. This is the reason it is essential to understand the intricacies of these metabolic and chemical processes.

References

1. Kuhn C, Werdan K: Hemodynamic monitoring. In Holzheimer RG, Mannick JA, editors: *Surgical treatment: evidence-based and problem-oriented*, Munich, 2001, Zuckschwerdt.
2. Shapiro BA: The history of pH and blood gas analysis, *Respir Care Clin N Am* 1(1):1–5, 1995.
3. Astrup P, Jorgensen K, Siggaard-Andersen O, Engel K: The acid-base metabolism. A new approach, *Lancet* 1:1035–1039, 1960.
4. Paulev PE, Zubieta-Calleja GR: Essentials in the diagnosis of acid base disorders and their high altitude applications, *J Phys and Pharm* 56(4):155–170, 2005.
5. Severinghaus JW: The invention and development of blood gas analysis apparatus, *Anesthesiology* 97:253–256, 2002.
6. Hess W: Affinity of oxygen for hemoglobin—its significance under physiological and pathological conditions, *Anaesthesist* 36(9):455–467, 1987.
7. Hasan A: *Handbook of blood gas/acid base balance*, ed 2, London, 2013, Springer-Verlag, pp 12–14.
8. Allen M: Lactate and acid base as a hemodynamic monitor and markers of cellular perfusion, *Pediatr Crit Care Med* 12(4 Suppl):S43–S49, 2011.
9. Husain FA, Martin MJ, Mullenix PS, et al.: Serum lactate and base deficit as predictors of mortality and morbidity, *Am J Surg* 185:485–491, 2003.
10. West JB, Dollery CT, Naimark A: Distribution of blood flow in isolated lung; relation to vascular and alveolar pressures, *J Appl Physiol* 19:713–724, 1964.
11. Hammond S: Oxygen saturation a guide to laboratory assessment, *CLN* 32(2):10–12, 2006.
12. Al-Otaibi HM, Hardman JG: Prediction of arterial oxygen partial pressure after changes in FIO_2: validation and clinical application of a novel formula, *Br J Anaesth* 107 (5):806–812, 2011.
13. De Koninck AS, De Decker K, Van Bocxlaer J, et al.: Analytical performance evaluation of four cartridge-type blood gas analyzers, *Clin Chem Lab Med* 50(6):1083–1091, 2012.
14. Martin DS, Grocott MPW: Oxygen therapy in critical illness: precise control of arterial oxygenation and permissive hypoxemia, *Crit Care Med* 41(2):423–432, 2013.
15. The Acute Respiratory Distress Syndrome Network: Ventilation with lower tidal volumes as compared with traditional tidal volumes for acute lung injury and the acute respiratory distress syndrome, *New Engl J Med* 342(18):1301–1308, 2000.
16. Task F, Ranieri VM, Rubenfeld GD, et al.: Acute respiratory distress syndrome: the Berlin definition, *JAMA* 307(23):2526–2533, 2012.

17. Bernard GR, Artigas A, Brigham KL, et al.: American-European consensus conference on ARDS, *Am J Respir Crit Care Med* 149:818–824, 1994.
18. Ferguson E, Fan L, Camporota M, et al.: The Berlin definition of ARDS: an expanded rationale, justification, and supplementary material, *Intensive Care Med* 38(10):1573–1582, 2012.
19. Barker SJ: Arterial blood-gas analysis interpretation and application for the nonchemist, *ASA Refresher Courses Anesthesiol* 39(1):1–5, 2011.
20. Esan A: Severe hypoxemic respiratory failure: part 1-ventilatory strategies, *Chest* 137 (5):1203–1216, 2010.
21. Hingston DM: A computerized interpretation of arterial pH and blood gas data: do physicians need it? *Respir Care* 27:809–815, 1982.
22. Gilfix BM, Bique M, Magder S: A physical chemical approach to the analysis of acid-base balance in the clinical setting, *J Crit Care* 8:187–197, 1993.
23. Kaplan JL, Kellum JA: Fluids, pH, ions and electrolytes, *Curr Opin Crit Care* 16:323–331, 2010.
24. Weiner DI, Verlander JW: Role of NH3 and NH4 transporters in renal acid-base transport, *AJP Renal Physiol* 300:11–23, 2011.
25. Hamm LL, Hering-Smith KS, Nakhoul NL: Acid-base and potassium homeostasis, *Semin Nephrol* 33(3):257–264, 2013.
26. Da Poian AT, El-Bacha T, Luz M: Nutrient utilization in humans: metabolism pathways, *Nature Education* 3(9):11, 2010.
27. Nakamura K, Inokuchi R, Doi K, et al.: Septic ketoacidosis, *Internal Med* 53(10):1071–1073, 2014.
28. Reddy P, Mooradian AD: Clinical utility of anion gap in deciphering acid-base disorders, *Int J Clin Pract* 63(10):1516–1525, 2009.
29. Moviat M: Stewart analysis of apparently normal acid-base state in the critically ill, *J Crit Care* 28 (6):1048–1054, 2013.
30. Finfer S: Clinical controversies in the management of critically ill patients with severe sepsis: resuscitation fluids and glucose control, *Virulence* 5(1):200–205, 2014.
31. Balasubramanyan N, Havens PL, Hoffman GM: Unmeasured anions identified by the Fencl-Stewart method predict mortality better than base excess, anion gap, and lactate in patients in the pediatric intensive care unit, *Crit Care Med* 27:1577–1581, 1999.
32. Kishen R, Honore PM, Jacobs R, et al.: Facing acid-base disorders in the third millennium - the Stewart approach revisited, *Int J Nephrol Renovasc Dis* 7:209–217, 2014.
33. Hughes R, Brain MJ: A simplified bedside approach to acid–base: fluid physiology utilizing classical and physicochemical approaches, *Anaesthesia Intensive Care Med* 14(10):445–452, 2013.

Venous Oxygen Saturation Monitoring

7

Barbara "Bobbi" Leeper

In recent years, with the aging of the population, many patients in critical care have multiple comorbidities complicating their medical condition that resulted in the hospital admission. Additionally, patients in the adult critical care unit have much higher risks of adverse events, death, or both. One of the primary contributors to these adverse events or death is when a critical illness or injury compromises the cardiopulmonary system, including oxygen delivery to tissues and the cellular uptake and utilization of oxygen. Several pathophysiologic events may contribute to global or tissue hypoxia and to patient demise.

For cells in the body to survive, the amount of oxygen delivered to tissues must be adequate to meet their metabolic demands. When demands exceed supply or supply is reduced, cells soon convert to anaerobic metabolism and begin to accumulate an oxygen debt, which is associated with increased adverse events and mortality. Unfortunately, our traditional measures for assessing tissue oxygenation, including vital signs and urine output, have been shown to be poor indicators of ongoing tissue hypoxia.[1] This chapter covers the basics of oxygen delivery and consumption and the two parameters (mixed venous oxygen saturation and central venous oxygen saturation) used to provide information about the balance between oxygen delivery and oxygen demand at the cellular level.

Physiology of Oxygen Delivery and Consumption

Gas Exchange in the Lungs

The primary purpose of the cardiopulmonary system is to regulate the transport of carbon dioxide (CO_2) and oxygen (O_2) to and from the tissues. The pulmonary system is responsible for gas exchange (CO_2 and O_2) in the alveoli and at the tissue level (respiration). The movement of oxygen and carbon dioxide across the alveolar membrane occurs by diffusion, moving from an area of high partial pressure and concentration to an area of low partial pressure and concentration. In the lungs, the alveolar partial pressure of oxygen (PO_2) is approximately 100 mm Hg compared with a PO_2 of 40 mm Hg in venous blood returning to the lungs. This difference creates a pressure gradient contributing to the diffusion of oxygen across the alveolar capillary membrane into blood. The partial pressure of carbon dioxide (PCO_2) is approximately 46 mm Hg in venous blood and 40 mm Hg in the alveolus. This pressure gradient contributes to the movement of carbon dioxide from venous blood across the alveolar capillary membrane into the alveolus.

At the tissue level, gas exchange is reversed. By the time arterial blood reaches tissues, the PO_2 of the capillary blood is approximately 45 mm Hg compared with a PO_2 in the cells of 2 mm Hg. The pressure difference between the two values, drives the oxygen into the cells. In contrast, the PCO_2 in peripheral tissues is approximately 50 mm Hg and 40 mm Hg in the arterial blood entering the capillary system. This pressure gradient drives the CO_2 to diffuse into the capillaries. This process is very efficient. The amount of oxygen diffusing into the tissues and the amount of carbon dioxide released from the tissues are regulated by tissue activity, that is, the metabolic demands of the tissues. Figure 7-1 illustrates this process.

Oxygen Delivery

Oxygen delivery (DO_2) comprises three steps: (1) gas exchange at the alveolar–capillary bed in the lungs; (2) transport to tissues; and (3) cellular uptake of oxygen (O_2). Ninety-eight percent of the oxygen diffusing across the alveolar capillary membrane combines with hemoglobin to form oxyhemoglobin. One gram (g) of hemoglobin that is fully saturated, that is, all of the binding sites have O_2 molecules attached to them, carries 1.38 milliliters (mL) of oxygen.

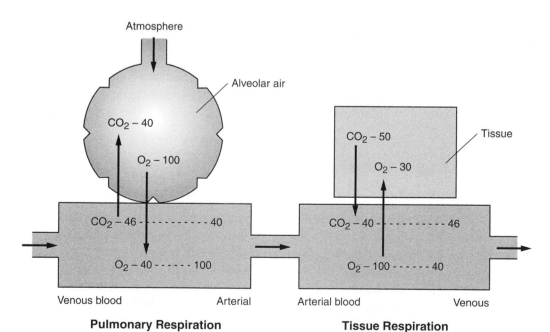

FIGURE 7-1 Exchange of oxygen and carbon dioxide in the lungs and tissues. (Courtesy of Edwards LifeSciences.)

The saturation of arterial oxygen (SaO_2) is a reflection of the percentage of hemoglobin binding sites carrying oxygen. The amount of hemoglobin bound oxygen (HbO_2) known as oxyhemoglobin, is calculated by using the following equation:[2]

$$HbO_2 = Hb \times 1.38 \times SaO_2$$

The remaining 2% of the oxygen that has diffused across the alveolar capillary membrane is dissolved in blood serum. Measurement of this is reflected in the PO_2 in the arterial blood (PaO_2) in mm Hg. The total dissolved volume is calculated using the following equation:

$$\text{Dissolved } O_2 = PaO_2 \times 0.0031$$

Arterial oxygen content (CaO_2) reflects the amount of oxygen in the arterial blood. Contributors to CaO_2 include Hb, SaO_2, and the partial pressure of arterial oxygen (PaO_2). The calculation of this volume is based on the following equation:

$$CaO_2 \text{ mL/Liter of blood} = Hb \times 1.38 \times (SaO_2 + PaO_2) \times 0.0031$$

However, in clinical practice, most clinicians will only include the bulk transport of oxygen, that is, the amount being transported by Hb because the dissolved oxygen represents only a small amount of the total oxygen being transported in the body.[3]

DO_2 is defined as the total amount of oxygen delivered to the tissues in 1 minute. Key components of DO_2 include the Hb, SaO_2, and cardiac output (CO) (Figure 7-2). Arterial oxygen delivery is calculated by the following:

$$DO_2 \text{ mL/min} = Hb \times 1.38 \times SaO_2 \times CO \times 10$$

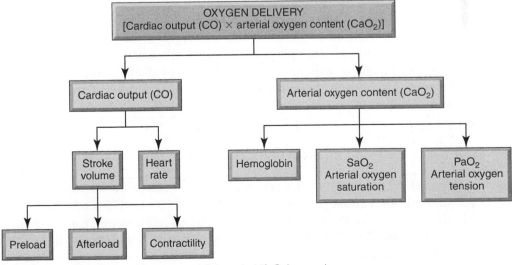

FIGURE 7-2 Oxygen delivery. (Courtesy of Edwards LifeSciences.)

Ten is the multiplier used to convert the CaO_2 from milliliter per liter (mL/L) to milliliter per minute (mL/min). Normally, 1000 mL/min of oxygen is delivered to tissues. If a value based on body size is required, substitute cardiac index (CI) for cardiac output in the equation above.

Venous Oxygen Content

Venous oxygen content is the amount of oxygen remaining in the bloodstream after the blood passes through tissues. At rest the tissues extract approximately 25% of the delivered oxygen at the cellular level, leaving approximately 75% remaining in venous blood. Mixed venous oxygen saturation (SvO_2), the oxygen saturation of the blood in the pulmonary artery, is used to calculate this amount:

$$\text{Venous oxygen content mL/min} = Hb \times 1.38 \times SvO_2 \times CO \times 10$$

Approximately 750 mL/min of oxygen remains in venous blood as it returns to the right atrium. This, too, can be indexed to body size using the CI.

The venous oxygen content represents the oxygen reserve for the body. If demand increases or if delivery is decreased, the body compensates by increasing oxygen extraction at the cellular level. Instead of extracting 25%, the cells may extract 40% or more, depending on the situation. The greater the volume of oxygen extracted by the cells, the less remaining in the venous blood causing the venous oxygen content to be lower.

Oxygen Consumption

Oxygen consumption (VO_2) is commonly used to refer to oxygen extraction. It is defined as the amount of oxygen consumed by the cells in 1 minute. As stated previously, this is normally 25% of oxygen delivery while at rest. Direct measurement of VO_2 in a critically ill patient may be difficult depending on the condition of the patient. For the patient who is intubated and on a ventilator, a gas analyzer can be inserted as an attachment between the endotracheal tube and the ventilator. The gas analyzer obtains physiologic measurements to calculate VO_2. This process is often referred to as using a "metabolic cart" and is not available in many facilities. A more common approach is to obtain mixed venous (SvO_2) blood gas samples from the pulmonary artery with a pulmonary artery catheter in place. Therefore, VO_2 is calculated by using:

$$VO_2 \text{ mL/min} = CO\,(SaO_2 - SvO_2) \times Hb \times 1.38 \times 10$$

Normal VO_2 is 200 to 250 mL/min or, as before, the cardiac index may be substituted for cardiac output so that VO_2 is 125 to 175 mL/min/m^2. Refer to Figure 7-3 depicting the process of oxygen delivery, consumption, and venous oxygen transport. Table 7-1 reflects the calculations and normal values for all these parameters using both CO and CI.

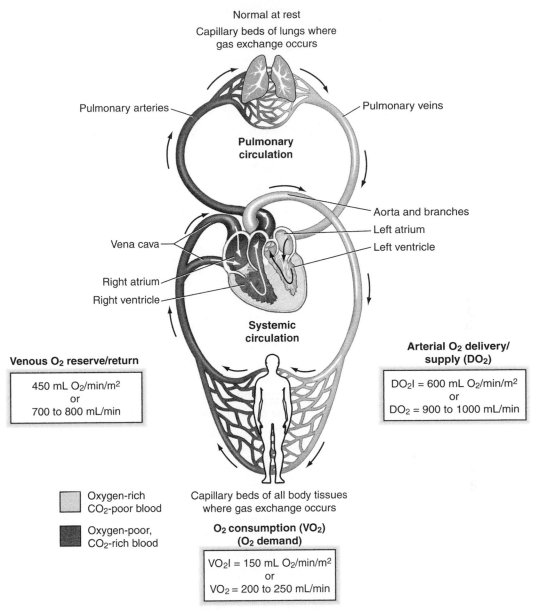

FIGURE 7-3 Normal oxygen supply–demand balance at rest.

Mixed Venous Oxygen Saturation

Mixed venous oxygen saturation monitoring requires the placement of a fiberoptic pulmonary artery catheter (PAC). Refer to Figure 7-4. SvO_2 can be monitored continuously using a fiberoptic PAC or, if a standard PAC is used, blood samples from the

TABLE 7-1	Normal Values	
PARAMETER	**EQUATION**	**NORMAL RANGE**
Arterial oxygen content (CaO_2)	$Hb \times 1.38 \times (SaO_2 + PaO_2) \times 0.0031$	16-22 mL/dL
Oxygen delivery (DO_2)	$Hb \times 1.38 \times SaO_2 \times CO \times 10$ $Hb \times 1.38 \times SaO_2 \times CI \times 10$	DO_2: 1000 mL/min DO_2I: 500-600 mL/min/m^2
Venous oxygen content	$Hb \times 1.38 \times SvO_2 \times CO \times 10$ $Hb \times 1.38 \times SvO_2 \times CI \times 10$	750 mL /min
Oxygen consumption (VO_2)	$CO\,(SaO_2 - SvO_2) \times Hb \times 1.38 \times 10$ $CI\,(SaO_2 - SvO_2) \times Hb \times 1.38 \times 10$	VO_2: 200-250 mL/min VO_2I: 120-160 mL/min/m^2
Mixed venous oxygen saturation (SvO_2)		60%-80%

CI, Cardiac index; *CO*, cardiac output; *Hb*, hemoglobin; *PaO₂*, partial pressure of arterial oxygen; *SaO₂*, saturation of arterial oxygen.

pulmonary artery may be obtained from the distal port of the catheter providing intermittent measurements. Continuous SvO_2 monitoring with a fiberoptic PAC uses reflectance spectrophotometry technology. When connected to the SvO_2 monitor, a light source from the optical module is transmitted to the tip of the PAC, where the oxyhemoglobin molecules absorb the light and reflect it back through the PAC to the light detector (photodetector) within the optical module. Refer to Figure 7-5.

Intermittent SvO_2 measurements require obtaining mixed venous blood samples. The blood is drawn from the distal port of the PAC. It is important that the blood sample be withdrawn slowly to avoid obtaining arterialized blood that will overestimate the SvO_2 value. The obtained blood gas sample should be managed using the same methods as an arterial blood gas sample. The mixed venous blood gas should be measured using a co-oximeter in the laboratory. If the co-oximeter laboratory value of measured SvO_2 varies by more than 5% from the value reflected on the SvO_2 monitor, the bedside PAC fiberoptic system should be recalibrated.

SvO_2 provides information about the venous oxygen content, indicating the amount of oxygen remaining in blood after it has passed through the tissues. Therefore, it provides information about the oxygen reserve reflecting the balance between oxygen supply and oxygen demand at the cellular level. SvO_2 is considered a global parameter. It does not provide specific information about oxygen balance within a particular organ or system but, instead, is reflective of the overall balance between oxygen supply and demand. Of interest, clinicians believed SvO_2 might serve as in indicator of cardiac output and therefore, it was often referred to as a "poor man's cardiac output." Through years of use, it has been shown that the correlation of SvO_2 with cardiac output is not reliable because oxygen delivery may be impacted by changes in hemoglobin, arterial oxygen saturation and oxygen consumption.[3,4] Refer to the first case study at the end of the chapter for a demonstration of a low cardiac output in the setting of a normal SvO_2.

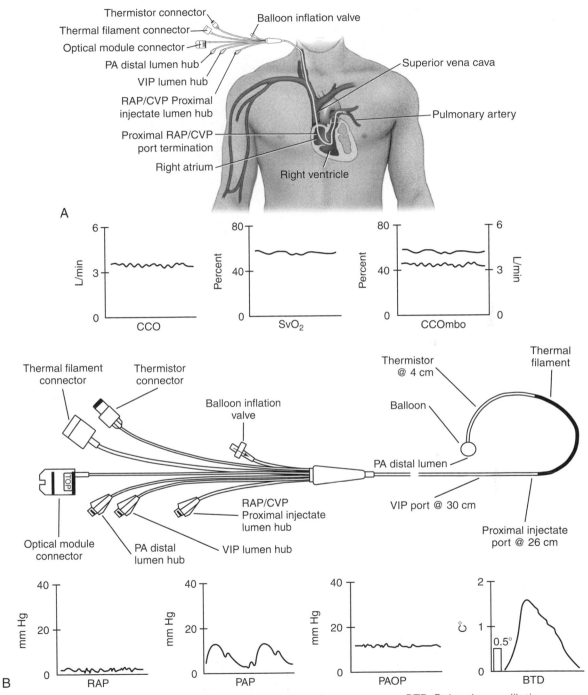

FIGURE 7-4 Fiberoptic pulmonary artery catheter in the pulmonary artery. *BTD,* Bolus thermodilution; *C°,* Centigrade; *CCO,* continuous cardiac output; *CCOmbo,* combination CCO and SvO$_2$; *cm,* centimeters; *CO,* cardiac output; *L/min,* liters per minute; *mm Hg,* millimeters of mercury; *PA,* pulmonary artery; *PAOP,* pulmonary artery occlusion pressure; *PAP,* pulmonary artery pressure; *RAP,* right atrial pressure; *SvO$_2$,* mixed venous oxygen saturation; *VIP,* venous infusion port. (Part B Courtesy of Edwards LifeSciences.)

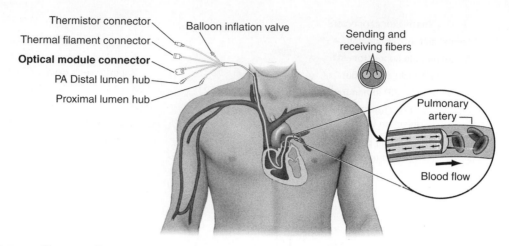

FIGURE 7-5 Two-way fiberoptic transmission of light through the pulmonary artery catheter in the pulmonary artery.

A normal SvO_2 range is 60% to 80%. However, a normal SvO_2 may not be a reliable indicator of the patient's demand–supply balance. Case study #1 reflects this situation. It is more important to monitor the SvO_2 trend. Specifically, a clinically significant change in the SvO_2 is present when the SvO_2 value increases or decreases by 5% to 10% lasting longer than 3 to 5 minutes.

Specific determinants of SvO_2 include the three components of DO_2 and VO_2. (See Figure 7-6.) A change in any one of these components may be associated with a change in the SvO_2. Although, keep in mind that the body uses compensatory mechanisms to

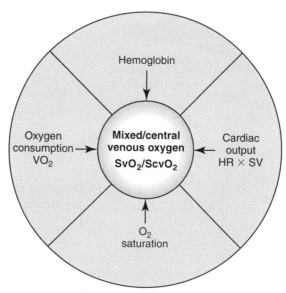

FIGURE 7-6 Determinants of saturation of venous oxygen.

respond to pathophysiologic conditions and the anticipated response may not always be present. Generally, a decrease in the SvO_2 indicates more oxygen is being extracted at the cellular level. This situation is caused by any condition that decreases oxygen delivery or increases oxygen demand reflecting an increase in VO_2. An increase in the SvO_2 indicates that less oxygen is being extracted. This may be caused by interventions to increase oxygen delivery or reduce oxygen demand. SvO_2 will also increase with end-stage sepsis when the microcirculation is impaired thereby interfering with cellular gas exchange. SvO_2 will increase when a pulmonary artery catheter is "wedged," purposefully or when spontaneous migration of the PAC occurs; the SvO_2 value will increase abruptly by approximately 10% to 20%. See Figure 7-7. This is caused by the obstruction of blood flow through the vessel and the fiberoptics "looking" at blood that has participated in gas exchange. It is extremely important that the pulmonary artery waveform be monitored continuously for the purpose of identifying if the catheter has migrated further out into the vessel and is occluding blood flow, as this may result in a pulmonary infarction. The abrupt increase in the digital SvO_2 reading has often served as the first indicator of spontaneous wedging in a critically ill patient. Table 7-2 provides a summary of clinical situations that may cause changes in the SvO_2. When the SvO_2 is changing, it is important for the clinician to assess the patient for all factors that potentially impact the SvO_2 value.

Oxygen Extraction Ratio

Oxygen extraction ratio (O_2ER) represents the percentage of oxygen delivery extracted by tissues as blood flows through the capillary bed. It can be expressed as follows:

$$O_2ER = VO_2 \div DO_2$$

Another method to estimate the O_2ER is by by simply calculating $SaO_2 - SvO_2$. As stated previously, normally, 25% of the oxygen is extracted when a person is at rest.

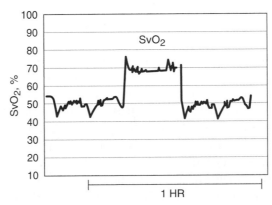

FIGURE 7-7 Effect of pulmonary artery catheter wedge pressure on the saturation of venous oxygen (SvO_2) value.

TABLE 7-2   Examples of Clinical Situations That May Impact the Saturation of Venous Oxygen (SvO$_2$)

Decreasing SvO$_2$

DECREASED OXYGEN DELIVERY	INCREASED OXYGEN DEMANDS
↓ Cardiac output	Seizures, shivering
↓ Hemoglobin	Pain, hyperthermia
↓ Arterial oxygen saturation	↑ Activity levels

Increasing SvO$_2$

INCREASED OXYGEN DELIVERY	DECREASED OXYGEN DEMANDS
↑ Fraction of inspired oxygen (FiO$_2$)	Hypothermia
Administration of blood products	Anesthesia
↑ Cardiac output	Relief of pain

Abrupt increase in SvO$_2$ value: assess waveform for spontaneous "wedging" of pulmonary artery catheter.

If DO$_2$ falls or demand increases, a larger percentage is extracted as a compensatory mechanism. The normal range for O$_2$ER is 22% to 30%. If O$_2$ER is greater than 30%, this indicates that an imbalance exists between supply and demand and that the metabolic requirements of tissues are not being met. An O$_2$ER of less than 22% indicates that the metabolic demands are being met or patient is in the end stage of septic shock. Table 7-3 demonstrates the impact of activities and clinical conditions on the O$_2$ER.

Imbalance between Oxygen Delivery and Oxygen Consumption

Typically, the body will initiate compensatory mechanisms whenever an imbalance exists between oxygen supply and demand. The first mechanism is mediated through activation of the sympathetic system, causing an increase in heart rate and myocardial contractility resulting in an increased cardiac output. Cardiac output may increase up to three to five times the normal value in this situation. The second compensatory mechanism is autoregulation, which is manifested by peripheral vasoconstriction and redistribution of blood flow to the vital organs. Keep in mind that if the patient is receiving sodium nitroprusside or is in hyperdynamic septic shock with a low systemic vascular resistance, this mechanism will be impaired. Last, the third mechanism is the increased oxygen extraction by the tissues increasing the O$_2$ER. Causes of DO$_2$-VO$_2$ imbalance are listed in Table 7-4. Table 7-5 provides information about the impact of some nursing interventions on DO$_2$ and VO$_2$.

TABLE 7-3 Impact of Determinants of Oxygen Delivery (DO_2) on Oxygen Extraction Ratio (O_2ER)

CLINICAL EXAMPLE	COMPONENT VALUES	DO_2	OXYGEN CONSUMPTION (VO_2)	O_2ER
Normal	CO: 5 L/min SaO_2: 98% Hb:15 g SvO_2: 75%	$CO \times Hb \times 1.38 \times 10 \times SaO_2$ $= 5 \times 15 \times 1.38 \times 10 \times 0.98$ $= 1014\,mL\,O_2/min$	$CO \times Hb \times 1.38 \times 10\,(SaO_2 - SvO_2)$ $= 5 \times 15 \times 1.38 \times 10\,(0.98 \times 0.75)$ $= 238\,mL\,O_2/min$	24%
With exercise	CO: 20 L/min SaO_2: 98% Hb: 15 g SvO_2: 60%	$CO \times Hb \times 1.38 \times 10 \times SaO_2$ $= 20 \times 15 \times 1.38 \times 0.98 \times 10$ $= 4057\,mL\,O_2/min$	$CO \times Hb \times 1.38 \times 10\,(SaO_2 - SvO_2)$ $= 20 \times 15 \times 1.38 \times 10\,(0.98 - 0.60)$ $= 1573\,mL\,O_2/min$	39%
Hypoxia	CO: 5 L/min SaO_2: 85% Hb: 15 g SvO_2: 60%	$CO \times Hb \times 1.38 \times 10 \times SaO_2$ $= 5 \times 15 \times 1.38 \times 10 \times 0.85$ $= 880\,mL\,O_2/min$	$CO \times Hb \times 1.38 \times 10\,(SaO_2 - SvO_2)$ $= 5 \times 15 \times 1.38 \times 10\,(0.85 - 0.60)$ $= 259\,mL\,O_2/min$	29%
Anemia	CO: 5 L/min SaO_2: 98% Hb: 8 g/dL SvO_2: 50%	$CO \times Hb \times 1.38 \times SaO_2 \times 10$ $= 5 \times 8 \times 1.38 \times 10 \times 0.98$ $= 540\,mL\,O_2/min$	$CO \times Hb \times 1.38 \times 10\,(SaO_2 - SvO_2)$ $= 5 \times 8 \times 1.38 \times 10\,(0.98 - 0.50)$ $= 265\,mL\,O_2/min$	49%
Ventricular failure	CO: 1.6 L/min SaO_2: 98% Hb: 15 g SvO_2: 31%	$CO \times Hb \times 1.38 \times 10 \times SaO_2$ $= 1.6 \times 15 \times 1.38 \times 10 \times 0.98$ $= 325\,mL\,O_2/min$	$CO \times Hb \times 13.8\,(SaO_2 - SvO_2)$ $= 1.6 \times 15 \times 1.38 \times 10\,(0.98 - 0.31)$ $= 222\,mL\,O_2/min$	68%
Severe sepsis	CO: 15 L/min SaO_2: 98% Hb: 15 g SvO_2: 88%	$CO \times Hb \times 1.38 \times 10 \times SaO_2$ $= 15 \times 15 \times 1.38 \times 10 \times 0.98$ $= 3043\,mL\,O_2/min$	$CO \times Hb \times 1.38 \times 10\,(SaO_2 - SvO_2)$ $= 15 \times 15 \times 1.38 \times 10\,(0.98 - 0.88)$ $= 311\,mL\,O_2/min$	10%

CO, Cardiac output; *g*, gram; *g/dL*, grams per deciliter; *Hb*, hemoglobin; *L/min*, liters per minute; *mL O_2/min*, milliliters of oxygen per minute; *SaO_2*, saturation of arterial oxygen; *SvO_2*, saturation of venous oxygen.
Courtesy of Edwards Lifesciences.

TABLE 7-4   Causes of Imbalance between Oxygen Delivery (DO_2) and Oxygen Consumption (VO_2)

DECREASED SUPPLY (↓ DO_2):	INCREASED DEMAND (↑ VO_2 and ↑ O_2ER)
Inadequate pulmonary gas exchange (↓ SaO_2)	Surgical trauma: 10% to 30%
Inadequate oxygen carrying capacity (↓ Hb)	Severe sepsis: 50% to 100%
Inadequate cardiac output (↓ CO)	Critically ill in the emergency department: 60%
Leftward shift of oxyhemoglobin dissociation curve	Head injury, not sedated: 138% Head Injury, sedated: 89%
Loss of autoregulation	Severe burns: 100%

CO, Cardiac output; *Hb*, hemoglobin; *O_2ER*, oxygen extraction ratio; *SaO_2*, saturation of arterial oxygen.

TABLE 7-5   Additional Clinical Factors in the Critical Care Unit that Increases Oxygen Demands

ACTIVITY	PERCENT INCREASE IN DEMAND
Dressing change	10%
Bath	23%
Position change (each time)	31%
Work of breathing	40%
Shivering	50%–100%
Endotracheal suctioning	27%–70%
Chest radiography	25%
Weight on a sling scale	36%
Agitation	16%
Getting out of bed	39%
Body temperature: 10%–13% ↑ in oxygen demand per degree Centigrade rise in temperature above normal	
MEDICATIONS	
Norepinephrine (0.10–0.31 mcg/kg/min)	10%–21%
Dopamine (5 mcg/kg/min)	6%
Dopamine (10 mcg/kg/min)	15%
Dobutamine	19%
Epinephrine (0.10 mcg/kg/min)	23%–29%

mcg/kg/min, Microgram per kilogram per minute.

Monitoring Technical Issues in Saturation of Venous Oxygen

Calibration

Ideally, the SvO_2 monitor should be plugged in and turned on prior to the insertion of the PAC, allowing the system to warm up. An in vitro or preinsertion calibration should be performed prior to insertion. The purpose is to standardize or calibrate the light source to the catheter.[5] This is done by attaching the optical module to the monitoring cable, keeping the rest of the catheter intact within the sterile package. The tip of the PAC is positioned in a calibration cup within the sterile section of the package. Once this calibration is performed, the PAC is flushed and prepared for insertion. Note that if the clinical situation requires emergent insertion of the fiberoptic PAC, it is not necessary to perform an in vitro calibration prior to insertion. Once the catheter is in the correct position and if time permits, an in vivo calibration is performed. Most manufacturers recommend performing an in vitro calibration every 24 hours or if any doubt exists about the displayed SvO_2 value. The in vivo calibration verifies the accuracy of the computer and the displayed value on the SvO_2 monitor. It is recommended that the information regarding the hemoglobin level be updated if a change occurs (≥ 1.8 grams per deciliter [g/dL]; ≥ 1.1 millimoles per liter [mmol/L]) and hematocrit ($\geq 6\%$). A change in hemoglobin may also affect the quality of the signal. Some manufacturers provide for a hemoglobin update to resolve problems with the signal quality.

Performing an in vitro calibration requires drawing a mixed venous blood sample from the distal port of the PAC. The rate of the blood draw should be slow, at a rate of 2 mL over 30 seconds. Drawing the sample too rapidly may result in aspiration of air into the barrel of the syringe, which would contribute to overestimation of the measured SvO_2 value. Also, too rapid drawing of the sample may result in obtaining some arterialized blood in the sample, again contributing to overestimation of the measured value.

Signal Quality or Light Intensity

The signal quality or light intensity verifies that the reflection of the light signals is adequate.[5] If the tip of the catheter is positioned against the wall of the pulmonary artery, which is white, the intensity will be high, overestimating the SvO_2. If the catheter becomes kinked, the emission of the light will be interrupted causing the signal to be too low.

Dysfunctional Hemoglobins

Carboxyhemoglobin and methemoglobinemia will cause abnormal SvO_2 values. Carbon monoxide binds 240 times faster to the hemoglobin molecule forming carboxyhemoglobin and will produce an overestimation of the SvO_2. Methemoglobinemia may be caused by anesthetic agents (e.g., benzocaine); nitric oxide; and some medications, including sodium nitroprusside, nitroglycerine, sulfonamides, and some antibiotics.[6] Again, the SvO_2 value could be overestimated. This emphasizes the importance of using a co-oximeter for the measurement of all blood gases, regardless of the origin of the sample.

Clinical Applications of Monitoring of Saturation of Venous Oxygen

Bleeding

Hemoglobin is an important component of oxygen delivery, since it carries approximately 98% of the oxygen being transported to the tissues. If bleeding occurs, heart rate increases to maintain an adequate cardiac output. Table 7-3 demonstrates the impact of low hemoglobin on the oxygen demand–supply balance. In the clinical setting, an SvO_2 less than 50% and tachycardia are often the earliest clues to hemorrhage. Refer to the second case study at the end of the chapter for an example of this situation.

Pulmonary Issues

Application of positive end-expiratory pressure (PEEP) in patients on mechanical ventilation is for the purpose of improving the patient's hypoxemia. The application of PEEP may be associated with a decline in cardiac output. Subsequently, the SvO_2 may fall. This occurs because the increased intrathoracic pressure associated with the PEEP is transmitted to the vessels and increases myocardial afterload. The cardiac output falls as a result. Figure 7-8 is an example of this clinical situation.

Patient position may be associated with a change in the SvO_2. Figure 7-9 demonstrates the falling SvO_2 when the patient was turned. The lower SvO_2 value could reflect the increase in oxygen demand with the change in position. This also may reflect

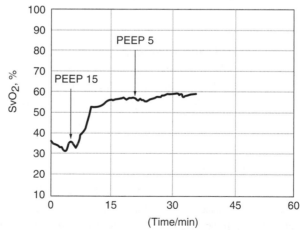

FIGURE 7-8 Changes in the Saturation of Venous Oxygen (SvO_2) with Positive End-Expiratory Pressure (PEEP). Higher levels of PEEP (15 cm) are associated with lower levels of SvO_2. By decreasing the amount of PEEP added to the ventilator, cardiac output and oxygen delivery are increased, thus meeting the metabolic demands of the tissues. (From Fahey PJ: Continuous measurement of blood oxygen saturation in the high risk patient: Theory and practice in monitoring mixed venous oxygen saturation (vol 2), San Diego, 1985, Beach International Inc., p. 22.)

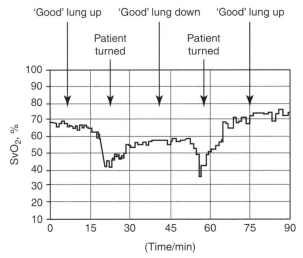

FIGURE 7-9 Effect of Turning a Patient on the Saturation of Venous Oxygen (SvO₂) Value. Initially the healthy "good lung" is uppermost and SvO₂ is approximately 65%-68%. When the patient is turned to the other side and the "good lung" is in a dependent position, the SvO₂ falls to 55-58%. About 30 minutes later when the patient is repositioned so that the "good lung" is uppermost, and gas exchange and perfusion are matched, the SvO₂ increases to 70%-75%.

that the "good lung" was down. The "good lung" is a term used to describe a lung that has effective gas exchange whereas the "bad lung" has impaired gas exchange which may be caused by a variety of factors including single-lung atelectasis, pneumonia or contusions from trauma. When the patient is turned on their side, so that the healthy "good" lung is upward, gas exchange and perfusion are matched and the SvO₂ value rises. When the patient is turned on the opposite side where the healthy "good" lung is downward, the resulting mismatch between good perfusion and poor gas exchange causes SvO₂ to decline as seen in Figure 7-9. This would be a clinical indication for the clinician to increase the patient's fraction of inspired oxygen (FiO₂) briefly prior to turning. When the patient is repositioned with the good lung up, note the increase in the SvO₂ (Figure 7-9).

Ventricular Septum Perforation

The SvO₂ value is very helpful in the case of a patient who has had an anteroseptal myocardial infarction and subsequently perforation of the intraventricular septum. This dreaded complication is diagnosed by looking for an "oxygen step-up" as the pulmonary artery catheter is advanced from the right atrium into the right ventricle. Normally, the oxygen saturation of the venous blood in the right atrium and right ventricle is 60% to 80%. If a perforated intraventricular septum is present, right ventricular blood will have an oxygen saturation that is much higher than that in the right atrium. Figure 7-10 is an example of the oxygen "step-up" associated with ventricular septal rupture.

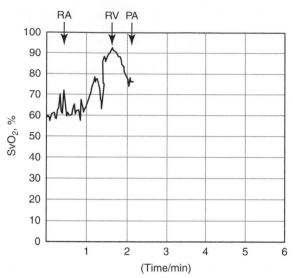

FIGURE 7-10 Oxygen Step-Up Associated with Perforated Intraventricular Septum. The oxygen saturation of the venous blood returning to the right atrium and right ventricle is normally 60% to 80%. Note the above oxygen saturation of the blood in the right atrium is 60%. As the pulmonary artery catheter is advanced across the tricuspid valve into the right ventricle, the oxygen saturation abruptly increases to 90%, which is a reflection of arterialized blood coming the a perforated ventricular septum into the right ventricle. (From Fahey PJ: Continuous measurement of blood oxygen saturation in the high risk patient: Theory and practice in monitoring mixed venous oxygen saturation (vol 2), San Diego, 1985, Beach International Inc., p. 22.)

Clinical Reasoning Pearl

- SvO_2 provides information about the balance between oxygen supply and oxygen demand in the body. The tissues extract approximately 25% of the delivered oxygen at the cellular level when the body is at rest. This leaves approximately 75% of the oxygen remaining in venous blood. The amount of oxygen remaining in venous blood represents the oxygen reserve for the body.

- If cellular oxygen demands increase or oxygen delivery is impaired, the tissues will extract a larger percentage, resulting in a smaller percentage of oxygen remaining in venous blood. A decline in the SvO_2 value indicates the cells are extracting a larger percentage of oxygen to sustain anaerobic metabolism. This represents an important compensatory mechanism. An increase in the SvO_2 value indicates less oxygen is being extracted. This situation may be caused by interventions to increase oxygen delivery or reduce O_2 demand.

- The Oxygen extraction ratio (O_2ER) represents the percentage of the oxygen extracted by the tissues as blood flows through the capillary bed. One method to estimate the O_2ER is calculating $SaO_2 - SvO_2$. If oxygen delivery decreases or tissue oxygen demand increases, a larger than normal percentage is extracted as a compensatory mechanism to meet the metabolic demands of the tissues. The normal range for the O_2ER is 22% to 30%. An O_2ER is greater than 30% indicates an imbalance between supply and demand and that the metabolic requirements of the tissues are not being met. An O_2ER of less than 22% indicates that the metabolic demands are being met or patient may be in the end stage of septic shock.

- If spontaneous migration of the PAC occurs, the SvO_2 value increases abruptly by approximately 10% to 20%. This increase is caused by the obstruction of blood flow through the vessel and the fiberoptics "looking" at arterialized blood that has participated in gas exchange. It is extremely important that the pulmonary artery (PA) waveform be monitored continuously for the purpose of identifying if the catheter has migrated further out into the vessel and is occluding blood flow, which may result in a pulmonary infarction. The abrupt increase in the digital SvO_2 value has often served as the first indicator of spontaneous wedging.

- In vitro calibration of the SvO_2 monitor should occur prior to insertion of the catheter. Most manufacturers recommend performing an in vivo calibration every 24 hours or when a question exists about the displayed value. Performing an in vivo calibration requires drawing a mixed venous blood sample from the distal port of the PAC. The rate of the blood draw should be slow, at a rate of 2 mL over 30 seconds. Drawing the sample too rapidly may result in aspiration of air into the barrel of the syringe, which would contribute to overestimation of the measured SvO_2 value. Also, too rapid drawing of the sample may result in obtaining some arterialized blood in the sample, again contributing to overestimation of the measured value.

- Carboxyhemoglobin and methemoglobinemia cause an abnormal SvO_2 value. Methemoglobinemias are caused by anesthetic agents (e.g., benzocaine); nitric oxide; and by some medications; including sodium nitroprusside, nitroglycerin, sulfonamides, and some antibiotics. The SvO_2 value could be overestimated, and this emphasizes the importance of using a co-oximeter for the measurement of all blood gases, regardless of the origin of the sample.

Central Venous Oxygen Saturation

Central venous oxygen saturation ($ScvO_2$) is the measurement of the oxygen saturation of the blood in the superior vena cava just above the right atrium. In recent years, this parameter has become clinically significant when used in a study demonstrating improvement in survival rates in patients with severe sepsis.[7] The investigator used a triple lumen central venous catheter that had been modified with fiberoptics providing a continuous $ScvO_2$ measurement. Studies have shown that the relationship between SvO_2 and $ScvO_2$ will vary depending on the health of the individual.[8–12] Mixed venous oxygen saturation reflects the total body SvO_2 of venous blood returning from all areas of the body, including the heart, whereas $ScvO_2$ reflects the oxygen saturation of venous blood returning from the head and upper extremities.[13] In healthy individuals the SvO_2 is higher than $ScvO_2$. The rationale for this is that the kidneys receive a larger proportion of the CO and use less oxygen, which causes more oxygen to return from the lower portion of the body and increases the oxygen saturation in the inferior vena cava. Figure 7-11 depicts the oxygen saturation of venous blood as it

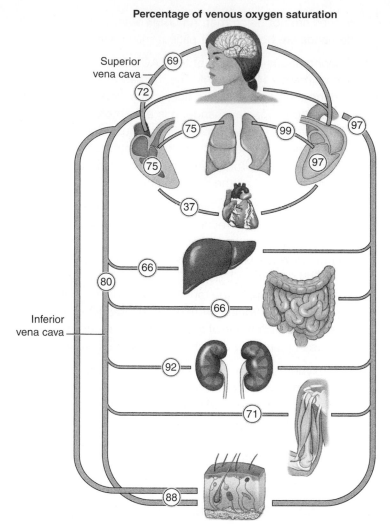

Percentage of venous oxygen saturation

FIGURE 7-11 This reflects the oxygen saturation of venous blood as it leaves various organs and returns to the right side of the heart. (Modified from Bloos F, Reinhart K: Venous oximetry, *Intensive Care Med* 31(7): 911–913, 2005.)

leaves various organs and returns to the right side of the heart.[13] However, in pathologic states, this relationship changes, and $ScvO_2$ is consistently higher than SvO_2 by 5% to 13%, the average being 7.5%. This is accounted for by the fact that blood is shunted to the brain and the heart in pathologic states, causing venous saturation in the inferior vena cava to be lower and resulting in a higher $ScvO_2$.

Although $ScvO_2$ and SvO_2 do not correlate in pathologic states, $ScvO_2$ has been shown to trend with SvO_2 (Figure 7-12) and is often being used as a surrogate for SvO_2. One must use caution when monitoring $ScvO_2$, as studies suggest that a low $ScvO_2$ indicates an even lower SvO_2.[13]

The clinical application of $ScvO_2$ monitoring is similar to that of SvO_2 monitoring. The components of oxygen delivery and oxygen consumption impact $ScvO_2$ in the

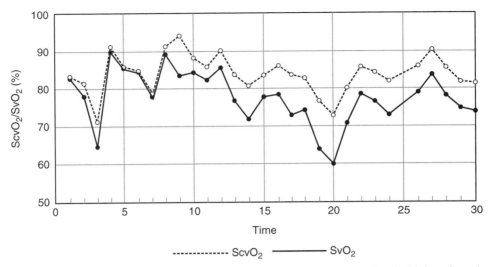

FIGURE 7-12 The central venous oxygen saturation (ScvO$_2$) value is slightly higher than the saturation of venous oxygen (SvO$_2$) value. Note that ScvO$_2$ trends in the same direction as SvO$_2$. (From Reinhart K, Eyrich K (eds.): *Clinical Aspects of O$_2$ Transport and Tissue Oxygenation*, Berlin, 1989, Springer.)

same manner as they do SvO$_2$. Blood must be drawn slowly from this distal port of the central venous catheter when obtaining a sample for laboratory measurement of central venous oxygen saturation.

Use of a femoral central venous catheter to monitor ScvO$_2$ is not valid. ScvO$_2$ and femoral venous oxygen saturation (SfvO$_2$) have been found to vary by more than 5%. Therefore, femoral-based venous oxygen saturation is not a reliable surrogate for ScvO$_2$.[14]

Central venous oxygen saturation has been used in a variety of clinical situations in addition to severe sepsis and septic shock. These include acutely decompensated heart failure, cardiac arrest and post-resuscitation following cardiac arrest, trauma, and hemorrhagic shock and in high-risk surgical patients.[15–18]

Relationships between Oxygen Delivery and Oxygen Consumption

Normally oxygen consumption is determined by the metabolic requirements of cells. If cellular demand increases, VO$_2$ increases. If cellular demand is reduced, VO$_2$ decreases. Therefore, oxygen consumption is independent of oxygen delivery. This is often referred to as *delivery-independent* or *supply-independent VO$_2$*. However, when oxygen delivery begins to fall, cells will extract a larger percentage of the available DO$_2$ as reflected in the O$_2$ER. As oxygen delivery continues to decline, the O$_2$ER will increase until the compensatory mechanisms fail to meet tissue requirements. This point has been called the "critical DO$_2$" or the "anaerobic threshold." At this point, the VO$_2$ follows the declining DO$_2$. This situation is referred to as *delivery-dependent* or *supply-dependent VO$_2$* and is associated with the onset of anaerobic metabolism and an increase in lactate production. Figure 7-13 depicts this situation.

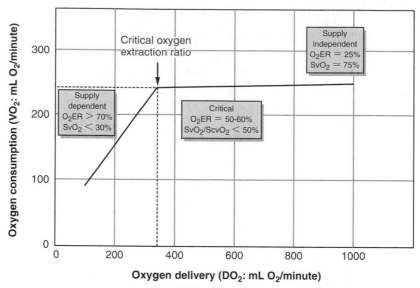

FIGURE 7-13 Conceptual Relationship between oxygen delivery (DO$_2$) and oxygen consumption (VO$_2$). As DO$_2$ falls, VO$_2$ is maintained for a period, but note that the oxygen extraction ratio (O$_2$ER) is increasing and the saturation of venous oxygen (SvO$_2$) is falling. When delivery falls below a critical point, VO$_2$ is driven by DO$_2$ and not by the metabolic demands of tissues. Management of this situation is to increase DO$_2$ (VO$_2$ will increase simultaneously) until the oxygen debt has been paid and the VO$_2$ "levels off" in spite of the increasing DO$_2$. (Modified from Nichols D, Nielsen N: Oxygen delivery and consumption: A macrocirculatory perspective, *Critical Care Clinics* 26(2): 239-253, 2010.)

Approaches to the management of supply dependent VO$_2$ are determined by the underlying pathologic condition of the patient. Successful efforts to increase oxygen delivery will be associated with a normalized VO$_2$ facilitating a return to oxygen delivery-independent consumption, where tissue oxygen demands drive VO$_2$. Many studies have examined therapeutic strategies to reverse delivery-dependent oxygen consumption. Early on, a few researchers focused on increasing DO$_2$ to supranormal levels with a cardiac index of 4.5 L/min/m², DO$_2$ of 600 mL/min/m² or greater, and VO$_2$ of 170 mL/min/m² or greater.[19] Although some of these studies were associated with reductions in mortality, other researchers were unable to replicate the results. More recently, researchers have demonstrated the effectiveness of intervening aggressively with goal-directed therapy in patients with severe sepsis or septic shock, as well as in high-risk surgical patients.[15–18]

Clinical Reasoning Pearl

- ScvO$_2$ also provides information about the balance between oxygen supply and oxygen demand in the body. Recall that the tissues extract approximately 25% of the delivered oxygen at the cellular level when the body is at rest. This leaves approximately 75% of the oxygen remaining in venous blood. The amount of oxygen remaining in venous blood represents the oxygen reserve for the body.

- If cellular oxygen demands increase or oxygen delivery is impaired, tissues will extract a larger percentage, which would result in a smaller percentage of oxygen remaining in venous blood. If the $ScvO_2$ values decline, this indicates that cells are extracting a larger percentage of oxygen to sustain anaerobic metabolism. This represents an important compensatory mechanism. An increase in the $ScvO_2$ indicates that less oxygen is being extracted. This situation may be caused by interventions to increase oxygen delivery or reduce oxygen demand.

- As was seen with SvO_2, the oxygen extraction ratio (O_2ER represents the percentage of the oxygen extracted by tissues as blood flows through the capillary beds. The O_2ER may also be estimated by using the equation: SaO_2-ScvO_2.

- In vitro calibration of the $ScvO_2$ monitor should occur prior to insertion of the catheter. Most manufacturers recommend performing an in vivo calibration every 24 hours or when a question exists about the displayed value. Performing an in vivo calibration requires drawing a central venous blood sample from the distal port of the central venous catheter. The rate of the blood draw should be slow, at a rate of 2 mL over 30 seconds. Drawing the sample too rapidly may result in aspiration of air into the barrel of the syringe, or pulling venous blood returning from the coronary sinus. Aspiration of air will result in the overestimation of $ScvO_2$. Venous blood from the coronary sinus will cause underestimation of $ScvO_2$ value.

- Carboxyhemoglobin and methemoglobinemia may cause unreliable $ScvO_2$ values, as seen with SvO_2. The $ScvO_2$ value could be overestimated, and this emphasizes the importance of using a co-oximeter for the measurement of all blood gases, regardless of the origin of the sample.

- If $ScvO_2$ is being used as part of the resuscitation for patients with severe sepsis or septic shock, the recommended resuscitation target is a value greater than 70%.

Case Study #1
Normal Saturation of Venous Oxygen with Low Cardiac Output

A 72-year-old female with insulin-dependent diabetes, renal insufficiency, and coronary artery disease underwent coronary artery bypass × 5. Coming off cardiopulmonary bypass surgery, she experienced an anaphylactic response when given protamine to reverse the heparin. Postoperatively, she had an intra-aortic balloon pump (IABP) with 1:1 assist, with continuous infusions of dopamine 2.5 micrograms per kilogram per minute (mcg/kg/min), epinephrine 0.02 mcg/kg/min, and dobutamine 5.0 mcg/kg/min. The following morning (08:00), she was maintained on mechanical ventilation and sedation. The IABP remained on 1:1 augmentation.

Continued

Case Study #1
Normal Saturation of Venous Oxygen with Low Cardiac Output—cont'd

PARAMETERS	08:00	16:00
Heart rate (beats/min)	95	98
Respiratory rate (ventilator rate)	10	10
Blood pressure (mm Hg)	94/56	95/58
PA (mm Hg)	45/20	42/18
PA occlusion pressure (PAOP) (mm Hg)	20	18
RAP/CVP (mm Hg)	10	10
CO (L/min)	1.4	2.2
CI (L/min/m^2)	0.8	1.4
SvO$_2$	72%	56%
SaO$_2$	97%	97%
Systemic vascular resistance (SVR) (dynes·sec/cm^5)	3000	1450
DO$_2$ (L/min)	169	261
VO$_2$ (mL/min)	45	115
O$_2$ER	27%	44%
Hb (g)	9	9

At 08:00, note that her SvO$_2$ is normal in spite of the extremely low cardiac output, and cardiac index, and DO$_2$. She is maximally vasoconstricted, as indicated by her very high systemic vascular resistance (SVR). The intense vasoconstriction undoubtedly limited tissue perfusion, so that oxygen was not extracted from the microcirculation; this may account for the normal SvO$_2$, for the very low VO$_2$, and the normal O$_2$ER. An additional concern was the impact of the high SVR on her myocardial workload, which contributed to her low cardiac output and cardiac index. The decision was made to initiate a sodium nitroprusside infusion at 0.2 mcg/kg/min.

By 16:00, her SVR level was decreased by half, effectively reducing the myocardial workload, improving contractility, and increasing cardiac output, cardiac index, and DO$_2$ while maintaining the same blood pressure. Note the lower SvO$_2$ at 56%. Although this value is lower than the normal range, it is acceptable on the basis that she is now vasodilated and

Case Study #1
Normal Saturation of Venous Oxygen with Low Cardiac Output—cont'd

has improved tissue perfusion, with increased oxygen extraction reflected by the higher VO_2 and O_2ER.

This is an example of how the SvO_2 does not always mirror the cardiac output and cardiac index. In this situation, at 08:00, the normal SvO_2 validated the poor tissue perfusion. Later, at 16:00, the SvO_2 reflected the high oxygen uptake at the tissue level as the cells attempted to make up their oxygen debt. ◼

Case Study #2
Occult Bleeding

A 57-year-old male was admitted to the critical care unit following coronary artery bypass × 3. He had no significant preoperative history of hypertension, left ventricular failure, chronic obstructive pulmonary disease (COPD), or valvular abnormality. The initial readings are taken 4 hours following surgery. The patient is receiving sodium nitroprusside 0.5 mcg/kg/min.

PARAMETERS	14:00	15:00	16:00	15:00	15:40	16:00
Temperature (°C)	35.3	35.8	36.8	38.4	38.8	38.6
Heart rate	96	98	120	128	132	116
Blood pressure	137/80	144/77	102/51	120/50	48/23	100/55
PA	24/17	23/16	29/19	28/15	—	22/13
PAOP	16	—	14	—	—	—
RAP /CVP	12	10	14	12	—	12
CO	3.9	6.4	7.4	6.7	—	5.5
CI	1.7	2.8	3.0	2.8	—	2.3
SvO_2	64%	58%	42%	44%	38%	50%
SVR	1380	1118	625	604	—	1292

The climbing HR and the downward trending of SvO_2 were the signs that indicated the patient was bleeding, even though the chest tube drainage was not significant. At 15:40, the surgeon was called to the bedside, the chest was opened, and an occult bleed was found. ◼

Patient Safety

- ### SvO$_2$ Monitoring:

  - Monitor the PA waveform for spontaneous migration and "wedging." The waveform will abruptly change from a PA waveform to a PAOP waveform.

  - If the SvO$_2$ value increases abruptly, check the PA waveform to determine if it is a PAOP waveform. An abrupt increase in the SvO$_2$ value is an early warning sign of spontaneous migration to a PAOP position.

  - The rate of the blood draw for obtaining a mixed venous blood gas sample should be slow, at a rate of 2 mL over 30 seconds. Drawing the sample too rapidly may result in aspiration of air into the barrel of the syringe, and this would contribute to overestimation of the measured SvO$_2$ value. Also, too rapid drawing of the sample may result in obtaining some arterialized blood in the sample, which again contributes to overestimation of the measured value.

- ### ScvO$_2$ monitoring:

  - The rate of the blood draw for obtaining a central venous blood gas sample should be slow, at a rate of 2 mL over 30 seconds. Drawing the sample too rapidly may result in aspiration of venous blood coming from the coronary sinus, resulting in underestimation of the ScvO$_2$ value.

- Maintain the integrity of the closed system by preventing introduction of air into the catheter.

- Ensure that all stopcocks are turned in the appropriate direction, and verify that the Luer lock connections are tight. These should be checked at the beginning of every shift.

Conclusion

Both SvO$_2$ and ScvO$_2$ monitoring allow for more precise monitoring on the oxygen delivery–demand balance. Both have been shown to be effective resuscitation targets for the management of severe sepsis or septic shock and in other situations as well. Research has shown that SvO$_2$ allows more rapid termination of pharmacologic interventions and reduces the incidence of manipulation of the mechanical ventilator.[4] It has been reported that critical care unit length of stay may be shorter with the use of this information. Some have questioned the added cost of using the continuous parameters of SvO$_2$ and ScvO$_2$ and prefer to obtain intermittent measurements instead. Certainly, the presence of continuous information allows for faster identification of changes in the patient's condition, quicker intervention, and potentially improved outcomes. The risk of obtaining intermittent measurements is associated with increased risk of central line bloodstream infections, which is a dreaded adverse event that all health care providers strive to prevent. In general, the importance of using either SvO_2 or $ScvO_2$ in the management of the critically ill patient can be summed up by the axiom: prompt restoration of tissue oxygen delivery is the major factor that improves patient outcomes.

References

1. Rady MY, Rivers EP, Norwalk RM: Resuscitation of the critically ill in the ED: Response of blood pressure, heart rate, shock index, central venous oxygen saturation and lactate, *Am J Emerg Med* 14:218–225, 1996.
2. Marini PL: *The ICU book*, ed 3, Philadelphia, 2007, Lippincott Williams & Wilkins.
3. Nichols D, Nielson ND: Oxygen delivery and consumption: a macrocirculatory perspective, *Crit Care Clin* 26:239–253, 2010.
4. Ahrens T: Continuous mixed venous (SvO2) monitoring: too expensive or indispensible? *Crit Care Nurs Clin North Am* 11(1):33–48, 1999.
5. Headley J: Continuous venous oxygen saturation monitoring. In Wiegand DLM, editor: *AACN procedure manual for critical care*, Philadelphia, 2011, Saunders, pp 113–120.
6. Rehman HU: Methemoglobinemia, *West J Med* 175(3):193–196, 2001.
7. Rivers EP, Nguyen B, Havstad S, et al.: Early goal directed therapy in the treatment of severe sepsis and septic shock, *N Eng J Med* 345(19):1368–1377, 2001.
8. Reinhart K, Huhn HJ, Hartog C, et al.: Continuous central venous and pulmonary artery oxygen saturation monitoring in the critically ill, *Intensive Care Med* 30:1572–1578, 2004.
9. Lee J, Wright F, Barber R, et al.: Central venous oxygen saturation in shock: a study in man, *Anesthesiology* 36:472–478, 1972.
10. Scheinman MM, Brown MA, Rapaport E: Critical assessment of use of central venous oxygen saturation as a mirror of mixed venous oxygen saturation in severely ill cardiac patients, *Circulation* 40:165–170, 1969.
11. Dahn MS, Lange MR, Jacobs LA: Central mixed and splanchnic venous oxygen saturation monitoring, *Intens Care Med* 14:373–378, 1988.
12. Rivers EP, Ander DS, Powell D: Central venous oxygen saturation monitoring in the critically ill patient, *Curr Opin Crit Care* 7:204–211, 2001.
13. Goodrich C: Continuous central venous oximetry monitoring, *Crit Care Nurs Clin NA* 18 (2):203–209, 2006.
14. Davison DL, Chawla LS, Selassie L, et al.: Femoral-based central venous oxygen saturation is not a reliable substitute for subclavian / internal jugular-based central venous oxygen saturation in patients who are critically ill, *Chest* 138(1):76–83, 2010.
15. Donati A, Loggi S, Preiser JC, et al.: Goal-directed intraoperative therapy reduces morbidity and length of hospital stay in high-risk surgical patients, *Chest* 132:1817–1824, 2007.
16. Hamilton MA, Cecconi M, Rhodes A: A systematic review and meta-analysis on the use of preemptive hemodynamic intervention to improve postoperative outcomes in moderate and high-risk surgical patients, *Anesth Anal* 112(6):1392–1402, 2011.
17. Rhodes A, Cecconi M, Hamilton M, et al.: Goal-directed therapy in high-risk surgical patients: a 15-year follow-up study, *Intens Care Med* 36(6):1327–1332, 2010.
18. Lees N, Hamilton M, Rhodes A: Clinical review: goal-directed therapy in high risk surgical patients, *Crit Care* 13(5):4–8, 2009.
19. Shoemaker WC, Appel PL, Kram HB, et al.: Prospective trial of supranormal values of survivors as therapeutic goals in high risk surgical patients, *Chest* 94:1176–1186, 1988.

Capnography Monitoring

Sagarika Ponnuru and Bhavani Shankar Kodali

8

Capnography is a noninvasive monitoring technique that detects the presence and concentration of carbon dioxide (CO_2) during exhalation, through the use of infrared technology. Since capnography was first introduced several decades ago, it has gained widespread use, and today it is an extremely valuable tool for anesthesiologists and critical care providers. Capnography directly measures the elimination of CO_2 by the lungs, and it indirectly measures the transport of CO_2 by the circulatory system and the production of CO_2 by tissues in the body. An abnormality in the numerical value of the partial pressure of end-tidal CO_2 ($PetCO_2$) or the waveform may be a warning sign of a pathologic process in the pulmonary system, cardiovascular system, or metabolism. Capnography also detects malfunctions or disconnections within the breathing apparatus, ventilator, and anesthesia machine. Therefore, capnography plays a crucial role in preventing adverse events and potentially irreversible patient injury. Although capnography has been used as a standard of care in the operating room for many years, it has more recently found a place in other locations where sedation is used including endoscopy, electrophysiology, interventional radiology, critical care, in the emergency department, and during cardiopulmonary resuscitation (CPR).[1–5]

> **Clinical Reasoning Pearl**
>
> Capnography provides continuous, real-time, noninvasive measurement of exhaled (end-tidal) CO_2. It plays a critical role in preventing adverse events and ensuring patient safety. It provides an early warning sign of a change in respiratory status, as well problems with ventilation equipment such as a malfunction or disconnection from the ventilator. Indications for capnography include verification of endotracheal tube or nasogastric tube placement, assessment of cardiopulmonary status, management of mechanical ventilation and during cardiopulmonary resuscitation.

Respiratory Physiology

Normally, CO_2 is produced by tissues and transported to the lungs by the venous circulation via the right heart to the pulmonary circulation. In the lungs, gas exchange occurs whereby CO_2 diffuses into alveoli from blood and oxygen diffuses into blood from alveoli. Alveolar CO_2 is eliminated through pulmonary breathing. Therefore, CO_2 output, measured at the mouth or nares, is indirectly reflective of CO_2 production in tissues and CO_2 transport to the lungs (cardiac output) and is directly reflective of CO_2 elimination (breathing).

Carbon Dioxide Measurement Devices

Infrared technology is the common method of CO_2 analysis. CO_2 is a polyatomic gas and absorbs infrared light at 4.3 millimicrons. Figure 8-1 shows the schematic principle of CO_2 measurement. An infrared beam from a source passes through the respiratory gases. Because CO_2 molecules absorb infrared light, the remaining light is detected by the infrared detector and computed to display the CO_2 waveform and CO_2 concentration. CO_2 concentration can be also displayed as millimeters of mercury (mm Hg) when atmospheric pressure is known.

Sidestream Capnography

Sidestream capnography (Figure 8-2) is the most widely used method for continuous CO_2 monitoring in the operating room. It involves the use of disposable tubing (6 feet long) and a T-piece adapter, which is inserted between the breathing circuit and the endotracheal tube or other airway device. The tubing is connected from the side port on the adapter to a separate monitor unit, which contains the CO_2 sensor. A sample of gas is aspirated through this disposable tubing during the respiratory cycle into the capnometer for measurement. Because this gas sample must travel through the tubing to the CO_2 sensor before it is processed, a slight delay occurs in the display of the CO_2 waveform. One of the main advantages of sidestream capnography is that it can be used in nonintubated patients. For example, modified nasal cannulas allow the sampling of expired gases even while supplemental oxygen is administered. A drawback of sidestream capnography is that the tubing may become blocked by water vapor or secretions. The use of a filter between the tubing and the unit containing the CO_2 sensor minimizes this problem. Keeping the sample tubing antigravity may also minimize contamination from water vapor or secretions.[2]

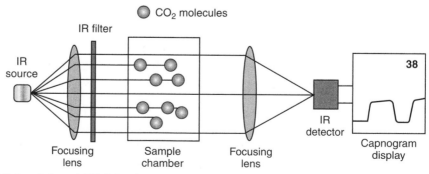

FIGURE 8-1 Infrared (IR) light absorption by the carbon dioxide (CO_2) molecules.

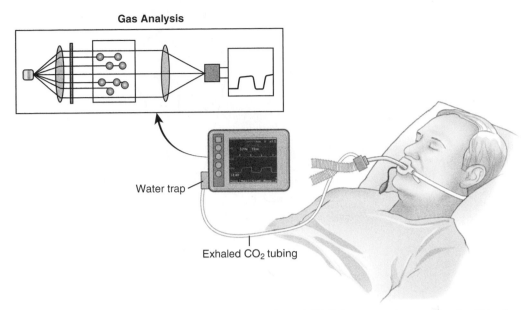

Gas Analysis

Water trap

Exhaled CO_2 tubing

FIGURE 8-2 Sidestream Capnography. The infrared (IR) light sensor is contained within the capnometer, not in the airway circuit.

Mainstream Capnography

Mainstream capnography (Figure 8-3) involves the use of an adapter between the breathing circuit and the endotracheal tube. In this method, a lightweight infrared sensor is attached directly to the adapter. The sensor emits infrared light to a photodetector on the other side of the adapter. During the respiratory cycle, respiratory gases flow through the adapter, and the amount of CO_2 in the sample is measured immediately. No extra tubing is required, and no delay occurs in the display of the waveform. The mainstream sensor is heated above body temperature, which prevents condensation and allows the sensor to function in high-moisture environments. Condensation of moisture may interfere with the functioning of the unit. The earlier generations of mainstream capnometers had significant disadvantages, including bulky sensors requiring sterilization after each use and a risk of facial burns from the heated sensor. Newer versions, however, are more lightweight and have disposable adaptors. The temperature of the sensors is lower with better shielding to minimize the risk of facial burns. Further advances in mainstream capnography have produced smaller lighter weight adapters for use in nonintubated patients also. These units attach directly to the oxygen facemask or nasal cannula, allowing for CO_2 monitoring in a spontaneously breathing patient receiving sedation.[2]

Colorimetric Devices

Colorimetric devices are portable, disposable, single-use devices that contain a pH-sensitive chemical indicator, which changes color on exposure to CO_2. Similar to the mainstream capnometer placement, this device is connected between the circuit and

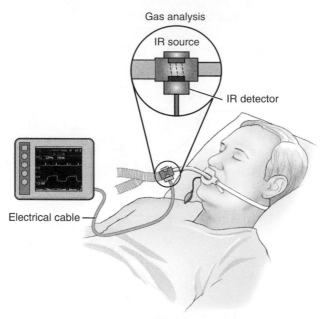

FIGURE 8-3 Mainstream Sensor Capnography. The infrared (IR) light sensor is positioned within the airway circuit.

the endotracheal tube. The indicator changes from purple to yellow when exposed to a sufficient concentration of CO_2 as a chemical reaction. The range of possible colors and the corresponding CO_2 concentrations are listed in Table 8-1. Often it is difficult to evaluate the colors, which poses challenges in predicting the CO_2 concentration in the expired gases. If the color changes to yellow during every exhaled breath, the CO_2 concentration can be estimated to be more than 2%, or over 16 mm Hg. If the color change is not yellow, the expired CO_2 level is less than desirable (Table 8-1).

Although colorimetric devices are used frequently by critical care providers and paramedics to confirm the presence of CO_2 after endotracheal intubation, these devices have their limitations. For example, acidic contents in the stomach may turn the indicator yellow, giving a false-positive reading. Also, a patient who is intubated during cardiac arrest may not expel sufficient CO_2 because of the lack of circulation, and the indicator would not change colors even with the endotracheal tube in the correct place.[2]

TABLE 8-1	Exhaled CO_2 Detection by Colorimetric Device
COLOR	**CO_2 CONCENTRATION**
Purple	<0.5%
Tan	0.5%–2%
Yellow	>2%

The current recommendation from the American Heart Association is to use waveform capnography instead of colorimetric devices even for emergency intubations, as well as during cardiopulmonary resuscitation.[1]

Waveform Analysis

Normal Capnogram

CO_2 concentration (Figure 8-4) can be plotted against time (time capnogram), or expired volume (volume capnogram). A time capnogram is commonly used in clinical practice (see Figure 8-4). It is similar in shape in all healthy adults. Any abnormal shape other than the normal capnogram requires full investigation to determine if the alteration in the shape is caused by a physiologic or pathologic abnormality.

To understand the components of a capnogram, a basic understanding of lung anatomy and physiology is essential. The trachea divides into the right and left main bronchi, the right side being shorter, wider, and more vertical. The implication is that a mainstem intubation is more likely to occur with the tube in the right main bronchus rather than in the left. Each mainstem bronchus divides into lobar bronchi, two on the left and three on the right. These bronchi further divide multiple times and eventually end in terminal bronchioles, each of which gives rise to respiratory bronchioles and alveoli. The conductive airways include everything from the trachea to the terminal bronchioles. The portion of lung past the terminal bronchioles, composed of the respiratory bronchioles and alveoli, participates in gas exchange. The alveolus is the most important structure participating in gas exchange, and the contribution of each alveolus to the capnogram depends on its ventilation and perfusion. Air flow and blood flow are not distributed evenly within the lung. The alveoli in the apex of the lung have high ventilation–perfusion (V/Q) ratios (more ventilation, less perfusion), and they contain relatively less CO_2 after gas exchange. In contrast, the alveoli in the lower portions of the lung have low V/Q ratios (less ventilation, more perfusion), and they contain CO_2-rich gas. During expiration, the CO_2 from all alveoli moves through the respiratory tract to exit the trachea, or the endotracheal tube, to the measuring sensor (Figure 8-5).[1,2,6]

A time-based capnogram is a graphic depiction of the partial pressure of end-tidal CO_2 ($PetCO_2$) over time during a ventilatory cycle. It includes both inspiratory and expiratory segments, which allows for monitoring of the dynamics of inspiration and expiration.

> **Clinical Reasoning Pearl**
>
> Never assume the partial pressure of exhaled carbon dioxide $PetCO_2$ values reflect partial pressure of arterial CO_2 ($PaCO_2$) values without waveform analysis. Any change in the waveform could be an indication of a change in the patient's pulmonary status and warrants further evaluation. Loss of the waveform may signal loss of effective respirations.

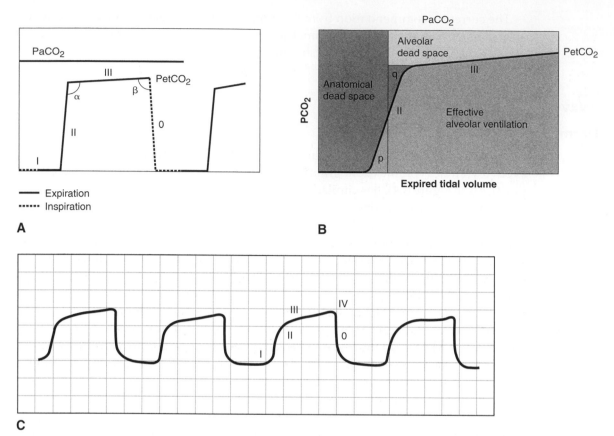

FIGURE 8-4 A, Time capnogram showing segments, phases, and angles. Inspiratory segment is phase 0, and expiratory segment is divided into three phases: I, II, and III. Maximum value of carbon dioxide (CO_2) at the end of the breath is designated as partial pressure of end-tidal carbon dioxide (PetCO$_2$) and is about 35 to 36 mm Hg. It is lower than the partial pressure of arterial CO_2 (PaCO$_2$, 40 mm Hg) by about 5 mm Hg. **B,** Volume capnogram (PCO$_2$ versus expired volume): Volume capnogram showing subdivisions of tidal volume. Area under the CO_2 curve is effective alveolar ventilation. Area above the CO_2 curve and the arterial PaCO$_2$ line indicates physiologic dead space. A vertical line is drawn across phase II such that the two triangles *p* and *q* are equal in area. This divides physiologic dead space into anatomic and alveolar dead spaces. **C,** A time capnogram recorded during cesarean delivery general anesthesia showing phase IV. (From Kodali BS: Capnography outside of the operating rooms, *Anesthesiology* 118(1):192–201, 2013.)

The inspiratory segment consists of phase 0, where a sharp decline in CO_2 occurs, compared with the end of expiration (see Fig 8-4, *A*). The expiratory segment is divided into three segments. It begins with phase I, which represents CO_2-free gas being expelled from the conducting airways and breathing apparatus. Since this anatomic dead space does not participate in gas exchange, the CO_2 concentration is initially zero at the beginning of expiration. Phase II consists of a rapid upstroke in CO_2 concentration. In this segment, mixing of expired air from anatomic dead space and alveoli occurs to produce a positive deflection in the graph. Phase III is a plateau with a slightly

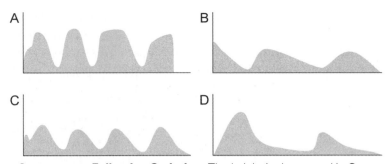

FIGURE 8-5 Capnograms Following Sedation. The height is decreased in **C** compared with **A**, and respiratory rate is decreased in **D** compared with **B**. (From Kodali, BS: Capnography outside the operating rooms, *Anesthesiology* 118(1):192-201, 2013.)

positive slope that represents CO_2-rich gas from alveoli. As stated above, inspiration yields no CO_2 as long as no rebreathing occurs, and this accounts for the rapid drop in CO_2 concentration from phase III to zero. A normal tracing always returns to baseline prior to the next expiratory cycle.

The alpha-angle is the angle between phase II and phase III, and it is affected by changes in the slope of phase III. The clinical implication of this angle is that it is an indirect indication of V/Q mismatch in the lungs. The beta-angle is the angle between phase III and the descending segment of the capnogram, or the beginning of phase 0. The beta-angle is usually 90 degrees.[1] The maximum concentration of CO_2 at the end of the breath is designated as $ETCO_2$. If measured in millimeters of mercury, it is designated as $PetCO_2$. It is usually about 35 to 36 mm Hg and lower than $PaCO_2$ by about 4 to 5 mm Hg. The difference between $PetCO_2$ and $PaCO_2$ represents alveolar dead space ($PaCO_2 - PetCO_2$).

Clinical Reasoning Pearl

In a patient who is hemodynamically stable, the $PetCO_2$ value can be used to estimate the arterial value of $PaCO_2$, with the $PetCO_2$ levels 1 to 5 mm Hg less than the $PaCO_2$ levels.

Causes of *increased* $PetCO_2$ values include situations in which CO_2 production is increased, for example, hyperthermia, sepsis, and seizures, or situations in which alveolar ventilation is decreased, for example, respiratory depression.

Causes of *decreased* $PetCO_2$ values include situations in which CO_2 production is decreased, for example, hypothermia, cardiac arrest and pulmonary embolism, or situations in which alveolar ventilation is increased, for example, hyperventilation.

Capnograms in Nonintubated Patients

Distinct capnograms as described above may not be present in patients breathing spontaneously without an endotracheal tube. In the spontaneously breathing patient without an endotracheal tube, nasal sampling or sampling via a facemask may result in capnograms shown in Figure 8-6. These variations in shapes of capnograms are caused by the dilution of expiratory gases with atmospheric air or by supplemental oxygen administered via the mask. These capnograms can be considered normal variants in spontaneously breathing patients. Changes from baseline capnograms may reflect the effect of sedation on breathing.

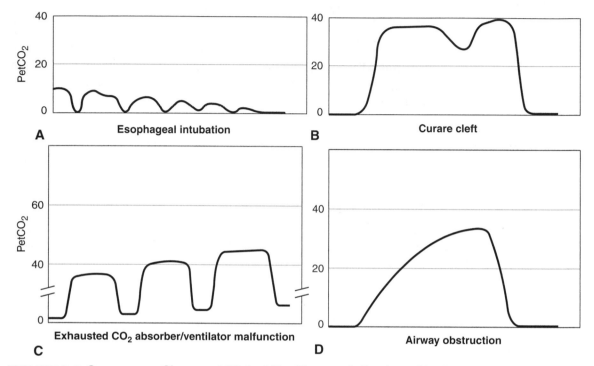

FIGURE 8-6 Capnograms Shape and Clinical Significance. A, Esophageal intubation. In esophageal intubation, the carbon dioxide (CO_2) trace may have zero line or few blips of CO_2 waveforms, depending on the concentration of CO_2 in the esophagus. The presence of CO_2 is caused either by swallowing of respiratory gases or by expiratory gases being pushed into the stomach during positive pressure ventilation via mask. However, with few ventilatory breaths, the CO_2 concentration decreases to zero resulting in a flat line. **B,** Curare cleft. A sudden dip during phase III, or the expiratory plateau, indicates spontaneous respiratory effort during mechanical ventilation. It may occur with surgical manipulation or any other cause of brief external compression of the abdomen. It also indicates recovery from neuromuscular relaxant agents.[2] **C,** Rebreathing. An elevation from the baseline is usually caused by an exhausted CO_2 absorber, which results in rebreathing of CO_2 during inspiration. As explained above in the analysis of the time capnogram, the CO_2 concentration decreases to zero at the end of the alveolar plateau, reflecting the beginning of inspiration of CO_2-free fresh gases. If rebreathing occurs, the downstroke will not reach the zero line and thus is elevated. During anesthesia, when controlled ventilation is used with closed circuit, elevation of baseline suggests inadequate CO_2 absorption and exhausted soda lime. A defect in inspiratory and/or expiratory valve malfunction produces increases in the beta-angle, and/or elevation of the baseline. When a mechanical ventilator is used, an elevation from baseline indicates malfunction within the ventilator (faulty ventilator valves).[6] **D,** Airway obstruction. An increase in the alpha-angle and an increase in the slope of phase III indicate airway obstruction. If severe enough, phase II may also be prolonged. The most common causes are kinking of the endotracheal tube, bronchospasm, asthma, or chronic obstructive pulmonary disease (COPD) or emphysema. Because of the airway obstruction, CO_2 is expired at a slower rate, which is reflected by the more gradual increase in CO_2 concentration.[2]

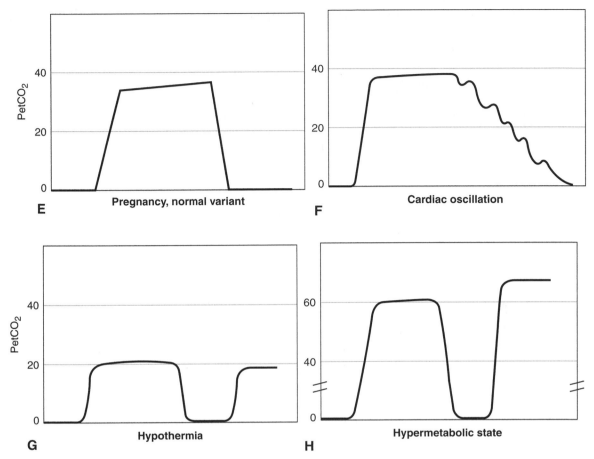

FIGURE 8-6, cont'd E, Normal variant of capnogram in pregnancy. The slope of phase III may be slightly increased in pregnant women undergoing general anesthesia. Although phase III in this figure looks similar to airway obstruction, phase II remains normal. This can be a normal physiologic variation in pregnancy.[6] Hemodilution and increases in cardiac output produces better perfusion of alveoli thereby decreasing alveolar dead space. This brings the partial pressure of end-expiratory CO_2 (PetCO_2) closer to the partial pressure of arterial CO_2 (PaCO_2), and the difference between the two is less than in nonpregnant subjects. However, regional variation occurs in ventilation-to-perfusion (V/Q) ratios because of the pressure of the growing uterus toward the diaphragm. This results in alveoli with a lower V/Q ratio containing relatively more CO_2 compared with the alveoli in the upper portions of the lung. The late emptying of the alveoli with higher CO_2 concentration from the lower portions of the lung results in the increase slope of the phase III, or the alveolar plateau. **F,** Cardiogenic oscillations. The ripple effect at the end of phase III occurs during low-frequency mechanical ventilation. Each heartbeat creates rhythmic lung compression that moves the respiratory gases back and forth. The sensor sampling site detects these changes in CO_2 to produce a ripple effect.[6] **G,** Hypothermia. A decrease in end-tidal CO_2 (PetCO_2) occurs during periods of hypothermia, reduced metabolism, and low cardiac output. The height of the waveform is shorter, but other characteristics remain unchanged.[6] **H,** Hypermetabolic state. A gradual rise in CO_2 concentration may be caused by a hypermetabolic state. Rising PetCO_2 is considered an ominous sign of malignant hyperthermia. A similar tracing may be seen with hypoventilation.[6]

Continued

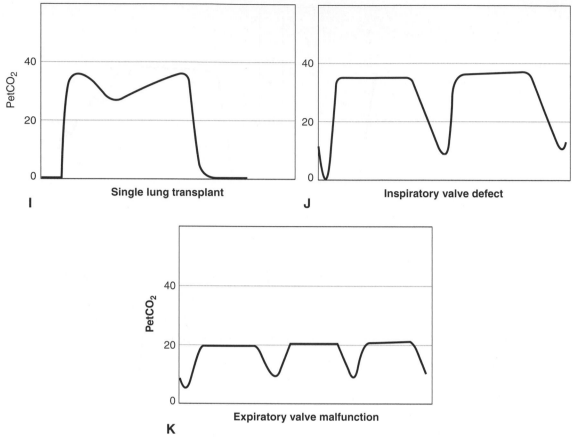

FIGURE 8-6, cont'd I, Lung transplantation. A biphasic capnogram is seen in a patient that has had single lung transplantation. The initial peak in the waveform represents the transplanted, healthy lung, which has normal compliance and ventilation/perfusion (V/Q) ratio. The delayed, second peak of the waveform represents the native, diseased lung, which has poor compliance and significantly greater V/Q mismatch. The native lung takes longer to expel CO_2 and mimics a capnogram from a patient with chronic obstructive pulmonary disease (COPD). The differing capnograms produced by each lung produces a dual peak capnogram. A similar capnogram may be seen when a partial disconnection or leak occurs within the apparatus.[6] **J,** Inspiratory valve malfunction. Malfunction of the inspiratory valve leads to rebreathing of carbon dioxide (CO_2) during inspiration. The waveform shows a slow decline in CO_2 during inspiration and the tracing may not return to baseline prior to the next expiratory cycle, and the beta-angle is greater than the usual 90 degrees.[6] **K,** Expiratory valve malfunction. Malfunction of the expiratory valve produces a shallow tracing that does not return to baseline with subsequent breaths. Phase II and phase 0 are abnormal because of mixing of inspiratory (CO_2-free) and expiratory (CO_2-containing) gases.[6] (From Kodali, BS: Capnography outside the operating rooms, *Anesthesiology* 118(1):192–201, 2013.)

Applications of Capnography in Clinical Practice

Clinical information can be obtained from three important components of capnography:

1. *Numerical end-tidal values:* End-tidal values provide information about the overall CO_2 status of the patient. In addition, acute changes in $PetCO_2$ values help with differential diagnosis when an abnormal clinical situation is encountered. Table 8-2 provides a list of factors that should be considered when abrupt changes occur in $PetCO_2$ values.

TABLE 8-2 Causes of Abnormal Partial Pressure of End-Expiratory Carbon Dioxide (PetCO$_2$)

	INCREASE IN PetCO$_2$ MALIGNANT HYPERTHERMIA	DECREASE IN PetCO$_2$ HYPOTHERMIA
Metabolic	Severe sepsis	Metabolic acidosis
	Thyroid storm	
Circulatory		Pulmonary embolism
		Profound hypovolemia
		Cardiogenic shock
		Intracardiac shunt
Respiratory	Hypoventilation	Hyperventilation
	Asthma	Intrapulmonary shunt
	Chronic obstructive pulmonary disease (COPD)	Pulmonary edema
Technical	Exhausted CO$_2$ absorber	Disconnection
		Blockage in tubing

2. *Shape of capnogram:* The morphological shape of the capnogram offers substantial information beyond simply analyzing numbers. In capnography waveform analysis, five important characteristics of the waveform need to be evaluated: height, shape, frequency, rhythm, and baseline. All healthy adults have identical waveforms, and any deviation from the normal capnogram should be investigated, as it usually indicates the presence of a pathologic condition, a technical problem, or a physiological variant.[6] The clinical significance of various shapes of abnormal capnograms is illustrated in Figure 8-6.

3. *PaCO$_2$–PetCO$_2$ gradient as an indicator of physiologic dead space:* PetCO$_2$, obtained by capnography, reflects the status of the alveoli that empty last. The normal PetCO$_2$ values range between 35 and 40 mm Hg. The only way to measure PaCO$_2$ is by obtaining a sample of arterial blood. However, in healthy subjects, PetCO$_2$ is usually 2 to 5 mm Hg lower than PaCO$_2$ because of alveolar dead space (regions where ventilation occurs but not perfusion). The conductive airways contribute to anatomic dead space, whereas disease processes in the lungs or V/Q mismatch contribute to alveolar dead space. Physiologic dead space comprises both anatomic and alveolar dead space. Because anatomic dead space is relatively constant, a change in PetCO$_2$ usually reflects a change in alveolar dead space. As alveolar dead space increases, as in states of low cardiac output or pulmonary embolism, PetCO$_2$ decreases, and the difference between PetCO$_2$ and PaCO$_2$ increases.[7] Other factors that increase PaCO$_2$–PetCO$_2$ include age and emphysema. Pregnant patients and children, have a slightly decreased PaCO$_2$–PetCO$_2$ gradient.[5]

A change in the PaCO$_2$–PetCO$_2$ gradient is a surrogate marker for a change in alveolar dead space only if phase III in the capnogram is flat or has a minimal slope (normal phase III shown in Figure 8-4, *A*). When a significant increase occurs in the slope of phase III, PetCO$_2$ approaches PaCO$_2$, and the difference between the two values may be minimal even though a substantial amount of alveolar dead space exists.[1,6]

Clinical Application

Endotracheal Intubation

Time capnography is more commonly used in clinical practice than volume capnography. The most widespread use of time capnography involves confirmation of endotracheal tube placement. Although capnography was first introduced in the 1940s, it did not become the standard of care for confirmation of tube placement and monitoring under anesthesia until several decades later. An endotracheal tube in the correct position, that is, 2 to 4 centimeters (cm) above the carina, will generate a normal capnogram waveform that is sustained over multiple ventilatory cycles. The exception is a patient with severely compromised cardiac output and reduced pulmonary blood flow, as in cardiac arrest or major pulmonary embolism, when the patient will not have a normal PetCO$_2$ or waveform, even with the endotracheal tube in the correct position.[1]

Before capnography became the standard of care for confirmation of endotracheal tube placement, accidental esophageal intubation was a significant cause of morbidity and mortality during the perioperative period.[6] In the present day, the combination of capnography and auscultation of breath sounds provides the most efficient and practical way to detect esophageal intubations, both in the operating room and other locations. Esophageal intubation usually produces minimal to no PetCO$_2$. The presence of esophageal or gastric CO$_2$, for example, in a patient who has consumed carbonated beverages prior to intubation, may produce a significant spike in CO$_2$ initially, but this will not be sustained over multiple ventilatory cycles.[1,2,6]

Capnography is also useful during other intubation techniques such as blind nasal intubation or double-lumen endotracheal tube placement. For blind nasal intubation, attachment of a sidestream capnography monitor to the proximal end of the nasal endotracheal tube allows continuous PetCO$_2$ monitoring in a patient with spontaneous respirations. As the tube is advanced through the nasal cavity and into the larynx, continued PetCO$_2$ readings indicate that the endotracheal tube is following the airway flow pathway into the larynx. If the tube deviates from this airway flow path or goes into the esophagus, PetCO$_2$ will decrease or disappear. For positioning and monitoring of a double-lumen endotracheal tube, capnography measurements of each lumen provide valuable information on the ventilatory status of each lung. In this case, sidestream tubing is attached to the proximal end of each lumen, which may be connected to a three-way stopcock. This type of setup precludes the need for two separate capnography monitors (Figure 8-7).[2,8]

Monitoring the Integrity of the Anesthetic Apparatus or Ventilators in Critical Care Units

Capnography plays an important role in monitoring the integrity of various components of the breathing apparatus, whether it is the breathing circuit, the anesthesia machine, or

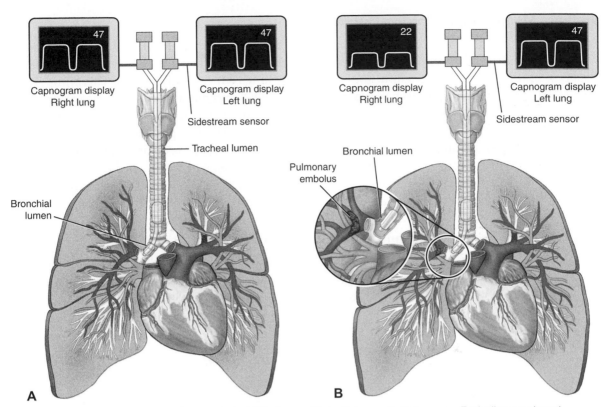

FIGURE 8-7 A, Normal lung: exhaled CO_2 is equal in both lungs. **B,** Pulmonary Embolism: reduced levels of CO_2 (22 mm Hg) in the lung with a pulmonary embolism, compared with the healthy lung (47 mm Hg).

the critical care unit ventilator. Changes in $PetCO_2$ and changes in the waveform not only indicate clinical abnormalities but also technical problems. Disconnections at any point along the breathing apparatus will yield a flat line on the capnography tracing, immediately allowing quick detection of the problem. Large circuit leaks will be detected through other mechanisms and alarms in the ventilator, but these same alarms may not be sensitive enough to detect a small circuit leak. With a small circuit leak, capnography will show a gradual rise in $PetCO_2$. Another cause of gradually increasing $PetCO_2$ is an exhausted CO_2 absorber or a defective ventilator. A kink or blockage in the breathing apparatus, if significant enough, will also lead to changes in $PetCO_2$. More importantly, the capnography waveform demonstrates an increased slope of phase III and an increase in the alpha-angle during airway obstruction, as with a kinked or partially blocked endotracheal tube.[1,2,6] This application is probably the most important use of capnography in the critical care unit despite the presence of ventilator alarms. A change in the shape of capnogram, $PetCO_2$, or both should alert the clinician to determine the cause of this change. It is prudent to observe the CO_2 waveform whenever the patient is turned from side to side to monitor whether integrity of the airway, ventilation, or cardiovascular hemodynamics is compromised during patient movement. Death caused by dislodgement of a tracheostomy tube while the patient was being turned has been reported.[1,9]

Indirect Monitoring of Cardiac Output

Normal cardiac output is approximately 5 liters per minute (L/minute). In a healthy patient and in the absence of significant intracardiac or intrapulmonary shunting, the entire cardiac output goes through the lungs with every heartbeat. This is important for adequate gas exchange at the level of alveoli and pulmonary capillaries. A decrease in cardiac output results in a decrease in pulmonary blood flow, resulting in more alveoli with high V/Q ratios. The areas that receive little or no perfusion cannot participate in gas exchange, and the excretion of CO_2 into the lungs is compromised. In this case, $PetCO_2$ decreases, but $PaCO_2$ remains normal or elevated because the body continues to produce CO_2. Therefore, a sudden decrease in $PetCO_2$ without any changes in ventilation may be an indication that cardiac output has declined.[1–3,5,6]

Indirect Monitoring of Carbon Dioxide Production

Hypermetabolic states such as malignant hyperthermia, thyroid storm, or severe sepsis all lead to increased production of CO_2. With the use of continuous capnography, a steady rise in $PetCO_2$ may be an early indication of a hypermetabolic crisis. Malignant hyperthermia is a rare, life-threatening condition that may develop after exposure to certain anesthetic agents such as volatile anesthetics or succinylcholine. Malignant hyperthermia is an autosomal dominant disorder involving a mutation in the calcium channel of skeletal muscle. When a patient with this disorder is exposed to a triggering medication, widespread and unopposed release of calcium from the sarcoplasmic reticulum of skeletal muscle occurs, causing profound contractures. In addition to muscle rigidity, other clinical signs of malignant hyperthermia include increased temperature, tachycardia, hypertension, and tachypnea. From the time of exposure to the triggering agent, the onset of clinical signs may be immediate or delayed up to 24 hours. The use of capnography plays an important role in the perioperative period because an increase in $PetCO_2$ is one of the earliest signs of malignant hyperthermia, and prompt diagnosis and treatment are critical in the management of this life-threatening condition.[6]

Nasogastric Tube Placement

Currently, most guidelines recommend confirming the position of an enteral feeding tube with radiography prior to use. Unintentional and unrecognized insertion of the tube into the trachea and bronchus may be detrimental or even fatal. An alternative method to imaging is to attach a capnography device to the feeding tube during insertion. Once the feeding tube is inserted to approximately 30 cm, capnography will show a normal waveform if the feeding tube is in the trachea, and it will not detect CO_2 if it is correctly placed into the esophagus. As long as CO_2 is not detected with capnography, the feeding tube should be advanced to approximately 50 cm. At this point, identification of the feeding tube in the stomach can be accomplished with epigastric auscultation and insufflation. If the auscultation is inconclusive, radiography should be performed to confirm the correct position of the tube. With this method of nasogastric tube placement, radiography is performed only about 10% of the time according to a recent study.[10]

Specialty Applications

Critical Care Unit

Although continuous capnography has become the standard of care in operating rooms, the extent of the use of capnography in critical care units varies widely among hospitals.[1] Most hospitals use capnography for intubation, but the majority of critical care units do not use continuous capnography in mechanically ventilated patients. Recent data from the United Kingdom shows that only 25% of critical care units use capnography for continuous monitoring of patients requiring mechanical ventilation.[11] Continuous capnography offers several benefits in this subset of patients. As outlined above, in the critical care unit, intubated patients are turned frequently for position changes, dressing changes, and bathing. Some of these patients also need to be transported out of the critical care unit for diagnostic studies or minor procedures. The use of continuous capnography offers immediate detection of a partially kinked endotracheal tube, blockage within the tube from secretions, or a completely dislodged tube resulting in inadvertent extubation. Continuous pulse oximetry does not offer the same rapid detection of airway mishaps because of the delay in oxygen desaturation, especially if the patient has been ventilated with a high fraction of inspired oxygen (FiO_2). Early detection of an airway mishap is crucial as it gives the clinician more time to re-secure the airway before onset of hypoxia in a patient. Since most critically ill patients do not have the pulmonary reserve to maintain their oxygen saturation for long periods, early detection is even more urgent in this group of patients.[1,11]

Another benefit to using continuous capnography in mechanically ventilated patients is that $PetCO_2$ and the corresponding waveform function as surrogate markers of ventilation, circulation, and metabolism.[1]

In the operating room, anesthesiologists rely on capnography and pulse oximetry to monitor ventilation and oxygenation of the patient. Arterial blood gas (ABG) samples are obtained, as needed, depending on the clinical situation and the status of the patient. In the critical care unit, however, it is common practice to obtain frequent ABG samples in virtually all intubated patients. One of the main reasons for this frequent sampling is to monitor the ventilation and oxygenation of the patient. However, not all intubated patients have arterial lines, and it is difficult to obtain an ABG sample in some of these patients because of their condition. Capnography and pulse oximetry offer an alternative, noninvasive method of routine monitoring in these patients. It is prudent to obtain a baseline ABG value to determine the $PaCO_2$–$PetCO_2$ gradient (a-ET gradient), which represents the amount of alveolar dead space and the relationship between $PetCO_2$ and $PaCO_2$. Subsequent ABG assessments may be necessary, depending on the clinical status of the patient, but capnography can certainly be used to replace routine ABG assessment to monitor ventilation. Furthermore, because capnography offers continuous monitoring, it allows for more efficient management of the ventilator, as the clinician does not have to wait for a laboratory result, or use a point of care ABG test to know the effect of a given change in ventilator settings.[1,2]

Morphology of Carbon Dioxide Waveforms

As described in the clinical application section, the morphology of CO_2 waveforms provides immediate diagnostic clues and the ability to determine the effectiveness of therapies in the clinical management of critically ill patients. The CO_2 waveform is identical in every individual with healthy lungs. Any deviation from the normal must be investigated for a physiologic or pathologic cause. Apart from circuit disconnections and ventilatory failures resulting in apneic capnograms, capnography waveforms provide dynamic information about airway caliber. An important application of capnography in asthma (prolonged phase II and phase III) is establishing effectiveness of bronchodilators in normalizing the capnogram shape. Capnography is also useful in the weaning of patients from mechanical ventilation. A close similarity between spontaneous ventilation capnograms and intermittent mandatory breath capnograms suggests the possibility of return of adequate spontaneous respiratory effort. In addition, capnography also facilitates monitoring of adequacy of spontaneous ventilation after weaning.[6]

Percutaneous Dilatational Tracheostomy

Percutaneous tracheostomy is increasingly performed in critical care units. The critical care units have developed their own guidelines to minimize complication rates. These guidelines focus on preoperative risk assessment, including levels of ventilatory support, anatomic considerations, experience level of staff, use of bronchoscopy, correction of coagulopathies, and use of capnography. In a study utilizing these guidelines, an immediate decrease in major and minor complications during and following the percutaneous tracheostomy procedure was reported.[12] In another study, the authors used capnography in 26 patients and bronchoscopy in 29 patients to confirm needle placement for percutaneous tracheostomy using the Blue Rhino kit. The operating times and the incidence of perioperative complications were similar for both groups. They concluded that capnography proved to be as effective as bronchoscopy in confirming correct needle placement.[13] Capnography has also been used to reliably confirm intratracheal cannula placement prior to percutaneous dilatational tracheostomy.[14] These studies support the value of capnography in percutaneous dilatational tracheostomy even in the absence of bronchoscopy.

Dead Space Indices. Ongoing studies are evaluating the utility of derived dead space indices to predict survival in mechanically ventilated patients with acute respiratory distress syndrome (ARDS). In one prospective observational study, researchers calculated dead space indices at admission, at 24 hours and at 48 hours in 36 patients with ARDS. The alveolar ejection volume (V_{AE})/tidal volume (Vt) ratio (V_{AE}/Vt) was the best predictor of outcome at admission and after 48 hours [$p = 0.013$], with a sensitivity of 82% and a specificity of 64%.[15]

Dead Space/Tidal Volume Ratio (Vd/Vt) and Gas Exchange Variables. There is ongoing interest in using capnography and oxygenation measurements as part of a bundle of physiologic measures to predict patient outcome. PaO_2, $PaCO_2$, PaO_2/FiO_2, arterial/alveolar oxygen tension ratio (PaO_2/PAO_2), alveolar–arterial oxygen tension difference/arterial oxygen tension ratio (P(A-a)O_2/PaO_2), CO_2 production (VCO_2), ventilation index ([PaCO_2 × peak inspiratory pressure × mechanical respiratory rate]/1000), and oxygenation index ([mean airway pressure × FiO_2 × 100]/PaO_2), are being investigated in children with early-stage obstructive acute respiratory failure. In one study, the measurements were derived using volumetric capnography and ABG analysis. Results suggest a significant association between an increase in Vd/Vt, severity of lung injury, and disturbances of oxygenation. Further evaluation of the usefulness of serial measurement of the dead space/tidal volume (Vd/Vt) ratio as a marker of disease severity in severe acute bronchiolitis and other causes of respiratory failure are warranted.[16]

Single Breath Tracing. Investigators are also evaluating single breath tracing of CO_2 in severe sepsis with tissue hypoxia. Single breath tracing for carbon dioxide (SBT-CO_2, volume capnogram) was analyzed in an observational study of 18 patients with sepsis. All patients were mechanically ventilated in a controlled mode; all had a pulmonary artery catheter inserted to calculate cardiac output. Using the Hill formula, all tracings were analyzed point by point to obtain the time required for CO_2 to achieve 50% maximal value and the fractional expiratory time 50 (FET$_{0.5}$). Nine of the patients had tissue hypoxia events. In the hypoxic group, CO_2 clearance and FET$_{0.5}$ values were higher than those in the nonhypoxic group. Furthermore, CO_2 clearance correlated with arterial lactate and base excess in the hypoxic patients.[17]

Capnography in the Post-Anesthesia Care Unit

During the initial postoperative period, the patient is transported from a highly monitored environment in the operating room to a significantly less monitored area in the post-anesthesia care unit (PACU). Some patients also receive substantial doses of opioids in the PACU, and these medications often cause respiratory depression. In the PACU, the patient may be left unattended for certain periods, and although continuous pulse oximetry is used routinely in the PACU, it does not detect respiratory depression and hypoventilation early enough.[1] By the time hypoxia is detected by pulse oximetry, the clinician has limited time to manage the situation. Capnography in the PACU would be an easy, noninvasive, and continuous method of monitoring patients who are vulnerable to respiratory depression in the early postoperative period.[2] In our institution, we are implementing capnography in the PACU to monitor patients who have received moderate amounts of opioids for pain relief.

Capnography in Out-of-Operating Room Locations

In recent times, more and more surgical procedures and interventions requiring sedation are being performed outside the main operating room. These locations include endoscopy, interventional radiology, radiation oncology, magnetic resonance imaging (MRI) units and physicians' offices. For these procedures, many patients receive intravenous sedation administered by a nurse or an anesthesia provider. In nonintubated patients receiving sedation, sidestream capnography tubing can be inserted directly into the oxygen facemask. Specific nasal cannulas with a connection for capnography

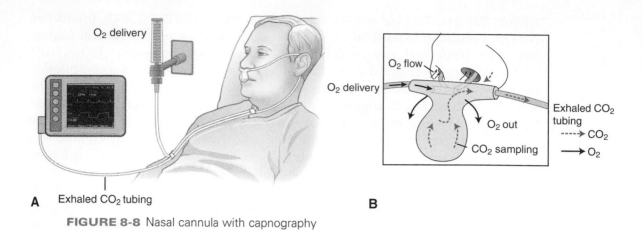

A Exhaled CO$_2$ tubing

B

FIGURE 8-8 Nasal cannula with capnography

tubing are also available (Figure 8-8). The capnographic waveform appears different because the expired air from the lungs mixes with supplemental oxygen and room air in the oxygen mask. Because it is not a closed system, often no phase III plateau occurs, which means that the numerical value of PetCO$_2$ is not an accurate measure of lung ventilation and is not a surrogate marker for PaCO$_2$. Rather, the PetCO$_2$ value indicates that the patient is maintaining spontaneous respirations, and the height of the waveform is a rough indication of the size of the breaths. Respiratory rate is easily measured as well.[1,4]

Patient Safety

Patient-controlled analgesia (PCA) is widely used for postoperative opioid administration. However, it has been associated with potentially fatal respiratory depression. Therefore, detecting a patient's declining respiratory status is crucial to patient safety. Postoperative patients typically are monitored by visual inspection and pulse oximetry; however, accumulating evidence shows that capnography is more accurate and provides earlier and more reliable warning of respiratory depression. Pulse oximetry provides an assessment of oxygenation and not ventilation; thus, by the time a change in the pulse oximetry readings occurs, the patient is often in respiratory distress and in need of intubation. Capnography is a useful adjunct to physical assessment in the identification of patients at risk for opioid-induced respiratory depression, particularly in high-risk patients such as those with underlying cardiac or pulmonary disease, morbid obesity, or sleep apnea. Frequent assessment prevents adverse events. Several organizations, including the American Society for Pain Management Nursing, the Anesthesia Patient Safety Foundation, and the Institute for Safe Medication Practices (ISMP) have recommended the use of capnography for the patients receiving postoperative opioids.[18,19]

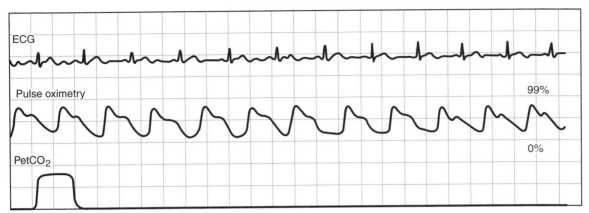

FIGURE 8-9 Pulse oximetry may not show decreases in oxygen saturation during initial phases of apnea.

Light sedation, deep sedation, and general anesthesia lie on a continuous spectrum, and a given medication does not have the same effect on each patient. Hypnotic agents such as propofol are being used more frequently in same-day or out-patient procedures to achieve faster patient recovery and discharge. With certain medications and combinations of medications, even highly skilled providers may encounter periods of apnea in their patients. As in the PACU environment, pulse oximetry is routinely used, but capnography has not become a standard of care. Considering the fact that sedated patients always receive supplemental oxygen, detection of hypoxia by pulse oximetry is even more delayed. The advantage of capnography in these cases involves rapid detection of hypoventilation and apnea before the occurrence of hypoxia (Figure 8-9) and the ability to titrate medications more efficiently. Capnography not only shows the size and shape of the waveform, but it also displays the respiratory rate. All of these factors are valuable in determining the dose and timing of medications to achieve a steady state of sedation without apnea. Patients receiving appropriate doses of sedation may still have airway obstruction. In the event of obstruction or apnea, the rapid decline or lack of PetCO$_2$ immediately alerts the clinician to perform the appropriate maneuvers. Usually, simple maneuvers such as chin lift or jaw thrust will prompt the patient to start breathing again, but sometimes more advanced airway management is necessary (see Figure 8-6).[3-5]

Patient Education

As with any technology, it is important to explain to the patient and the family the purpose of capnography. When used in the nonintubated patient, the patient is required to wear a nasal cannula. The cannula serves two purposes: It provides oxygen for those patients requiring supplemental oxygen, and it measures the patient's exhaled CO$_2$ and respiratory rate.

The cannula is bulky, and some patients do not want to wear it, particularly those who do not require supplemental oxygen. Compliance is critical, and explaining how important these measurements are for patient safety usually increases compliance. It is essential to provide this information to surgical patients before surgery as part of the routine preoperative teaching. For example, the reason for capnography is to provide additional monitoring of breathing because of the underlying medical condition or because the sedative or pain medications may depress the ability to breathe. It is important to explain that an alarm will sound if the breathing is too shallow or too slow and that the alarm is a signal to take a deep breath.

The patient should be instructed that the nasal cannula should not be worn while eating. The monitor can be placed on standby to avoid the continual sounding of the alarm. The cannula does not need to be worn during ambulation. The patient should be told how long he or she is expected to wear the cannula. Although the time varies, for postoperative surgical patients on patient controlled analgesia (PCA), capnography monitoring is often limited to the first 24 hours after surgery.

Cardiopulmonary Resuscitation

The American Heart Association (AHA) updated the Advanced Cardiac Life Support (ACLS) guidelines in 2010, and one of the new recommendations involves the use of continuous waveform capnography during cardiopulmonary resuscitation (CPR). Capnography plays an important role in monitoring the effectiveness of chest compressions and detecting the return of spontaneous circulation. During a cardiac arrest, pulmonary blood flow stops, and $PetCO_2$ may be absent even with the endotracheal tube in the correct position. Closed chest compressions are the most important component of CPR, but not all compressions are effective in circulating blood throughout the body. Ineffective chest compressions may produce a small amount of $PetCO_2$, but a sustained value of $PetCO_2$ greater than 10 mm Hg indicates adequate chest compressions. Even with effective chest compressions, $PetCO_2$ will be lower than normal. The decrease in pulmonary blood flow combined with a relatively large tidal volume delivered by bag-mask ventilation creates a large V/Q mismatch, as many alveoli receive ventilation but no perfusion. When spontaneous circulation returns, an abrupt increase in $PetCO_2$ (35–45 mm Hg) occurs from increased cardiac output and pulmonary blood flow (Figure 8-10).[1,3,20] It is the practice at our institution to make capnography available for all codes (Figure 8-11).

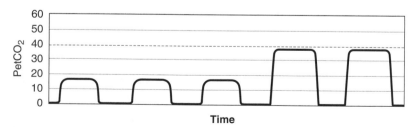

FIGURE 8-10 Return of spontaneous circulation is demarcated by abrupt increase in partial pressure of end-expiratory carbon dioxide ($PetCO_2$) during cardiopulmonary resuscitation.

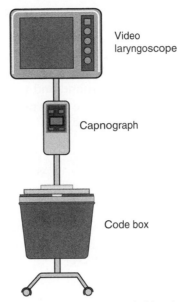

Video
laryngoscope

Capnograph

Code box

FIGURE 8-11 A stand equipped with capnometer and video laryngoscope is wheeled to all codes.

Transcutaneous Partial Pressure of Carbon Dioxide

Transcutaneous monitoring of CO_2 is an alternative method of indirectly monitoring the amount of CO_2 being produced by the body. Both capnography and monitoring of partial pressure of transcutaneous CO_2 ($PtcCO_2$) are continuous, noninvasive, surrogate measures of $PaCO_2$. In general $PtcCO_2$ values exceed $PaCO_2$ by about 3 to 5 mm Hg. The $PtcCO_2$ monitoring device contains an electrochemical sensor, which is placed on an area of intact skin. The sensor is heated, and on contact with skin, an increase occurs in blood flow to that area. CO_2 passively diffuses from these blood vessels into subcutaneous tissue and skin, and the sensor is able to measure CO_2 in this manner. Most sensors require periodic calibration and replacement of the membrane for optimal function, but recent technology has made this process simple and quick. Like capnography, $PtcCO_2$ devices may be used to approximate $PaCO_2$ or monitor trends, but they do not provide much information with regards to cardiac output or pulmonary blood flow. Some $PtcPCO_2$ devices can also measure the partial pressure of transcutaneous oxygen ($PtcO_2$) and thus provide a surrogate measure of PO_2 in addition to PCO_2.[21]

In the critical care unit $PtcCO_2$ monitoring is particularly useful in patients receiving high-frequency ventilation or noninvasive ventilation, as capnography does not provide reliable measurements in these patients. The $PtcCO_2$ monitoring device does have some technical limitations in certain patients because of significant edema, poor skin integrity, or profound peripheral vasoconstriction.[21]

Conclusion

In summary, capnography should be a key component in the monitoring standards in the operating room and used for optimization of mechanical ventilation in the critical care unit.[22] Once the science around and within CO_2 waveforms is understood by clinicians, this device will become indispensable, as it provides critical data about patients' cardiorespiratory status.

Case Study

Mr. J is a 72-year-old male who is obese. He has a long history of chronic obstructive pulmonary disease (COPD) associated with smoking three packs of cigarettes a day for 50 years. Over the past week, Mr. J has experienced a "flu-like" illness with fever, chills, malaise, and a productive cough with thick, greenish, purulent sputum. He was admitted to the critical care unit with respiratory insufficiency and pneumonia. Mr. J continued to deteriorate and was intubated and ventilated with a manual resuscitation bag. Initial breath sounds were absent, and the colorimetric end-tidal CO_2 (ETCO$_2$) detector remained purple. The endotracheal tube was removed, as it was thought to be in the esophagus, and Mr. J was reintubated. This time, bilateral breath sounds were present, and the colorimetric ETCO$_2$ detector changed color to yellow, indicating the presence of CO_2. Chest radiography confirmed correct placement of the endotracheal tube in the trachea, 3 cm above the carina.

Mr. J was placed on the ventilator. Antibiotics were administered and sedation initiated to manage continued agitation. Continuous pulse oximetry and mainstream capnography were initiated per unit standard. Mr. J's PetCO$_2$ level was 48 mm Hg with a normal capnogram and his PaCO$_2$ level was 50 mm Hg via ABG analysis. Over the next several hours, the capnogram changed its shape from a plateaued phase III to a sloped phased III. Mr. J's inspiratory pressures also rose and his breath sounds were significantly diminished on the left side. Chest radiography revealed substantial left upper and lower lobe atelectasis. Bronchoscopy was performed, and a large mucus plug was removed from the left main stem bronchus. The capnogram returned to a normal plateau shape once the mucus plug was removed. ▪

References

1. Kodali BS: Capnography outside the operating rooms, *Anesthesiology* 118(1):192–201, 2013.
2. www.capnography.com. Accessed July 2014.
3. Whitaker DK: Time for capnography—everywhere, *Anaesthesia* 66:544–549, 2011.
4. Gerstenberger PD: Capnography and patient safety for endoscopy, *Clin Gastroenterol Hepatol* 8:423–425, 2010.
5. Galvagno SM, Kodali BS: Critical monitoring issues outside the operating room, *Anesthesiol Clin* 27:141–156, 2009.

6. Bhavani-Shankar K, Moseley H, Kumar AY, Delph Y: Capnometry and anaesthesia, *Can J Anaesthesia* 39:617632, 1992.

7. McSwain SD, Hamel DS, Smith PB, et al.: End-tidal and arterial carbon dioxide measurements correlate across all levels of physiologic dead space, *Respir Care* 55:288–293, 2010.

8. Shankar KB, Russell R, Aklog L, Mushlin PS: Dual capnography facilitates detection of a critical perfusion defect in an individual lung, *Anesthesiology* 90:302–304, 1999.

9. Cantwell R, Clutton-Brock T, Cooper G, et al.: Saving Mothers' lives: reviewing maternal deaths to make motherhood safer: 2006-2008. The Eighth Report of the Confidential Enquiries into Maternal Deaths in the United Kingdom, *Br J Obstet Gynaecol* 118(Suppl 1):1–203, 2011.

10. Ioos V, Galbois A, Chalumeau-Lemoine L, et al.: An integrated approach for prescribing fewer chest x-rays in the ICU, *Ann Intensive Care* 1:4, 2011.

11. Georgiou AP, Gouldson S, Amphlett AM: The use of capnography and the availability of airway equipment on intensive care units in the UK and the Republic of Ireland, *Anaesthesia* 65:462467, 2010.

12. Cosgrove JE, Sweenie A, Raftery G, et al.: Locally developed guidelines reduce immediate complications from percutaneous dilatational tracheostomy using the Ciaglia Blue Rhino technique: a report on 200 procedures, *Anaesth Intensive Care* 34:782–786, 2006.

13. Mallick A, Venkatanath D, Elliot SC, et al.: A prospective randomised controlled trial of capnography vs. bronchoscopy for Blue Rhino percutaneous tracheostomy, *Anaesthesia* 58:864–868, 2003.

14. Coleman NA, Power BM, van Heerden PV: The use of end-tidal carbon dioxide monitoring to confirm intratracheal cannula placement prior to percutaneous dilatational tracheostomy, *Anaesth Intensive Care* 28:191–192, 2000.

15. Lucangelo U, Bernabe F, Vatua S, et al.: Prognostic value of different dead space indices in mechanically ventilated patients with acute lung injury and ARDS, *Chest* 133:62–71, 2008.

16. Almeida-Junior AA, da Silva MT, Almeida CC, Ribeiro JD: Relationship between physiologic deadspace/tidal volume ratio and gas exchange in infants with acute bronchiolitis on invasive mechanical ventilation, *Pediatr Crit Care* 8:372–377, 2007.

17. Zatelli R: Single breath tracing for carbon dioxide in septic patients with tissue hypoxia, *Adv Exp Med Biol* 599:207–212, 2007.

18. Jarzyna D, Junqquist CR, Pasero C, et al.: Guidelines on monitoring for opioid-induced sedation and respiratory depression, *Pain Manag Nurs* 12(3):118–145, 2011.

19. Joint Commission: Safe use of opioids in hospitals. *Sentinel Event Alert Issue 49* 2012. http://www.jointcommission.org/assets/1/18/SEA_49_opioids_8_2_12_final.pdf. Accessed March 20, 2014.

20. Pokorná M, Nečas E, Kratochvíl J, et al.: A sudden increase in partial pressure end-tidal carbon dioxide ($P_{ET}CO_2$) at the moment of return of spontaneous circulation, *J Emerg Med* 38:614–621, 2010.

21. Eberhard P: The design, use, and results of transcutaneous carbon dioxide analysis: current and future directions, *Anesth Analg* 105(6 Suppl):S48–S52, 2007.

22. Walsh BK, Crotwell DN, Restrepo RD: Capnography/Capnometry during mechanical ventilation: 2011, *Resp Care* 56(4):503–509, 2011.

Vasoactive Medications

Rosemary A. Timmerman

9

Critically ill patients often require intravenous (IV) infusions of vasoactive medications to restore tissue perfusion and aerobic cellular metabolism. A variety of pharmacologic agents are available to manage different types of shock. Vasopressors are administered to increase blood pressure by increasing systemic vascular resistance, and positive inotropes are used to increase myocardial contractility and cardiac output. Vasodilators decrease arterial vascular tone and systemic vascular resistance (SVR), thus improving cardiac output by reducing the resistance for left ventricular ejection. This chapter focuses on the pharmacologic actions of the various categories of vasoactive medications.

Adrenergic Receptors

Alpha-1 receptors are located in arterial smooth muscle and, when stimulated, cause vasoconstriction, which increases blood pressure by increasing SVR. Although this vasoconstriction has been shown to increase coronary and cerebral perfusion, it may also reduce regional blood flow to the skin, kidneys, and abdominal viscera.[1,2]

Alpha-2 receptors are located on presynaptic nerve endings and when stimulated prevent the release of endogenous norepinephrine causing vasodilation and a reduction of blood pressure and afterload. Stimulation of beta-1 receptors located on the heart exerts positive inotropic (increased contractility), chronotropic (increased heart rate), and dromotropic (increased conduction velocity through the atrioventricular node) effects.

Beta-2 receptors are located within the bronchi and vasculature of skeletal muscles and mediate bronchodilation and vasodilation, respectively. Vasodilation of mesenteric and renal arteries occurs when D_1 and D_2 dopaminergic receptors are stimulated and results in an increase in blood flow to these areas.[3]

Vasopressin receptors help raise blood pressure through several mechanisms. V-1 receptors are located on arterial smooth muscle and directly produce vasoconstriction by increasing intracellular calcium.[3-5] When V-2 receptors, which are located on renal tubules, are stimulated, they increase circulating volume by inhibiting diuresis.[3-5]

TABLE 9-1   Adrenergic Receptors

RECEPTOR	LOCATION	ACTION
Alpha-1	Vascular smooth muscle	Vasoconstriction Increased afterload Decreased heart rate (baroreflex) Increased coronary and cerebral blood flow
Alpha-2	Presynaptic nerve endings	Inhibition of norepinephrine release; peripheral vasodilation
Beta-1	Atrial and ventricular muscle Cardiac conduction system	Increased contractility Increased heart rate Increased conduction Increased automaticity
Beta-2	Bronchial smooth muscle Vascular smooth muscle of skeletal blood vessels	Bronchodilation Vasodilation
Dopaminergic	Mesenteric, renal, coronary, and cerebral blood vessels	Vasodilation and natriuresis

Although many hemodynamic medications have similarities, each has a unique pharmacologic profile and an assorted range of therapeutic effects. In particular, catecholamine agents have varying effects because affinity for different adrenergic receptors is medication specific (Table 9-1 and Figure 9-1). Therefore, certain vasoactive agents are better suited to manage specific cardiovascular conditions. It is important for clinicians to have clear understanding of hemodynamics, the pathophysiology of different cardiovascular disease states, and the pharmacologic profile of each agent so that appropriate medications can be selected for different hemodynamic derangements. See Figure 9-2 for an illustration of how the properties of different medications impact blood flow and pressure.

Vasopressor Medications

As blood pressure decreases, neural and hormonal autoregulatory mechanisms may become compromised, causing tissue bed perfusion to become solely reliant on the maintenance of adequate blood pressure for a sufficient supply of oxygenated blood. Consequently, medications with vasopressor properties are often used to restore blood pressure and perfusion in states of hypotension and shock. Data from a large multicenter, descriptive study in the United States revealed that almost one quarter of adults admitted to a critical care unit require at least one vasoactive infusion, and more than a third of patients in cardiovascular surgery units require vasopressor support.[6]

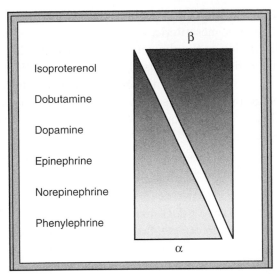

FIGURE 9-1 Alpha (α)- and beta (β)-adrenergic effects of vasoactive catecholamines. (Modified from Hollenberg SM: Inotrope and vasopressor therapy of septic shock, *Crit Care Clin* 25(4):781–802, 2009.)

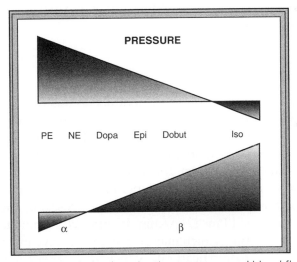

FIGURE 9-2 Effects of vasoactive catecholamines (α, β) on pressure and blood flow. *NE*, Norepinephrine; *PE*, phenylephrine. (Modified from Hollenberg SM: Inotrope and vasopressor therapy of septic shock, *Crit Care Clin* 25(4):781–802, 2009.)

Most vasoactive agents are catecholamines, or adrenergic agonists. They mimic the effects of the sympathetic nervous system by stimulating alpha-, beta-, and other vascular receptors. They are administered intravenously, have a half-life of 1 to 2 minutes and reach their peak effect within 10 minutes.[1,7] As a result, they can be quickly titrated to manage hemodynamic instability.

The majority of catecholamines increase blood pressure by stimulating alpha-1 adrenergic receptors in vascular smooth muscle. It is important to evaluate clinical signs of adequate tissue perfusion while administering these medications, particularly at higher doses, as the resultant vasoconstriction may adversely reduce perfusion to vulnerable cutaneous, mesenteric, and renal tissue beds. See the Clinical Indications section for a discussion on the clinical signs of perfusion. Medications with strong vasoconstrictive properties should be used cautiously in patients with compromised myocardial function, as the increase in afterload may impede cardiac output and increase myocardial oxygen demand. Use of vasoactive agents in the setting of hypovolemia does not markedly improve cardiac output and may worsen microcirculatory flow because of vasoconstriction.

Clinical Reasoning Pearl

Administering vasoactive medications to patients with hypovolemia does not improve tissue perfusion and may induce tachycardia. Therefore, volume status should be assessed, and when appropriate, fluids should be administered prior to starting these agents. Under certain circumstances, functional hemodynamics such as stroke volume variation (SVV) may help evaluate whether a fluid bolus is warranted.

The names, properties, and usual dose ranges of commonly used vasopressors are listed in Table 9-2. Also, see Box 9-1 for a discussion of the differences and similarities of three specific vasopressors.

Dopamine

Dopamine (*Intropin*) is an endogenous central nervous system neurotransmitter that is a direct precursor of norepinephrine and epinephrine. Once metabolized, it stimulates the sympathetic nervous system. The effects of exogenously administered dopamine are dose dependent. Dopamine primarily has dopaminergic properties at low doses of 2 micrograms per kilogram per minute (mcg/kg/min), and beta-1 properties at doses between 2 and 10 micrograms per kilogram per minute.[8] See the Positive Inotropes section for a discussion on the inotropic, vascular, and kidney effects of dopamine. At doses over 10 mcg/kg/min, it primarily stimulates alpha-1 receptors and causes vasoconstriction, which may negate the positive inotropic effects.[8] It may also cause a marked increase in heart rate, which may increase myocardial oxygen demand and reduce cardiac output by shortening diastolic filling time. Dopamine may be used to manage hypotension of unknown origin and is titrated to achieve a desirable blood pressure. Appropriate circulating volume must be ensured prior to starting dopamine because it has a high propensity for causing tachycardia in hypovolemic patients. Dopamine may be considered for the management of hypoperfusion in the setting of septic shock when the patient is exhibiting relative or absolute bradycardia and is not likely to develop a tachydysrhythmia.[9] Soft tissue ischemia and necrosis will result from extravasation of dopamine or other vasopressors. Consequently, it is preferable to infuse these medications in a central venous catheter.[7] If infiltration does occur, phentolamine is the treatment of choice and is discussed further in the section on Alpha Blockers.

TABLE 9-2 **Vasopressor Medications**				
MEDICATION	**RECEPTORS**	**ACTIONS**	**USUAL DOSE RANGE**	**TITRATION**
Dopamine Low dose:	D_1 & D_2	Vasodilation of renal and mesenteric blood vessels	0.5–2 micrograms per kilogram per minute (mcg/kg/min)	Low dose not usually titrated
Moderate dose:	Beta-1	↑ Myocardial contractility and heart rate	2–10 mcg/kg/min	1–3 mcg/kg/min. every 10 min
High dose:	Alpha-1	Vasoconstriction	10–20 mcg/kg/min	
Phenylephrine	Alpha-1	Vasoconstriction	Bolus: 100 mcg over 1 min Infusion: 20–200 mcg/min. Max: 300 mcg/min	20 mcg/min. every 10 min
Norepinephrine	Strong Alpha-1 Weak Beta-1	Strong vasoconstriction Weak ↑ myocardial contractility	2–12 mcg/min Max: 30 mcg/min	0.5 mcg/min. every 10 min
Epinephrine	Beta-1 Beta-2 Alpha-1	Strong ↑ myocardial contractility and heart rate, bronchodilation, and vasoconstriction	2–10 mcg/min. Max: 30 mcg/min	0.5 mcg/min. every 10 min
Vasopressin	V1 & V2	Vasoconstriction	0.01–0.04 units/min (commonly fixed dose of 0.03 units/min) Max: 0.1 units/min	

D, Dopaminergic receptor; *mcg/kg/min*, micrograms per kilogram per minute; *mcg/min*, micrograms per minute.

Phenylephrine

Phenylephrine (Neo-Synephrine) is a synthetic catecholamine that is a pure alpha-1 agonist that causes vasoconstriction. Phenylephrine has no beta-adrenergic agonist activity, has no direct effect on the myocardium, and does not increase heart rate. Phenylephrine may be used to restore blood pressure for neurogenic shock and hypotension caused by medications or vagal stimulation. In light of the lack of myocardial effect, it may be used for septic shock when norepinephrine is associated with tachydysrhythmia or if cardiac output is known to be high with a persistently low blood pressure.[9] A bolus dose of 0.1 to 0.5 micrograms may be given every 10 to 15 minutes for precipitous decreases in blood pressure.[4] Side effects of phenylephrine include increased afterload, reflex bradycardia, and peripheral ischemia.

BOX 9-1   Comparison of Dopamine, Norepinephrine, and Epinephrine

Dopamine, norepinephrine, and epinephrine stimulate alpha- and beta-adrenergic receptors and cause an increase in blood pressure and cardiac output. However, their clinical effect may be somewhat variable, possibly making some of these medications more advantageous in certain circumstances. Although far from conclusive, some data exist to help clinicians select the best vasopressor for treating shock.

As noted in the text, dopamine is primarily a positive inotrope at moderate doses and does not exert its vasoconstrictive effects until it is infused at higher doses. Although controversy exists as to whether dopamine produces a more marked increase in cardiac output compared with norepinephrine, some evidence indicates that it does cause more tachydysrhythmias.[2,43] Even though a large multicenter, randomized clinical trial comparing dopamine and norepinephrine for shock showed similar mortality rates for both groups, the death rate was significantly higher ($p = 0.03$) in a subgroup of patients with cardiogenic shock who received

dopamine, possibly signifying a relationship between the higher heart rates and more ischemic events. A meta-analysis of studies comparing dopamine and norepinephrine for the treatment of septic shock also revealed a significantly higher mortality rate ($p = 0.35$) for study participants who received dopamine.[10]

Although epinephrine and norepinephrine both increase blood pressure, at higher doses, epinephrine has a stronger affinity for beta-receptors and produces a higher increase in cardiac output.[11] Epinephrine, however, has been shown to cause more deleterious side effects compared with norepinephrine. A large multicenter, double-blind study comparing these medications for the management of different types of shock demonstrated no significant difference in the mortality rate ($p = 0.49$) or the time that they took to achieve a target mean arterial pressure ($p = 0.26$).[44] Yet, the study participants who received epinephrine had to have the infusion stopped more frequently because of clinically relevant side effects such as tachycardia and lactic acidosis.

Data from De Backer D, Biston P, Devriendt J, et al.: Comparison of dopamine and norepinephrine in the treatment of shock, *N Engl J Med* 362(9):779–789, 2010; De Backer D, Aldecoa C, Njimi H, Vincent J-L: Dopamine versus norepinephrine in the treatment of septic shock: a meta-analysis, *Crit Care Med* 40(3):725–730, 2012; Neumar RW, Otto CW, Link MS, et al.: Part 8: Advanced cardiovascular life support: 2010 American Heart Association guidelines for cardiopulmonary resuscitation and emergency cardiovascular care, *Circulation* 122(18 Suppl 3):S729–S767, 2010.43. De Backer D: Treatment of shock, *Acta Clin Belg* 66(6):438–442, 2011; and Myburgh JA, Higgins A, Jovanovska A, et al.: A comparison of epinephrine and norepinephrine in critically ill patients, *Intens Care Med* 34(12): 2226–2234, 2008.

Norepinephrine

Norepinephrine (*Levophed*), an endogenous neurotransmitter, is a potent alpha-1 agonist with mild beta-1 properties and no beta-2 activity. Therefore, it is a relatively weak positive inotrope and a potent vasoconstrictor, as its alpha-1 properties are unopposed. Norepinephrine is indicated for hypotension caused by vasodilatory shock states. In particular, it is recommended as a first-line agent in the setting of septic shock and should be titrated to increase the mean arterial blood pressure to 65 millimeters of mercury (mm Hg).[9,10] Side effects of norepinephrine include tachycardia, dysrhythmias, myocardial ischemia, and, at higher doses, decreased organ and peripheral perfusion.

Not all forms of shock are amenable to treatment with norepinephrine, which should not be started late in the course of cardiogenic shock because it increases afterload and decreases cardiac output.

Epinephrine

Epinephrine, also referred to as *adrenaline* in many countries, is an endogenous catecholamine that has strong beta-1 and beta-2 adrenergic properties that may cause a marked increase in cardiac output and heart rate, as well as bronchodilation. Although it increases blood flow to skeletal muscle beds, its potent alpha-1 agonist and vasoconstriction properties moderate the vasodilation from beta-2 receptor stimulation. Epinephrine also stimulates cardiac muscle cells to release a local vasodilator that increases coronary blood flow. A bolus dose of 1 milligram (mg) of epinephrine is indicated for cardiac arrest because of its ability to increase perfusion pressure to the coronary and cerebral blood vessels.[11] It is sometimes used for vasodilatory hypotension and cardiogenic shock when other agents do not produce the desired outcomes. Epinephrine may also be used as a second line of therapy for bradycardia and heart block associated with hypotension. Its bronchodilatory effects make it useful for anaphylaxis and severe asthma that is unresponsive to other therapies. When patients with septic shock remain hypotensive, epinephrine may be added to or substituted for norepinephrine.[9] Because of its potent effects, epinephrine should be started at low doses and carefully titrated to achieve a desirable response. Side effects of epinephrine include tachycardia and increased myocardial oxygen consumption. Therefore, it is generally regarded as a second-line therapy and reserved for treatment of profound shock because of its potential for inducing myocardial ischemia and tachydysrhythmia. Regional perfusion deficits may be caused by its strong alpha-1 effects. Because it is a stress hormone, epinephrine may stimulate gluconeogenesis and insulin resistance, which result in hyperglycemia.

Vasopressin

Vasopressin, a synthetic antidiuretic hormone, is a unique vasopressor that does not stimulate adrenergic receptors. Instead, it stimulates the V1 and V2 receptors, causing potent vasoconstriction and increased blood volume, respectively. Other mechanisms that promote vasoconstriction are thought to be related to vasopressin's ability to reduce nitric oxide production and to attenuate adrenergic receptor downregulation, which results in an enhancement of the body's response to catecholamines.[4,5] An IV infusion of vasopressin is indicated for treating refractory vasodilatory shock. Vasopressin may be particularly helpful in hypoxic and acidotic states when adrenergic agonists are less effective. An infusion of 0.03 units per minute (units/min) is recommended as a second-line treatment for septic shock to either increase the mean arterial pressure or to decrease the dose and potential adverse effects of norepinephrine.[5,9] The infusion dose is constant. It is not titrated, as it is administered as a replacement for a relative deficiency of endogenous vasopressin hormone. Vasopressin may also be beneficial for those who experience vasoplegic shock after cardiopulmonary bypass surgery.[4,12] A single IV dose of 40 units may be given for asystole, pulseless electrical activity, shock, refractory ventricular fibrillation, and pulseless ventricular tachycardia.[11]

Vasodilator Medications

Direct-acting vasodilators stimulate the formation of nitric oxide by the vascular endothelium, which, in turn, activates cyclic guanosine monophosphate. This substance facilitates smooth muscle relaxation by preventing cross-bridging of myosin with actin. Vasodilators are typically used to manage severe increases in blood pressure and may also be used in conditions in which excessive afterload impedes cardiac output. The venous system, which is able to distend, can accommodate large volumes of blood under low pressure. Medications that dilate veins further increase venous capacitance, and reduce venous return to the heart, thus reducing cardiac preload. Patients with acute decompensated heart failure with pulmonary congestion and dyspnea at rest may benefit from a vasodilator as long as their blood pressure is adequate.[13,14] See Table 9-3 for commonly used vasodilators with their mechanisms of action, dose ranges, and usual titration doses.

Nitroprusside

Nitroprusside (Nipride), a potent and rapid-acting direct arterial and venous vasodilator, is used to manage severe hypertension. It may also be used to reduce afterload in patients with acute decompensated heart failure, particularly when they are

TABLE 9-3   Vasodilating Medications

MEDICATION	MODE OF ACTION	USUAL DOSE RANGE	TITRATION
Nitroprusside	Direct vascular smooth muscle relaxant	0.1–4 micrograms per kilogram per minute (mcg/kg/min) Maximum dose: 10 mcg/kg/min	0.01 mcg/kg/min every 3–5 min
Nitroglycerin	Dilates coronary arteries Venous dilation at lower doses Arterial dilation at higher doses	5–200 mcg/min	5–10 mcg/min every 5 min
Hydralazine	Direct vascular smooth muscle relaxant	Injection: 10–20 milligrams (mg)	
Nicardipine	Calcium channel blocker	5–15 milligrams per hour (mg/hr) Maintenance dose: 3–5 mg/hr	2.5 mg/hr every 5–15 min

mcg/kg/min, Micrograms per kilogram per minute; *mcg/min*, micrograms per minute; *mg, milligrams*; *mg/hr*, milligrams per hour.

hypertensive or have mitral valve regurgitation.[14] The onset of its action is almost immediate, and the effects dissipate moments after it is discontinued. Nitroprusside is sensitive to light and must be protected with an opaque covering to prevent break-down. It should be carefully titrated to achieve the desired blood pressure, which occurs with decreased SVR. Because of its short half-life and powerful effects, care should be taken to avoid any deleterious swings in blood pressure.

The side effects of nitroprusside include hypotension, decreased platelet aggregation, flushing, diaphoresis, and rash. Hypoxemia with ventilation–perfusion mismatch may also occur when pulmonary arterioles in nonventilated areas dilate. Nitroprusside has been associated with increases in intracranial pressure caused by alterations in cerebral autoregulation.[15] Cyanide and thiocyanate, which are metabolites of nitroprusside metabolism, may cause toxic effects after exposure to high doses for prolonged periods. Cyanide causes metabolic acidosis by interfering with aerobic metabolism. The body has a limited supply of rhodanase, the enzyme needed to convert cyanide to thiocyanate. Originally, it was thought that if the amount of administered nitroprusside exceeded this limit, toxic levels of cyanide would accumulate and result in lactic acidosis. This premise led the U.S. Food and Drug Administration (FDA) to issue its strongest level of warning—a black box warning—to avoid nitroprusside doses greater than 2 mcg/kg/min. More recently, new data have suggested that additional enzymes and other chemical pathways for nitroprusside metabolism exist.[16] Accordingly, higher doses of nitroprusside may be safe but warrant vigilant monitoring. Signs of cyanide toxicity include mental confusion, tinnitus, blurred vision, nausea, weakness, hyperreflexia, metabolic acidosis, and death. The maximum dose of 10 microgram per kilogram per minute should not be infused for more than 10 minutes.[8] Nitroprusside infusions lasting more than 9 days should be avoided to prevent the accumulation of thiocyanate. Although thiocyanate is much less toxic than cyanide, prolonged exposure may cause neurologic derangements manifesting as confusion, hallucinations, seizures, and coma.[16] Individuals with kidney insufficiency may suffer these toxic effects in as little as 3 days. Consequently, other antihypertensives should be considered when adequate blood pressure control is not achieved within this timeframe or as high doses are approached.

Nitroglycerin

Nitroglycerin (Tridil) causes vasodilation by generating nitric oxide in vascular smooth muscle. It is considered the drug of choice for angina and acute coronary syndrome because it dilates the coronary arteries and helps improve collateral blood flow to the ischemic areas of the myocardium. Nitroglycerin may be administered as a sublin-gual tablet or spray, transdermally, or intravenously. When administered intrave-nously at lower doses, it dilates the veins and reduces ventricular preload by reducing venous return to the heart. The reduction of intracardiac volume reduces ven-tricular wall stress and myocardial oxygen consumption. Therefore, nitroglycerin is also recommended for normotensive patients in acute heart failure when they are unre-sponsive to the usual therapies.[14] At doses over 150 mcg/min, nitroglycerin decreases blood pressure and afterload by dilating the peripheral arteries.[8] The side effects of nitroglycerin include hypotension, especially if the patient is volume depleted. Syncope and orthostatic hypotension may occur in patients sensitive to the medication. It is important to avoid using nitroglycerin in patients with right ventricular failure, as the right ventricle is reliant on sufficient venous return to maintain adequate cardiac output. Headache is another common side effect, and tolerance, which may necessitate escalation of doses to achieve the same clinical effect, may occur with prolonged use. Although the exact mechanism for this phenomenon is not completely understood, it is believed that nitric oxide production is reduced, whereas clearance is increased.[17] Other proposed mechanisms include an increased sensitivity to vasoconstrictors and activation of the renin–angiotensin–aldosterone system, which oppose the effects of the remaining nitric oxide that is produced.[17]

Interactions with other medications are a concern. Patients who have taken a 5'phophosdiasterase inhibitor within the last 24 to 48 hours should not be given nitroglycerin because the combination may cause severe hypotension.[8]

The onset of action is 1 to 2 minutes, so the patient's blood pressure should be closely monitored while initiating and titrating nitroglycerin. Nitroglycerin is titrated to achieve the desired clinical effects, which typically include elimination of anginal pain, reduction in pulmonary congestion, or decrease in blood pressure. Decrease of the systolic blood pressure below 90 mm Hg should be avoided to prevent a reduction in myocardial perfusion. Hypertensive individuals should not have a decrease of more than 25% in their blood pressure over several minutes to 1 hour.[8]

Hydralazine

Hydralazine (Apresoline) is an antihypertensive that causes arterial vasodilation by altering the movement of calcium within vascular smooth muscle. The peripheral vasodilation decreases peripheral vascular resistance with a resultant rise in stroke volume. Hydralazine has minimal effect on the veins and does not alter preload. Its propensity for inducing reflex tachycardia limits its usefulness, but this effect may be ameliorated by adding a beta-blocker. A slow IV injection of 10 to 20 mg may be administered for hypertensive crisis or for severe hypertension associated with preeclampsia or eclampsia.[8,18] Subsequent doses should be administered cautiously after 15 minutes when the maximal blood pressure decrease can be determined. Side effects of hydralazine include headache, palpitations, flushing, and exacerbation of angina.

Nicardipine

Nicardipine (Cardene) is a dihydropyridine calcium channel blocker that causes arterial vasodilation and reduces systemic vascular resistance by blocking the influx of calcium in vascular smooth muscle. It is used for the short-term management of hypertension and is particularly useful in patients who have experienced an ischemic stroke.[15,19] A systematic review comparing nicardipine and labetalol in the management of hypertensive crisis showed that while both agents had similar efficacy and safety profiles, nicardipine provided more consistent effects and required fewer dose changes.[20]

Nicardipine is contraindicated in those with advanced aortic stenosis. Its side effects include hypotension, tachydysrhythmia, headache, flushing, and dizziness.

Nesiritide

Nesiritide (Natrecor) is a recombinant form of human brain natriuretic peptide. When the heart becomes volume overloaded, the overstretched ventricular myocardium secretes the endogenous form of this hormone, which causes arterial and venous vasodilation. Accordingly, nesiritide is administered to patients with heart failure to alleviate pulmonary congestion and dyspnea by decreasing systemic afterload and venous return and by exerting a mild natriuretic effect. Natriuresis is a diuresis of urine with higher levels of sodium. An infusion of nesiritide for 24 to 48 hours is indicated in the management of dyspnea associated with acute decompensated heart failure, where it has been shown to decrease pulmonary artery occlusion pressure (PAOP), increase cardiac output, and improve diastolic function.[21]

If an endogenous brain natriuretic peptide level is needed for diagnostic purposes, it should be measured prior to starting a nesiritide infusion, as it cannot be reliably ascertained once the medication has been administered. Because the effects of nesiritide are not evident for several hours, dose changes are usually prescribed and performed no more frequently than every 3 hours. Nesiritide may cause hypotension, which usually occurs in the first hour and may last several hours. The initial bolus dose may be omitted to avoid hypotension in vulnerable individuals. If hypotension does occur, the infusion should be immediately stopped and a fluid bolus administered. Patients receiving nesiritide should be monitored for hypersensitivity reactions and anaphylaxis.[8] Other adverse effects include bradycardia, atrial fibrillation, and other tachydysrhythmia.

The Acute Study of Clinical Effectiveness of Nesiritide in Decompensated Heart Failure (ASCEND-HF), a large, randomized, double-blind clinical trial, demonstrated that although nesiritide is relatively safe and confers a small, yet nonsignificant ($p=0.007$), benefit on subjective reports of dyspnea, it did not significantly reduce the composite endpoint of heart failure re-admission or 30-day mortality ($p=0.31$).[22] Additionally, the use of nesiritide did not reduce the risk of kidney dysfunction. The study investigators recommended that nesiritide not be used in all patients with acute heart failure symptoms. Instead, it might be useful for selected individuals with volume overload, in whom a clinical benefit is observed.[23] Patients who have had their native ventricles removed for implantation of a total artificial heart and are not able to produce endogenous brain natriuretic peptide, may benefit from nesiritide in situations where resistance to diuretics has developed.[14]

Positive Inotropes

Positive inotropic agents are administered to increase cardiac output in patients with seriously altered cardiac function. Improvement in cardiac contractility may help relieve cardiopulmonary congestions associated with cardiac failure by promoting more complete emptying of the ventricles. Catecholamine agents that have beta-1 adrenergic properties increase myocardial contractility by increasing the levels of cyclic adenosine monophosphate and intracellular calcium available to bind myosin and actin filaments within myocytes.[3,4,24,25] Tachydysrhythmia and myocardial ischemia may be induced when positive inotropic agents are given to patients with inadequate preload. Therefore, it is important to administer appropriate fluid resuscitation prior to the administration of positive inotropic medications or simultaneously.[9] These agents should be used cautiously in patients with severe aortic valve stenosis and idiopathic hypertrophic subaortic stenosis, as these agents may exacerbate myocardial ischemia and worsen outflow tract obstruction.[7]

Dopamine

Dopamine (Intropin), at moderate doses of 2 to 10 micrograms per kilogram per minute (mcg/kg/min), primarily stimulates beta-1 adrenergic receptors, which increases cardiac contractility and heart rate.[8] At this dose range, dopamine may be used for treating cardiogenic shock and symptomatic bradycardia. At doses less than 2 mcg/kg/min, dopamine stimulates dopaminergic receptors causing renal and mesenteric vasodilation.[8] It also exerts a natriuretic effect at low doses, which results in loss of sodium and water in urine. Although these effects may increase urine output, several systematic reviews and one large randomized clinical trial revealed that it does not decrease the incidence of acute kidney injury, the need for renal replacement therapy, or mortality.[26–30] Furthermore, Dopamine may worsen kidney function in patients with marginal or inadequate volume status. Therefore, what was once known as 'renal dose' dopamine is no longer routinely used to improve kidney function.

A common side effect of dopamine is tachycardia, particularly when patients are hypovolemic. Therefore, clinicians should ensure adequate circulating volume before starting this medication. Dopamine increases myocardial cellular metabolism and oxygen consumption, which may result in myocardial ischemia and dysrhythmias. At higher doses, dopamine may inhibit microcirculatory flow because of vasoconstriction, thus limiting its usefulness in the later stages of shock. The vasoconstrictive effects may also increase afterload and decrease cardiac output. Therefore, it is imperative to assess peripheral perfusion at these doses and consider other inotropic agents. Alternatively, a reduction of dopamine to 7.5 mcg/kg/min and simultaneous administration of a second beta-1 agonist agent such as dobutamine may improve cardiac output without excessively increasing afterload and microcirculatory flow.[4]

Isoproterenol

Isoproterenol (Isuprel), a synthetic catecholamine, is a potent beta-adrenergic agent with minimal alpha-agonist properties. Although it has positive inotropic properties, this effect is attenuated by a decrease in afterload, which results in no marked change in cardiac output. Its usefulness in treating cardiogenic shock is limited because of its ability to increase cardiac impulse conduction and heart rate. Consequently, it is sometimes referred to as the *pharmacologic pacemaker* and may be used as a temporizing measure for atropine refractory symptomatic bradycardia and heart block until pacemaker therapy can be initiated. It is particularly useful in heart transplant recipients, who have symptomatic bradydysrhythmias and lack parasympathetic innervation of the myocardium. Isoproterenol has beta-2 adrenergic properties that cause bronchodilation and vasodilation of the pulmonary vasculature. Therefore, it may be used to treat refractory bronchospasms. The dose range for isoproterenol is 2 to 10 mcg/min.[8] Side effects include tachycardia, myocardial ischemia, ventricular dysrhythmias, anxiety, and flushing.

Inodilators

Inodilators (Table 9-4) are medications that decrease afterload by dilating arteries while also exerting a positive inotropic effect. The combination of increased contractility and vasodilation may be beneficial to patients experiencing cardiogenic shock with increased afterload caused by stimulation of the sympathetic nervous system. Inodilators are also indicated for short-term support to maintain end-organ perfusion in patients with acute heart failure with systolic dysfunction.[31]

TABLE 9-4 Inodilator Medications

MEDICATION	ACTION	USUAL DOSE RANGE	DOSE MANAGEMENT
Dobutamine	Catecholamine: beta-1 and beta-2	2–20 micrograms per kilogram per minute (mcg/kg/min)	Titrate by 0.5 mcg/min every 10 min
Milrinone	Phosphodiasterase 3 inhibitor	*Loading dose:* 50 mcg/kg over 10 minutes *Min:* 0.375 mcg/kg/min *Standard:* 0.5 mcg/kg/min *Max:* 0.75 mcg/kg/min	*Onset of action:* 15 min *Peak of action:* 2 hours (Wait at least 2 hours before increasing the dose) *Duration:* 3 to 6 hrs
Nesiritide	Recombinant brain natriuretic peptide promotes arterial and venous dilation	Bolus dose of 2 mcg/kg over 60 seconds, followed by an infusion of 0.01 mcg/kg/min Dose may be increased by 0.005 mcg/kg/min every 3 hours *Max:* 0.03 mcg/kg/min	*Onset:* 15 min *Peak effect:* 60 min *Half-life:* 20 min *Duration:* 3 hours Wait at least 3 hours before increasing the dose

mcg/kg/min, Micrograms per kilogram per minute; *mcg/min*, micrograms per minute.

Dobutamine

Dobutamine (*Dobutrex*) is a synthetic catecholamine with a strong affinity for beta-1 and beta-2 receptors. It is a potent positive inotrope with weak chronotropic activity. Its beta-2 activity causes vasodilation in the blood vessels in skeletal muscle, which decreases peripheral afterload. Although it has some alpha-1 properties, its affinity for beta-2 receptors is stronger, so the net effect favors mild vasodilation. Therefore, dobutamine does not markedly increase blood pressure. It is commonly used to treat cardiogenic shock. Because it increases myocardial metabolism and oxygen consumption, myocardial ischemia and dysrhythmias may occur. This agent may cause tachydysrhythmias, but they are usually much less pronounced than those that occur with dopamine. Dobutamine is recommended for patients with septic shock who have a low cardiac output despite an adequate preload and mean arterial pressure.[9] It is not advisable to use dobutamine to increase cardiac output to supraphysiologic levels for this patient population.

Milrinone

Milrinone (*Primacor*), a phosphodiesterase III inhibitor, produces a positive inotropic effect by inhibiting the enzyme that metabolizes cyclic adenosine monophosphate, which results in an increase in the availability of intracellular calcium in myocytes.[3,24,25] Its lusitropic effects, or the ability to facilitate diastolic ventricular relaxation, enhances diastolic filling, which optimizes preload. Increased levels of cyclic adenosine monophosphate in vascular smooth muscle cause a large vasodilatory effect on peripheral and pulmonary vessels, often more potent than dobutamine, and remain effective even when the patient is receiving beta-blockers. This combination of effects may result in a decrease in cardiac filling pressures, whereas blood pressure and heart rate remain relatively unchanged. Because it does not have beta-1 adrenergic properties, milrinone is indicated for treating heart failure associated with pulmonary congestion and hypoperfusion, particularly when catecholamine agents are no longer effective because of beta-receptor downregulation. Nausea, vomiting, cardiac ischemia, and tachydysrhythmia are side effects. Hypotension may also occur and persist, as the half-life of milrinone may be as long as 2 hours.[7] This longer half-life precludes rapid titration of the medication and may prolong the duration of adverse effects.

Beta-Blockers

Beta-adrenergic blockers (Table 9-5) compete with endogenous catecholamines for available beta-receptor sites and blunt the effects of the sympathetic nervous system. As a result, these medications reduce cardiac contractility and heart rate and inhibit bronchodilation and vasodilation. Some beta-blockers are more cardioselective and have minimal effect on beta-2 receptors. Therefore, they reduce myocardial work and oxygen consumption but are less likely to cause bronchoconstriction. In patients experiencing a

TABLE 9-5   Alpha- and Beta-Blockers

MEDICATION	CLASS	ONSET OF ACTION	DOSAGE
Metoprolol	Beta-1 blocker Weak beta-2 blocker	10 minutes (min)	5 milligrams (mg), intravenously (IV), every 5 min, up to 3 doses
Esmolol	Beta-1 blocker	Immediate	Loading dose of 500 milligrams per kilogram (mg/kg) over 1 min followed by an infusion of 50 micrograms per kilogram per minute (mcg/kg/min); may be titrated every 5 min to a maximum of 300 mcg/kg/min
Labetalol	Alpha-1 and Beta-blocker	5 min	20 mg, IV bolus, followed by an infusion of 2 to 8 mg/min Bolus dose may be repeated in 10 min

IV, Intravenous; *mcg/kg/min*, micrograms per kilogram per minute; *mg/kg*, milligrams per kilogram; *mg/min*, milligrams per minute.

myocardial infarction, beta-blockers have been shown to reduce the size of infarction, life-threatening ventricular dysrhythmia, cardiac remodeling, and other associated complications.[31,32] They are also used to manage hypertension and supraventricular tachy-dysrhythmia and have been shown to reduce mortality and hospitalizations in patients with heart failure.[13,31] Patients with hypertrophic cardiomyopathy may demonstrate improved diastolic filling when given beta-blockers because of the decrease in heart rate.[33] Some proposed mechanisms for their ability to lower blood pressure include improved vascular compliance and decreased heart rate and venous return.[33]

Beta-blockers have some important side effects. Noncardioselective beta-blockers may induce bronchoconstriction and should be avoided in patients with reactive airway disease. Because beta-blockers reduce cardiac contractility, they should not be given to patients with cardiogenic shock and should be used cautiously in individuals with left ventricular dysfunction. Beta-blockers should not be given to patients with prolonged first-degree or high-grade atrioventricular heart block. Signs of hypoglycemia, which are mediated through stimulation of the sympathetic nervous system, may be masked by beta-blockers.

Currently, *metoprolol* (*Lopressor*) and *esmolol* (*Brevibloc*) are the only two cardioselective beta-blockers that can be administered parenterally.

Metoprolol

Metoprolol has strong beta-1 blockade activity with a less potent effect on beta-2 receptors, which makes it useful in some individuals with reactive airway disease. It is recommended for the initial management of ST-elevated myocardial infarction in individuals who present with hypertension or are exhibiting ongoing ischemia because it reduces myocardial oxygen consumption and infarction size.[32]

Esmolol

Esmolol is a short-acting beta-1 selective blocker that is given to manage peri-operative hypertension and hypertensive emergencies, particularly those associated with tachycardia. It is given by administering a loading dose, followed by a continuous infusion that may be titrated to achieve the desired decrease in blood pressure. Adverse effects include hypotension, heart failure, heart block, bradycardia, flushing, and pulmonary edema. Phlebitis has been reported, and tissue necrosis may occur with extravasation, so this medication should be infused through a large vein.

Alpha-Blockers

Alpha-blockers (see Table 9-5) decrease blood pressure by blocking the effects of the sympathetic nervous system on peripheral blood vessels. Some agents block alpha-1 receptors, and others are alpha-2 agonists and inhibit the release of norepinephrine from presynaptic nerve endings in the central nervous system. Although alpha-1 blockers are not used as first-line treatment for hypertension, they may be used in combination with other antihypertensives. Prolonged use may cause fluid retention, which limits their usefulness in heart failure and makes it desirable to co-administer with a diuretic.[34]

Phentolamine

Phentolamine (Regitine) blocks alpha-1 and alpha-2 receptors and decreases blood pressure by causing arterial and venous vasodilation. It is used to control hypertension in patients with pheochromocytoma, an adrenal medulla tumor that secretes epinephrine. It is administered in the operating room and critical care unit as a slow IV injection in doses of 1 to 5 mg. It may cause orthostatic hypotension and drowsiness.

Phentolamine is administered subcutaneously after extravasation of vasopressors to prevent tissue ischemia. A dose of 5 to 10 mg diluted in 10 to 15 milliliters (mL) of normal saline should be injected around the infiltrated area to block vasoconstriction and tissue necrosis.[8]

Clonidine

Clonidine (Catapres) is a centrally acting sympathoplegic agent that stimulates alpha-2 receptors in the brainstem. It inhibits central sympathetic discharge by blocking the release of norepinephrine from presynaptic nerve endings, thus decreasing blood pressure by reducing the amount of endogenous catecholamines available to stimulate cardiovascular adrenergic receptors. Although it decreases SVR, it also reduces cardiac output by decreasing heart rate. Clonidine may be administered orally or as a transdermal patch. This drug should be gradually withdrawn to avoid rebound sympathetic activity with resultant anxiety, tachycardia, tremors, and hypertensive crisis. Clonidine is generally considered a fourth-line antihypertensive because of its side effects of sedation, dry mouth, and fatigue.[35]

Combined Alpha–Beta Blockers

Labetalol

Labetalol (Normodyne) (see Table 9-5) is a combined alpha-1 and noncardioselective beta-blocker that decreases blood pressure by decreasing heart rate and decreasing SVR. Its potent alpha-1 blocking action lowers the blood pressure, and its blockade of beta-1 receptors prevents reflex tachycardia and diminishes the rate of left ventricular pressure rise and aortic wall stress, which makes it suitable for the treatment of acute aortic dissection. It is also indicated in patients with hypertensive emergencies, peri-operative hypertension, and severe hypertension associated with pre-eclampsia and eclampsia.[15,18,33] Side effects include atrioventricular heart block, nausea, vomiting, and orthostatic hypotension. Bronchoconstriction may occur in individuals with chronic obstructive pulmonary disease (COPD) because of its beta-2 blocking properties. When administering labetalol, it is important to gradually lower the blood pressure to prevent cerebral and myocardial ischemia.

Clinical Implications

Hemodynamic monitoring is often employed to assess patient response to vasoactive medications. Blood pressure measured with the sphygmomanometer, a noninvasive blood pressure device, may be erroneous in hypotensive states. Therefore, invasive arterial pressure monitoring may be required to obtain more accurate blood pressure measures to achieve timely evaluation of the patient's response and titration of medications.[5] Mean arterial pressure serves as a surrogate for tissue perfusion, so vasoactive medications are generally titrated to keep this parameter above 60 mm Hg.[7,9,36]

> **Clinical Reasoning Pearl**
>
> Vasopressors are titrated to maintain a targeted mean arterial pressure, whereas vasodilators are administered to decreased afterload. In some cases these are the same medications infused at different dosages. Physical assessment findings should be monitored to ensure that tissue perfusion is restored to organs regardless of measured and calculated hemodynamic parameters.

Electrocardiography (ECG) is used to monitor the effect of the medications on the heart rate and rhythm.[24] Other forms of hemodynamic monitoring such as cardiac output and cardiac index, cardiac filling pressures, mixed venous oxygenation saturation, and functional hemodynamics, as well as systemic and pulmonary vascular resistance calculations, may be needed to evaluate the effectiveness of medications.[1,5] This monitoring is particularly needed when patients have more than one type of shock coexisting.

Although hemodynamic indices may be helpful, it is imperative to assess for physical signs and laboratory test results that indicate that tissue perfusion has been sufficiently restored. These signs include urinary output of 0.5 milliliters per kilogram per hour (mL/kg/hr), restoration of baseline mentation, warm and dry skin, normalization of serum lactate and arterial pH levels, and correction of acute kidney injury and liver dysfunction.[5,9,36] It is especially important to assess the physical signs of perfusion when vasopressors are infusing at high doses, as intense vasoconstriction may cause ischemia and necrosis of the digits. Perfusion to the abdominal viscera is also vulnerable with high doses of vasopressors; signs of poor perfusion to this area include gastric ulcers, intolerance of enteral nutrition, ileus, and bowel infarction.

Clinical Reasoning Pearl

High doses of vasoconstrictors may inhibit microcirculatory flow to vulnerable tissue beds in the skin, abdominal viscera, and kidneys. Vasoconstriction may also increase afterload and decrease cardiac output, especially for patients with myocardial dysfunction. Beta-1 agonists increase myocardial workload and may exacerbate myocardial ischemia and cause atrial and ventricular dysrhythmias. Because of these potent side effects, these medications should be started at low doses and titrated to appropriate clinical endpoints. Alternative medications should be considered if the patient exhibits deleterious side effects.

Therapeutic goals are tailored for individual patients. For example, a patient with a history of hypertension and atherosclerosis may require a mean arterial pressure higher than 65 mm Hg to restore the balance between oxygen delivery and demand in some tissues.[9] Although the optimal mean arterial pressure (MAP) in patients with neurogenic shock has not been established, there is some evidence of improved outcomes when it is maintained at 85 mm Hg.[37]

Medication Safety

Medication safety practices should be adhered to when administering vasoactive medications because of their potency and the unstable condition of patients receiving them. Bar code–assisted medication administration systems may prevent medication errors when initiating vasoactive infusion or when changing infusion containers.[38,39] Continuous infusions should be administered through an IV pump, and, when available, drug library and dose limit safety features should be used. Although this technology may help improve patient safety, it cannot prevent every medication error and should not replace other prudent medication administration practices. IV pumps should be checked at the start of each nursing shift and whenever medication containers are changed to ensure proper programming. An independent double-check should be performed when initiating or changing IV infusion containers that the health care organization has identified as a high-risk medication.[40] It may be useful to implement standardized IV bag labeling practices such as color coding or Tallman lettering to help avoid misidentification of medications that have similar names.

One patient weight should be used when calculating weight-based doses and programming IV pumps.[41] Typically, the patient's actual weight measured close to the time of the initiation of the medication is used. Ideal body weight may be used in patients weighing more than 200 pounds, since little is known about the volume distribution of many of these medications.[41] Ultimately, these medications should be titrated to the desired clinical effect, if possible.

Although the actions of these medications are well known, some patients may react differently. For this reason, medications may need to be started at the lowest recommended dose and slowly titrated until it is clear how a particular patient responds. The lowest effective dose is also desirable to avoid adverse effects.

Clinical Reasoning Pearl

When starting vasoactive agents, it is important to know the mechanism of action and time to onset of each medication so that the clinical effects can be anticipated. Not every patient responds to a particular medication in the same manner, especially when catecholamine agents are given to patients with adrenergic receptor downregulation. Hemodynamics should be monitored, and medications titrated carefully until it can be determined how the patient responds.

Ideally, one medication is titrated at a time so that the impact of the dose modifications can be clearly understood. Generally, the medication that impacts the altered hemodynamic parameter is titrated first. Patient response to catecholamines may be diminished in the setting of acidosis, hypoxemia, and relative adrenal insufficiency.[1,4] Therefore, these conditions are corrected, whenever possible. Corticosteroids have been shown to improve beta-receptor responsiveness to catecholamines, and may be considered for patients who remain dependent on vasopressors.[42] Alternative agents should be considered when selected medications do not result in the desired response. More concentrated solutions may need to be used when medications are infusing at high rates, especially in patients with fluid overload. In most circumstances, antihypertensives are discontinued when vasoconstrictor and positive inotropic agents are initiated. This recommendation is sometimes overlooked in emergency situations.

Patient Safety

- Carefully check the integrity of the IV infusion site. Medications that have vasoconstrictive properties may cause tissue ischemia and necrosis if the IV fluid infiltrates. Infusion via a large central vein may reduce the risk of infiltration. Know your facility's policy for managing infiltration of vasoconstrictive medications.

- Check medication compatibilities prior to infusing more than one medication through a single IV catheter. In general, catecholamine agents are not compatible with alkaline solutions.

- When infusing vasoactive medications, it is helpful to label the tubing of catheters at the distal connection site to prevent inadvertent injection of an incompatible medication or administration of a bolus dose of a vasoactive medication. If possible, reserve one IV catheter for administration of medications in the event of a cardiac arrest.

- Anticipate when the next IV container of a vasoactive medication will be needed. Many vasoactive medications have a short half-life, and if the IV container runs empty, the patient may experience hemodynamic deterioration.

When it is time to wean the patient off vasoactive infusions, it is important to start by reviewing the prescription as well as the hemodynamic goals. This review is an essential element of the hand-off report that occurs between clinicians. Generally, the patient is weaned off one medication at a time, using one of several strategies. Some clinicians first wean the patient off the infusion that impacts the most stable parameter, others will start with medications that are most likely to hinder microcirculatory flow, induce myocardial ischemia, or cause dysrhythmias. The infusion dose should be titrated down slowly until it can be determined how the patient responds. Goals and weaning plans should be reviewed and adjusted at least daily and as needed. Once the infusion has been stopped, the IV line should be cleared of the medication so that the patient does not receive a bolus dose the next time the IV line is used.

Patient Education

- Explain the intended actions and possible side effects of vasoactive medications to the patient and the family so that the patient can report any untoward effects such as headache and flushing (nitroglycerin) or tachycardia (dopamine, epinephrine).

- If a central venous catheter is being used, explain to the patient the rationale for using the catheter and provide information about the prevention and detection of catheter-related bloodstream infection.

Case Study

James Robertson is a 68-year-old man who presents to the emergency department (ED) with complaints of dyspnea. He states that he developed a productive cough of thick yellow mucus 1 week ago and that it has become progressively worse. Today, he woke up feeling very weak and tired and was unable to get out of bed because of shortness of breath. Consequently, he called 9-1-1 for medical assistance. Mr. Robertson is widowed, lives alone, and has two adult sons. He has a history of dyslipidemia, hypertension, and coronary heart disease. Nine months ago, he suffered a non–ST-segment elevated myocardial infarction (NSTEMI) and underwent a percutaneous coronary intervention (PCI) with angioplasty and placement of a drug-eluting stent. His home medications include metoprolol 100 mg twice a day, aspirin 325 mg daily, atorvastatin 10 mg daily, and clopidogrel 75 mg daily.

On physical examination, Mr. Robertson is pale, diaphoretic, tachypneic, and using his accessory muscles to breathe. He is lethargic and only able to speak a few words at a time because of his dyspnea. On auscultation, his heart tones are normal and his breath sounds have rhonchi and fine crackles. His abdomen is soft, and bowel sounds are hypoactive. Peripheral pulses are weak and thready. Vital signs are temperature 39°C (102.2°F); heart rate 142 beats/min; blood pressure 80/42 mm Hg; respiration rate 36 breaths/min; pulse oximeter oxygen saturation (SpO_2) 87%. Arterial blood gas results are pH 7.28; $paCO_2$ 57; PaO_2 53; and bicarbonate (HCO_3^-) 21.

He is intubated and placed on a mechanical ventilator with the following settings: Assist Control (AC), rate 14; V_T 550; FiO_2 0.7 (70%); and positive end-expiratory pressure (PEEP) 5 centimeters of water (cm H_2O). A large-bore peripheral IV is inserted, and a fluid bolus of 3.5 liters (L) of normal saline is rapidly infused. A urinary catheter is inserted with return of a small amount of dark amber urine. Blood and sputum cultures are collected and sent to the laboratory, and broad-spectrum antibiotics are administered.

Laboratory values are white blood cell (WBC) count 22,000 mm^3, hemoglobin 14.8 grams per deciliter (g/dL); hematocrit 36%; platelet count 145,000/microliter (μL); sodium 145 milliequivalents per liter (mEq/L); potassium 4.2 mEq/L; glucose 167 milligrams per deciliter (mg/dL); lactate 5.2 millimoles per liter (mmol/L); blood urea nitrogen (BUN) 26 mg/dL; and creatinine 1.8 mg/dL.

Critical Care Unit Admission (13:00). Mr. Robertson is admitted to the critical care unit with a diagnosis of community-acquired pneumonia and septic shock. Shortly thereafter, an arterial line with stroke volume variation (SVV) analysis technology and a central venous catheter (CVC) are inserted. He remains tachycardiac and hypotensive with a stroke volume 43 mL; SVV 17%; and SVR 590 dynes·sec/cm^5. A sample of venous blood is drawn from his central venous catheter and reveals a central venous oxygen saturation ($ScvO_2$) of 58%. Urine output is 15 mL during the first hour after admission. An additional IV bolus of 1 liter of normal saline is administered over 20 minutes.

Critical Care Unit (13:30). Hemodynamic parameters after the second fluid bolus are stabilizing with MAP 59 mm Hg; CVP 12 mm Hg, stroke volume 57 mL and SVV 11%.

A norepinephrine infusion is started at 0.5 mcg/min and titrated up to 7.5 mcg/min over the next hour to achieve a MAP of 65 mm Hg.

Critical Care Unit (14:30). Subsequently, his hemodynamic indices stabilize, his serum lactate drops to 1.8 mmol/L, and $ScvO_2$ rises to 72%. At this point, his urine output is

Continued

Case Study—cont'd

60 mL/hour, and his skin is pink and warm with capillary refill taking less than 3 seconds. Morphine and propofol are administered for pain and sedation. Enteral nutrition, peptic ulcer prophylaxis, and venous thromboembolus prophylaxis are started. A continuous insulin infusion is started and titrated to keep his blood glucose between 140 to 180 mg/dL.

	11:50 ED	13:00 CRITICAL CARE UNIT ADMISSION	13:30 CRITICAL CARE UNIT	14:30 CRITICAL CARE UNIT
Interventions	Fluid bolus 3.5 liters Intubated	A-line inserted CVC inserted Fluid bolus 1 liter	Norepinephrine 0.5–7.5 mcg/min	Norepinephrine 7.5 mcg/min
Heart rate (beats/min)	142	130	105	96
Respiratory rate breaths/min	36			
MV rate	14	14	14	14
Blood pressure mm Hg (cuff) S/D (MAP)	80/42 (cuff)	85/35 (51)	97/40 (59)	92/55 (67)
CVP		4	12	12
Cardiac output (L/min)		5.7	6.0	6.9
Cardiac index (L/min/m^2)		2.5	2.6	3.0
Stroke volume (mL)		43	57	72
SVV		17%	11%	11%
SVR dynes·sec/cm^5		590	606	795
ScvO$_2$		58%		72%
Lactate (mmol/L)	5.2			1.8

Critical Care Unit Day 2. On day 2, Mr. Robertson remains mechanically ventilated. He develops atrial fibrillation with a ventricular response of 145 beats/min and a resultant decrease in blood pressure to 88/50 mm Hg. A phenylephrine infusion is started and quickly titrated up to 120 mcg/min, while the norepinephrine is discontinued. Thirty minutes later, Mr. Robertson regains normal sinus rhythm, and his blood pressure stabilizes.

Critical Care Unit Day 4. By day 4 in the critical care unit, Mr. Robertson is hemodynamically stable, and is weaned off phenylephrine. His serum creatinine has decreased to 0.9 mg/dL. A sedation vacation is performed, and he is weaned from the mechanical ventilator and extubated. Antibiotics are continued as Mr. Robertson continues to improve. The next day, he is transferred to a telemetry progressive care unit. He is discharged home in stable condition 3 days later. ■

Conclusion

Currently, many different vasoactive medications that play an important role in restoring tissue perfusion are available for patients with hemodynamic alterations. It is important to select pharmacologic agents on the basis of the patient's underlying pathophysiology and the properties of each medication and then manage those agents to achieve the desired therapeutic endpoints. Hemodynamic monitoring, laboratory test results, and physical assessment findings should be used to guide the management of these agents. It is also imperative to monitor for potentially serious adverse effects and employ safe medication practices to protect patients from harm.

References

1. Piastra M, Luca E, Mensi S, et al.: Inotropic and vasoactive drugs in pediatric ICU, *Curr Drug Targets* 13(7):900–905, 2012.
2. De Backer D, Biston P, Devriendt J, Madl C, et al.: Comparison of dopamine and norepinephrine in the treatment of shock, *N Engl J Med* 362(9):779–789, 2010.
3. Bangash MN, Kong ML, Pearse RM: Use of inotropes and vasopressor agents in critically ill patients, *Br J Pharmacol* 165(7):2015–2033, 2012.
4. Overgaard CB, Dzavik V: Inotropic and vasopressors: review of physiology and clinical use in cardiovascular disease, *Circulation* 118(10):1047–1056, 2008.
5. Hollenberg SM: Inotrope and vasopressor therapy of septic shock, *Crit Care Clin* 25(4):781–802, 2009.
6. Lilly CM, Zuckerman IH, Badawi O, Riker RR: Benchmark data from more than 240,000 adults that reflect the current practice of critical care in the United States, *Chest* 140(5):1232–1242, 2011.
7. Cooper BE: Review and update on inotropes and vasopressors, *AACN Adv Crit Care* 19(1):5–15, 2008.
8. Gahart BL, Nazareno AR: *2014 intravenous medications*, St. Louis, MO, 2014, Mosby.
9. Dellinger RP, Levy M, Rhodes A, et al.: Surviving sepsis campaign: international guidelines for management of severe sepsis and septic shock, *Crit Care Med* 41(2):580–637, 2013.
10. De Backer D, Aldecoa C, Njimi H, Vincent J-L: Dopamine versus norepinephrine in the treatment of septic shock: a meta-analysis, *Crit Care Med* 40(3):725–730, 2012.

11. Neumar RW, Otto CW, Link MS, et al.: Part 8: Advanced cardiovascular life support: 2010 American Heart Association guidelines for cardiopulmonary resuscitation and emergency cardiovascular care, *Circulation* 122(18 Suppl 3):S729–S767, 2010.

12. Egi M, Bellomo R, Langenberg C, et al.: Selecting a vasopressor drug for vasoplegic shock after adult cardiac surgery: a systematic literature review, *Ann Thorac Surg* 83(2):715–723, 2007.

13. Ezekowitz JA, Hernandez AF, Starling RC, et al.: Standardizing care for acute decompensated heart failure in large megatrial: the approach for the acute studies of clinical effectiveness of Nesiritide in subjects with decompensated heart failure (ASCEND-HF), *Am Heart J* 157 (2):219–228, 2009.

14. Carlson MD, Eckman PM: Review of vasodilators in acute decompensated heart failure: the old and the new, *J Card Fail* 19(7):478–493, 2013.

15. Sarafidis PA, Georgianos PI, Malindretos P, Liakopoulos V: Pharmacological management of hypertensive emergencies and urgencies: focus on newer agents, *Expert Opin Investig Drugs* 21(8):1089–1106, 2012.

16. Lockwood A, Patka J, Rabinovich M, et al.: Sodium nitroprusside-associated cyanide toxicity in adult patients—fact or fiction? A critical review of the evidence and clinical relevance, *Open Access J Clin Trials* 2:133–148, 2010.

17. Sage PR, de la Lande IS, Stafford I, et al.: Nitroglycerin tolerance in human vessels: evidence for impaired nitroglycerin bioconversion, *Circulation* 102:2810–2815, 2000.

18. Committee on Obstetric Practice: Emergent therapy for acute-onset, severe hypertension with preeclampsia or eclampsia, *Obstet Gynecol* 118(6):1465–1468, 2011.

19. Jauch EC, Cucciara B, Adeoye O, et al.: Part 11: Adult stroke: 2010 American Heart Association guidelines for cardiopulmonary resuscitation and emergency cardiovascular care, *Circulation* 122(18 Suppl 3):S818–S828, 2010.

20. Peacock WF, Hilleman DE, Levy PD, Rhoney DH: A systematic review of nicardipine vs labetalol for the management of hypertensive crises, *Am J Emerg Med* 30(6):981–993, 2012.

21. Publication committee for the VMAC Investigators: Intravenous nesiritide vs nitroglycerin for treatment of decompensated congestive heart failure: a randomized controlled trial, *JAMA* 287(12):1531–1540, 2002.

22. Dandamudi S, Chen HH: The ASCEND-HF trial: An acute study of clinical effectiveness of Nesiritide and decompensated heart failure, *Expert Rev Cardiovasc Ther* 10(5):557–563, 2012.

23. Pleister AP, Baliga RR, Haas GJ: Acute study of clinical effectiveness of Nesiritide in decompensated heart failure: Nesiritide redux, *Curr Heart Fail Rep* 8(3):226–232, 2011.

24. Metra M, Bettari L, Carubelli V, Cas LD: Old and new intravenous inotropic agents in the treatment of advanced heart failure, *Prog Cardiovasc Dis* 45(2):97–106, 2011.

25. Hasenfuss G, Teerlink JR: Cardiac inotropes: current agents and future directions, *Eur Heart J* 32(15):1838–1845, 2011.

26. Bellomo R, Chapman M, Finfer S, et al.: Low-dose dopamine in patients with early renal dysfunction: A placebo-controlled randomized trial. Australian and New Zealand Intensive Care Society (ANZICS) Clinical Trials Group, *Lancet* 356(9248):2139–2143, 2000.

27. Friedrich JO, Adhikari N, Herridge MS, et al.: Meta-analysis: Low-dose dopamine increases urine output but does not prevent renal dysfunction or death, *Ann Intern Med* 142(7):510–524, 2005.

28. Kellum JA, Decker JM: Use of dopamine in acute renal failure: a meta-analysis, *Crit Care Med* 29(8):1526–1531, 2001.

29. Marik PE: Low-dose dopamine: a systematic review, *Intensive Care Med* 28(7):877–883, 2002.

30. Venkataraman R: Can we prevent acute kidney injury? *Crit Care Med* 36(Suppl):S166–S171, 2008.

31. Yancy CW, Jessup M, Bozkurt B, et al.: 2013 ACCF/AHA guideline for the management of heart failure: executive summary, *Circulation* 128:1810–1852, 2013.

32. O'Gara PT, Kushner FG, Ascheim DD, et al.: 2013 ACCF/AHA Guideline for the Management of ST-elevation myocardial infarction: A report of the American College of Cardiology Foundation/American Heart Association Task Force on Practice Guidelines, *Circulation* 127: e362–e425, 2013.

33. Frishman WH: Saunders E: β-adrenergic blockers, *J Clin Hypertens* 13(9):649–653, 2011.

34. Grimm RH, Flack JM: Alpha 1 adrenoreceptor antagonists, *J Clin Hypertens* 13(9):654–657, 2011.

35. Vongpatanasin W, Kazuomi K, Atlas SA, Victor RG: Central sympatholytic drugs, *J Clin Hypertens* 13(9):658–661, 2011.

36. Thompson CJ: Cardiovascular problems. In Whetstone Foster JG, Prevost SS, editors: *Advanced practice nursing of adults in acute care*, Philadelphia, 2012, F.A. Davis, pp 368–390.

37. Consortium for Spinal Cord Medicine: Early acute management in adults with spinal cord injury: a clinical practice guideline for health-care providers, *J Spinal Cord Med* 31(4):403–479, 2008.

38. Hassink JJ, Essenberg MD, Roukema JA, van den Bemt PM: Effect of bar-code-assisted medication administration on medication administration errors, *Am J Health Syst Pharm* 70(7):572–573, 2013.

39. Poon EG, Keohane CA, Yoon CS, et al.: Effect of bar-code technology on the safety of medication administration, *N Eng J Med* 362(18):1698–1707, 2010.

40. Parry A: Inotropic drugs and their uses in critical care, *Nurs Crit Care* 17(1):19–27, 2011.

41. Cooper B: Ask the experts: vasoactive medication dosage and daily weight changes, *Crit Care Nurse* 38(2):136–137, 2008.

42. Sprung CL, Annane D, Keh D, et al.: Hydrocortisone therapy for patients with septic shock, *N Engl J Med* 358(2):111–124, 2008.

Doppler Hemodynamic Monitoring

10

Rob Phillips

Doppler ultrasound has been used in clinical practice for over 50 years with a proven safety and effectiveness profile. Advances in Doppler technology and a high sensitivity to detect changes in hemodynamic variables make Doppler ultrasonography an attractive option for noninvasive and minimally invasive monitoring in both high-risk and low-risk patients.

Historical Milestones

The Doppler effect was first described in 1842 by Christian Doppler (1803–1853), when he observed the different color of the stars in the night sky and hypothesized that this difference in color was related to the different star velocities relative to a fixed observer.[1] It took more than 100 years after this initial observation for Doppler's principle to become a foundation for modern ultrasound practice.

In 1957, Shigeo Satomura described the first clinical application of a Doppler device for measuring cardiac blood flow.[2] In 1961, the first continuous-wave Doppler device was used for measurement of cardiac flow.[3] More recently, Doppler technology has been implemented for specialized applications such as detection of cardiac wall motion assessment.[4]

The first stand-alone Doppler device was proposed in 1983 when Lee Huntsman used transcutaneous pulsed ultrasound and continuous wave Doppler ultrasound to obtain measurements of cardiac output.[5] These findings led to the first commercial Doppler-based cardiac output measurement device: the Ultra Com. The Doppler monitoring concept was further advanced when Mark et al. (1986) reported the use of transesophageal Doppler for intraoperative monitoring of cardiac output.[6] The ultrasound transducer was introduced into the esophagus of an anesthetized surgical patient and orientated to sample the maximal flow in the descending thoracic aorta. The esophageal Doppler was described by Singer et al.,[7] and commercialized in 1990 by Deltex (Deltex Limited, Chichester, U.K.). The Deltex (CardioQ) Esophageal Doppler Monitor (EDM) uses descending thoracic aortic flow as a surrogate of cardiac output and stroke volume. Note the term ODM (Oesophageal Doppler Monitor) is used in many countries reflecting the different spellings of esophagus.

TABLE 10-1   Historical Milestones in Doppler Hemodynamic Monitoring

DATE	AUTHOR	DEVELOPMENT
1842	Doppler[1]	Description of Doppler effect
1957	Sotamura[2]	Doppler measurement of blood flow
1961	Franklin et al.[3]	CW Doppler measurement of cardiac flow
1983	Huntsman et al.[4]	Stand-alone M-Mode and CW Doppler monitor
1986	Mark et al.[5]	Transesophageal CW Doppler
1990	Singer[7]	Minimally invasive esophageal CW Doppler monitoring
2002	Phillips[8]	Noninvasive transcutaneous CW Doppler monitoring

CW, Continuous wave; *M-Mode*, motion mode.

Improvements in Doppler signal processing fostered development of noninvasive transcutaneous Doppler, where the ultrasound transducer is placed directly on the skin and the Doppler angled across the aortic valve or pulmonic valve to acquire a cardiac output signal.[8] The Ultrasonic Cardiac Output Monitor (USCOM) device, which was commercialized in 2002 by Uscom Ltd, Sydney, Australia, provides noninvasive cardiovascular assessment. Advances in Doppler technology are summarized in Table 10-1.

Key Physiologic Concepts

The most commonly measured reference measure to evaluate the effectiveness of the circulation is cardiac output (CO), or the volume of blood flowing from the heart per minute. Cardiac output is the product of the stroke volume (SV), the volume of blood pumped per stroke or beat, and the heart rate (HR). The stroke volume is the fundamental contractile outcome measure of heart function, and the parameter that Doppler ultrasound can measure with very high fidelity.

Although stroke volume, heart rate, and cardiac output are predominantly regulated by the autonomic nervous system, preload and afterload, or vascular tone, are the coupling factors, which feed back from via baroreceptors in the vessels and the heart, while chemoreceptors feed back to the brainstem and to the autonomic nervous system. The autonomic nervous system regulates heart rate, stroke volume, and cardiac output to preserve an equilibrated circulation, an adequate oxygen delivery (DO_2), and a stable blood pressure. Although hemodynamics by definition relates to blood flow, measurement of blood pressure, when coupled with stroke volume and cardiac output measurements, allows for quantitative assessment of vessel performance known as *systemic vascular resistance* (SVR) and arterial elastance (Ea), which

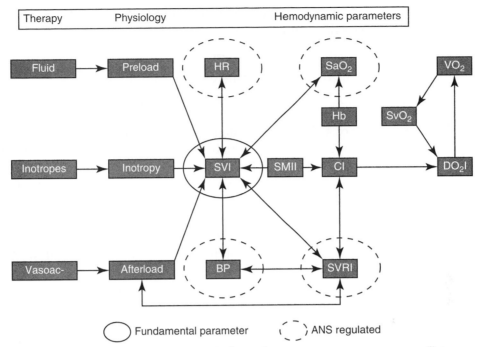

FIGURE 10-1 Simplified relationship of therapy (volume, inotropes, vasopressors, vasodilator medications), physiology, hemodynamics and oxygen demand (VO$_2$), and delivery (DO$_2$), demonstrating the central role of stroke volume index (SVI) as a hemodynamic target. The regulatory role of the autonomic nervous system is also demonstrated.

represents the ratio of pressure to volume (P/V), or dP/dV, in the cardiovascular system; (*d* refers to the Greek letter delta [δ] indicating change).

Normal circulation is dynamic and continually responsive to increases and decreases in blood pressure and DO$_2$, with predominant mediation by the extensive network of cardiovascular baroreceptors. The normal response to increased oxygen demand is an upregulation of cardiac output, stroke volume, and heart rate, as during exercise, whereas cardiac output, stroke volume, and heart rate are downregulated at rest when circulation is idle with only a baseline oxygen demand requirement (Figure 10-1).

Regulation of the Circulatory System

An understanding of the relationship and regulation of the circulatory system is fundamental to effective monitoring and interpretation of monitors and the application of hemodynamic monitoring to therapeutic management. The simplified model shown in Figure 10-1 isolates the action of different therapy classes. However, this simplified physiologic model is complicated by the autonomic nervous system as it regulates stroke volume, heart rate, and SVR from feedback, predominantly from the baroreceptors, to maintain the blood pressure in a narrow range. Current concepts of circulation are based on the Guyton's time averaged model of MAP = CO × SVR as represented by the following series of equations:[9]

$$MAP = CO \times SVR$$
$$CO = SV \times HR$$
$$CO = SV \times HR \times SVR$$

The application of a therapy that alters either stroke volume or SVR will result in a compensatory change in the other variable, as the autonomic nervous system acts to preserve blood pressure by regulation of the other two variables. Consequently, the autonomic nervous system masks changes in stroke volume or SVR by compensatory regulation of the counter variable to preserve the blood pressure. Measurements of both stroke volume and SVR are required to adequately identify circulatory abnormalities and guide interventions. This also ensures that measures of blood pressure alone are less sensitive to changes in hemodynamics, than measures of stroke volume and SVR.

The adoption of Doppler technologies, which measure real time stroke volume, provides instantaneous measurements of ventricular–arterial coupling such as arterial elastance (Ea) or dP/dV, and allows Guyton's law to be written as BP = SV × Ea.

Doppler Background

> ### Clinical Reasoning Pearl
>
> A Doppler examination will never overestimate flow velocity. However, a poorly positioned probe can under measure flow; therefore, operators should take the time to optimize Doppler flow profiles so that both stroke volume and cardiac output are correct and not underestimated.

Doppler Method

The Doppler method depends on a transducer transmitting ultrasound waves into the body at a known fixed frequency, which are then reflected by the tissues and cells, predominantly red blood cells, and the reflected ultrasound waves are measured by the Doppler system (Figure 10-2 and Box 10-1).

Doppler Equation

The Doppler equation allows for calculation of the blood velocity from measurement of the reflected Doppler signals. The frequency of the reflected waves is subtracted from that of the transmitted waves to calculate the frequency shift (df), and then the blood velocity (v), can be calculated according to the Doppler equation as shown in Box 10-1.[10]

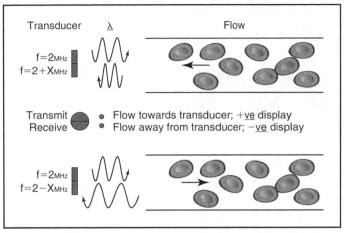

FIGURE 10-2 Ultrasound transmission frequency and reflected frequency after interaction with mobile red blood cells travelling toward the transducer (*upper image*) and travelling away from the transducer (*lower picture*). The perceived Doppler frequency is increased with blood flow toward the transducer, measured as 2+XMHz, and the perceived Doppler frequency is reduced, measured as 2−XMHz, when the blood is travelling away from the transducer.

BOX 10-1   Doppler Equation and The Bernoulli Equation

The Doppler Equation

The Doppler equation is as follows

$$df = 2fv \cos\varnothing/c$$

and

$$v = df \, c/2f \cos\varnothing$$

Where:

df = frequency shift
f = transmitted frequency
v = velocity of the reflector (unknown)
Cos Ø = angle of the incident beam to the flow
c = constant (speed of sound)

The Bernoulli Equation

In his treatise "Hydrodynamica", Daniel Bernoulli (1700–1782) provided the mathematical connection between velocity and pressure. Bernoulli demonstrated that the total energy in a steady fluid system is a constant along the flow path. Therefore, as the velocity increases, its pressure decreases.[10] He further proposed the "simplified Bernoulli equation," in which he made assumptions regarding flow and convective acceleration in relation to a known blood density, to calculate the pressure gradient from the measured velocity in any fluid.

The modified Bernoulli equation is as follows:

$$\Delta P = 4V^2$$

Where

ΔP = change in pressure
V = velocity

The combination of the Doppler equation, which allows calculation of velocity from Doppler shift, and the Bernoulli equation, which allows calculation of pressure from velocity, provides for integration of pressure and flow measurements. These equations provide the foundation on which modern Doppler hemodynamics are based.

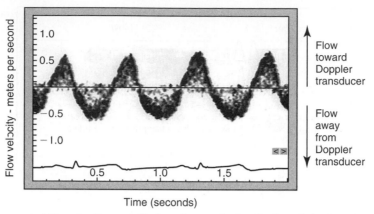

Time (seconds)

FIGURE 10-3 The spectral Doppler flow profile is a time–velocity display of the Doppler signal and displays the velocity of each red blood cell and the number of blood cells travelling at each velocity at any time. The higher the number of cells travelling at any velocity the more dense the signal.

Doppler Signal

The velocity of the reflectors, in this case red blood cells, can be plotted on a time–velocity display to generate a Doppler flow profile in which flow toward and away from the transducer is represented (Figure 10-3). The characteristic Doppler flow waveforms display the following:

1. Positive deflection, by convention representing blood flow toward the transducer
2. Negative deflection, representing blood flow away from the transducer

The intensity of the signal is also plotted and reflects the density of reflectors, in this case red blood cells. The greater the number of cells travelling at any velocity, the more dense the signal appears.

Doppler Flow Profile

The Doppler flow profile can be traced to derive an area under the curve, also known as a *velocity time integral* (vti), according to the standard echocardiographic method (Figure 10-4). The velocity time integral is the stroke distance (SD) or distance that a single red blood cell travels per stroke in centimeters and varies from about 25 cm when measured at the aortic valve, to 10 cm when measured in the descending thoracic aorta. To calculate flow volume the velocity time integral (vti) in centimeters (cm), is multiplied by the flow in a cross-sectional area in square centimeters to obtain a measurement of stroke volume in cubic centimeters,[11] as shown in Figure 10-5. The strength of the Doppler method is that it measures flow directly across the ventricular–arterial valves or within the aorta and measures each of the component variables directly from the Doppler flow profile, velocity time integral (vti) and heart rate with high precision. Therefore, calculations derived from these measurements are highly accurate as seen in Box 10-2.

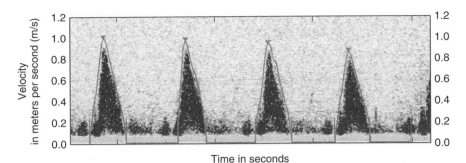

FIGURE 10-4 Spectral continuous wave Doppler display: demonstrating signal tracing through one complete cardiac cycle, from the opening valve "click" of systole, through systolic flow, through diastole, and continuing until the point of onset of the next systole. The area under the curve, also known as the velocity time integral (vti,), and the heart rate, can be directly measured from the screen.

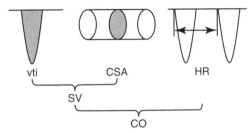

FIGURE 10-5 The component variables used in the Doppler ultrasound method to calculate stroke volume (SV) and cardiac output (CO). Heart rate (HR) and velocity time integral (vti) are directly measured from the velocity flow profile and cross-sectional area (CSA) can be directly measured from the valve or using an anthropometric algorithm.

Doppler Flow Volume Calculations

The accurate calculation of flow volume using the Doppler method requires that the cross-sectional area be measured at the point where the Doppler signal is acquired. For noninvasive transcutaneous ultrasound this is at the level of the aortic valve or pulmonic annulus, and for minimally invasive esophageal probes, the cross-sectional area is measured at the level of the descending thoracic aorta. Both methods use predictive algorithms for the calculation of the cross-sectional area. Despite differences between the device algorithms, comparative studies have demonstrated good agreement between the two methods.[12–14]

Therefore, despite different Doppler monitoring sites and different approaches to predicting flow cross-sectional area, both transcutaneous and esophageal Doppler methods can be used interchangeably, with the choice of preferred device based on the clinical application, patient needs, and operator comfort. This interchangeability of results suggests a robustness of the Doppler method.

BOX 10-2   Calculations for Stroke Volume and Cardiac Output

Stroke Volume Calculation

$$SV = vti \times CSA$$

Where

SV = stroke volume
vti = velocity time integral
CSA = cross-sectional area

Once stroke volume is determined, cardiac output can then be calculated by multiplying stroke volume by heart rate.

Cardiac Output Calculation

$$CO = SV \times HR$$

Where

CO = cardiac output
SV = stroke volume
HR = heart rate

The relationship of these measurements and calculations are illustrated in Figure 10-7.

Angle of Insonation

To accurately calculate flow velocity with Doppler ultrasound, the operator must align the beam along the flow toward or away from the transducer, at 0 or 180 degrees, so that the cos Ø component of the Doppler equation equates to "1" (Figure 10-6). Any nonparallel angulation will result in cos Ø being less than 1 and result in underestimation of the blood flow velocity. If the beam is directly perpendicular to flow, at 90 degrees, or 270 degrees, no Doppler shift will occur and no velocity can be detected. In clinical practice, Doppler beam angulation is not a limitation as any undermeasurement is usually small; in serial measures from the same point of insonation, the error is exactly repeated, so the monitoring function is unaffected. The Doppler

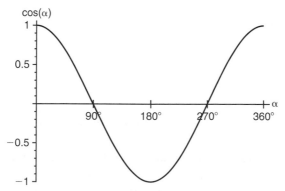

FIGURE 10-6 Cos Ø associated with different angles of insonation. As cos Ø is a function of the Doppler equation, the angle of insonation, Ø, defines the error in calculation of velocity by the Doppler equation. At 0 degree, 180 degrees, and 360 degrees, cos Ø = 1, so the values are accurate. At 90 degrees and 270 degrees, cos Ø = 0, so no Doppler shift is registered.

equation predicts an error in stroke volume velocity of less than 6% with an insonation angle of ±20 degrees. Thus, insonation within a 40-degree sector results in Doppler measurements of more than 94% reliability. Regardless, even if the insonation angle is greater than 20 degrees, if the angle remains unchanged between repeated measurements, the sensitivity to hemodynamic change remains 5% to 10% and is much more sensitive than other clinical monitoring methods.[15]

Doppler Parameters

By combining the Doppler velocity flow profile tracing (vti), the calculated velocity, and a proprietary algorithm, a number of hemodynamic parameters can be calculated. Further input of common physiologic variables of blood pressure, pulse arterial oxygen saturation, pulse oximetry (SpO_2), and central venous oxygen saturation ($ScvO_2$), allows calculation of additional physiologic variables. These variables can all be indexed to body surface area for comparison across sizes and ages.[16] Although all values can be determined for each single beat, they can also be averaged over a number of beats to provide a more representative reference measure. As most hemodynamic parameters are mathematically derived from stroke volume measurement, the clinical accuracy and effectiveness of these hemodynamic variables is dependent on the accuracy with which Doppler measures stroke volume, and Doppler has a proven capacity to accurately measure stroke volume and small changes in it.

Doppler Transducers

Doppler ultrasound transducers are constructed from piezoelectric materials that convert pressure to electricity (functioning as transmitters) and electricity to pressure (functioning as receivers). With the application of an alternating current, the transducer element expands and contracts at a high frequency related to the frequency of the current and the thickness of the piezoelectric crystal. In clinical practice this characteristic frequency is usually in the range of 2 to 10 megahertz (MHz). This high-frequency contraction and expansions transmits compression and rarefaction waves into any coupled tissue. Normal tissue, which is substantially composed of water, transmits these waves at approximately 1540 meters per second. With transcutaneous Doppler, a hydrophilic-soluble gel applied between the skin surface and the transducer augments acoustic coupling. This transmitted ultrasound wave passes through the body until it meets a reflector or acoustic interface (i.e., a solid organ), and is returned to the transducer, where the signal is reconstructed to form an ultrasound image. Air and bone are high-level reflectors of ultrasound waves and so return the majority of the ultrasound beam, casting acoustic shadows and preventing transmission and deeper tissue insonation. Broadly, four different ultrasound modalities exist: M-mode, two-dimensional (2D), three-dimensional (3D), and Doppler (Table 10-2), but only Doppler has been applied to hemodynamic monitoring.[17]

TABLE 10-2   Comparison of Doppler Hemodynamic Monitoring Technologies

	TRANSCUTANEOUS (USCOM)	ESOPHAGEAL (CardioQ-EDM)
Access	Transcutaneous	Transesophageal
Doppler modality	Continuous wave	Continuous wave
Measurement site	Aortic valve and pulmonary valve flow	Descending thoracic aortic flow
Algorithm	Anthropometry—height-based in adults and children, weight-based in neonates	Pulmonary artery catheter (PAC) database
Invasiveness	Noninvasive	Minimally invasive
Morphology	No	No
Monitoring	Yes	Yes
Auto-trace	Yes	Yes
Stroke volume sensitivity to detect a change in cardiac output	5%	4%
Advanced parameters and trending	Yes	Yes
Examination time	1 to 5 minutes	Less than 5 minutes after anesthesia induction or sedation administration
Validation	26 weeks to 110 years	0 to 99 years
Application	All	Peri-operative optimization
Training time	3 days	12 examinations
Complications	None	Risks associated with esophageal probe placement are similar to orogastric or nasogastric tube placement

Spectral Doppler Ultrasound

Doppler ultrasound can be further divided into spectral Doppler ultrasound, in which the velocity change is displayed across a time–velocity spectrum, and color Doppler, in which frequency shift is mapped as color-coded information on a 2D/3D B-mode image. High-velocity filters can be applied to measure high-velocity flow, usually blood flow, between 0.2 and 6 meter per second (m/s), and low-velocity flow, usually tissue motion, with a velocity that is usually less than 0.1 m/s. Both transcutaneous ultrasound and esophageal ultrasound utilize spectral Doppler imaging of moving blood.

The two different types of spectral Doppler ultrasound, continuous wave and pulse wave Doppler, have different properties, modes of generation, applications, and limitations. Pulse wave Doppler involves setting a sample volume in the insonation field to measure velocities at a fixed location in the body and pulsing ultrasound into the body in small wave clusters, usually in the order of two to three wavelengths. Continuous-wave Doppler involves uninterrupted streaming of the Doppler beam directed at the target, usually across the aortic valve or pulmonic valve. Both continuous-wave and pulse-wave Doppler have been demonstrated to be 96% to 98% accurate across the range of clinical velocities from −4 m/s to 4 m/s in phantoms.[18] The reproducibility of continuous wave Doppler approaches 98%. However, for pulse wave, where the location of the sample volume creates additional variability, the reproducibility is approximately 77%.[19,20] Therefore, continuous wave is the preferred method for measurement of transvalvular flow.[20] Both transcutaneous and esophageal Doppler monitoring devices use continuous wave Doppler.

Clinical Applications of Doppler Monitoring

Quantitating the hemodynamic response to fluids, inotropes, and vasoactive medications is crucial for patient management. Understanding of a number of key Doppler parameters and concepts is important when utilizing Doppler for clinical assessment. Because stroke volume is directly modulated by preload, contractility, and afterload, monitoring stroke volume provides simple quantitation of the effectiveness of circulatory therapeutic interventions.

Preload and Stroke Volume

Preload is the volume in the ventricle at end diastole, and it is this volume that increases ventricular myocyte stretch prior to contraction. Increasing the intravascular fluid volume and thus increasing preload volume results in increased stroke volume. Fluid responsiveness, defined as an increase in stroke volume associated with volume expansion, offers a very direct method for assessment of preload responsiveness and is demonstrated in Figure 10-7. Preload can either be increased with an intravenous (IV) fluid infusion or decreased with a diuretic.

Stroke Volume Variation

Stroke volume variation (SVV) represents the variability of the stroke volume across a respiratory cycle that occurs with breathing (Figure 10-8). SVV is the percentage variation of stroke volume, above and below the mean stroke volume, over one complete respiratory cycle. The SVV equation is:

$$SVV = (\{SV_{max} - SV_{min}\} \div SV_{mean}) \times 100$$

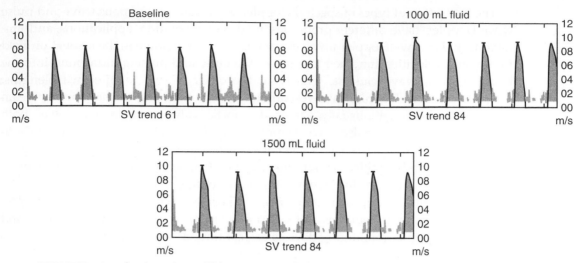

FIGURE 10-7 Stroke volume (SV) response to fluid infusion demonstrating fluid responsiveness from 61 milliliters (mL) to 84 mL. At the point of optimization (84 mL), infusing more fluid volume does not increase the stroke volume. *m/s*, Meters per second.

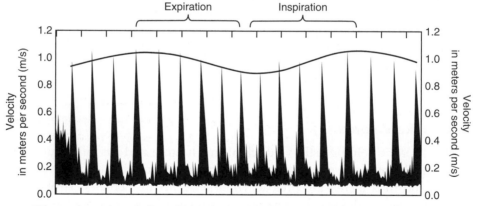

FIGURE 10-8 Fifteen-second aortic Doppler scan demonstrating normal stroke volume variation (SVV) <15%. The normal intrathoracic pressure changes associated with respiration vary the filling pressures, preload, and ultimately stroke volume to create the normal SVV. *m/s*, Meters per second.

Normal breathing and mechanical ventilation breathing both generate changes in intrathoracic pressure that influence cardiac preload and stroke volume. During spontaneous inspiration, the intrathoracic pressure decreases, and blood flows into the atria, increasing preload and stroke volume. During expiration, the intrathoracic pressure is increased, reducing the preload and lowering stroke volume.

Intrathoracic pressures are reversed in mechanical ventilation, where, during the positive pressure inspiratory phase, intrathoracic pressure increases, compressing the vena cava and reducing venous return to the right atrium, consequently reducing preload and stroke volume. During exhalation the opposite occurs. This variability is used to assess SVV. In practice, the lower the preload, the greater the SVV, so that an elevated SVV indicates more fluid responsiveness. Clinically when the SVV is greater than 15% the patient will respond favorably to a fluid bolus.[21,22] The use of a Doppler beat-to-beat auto-tracing and high-fidelity stroke volume measure allows accurate beat-to-beat quantitation of stroke volume during respiration as shown in Figure 10-8.

The use of SVV is not limited to one technology and is discussed in more detail in Chapters 3 and 12. There is further discussion about the impact of mechanical ventilation on venous return in Chapter 14.

Doppler Monitoring Devices

The Doppler method depends on the acquisition and measurement of the Doppler flow profiles, calculations, and interpretation of the results. Doppler technologies generate flow waves that demonstrate "how much" (stroke volume) and "how often" (heart rate) the heart beats.

Currently, two types of Doppler monitoring devices are available: noninvasive transcutaneous Doppler, and minimally invasive esophageal Doppler. Both transcutaneous and esophageal Doppler technologies use solid-state devices that do not require calibration.

Transcutaneous Doppler Monitoring

Transcutaneous Doppler Indications

Transcutaneous Doppler can be used in any clinical environment in which knowledge of the circulatory status is important, including sepsis, heart failure, hypertension, presurgical optimization, and postsurgical review. Because transcutaneous Doppler is noninvasive, its application ranges from intraoperative, critical care unit, general ward, clinical, through to home care settings. The principle applications are pediatrics, critical care, anesthesiology, obstetrics, and emergency medicine. The mean acquisition time for Doppler waveforms has been reported as 3.69 to 7.1 minutes from startup to signal read-out.[23,24] This technology can be reliably adopted in the critical care unit by nurse led implementation.[25] Competence in operating the technology can be achieved after 20 to 30 examinations.[25,26] This discussion is focused on the transcutaneous Ultrasonic Cardiac Output Monitor (USCOM), (Uscom Ltd, Sydney, Australia).

Transcutaneous Doppler Examination

Usually, transcutaneous Doppler ultrasonography is performed with the patient in the supine position or in the slightly left-lateral position with the Doppler directed across the aortic or pulmonic valve (Figure 10-9). If the patient has a tracheotomy and the suprasternal access to the aortic valve is obstructed, the parasternal window can be used and the pulmonic valve monitored. Transcutaneous Doppler is an intermittent monitoring method with signal acquired during hand-held acquisition.

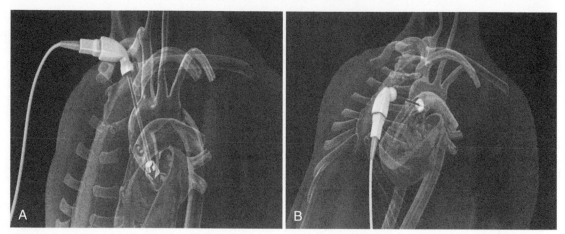

FIGURE 10-9 Transcutaneous Doppler access across the aortic valve (**A**) and pulmonic valve (**B**) from transcutaneous suprasternal and parasternal acoustic access, respectively. (Courtesy Uscom Ltd, Sydney, Australia)

Patient Education

- Transcutaneous Doppler devices require the acquisition of a baseline flow profile. The patient is asked to lie supine and relaxed without recent activity to obtain a resting physiologic baseline.

- Water-soluble ultrasound gel is applied to the transducer to obtain the best Doppler signal.

- The transcutaneous Doppler presses against the skin for a short period (usually less than 2 to 3 minutes)

Patient Safety

- The reusable transcutaneous Doppler transducer must be antiseptically cleaned between patients to prevent infection transmission. The institution usually determines the specific cleaning protocols.

- In low-risk settings, an alcohol wipe of the transducer and operator interface between patients is acceptable.

- In isolation settings, a more thorough approach to disinfection may be required. Some units have dedicated Doppler devices for specific patients to minimize the risk of cross-contamination.

Patient Comfort

Transcutaneous Doppler is a noninvasive technology. A simple reassuring explanation of the examination is essential, with every effort made to comfort the patient.

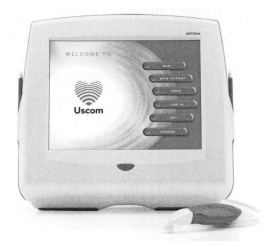

FIGURE 10-10 USCOM transcutaneous Doppler monitor. (Courtesy Uscom Ltd, Sydney, Australia)

Doppler Waveform

The hand-held transducer emits a continuous Doppler ultrasound wave through the skin and through the body and is directed across the cardiac valves. Moving red blood cells reflect the sound waves. The transducer detects and measures the returning ultrasound waves and determines the Doppler shift. The signal is optimized to the point of maximal waveform velocity, and the screen frozen (Figure 10-10). The Doppler waveform is then plotted as a time velocity (vti) wave profile that demonstrates the change in blood velocity across the aortic valve or pulmonic valve throughout the cardiac cycle. This Doppler waveform is automatically traced in real time to generate the quantitative parameters required to apply the Doppler method to clinical hemodynamic practice.

Transcutaneous Doppler Validation

Transcutaneous Doppler has been validated in subjects aged 26 gestational weeks to 110 years and is equally accurate at flow rates ranging from 0.12 liters per minute (L/min) to 18.7 L/min.[27,28] Doppler devices are used by physicians, nurses, and paramedics to achieve a fast and accurate assessment of the effectiveness of circulatory interventions such as fluid, inotropes, and vasoactive medications.[25,26] A meta-analysis of transcutaneous Doppler (USCOM) evidence demonstrates acceptable agreement with invasive methods such as the pulmonary artery catheter (PAC)[29] and true gold standard flow probes.[30]

Transcutaneous Doppler Monitor Algorithms

Transcutaneous Doppler measures flow directly across the aortic valve, via the sternal notch and the pulmonic valve, via the left parasternum (see Figure 10-9).

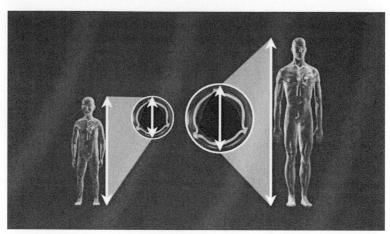

FIGURE 10-11 Principle for anthropometric determination of cardiac valvular annular diameters; "big hearts have big valves." Skeletal height best predicts cardiac valvular diameter allowing the derivation of anthropomorphic algorithms to predict valve diameters. (Courtesy Uscom Ltd, Sydney, Australia)

A linear relationship has been demonstrated between cardiac dimensions and body size, with body height identified as the best predictor of aortic dimensions.[31,32] Thus, the diameter of the cardiac valves can be estimated from the patient's body size. A proprietary height-referenced algorithm is used to determine annular diameters of the aortic valve and the pulmonic valve (Figure 10-11). This approach circumvents the complex and relatively inaccurate measurement of the aortic valve or the pulmonary valve by echocardiography.[11] Doppler data are then combined with this anthropometric prediction of valve diameters for the calculation of flow volumes. A height-referenced algorithm is used for adults and a weight-based algorithm for neonates.

Doppler flow time corrected (FTc) is a static indicator of fluid responsiveness and is the duration of ejection normalized to heart rate using the Bazett formula: $FTc = FT/\sqrt{(60/HR)}$.[33] FTc less than 360 milliseconds indicates preload depletion and preload responsiveness.[34] FTc is automatically calculated beat-to-beat to create a static measure of preload responsiveness from the Doppler flow profile on the USCOM device.

Transcutaneous Doppler Monitor Limitations

Transcutaneous Doppler requires hand-held operation and is an intermittent measurement device. In a small number of instances, especially immediately after cardiac surgery, or in patients with severe pulmonary disease, acoustic access may be difficult. Dermatologic conditions may preclude topical image acquisition in some patients. The features of the transcutaneous Doppler monitoring system (USCOM) are summarized in Table 10-3.

TABLE 10-3 **Ultrasound Modes and Their Application**

MODE	DESCRIPTION	APPLICATION
M-Mode	B-mode from single line of sight	Relative motion of structures
Two-dimensional (2D)	B-mode from multiple scanned lines of sight	High-resolution 2D morphology
Three-dimensional (3D)	Multiple B-mode planes reconstructed over time	3D structure
Doppler	Detects velocity shift from moving reflectors	Blood flow and tissue motion (Table 10-4)

TABLE 10-4 **Ultrasound Modes for Examination of the Motion of Blood and Cardiac Tissues**

DOPPLER	MODALITY	REFLECTOR	DESCRIPTION
Spectral	CW	Blood	Detects velocity shift from moving reflectors—RBCs without range discrimination
Spectral	PW	Blood	Detects velocity shift from moving RBCs with range discrimination
Spectral	PW	Tissue	Detects velocity shift from slow moving tissue
Color	PW	Blood	Detects velocity shift from moving RBCs and maps color coded velocity on 2D or M-Mode image
Color	PW	Tissue	Detects velocity shift from moving tissues and maps color coded velocity on 2D or M-Mode image

CW, Continuous-wave Doppler; *PW*, pulse-wave Doppler; *RBCs*, red blood cells.

Esophageal Doppler Monitoring

Esophageal Doppler Indications

Esophageal Doppler monitoring is a minimally invasive technology. A Doppler probe is inserted into the esophagus to intermittently measure flow in the thoracic aorta integrating an algorithm for calculation of descending thoracic aortic diameter. Indications include monitoring of cardiac output and fluid status during major or high-risk surgery, and in the critical care unit.[35] This discussion is focused on the esophageal CardioQ-EDM (Deltex Medical, UK).

Esophageal Doppler Examination

The Monitor is connected to a Doppler transducer mounted on a thin catheter (5-millimeter [mm] diameter) that is lubricated and inserted approximately

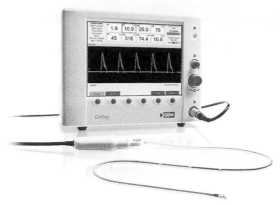

FIGURE 10-12 Esophageal probe demonstrating device controls, software interface, display and esophageal transducer. CardioQ-EDM (Courtesy Deltex Medical Ltd, U.K.).

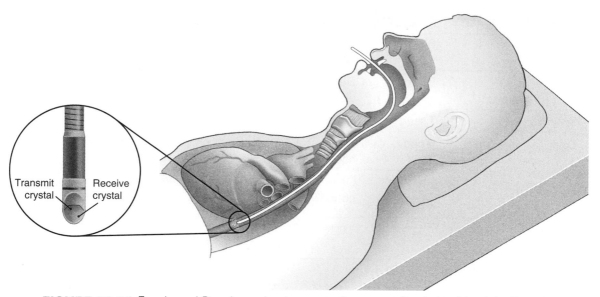

FIGURE 10-13 Esophageal Doppler probe demonstrating anatomic relationship of the Doppler beam to the descending aorta.

40 centimeters (cm) into the esophagus following sedation or anesthesia (Figure 10-12). Insertion and focusing of the probe optimally takes less than 5 minutes.

The Doppler transducer is positioned at the tip of the probe, at a 45-degree angle (Figure 10-13). The beam is positioned behind and to the left of the esophagus and the orientation of the beam is optimized to the descending thoracic aortic flow signal. The continuous wave Doppler beam is angled at 45 degrees to the long axis of the descending thoracic aortic flow, allowing the flow velocity to be measured accurately using the Doppler equation (Figure 10-14).

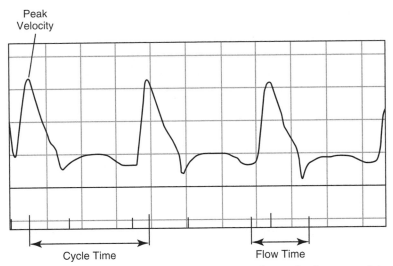

FIGURE 10-14 Esophageal Doppler waveform demonstrating major features of the descending thoracic aortic flow profile used for monitoring.

The descending thoracic aortic flow volume is calculated from a proprietary algorithm estimating the descending thoracic aortic diameter and applied to the thoracic aortic Doppler flow profile to allow calculation of cardiac output at the aortic valve.[22]

Patient Education

- The esophageal Doppler procedure usually involves sedation or anesthesia.

- Typically, patients who have an esophageal Doppler inserted are intubated and mechanically ventilated.

- More flexible esophageal Doppler probes can be used in patients who are awake.

- The esophageal Doppler probe is inserted through the nose or the mouth and is advanced into the esophagus with the transducer tip positioned where the esophagus and the descending aorta are side by side, within 1 cm of each other (thoracic vertebrae T5/T6). This proximity allows excellent Doppler assessment of blood flow in the aorta.

Patient Safety

- The esophageal Doppler transducer probe is for single use only. A water-based lubricant is liberally applied to the probe tip before insertion. Care should be taken to maintain an antiseptic environment during insertion and positioning of the probe. A setup tray and gloves are required.

Continued

Patient Safety—cont'd

- The adult probe is 50 cm in length and has markings at 30 cm, 35 cm, and 45 cm to guide the depth of probe insertion; which is 35-40 cm for oral insertion (from the lips), and 40-45 cm for nasal insertion (from the nares). Small depth adjustments are then made to acquire the best audible signal and waveform.

- The single-use critical care probe may remain in place for up to 10 days. The probe may require repositioning to acquire an optimal Doppler signal before each measurement. The optimal Doppler signal will have a clear and sharp waveform, a bright color around the edge and a dark center, with the tallest peak when the probe transducer tip is close and facing the descending aorta.

Patient Comfort

Many patients monitored with an esophageal Doppler are intubated and mechanically ventilated. Pain and sedation management or anesthesia management are not altered by the addition of an esophageal Doppler probe. Pain and sedation management are guided by current clinical practice guidelines for care of the ventilated patient.

More flexible, softer probes that require only local sedation are used in patients who are awake.

Esophageal Doppler Monitor Algorithms

Esophageal Doppler (CardioQ-EDM) uses a proprietary algorithm based on a database of pulmonary artery catheter (PAC) output measurements referenced to patient age, height, and weight and correlated to corresponding descending thoracic aortic diameters.

Esophageal Doppler Limitations

The catheter probe requires insertion into the esophagus, accompanied by sedation or anesthesia. The probes are single use and can remain inserted for up to 240 hours (10 days). The probe requires hands-on signal optimization prior to each repeated measure. A limitation of the esophageal technology may be the unpredictability and variability of the descending thoracic aortic diameter.[36] The diameter can vary because of thoracic aortic ectasia (dilation), and dynamic diameter changes associated with differing cardiac outputs and blood pressures.

Potential complications of esophageal Doppler are generally minor and uncommon. The esophageal probe cannot be inserted in patients undergoing esophageal surgery, head and neck surgery, or aortic surgery.[35] Other contraindications include upper gastrointestinal bleeding or perforation and esophageal pathology such as stricture, trauma, tumor, or fistula.

Esophageal Doppler risks are related to probe insertion and are similar to risks associated with insertion of a nasogastric or orogastric tube. Because the transducer element is in contact with the mucosal esophageal lining there may be a slight increase in local temperature of less than 1 degree centigrade, although this has not been reported to cause clinical problems.

Esophageal Doppler Validation

There are different esophageal probes for different clinical indications (intraoperative versus critical care) and for different ages. Esophageal Doppler is validated for patients 16 to 99 years weighing from 30 to 150 kg. The pediatric version is for patients 0-15 years, weighing 3-60 kg, with a height range of 50-170 cm.

The evidence for esophageal Doppler has predominantly focused on intraoperative fluid optimization in the surgical setting. In the United Kingdom (UK), the National Institute for Health and Care Excellence (NICE) produced a Medical Technology Guidance paper on esophageal Doppler and concluded that with the use of esophageal monitoring, "there is a reduction in postoperative complications, use of central venous catheters, and in-hospital stay (with no increase in the rate of re-admission or repeat surgery) compared with conventional clinical assessment with or without invasive cardiovascular monitoring. When esophageal Doppler (CardioQ) is used instead of a CVP catheter, the cost saving per patient is about $1850 (£1100) based on a 7.5-day hospital stay."[35,37]

In the United States the Centers for Medicare and Medicaid (CMS) endorse cardiac output monitoring using esophageal Doppler in mechanically ventilated patients in critical care and intraoperatively for patients who require fluid volume optimization.[38,39] The features of the esophageal Doppler monitoring system (CardioQ-EDM) are summarized in Table 10-3.

Clinician Education and Training

Effective use of all Doppler ultrasound technologies requires an understanding of how the technology is operated, how to acquire the signals, and ultimately how to manage the patient from these signals. Evidence demonstrates that with a half-day didactic training session and 20 to 30 clinical examinations, physicians, nurses, and paramedics can achieve acceptable competence in transcutaneous Doppler (USCOM) operation with reliable and reproducible results.[25,26] For the esophageal Doppler (CardioQ-EDM), there is evidence that 12 insertions are required for safe insertion and handling of the esophageal probe.[40] As with any monitoring technology, the more experienced the examiner, the more reliable the performance.

Achievement of the best results from these technologies requires a specialized monitoring team. The deployment of a group of specialized practitioners with interest, education, and skills in cardiovascular monitoring will ensure that optimal hemodynamic care is instituted. The group should include sufficient members to provide adequate coverage to ensure that a continuous Doppler monitoring hemodynamic optimization service can be provided.

Future Developments

Doppler has proven utility as a flow measuring technology for identifying hemodynamic abnormalities and optimization of fluids, inotropes, and vasoactive medications. However, the potential to input additional parameters provide the opportunity to expand this technology and create more physiologically centered goals. The addition of oximetry allows generation of beat-to-beat oxygen delivery data, and the addition of electrocardiography creates the opportunity for a specialized electrophysiology optimization device. Other potential features include a noninvasive blood pressure device and a specialized hypertension and heart failure device. Miniaturization will further extend the applications of Doppler hemodynamic monitors.

Case Study

Presentation. A 5-year-old child developed septic shock following bowel surgery and was transferred to a tertiary critical care unit.

Observations. Tachycardia—120 beats per minute; blood pressure 96/51 mm Hg (MAP 66 mm Hg), following 1 liter of fluid in the preceding 24 hours. A transcutaneous Doppler examination was performed to determine fluid responsiveness state.

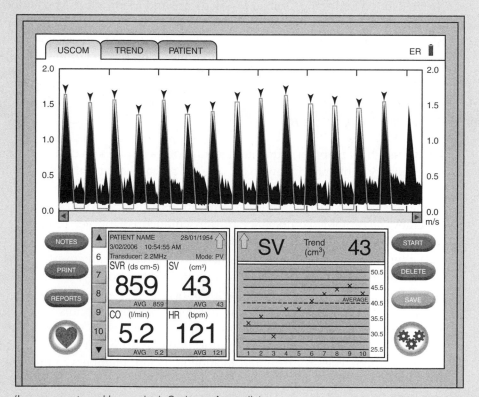

(Image courtesy Uscom Ltd, Sydney, Australia)

Case Study—cont'd

Diagnosis. Hypovolemia (low-normal stroke volume and high SVV). Given the patient has septic shock, stroke volume was expected to be elevated; however, it was low-normal consistent with preload depletion. Elevation of heart rate (121 beats per minute) was to preserve cardiac output and oxygen delivery despite the impaired stroke volume.

Intervention. Fluid bolus (150 mL over 10 minutes) while monitoring stroke volume response at 2.5-minute intervals (approximately 40-mL intervals) to identify stroke volume reserve and fluid responsiveness.

Outcome. SVV was 42% at first observation, indicating the patient was likely to be fluid responsive. SVV was reduced to 23% with fluid infusion, and stroke volume increased by 23%. Cardiac output also increased, and a decrease in heart rate and SVR was demonstrated on trend graphing. Fluid modulated stroke volume resuscitation resulted in an increased oxygen delivery in excess of 20%.

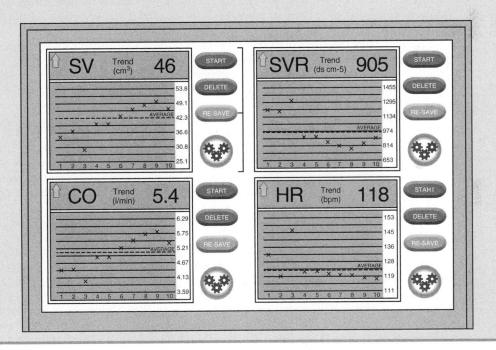

Conclusion

Doppler hemodynamic monitoring is an emerging standard of care, providing simple and accurate diagnosis of circulatory abnormalities and a reliable method for guiding therapy. The technology is safe and accurate and has proven outcome benefits. The devices can be operated by physicians, nurses, and paramedics and are validated from very low outputs to very high outputs after a short period of training. The effective application of hemodynamic Doppler devices requires an understanding of the technology, the physiologic information provided, and how to use this data to guide management. The physiologic insights Doppler monitoring provides allows for a direct and rational approach to cardiovascular diagnosis and management.

References

1. Doppler JC: Ueber das ferbige Licht der Dopplersterne und einiger anderer Gestirne des Himmels. Abhandlungen der Konigl, *Bohmischen Gesellschaft dert Wissenschaften* 2:465, 1842, 5th ser.
2. Sotamura S: Ultrasonic Doppler method for the inspection of cardiac functions, *J Acoust Soc Am* 29:1181–1185, 1957.
3. Franklin DL, Schlegel W, Rushmer RF: Blood flow measured by Doppler frequency shift of back scattered ultrasound, *Science* 134:564, 1961.
4. Donovan CL, Armstrong WF, Bach DS: Quantitative Doppler tissue imaging of the left ventricular myocardium: validation in normal subjects, *Am Heart J* 130(1):100–104, 1995.
5. Huntsman LL, Stewart DK, Barnes SR: Noninvasive Doppler determination of cardiac output in man: clinical validation, *Circulation* 67:593, 1983.
6. Mark JB, Steinbrook RA, Gugino LD, et al.: Continuous noninvasive monitoring of cardiac output with esophageal Doppler ultrasound during cardiac surgery, *Anesth Analg* 65 (10):1013–1020, 1986.
7. Singer M, Clarke J, Bennett ED: Changes in cardiac output measured by esophageal Doppler; validation using thermodilution as the reference technique, *Clin Sci* 74:31, 1988.
8. Phillips RA, Dadd MJ, Gill RW, et al.: Transcutaneous continuous wave Doppler cardiac output monitoring is feasible producing reliable and reproducible signals, *J Am Coll Cardiol* 39(Suppl B): 283B, 2002.
9. Guyton AC, Abernathy B, Langston JB, et al.: Relative importance of venous and arterial resistance in controlling venous return and cardiac output, *Am J Physiol* 196:1008–1014, 1959.
10. Bernoulli D: *Hydrodynamica sive de viribus et motibus fluidorum commentarii*, 1738.
11. Quinones MA, Otto CM, Stoddard M, et al.: Recommendations for quantification of Doppler echocardiography: a report from the Doppler quantification task force of the nomenclature and standards committee of the American Society of Echocardiography, *J Am Soc Echo* 15(2): 167–184, 2002.
12. Critchley LAH, Huang L: Cardiac output changes during robotic laparoscopic surgery, *Acta Anaesth Scand* 57(Suppl 120):11, 2013.
13. Critchley LA: Differences between Cardio-q and USCOM Doppler cardiac output readings in high risk surgical patients, *Br J Anaesth* 108(S2):ii113, 2012.
14. Phillips RA: *USCOM Doppler cardiovascular monitoring: concept, development, clinical validation and the future*, PhD thesis, September 2013, School of Medicine, The University of Queensland.
15. Boyd E: *The growth of the surface area of the human body*, 1935, University of Minnesota Press.
16. Thiel SW, Kollef MH, Isakow W: Non-invasive stroke volume measurement and passive leg raising predict volume responsiveness in medical ICU patients: an observational cohort study, *Crit Care* 39:666–688, 2009.
17. Gent R: *Applied physics and technology of diagnostic ultrasound*, Prospect South Australia, 1997, Milner Publishing.
18. Walker A, Olsson E, Wranne B, et al.: Accuracy of spectral Doppler flow and tissue velocity measurements in ultrasound systems, *Ultrasound Med Biol* 30(1):127–132, 2004.
19. Kusumoto F, Venet T, Schiller NB, et al.: Measurement of aortic blood flow by Doppler echocardiography: temporal, technician and reader variability in normal subjects and the application of generalizability theory in clinical research, *J Soc Echocardiogr Am* 8:647–653, 1995.

20. Moulinier L, Venet T, Schiller NB, et al.: Measurement of aortic blood flow by Doppler echocardiography: day to day variability in normal subjects and applicability in clinical research, *J Am Coll Cardiol* 17:1326–1333, 1991.

21. Zhang Z, Lu B, Sheng X, Jin N: Accuracy of stroke volume variation in predicting fluid responsiveness: a systematic review and meta-analysis, *J Anesth* 25(6):904–916, 2011.

22. Singer M: *Continuous haemodynamic monitoring by esophageal Doppler,* Doctor of Medicine thesis, April 1989, The University of London.

23. Siu CW, Tse HF, Lee K, et al.: Cardiac resynchronization therapy optimization by ultrasonic cardiac output monitoring (USCOM) Device, *Pacing Clin Electrophysiol (PACE)* 30(1):50–55, 2007.

24. Horster S, Stemmler HJ, Strecker N, et al.: Cardiac output measurements in septic patients: comparing the accuracy of USCOM and PiCCO, *Crit Care Res Prac* 2012, 5 pages. Epub 2012; article ID 270631, http://dx.doi.org/10.1155/2012/270631.

25. Corley A, Barnett AG, Mullany D, Fraser JF: Nurse-determined assessment of cardiac output. Comparing a non-invasive cardiac output device and pulmonary artery catheter: a prospective observational study, *Int J Nurs Studies* 46(10):1291–1297, 2009.

26. Dey I, Sprivulis P: Emergency physicians can reliably assess emergency department patient cardiac output using the USCOM™ continuous wave Doppler cardiac output monitor, *Emerg Med Aus* 17:193–199, 2005.

27. Phillips RA, Paradisis M, Evans NJ, et al.: Validation of USCOM CO measurements in preterm neonates by comparison with echocardiography, *Crit Care* 10(Suppl 1):144, 2006.

28. Su BC, Yu HP, Yang MW, et al.: Reliability of a new ultrasonic cardiac output monitor in recipients of living donor liver transplantation, *Liver Transpl* 14:1029–1037, 2008.

29. Chong SW, Peyton PJ: A meta-analysis of the accuracy and precision of the ultrasonic cardiac output monitor (USCOM), *Anaesthesia* 1365–2044, 2012.

30. Phillips RA, Hood SG, Jacobson BM, et al.: Pulmonary artery catheter (PAC) accuracy and efficacy compared with flow probe and transcutaneous Doppler (USCOM): an ovine validation, *Crit Care Res Prac,* 2012. 9 pages. Epub 2012; article ID 621496, http://dx.doi.org/10.1155/2012/621496.

31. Nidorf SM, Picard MH, Triulzi MO, et al.: New perspectives in the assessment of cardiac chamber dimensions during development and adulthood, *J Am Coll Cardiol* 19:983–988, 1992.

32. Sheil MLK, Jenkins O, Sholler GF: Echocardiographic assessment of aortic root dimensions in normal children based on measurement of a new ratio of aortic size independent of growth, *Am J Cardiol* 75:711–715, 1995.

33. Bazett HC: An analysis of the time-relations of electrocardiograms, *Heart* 7:353–370, 1920.

34. Yang SY, Shim JK, Song Y, et al.: Validation of pulse pressure variation and corrected flow time as predictors of fluid responsiveness in patients in the prone position, *Br J Anaesth* 110 (5):713–720, 2013.

35. UK National Institute for Health and Care Excellence MTG3: *CardioQ-ODM oesophageal Doppler monitor,* March 2011. http://www.nice.org.uk/guidance/MTG3. Accessed August 24, 2014.

36. Langewouters GJ, Wesseling KH, Goehard WJA: The static elastic properties of 45 human thoracic and 20 abdominal aortas in vitro and the parameters of a new model, *J Biomech* 17(6):425–435, 1984.

37. Lowe GD, Charmberlain BM, Philpott EJ, Willshire RJ:?, *Deltex Medical Technical Review,* Epub, 2011 http://www.deltexmedical.com/downloads/TechnicalReview.pdf. Accessed August 24, 2014.

38. Agency for Healthcare Research and Quality: *Technology assessment: esophageal Doppler ultrasound-based cardiac output monitoring for real-time therapeutic management of hospitalized patient: a review,* Rockville, MD, 2007, Economic Cycle Research Institute (ECRI) Evidence-based Practice Center (EPC) under contract to the Agency for Healthcare Research and Quality

(AHRQ) (Contract No. 290-02-0019). https://www.ecri.org/Documents/EPC/Esophageal_Doppler_Ultrasound-Based_Cardiac_Output_Monitoring.pdf. Accessed August 24, 2014.

39. Decision Memo for Ultrasound Diagnostic Procedures (CAF-00309R). Centers for Medicare and Medicaid Services. website http://www.cms.gov/medicare-coverage-database/details/nca-decision-memo.aspx?NCAId=196. Accessed August 24, 2014.

40. Lefrant JY, Bruelle P, Aya AG, et al.: Training is required to improve the reliability of esophageal Doppler to measure cardiac output in critically ill patients, *Intensive Care Med* 24 (4):347–352, 1998.

Ultrasonography-Based Hemodynamic Monitoring

11

Elizabeth E. Turner, Yasir Tarabichi, and Nitin Kumar Puri

Bedside ultrasonography, also known as *point-of-care ultrasonography*, *critical care ultrasonography*, or *focused ultrasonography*, has become increasingly important in the real-time evaluation of acutely and critically ill or injured patients. The use of bedside ultrasonography to guide procedures such as central venous catheterization, thoracentesis, and paracentesis is widely recognized as the preferred technique and, in some cases, the standard of care.[1–4] In recent years, a growing body of literature and acceptance has accumulated for bedside ultrasonography also having significant utility in the evaluation of cardiac function, pericardial tamponade, volume status, lung pathology, deep venous thrombosis (DVT), and abdominal pathology, to name a few. Emergency and critical care physicians, nurse practitioners, and physician assistants incorporate point-of-care ultrasonography into their evaluation, diagnosis, management, and ongoing monitoring of the critically ill or injured patient. This investigative and diagnostic modality has become a standard part of the training of emergency and critical care clinicians and has been proven to be not only a crucial skill to possess but also valid and reliable in the hands of nontraditional operators.[5–8]

Clinical Reasoning Pearl

Bedside ultrasonography is noninvasive and provides real-time information about the physiology of seriously ill patients. Time is a precious commodity for critically ill patients; therefore, expedited diagnosis helps caregivers understand at the point of care the therapeutic path that needs to be followed.

It is important to differentiate the goals of traditional ultrasonographic studies and formal echocardiography interpreted by radiologists and cardiologists, respectively. Goal-directed bedside ultrasonography aims to answer focused questions in real time and immediately impacts the management of the patient. The clinician who performs the examination also interprets the images and data, subsequently acting on the findings. This allows for a streamlined workflow and rapid delivery of appropriate

TABLE 11-1   **Comparison of Radiology, Cardiology, and Bedside Ultrasonography**

	RADIOLOGY	CARDIOLOGY	BEDSIDE ULTRASONOGRAPHY
Image acquisition	Radiology technician	Cardiac echocardiography technician	Treating physician
Image interpretation	Radiologist	Echocardiography physician	Treating physician
Time to action	Delayed	Delayed	Immediate
Goal	Anatomy	Anatomy + physiology	Physiology more than anatomy

treatment to benefit the patient by potentially reducing morbidity, mortality, and long-term disability. In addition, serial examinations may be readily performed to monitor the effectiveness of interventions and determine the need for changes in management strategy more expeditiously[9] (see Table 11-1). It is, therefore, of great importance that a clinician performing ultrasonography truly understand the implications, limitations, and all ultrasonographic findings before any clinical decisions are made on the basis of bedside ultrasonography.

Patient Education

Patients and families appreciate the hands-on approach that is needed for point-of-care ultrasonographic evaluations, and the interactions provide an opportunity for the understanding of the patient's condition with visual reinforcement. Anecdotal as well as actual evidence indicates that patient satisfaction with their provider and critical care unit experience is improved when bedside ultrasonographic evaluations are performed.[9a]

Several algorithms have been developed and validated to guide the organized approach to ultrasonography performed on a patient in the emergency or critical care setting.[10–13] For cardiac assessment, the focused assessed transthoracic echocardiography (FATE),[14] focused cardiac ultrasound (FOCUS), and focused echocardiography evaluation in life support (FEEL) protocols are widely utilized in the goal-directed evaluation of cardiac function in the critical patient. In addition, the rapid ultrasound in Shock (RUSH), bedside lung ultrasound evaluation (BLUE), and focused assessed sonography in trauma (FAST or eFAST) protocols are implemented for noncardiac evaluations (Table 11-2). Each of these will be discussed in more detail in subsequent sections of this chapter.

TABLE 11-2 Comparison of Common Bedside Ultrasonography Protocols

PROTOCOL	ABBREVIATION	VIEWS	GOALS
Focused Assessed Transthoracic Echocardiography	FATE	Cardiac: Subcostal, including inferior vena cava Parasternal Apical Pulmonary: Bilateral pleura Bilateral diaphragms	1. Identify obvious cardiac abnormalities 2. Chamber size and dimension 3. Contractility 4. Pleural pathology 5. Incorporate findings into clinical context
FOcused Cardiac Ultrasonography	FOCUS	Cardiac: Subcostal, including inferior vena cava Parasternal Apical	Same as FATE minus pleural evaluation
Focused Echocardiography Evaluation in Life Support	FEEL	Cardiac: Subcostal view between compressions for RV/ LV function, effusion, and volume status Pleura: Evaluation for tension pneumothorax	Evaluation for reversible causes of cardiac arrest during code blue situations
Focused Assessed Sonography in Trauma	FAST	1. Subcostal cardiac view 2. Bilateral diaphragms or upper quadrants 3. Retrovesicular	Rapid evaluation in trauma for free fluid indicative of hemorrhage
Extended Focus Assessed Sonography in Trauma	eFAST	FAST + bilateral pleura	Above + rule out pneumothorax
Rapid Ultrasonography in Shock	RUSH	FATE FAST Aorta	Evaluate pump, tanks, and pipes for origin of shock
Bedside Lung Ultrasound	BLUE	Lung pleura Lung artifacts (A- and B-lines) Bilateral diaphragms	Evaluate for etiology of respiratory failure

Image Acquisition and Interpretation of Structures in Ultrasonography

Knobology

An ultrasound machine has three major components; the transducer, the computer, and the display screen. Transducers have delicate piezoelectric crystals that turn electricity into sound waves that are directed at the areas of interest. These sound waves encounter anatomic structures and may be reflected back toward the probe in varying degrees, depending on the inherent motion and the physical makeup of the structures encountered. These reflected waves are sensed by the same piezoelectric crystals and interpreted by the processor to produce an image on the display. The way in which reflecting sound waves are interpreted and presented depends on the particular mode selected, as will be discussed in detail in this section.

> **Patient Safety**
>
> Ultrasonography is noninvasive, emits no ionizing radiation, and improves the time to diagnosis, thus allowing proper therapy to be administered early in the course of illness.

Probe Selection

Ultrasound probes are categorized by the frequency of emission or the wavelength of sound waves produced, as well as the physical shape of the end of the transducer, or "footprint" of the probe being utilized. Commonly, two types of probes are used to evaluate critically ill patients; these include the high-frequency (10–15 megahertz [MHz]) and low frequency (2–5 MHz) probes. The choice of probe depends on the depth of the anatomic structure that needs to be imaged and the quality of the image that needs to be obtained.

High-frequency probes are best used to image superficial structures such as blood vessels, nerves, and pleura, as the clarity and detail of these structures are important; in contrast, low-frequency probes are used to examine deeper structures such as the heart or the abdomen. Clarity and detail of deeper organs and structures are important; however, ultrasonographic technology and physics limit the ability to see objects clearly at these depths. This unfortunate setback is a function of the physical limitations of the ultrasound at longer wavelengths, and as yet, no method exists to overcome this. The frequency of the transducer determines the quality of the image that is able to be obtained; specific probe frequencies and footprints have been paired for practicality. For example, low-frequency, phased-array transducers are ideal to examine the heart because the probe footprint fits between the ribs and the ultrasound waves fan out as they travel into the body to provide a progressively widening field of view. However, the aforementioned image comes with the expense of decreased resolution at greater depths. In contrast, the linear high-frequency probe has a wide and flat footprint from which the ultrasound waves emanate in a straight line, providing higher resolution along the entire course of the view; however, the depth of the field of view is greatly reduced (Figure 11-1).

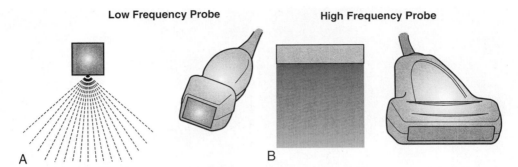

FIGURE 11-1 Two Types of Ultrasound Probes. A, Low-frequency phased-array probe for deep structures. **B,** High-frequency linear probe for superficial applications.

Gel

Air is considered the "enemy" of ultrasound as the presence of air significantly reduces the transmission of the ultrasound waves. To overcome this, ultrasound gel is used as a conduit to transmit sound energy between the patient and the transducer. Any viscous liquid can serve as a medium, but the specially designed gel is particularly useful, as it provides the best image quality with the least air interference. It is important to avoid the mouth of the gel bottle touching the patient or the probe to prevent contamination and transmission of infection to other patients.

Patient Comfort

Ultrasonography may cause temporary discomfort to the patient because of the need for the application of the water-based gel to the skin for the examination. It is important for patient comfort that the gel be fully wiped off with a soft washcloth after the examination. Occasionally, the patient's gown may need to be removed to facilitate the examination and replaced afterward to ensure comfort.

Image Optimization

When examining a patient, several adjustments are made by the operator to optimize the image obtained; these include gain, depth, and proper selection of mode options.

Gain

Gain is used to adjust the brightness of the acquired images. Optimizing gain is important to view structures adequately and accurately. Two common mistakes made when using gain are overgaining and undergaining. For example, when accessing a blood vessel under ultrasound guidance, the novice sonographer often underutilizes gain and significantly decreases the quality of the obtained images (Figure 11-2). Similarly, the overuse of gain when trying to obtain vascular access under ultrasound guidance may give the operator the false impression that a blood clot may exist because of the artifactual "smoky" appearance of the echogenic intravascular blood. Most machines have an auto-gain feature, which resets gain to a predetermined midrange

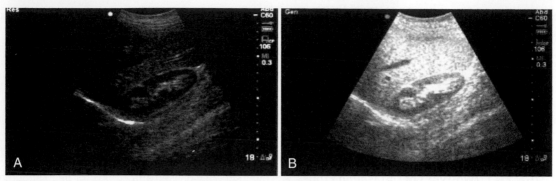

FIGURE 11-2 **Common Mistakes Made When Using Gain. A,** Undergained image. **B,** Overgained image.

level, which may be useful in circumstances when gain has been altered significantly by a prior user.[15]

Depth

The sonographer sets the image depth to adequately visualize structures. Standard practice is to start with a greater depth and decrease the field size to bring the structure of interest into the middle of the screen; this ensures that deep or distal pathology does not go unnoticed. It is important to have all critical anatomic structures visible when performing invasive procedures using bedside ultrasonography. For example, the diaphragm should be visualized when doing a thoracentesis for a pleural effusion to avoid a subdiaphragmatic puncture, and the accompanying artery should be visualized when cannulating central veins to avoid inadvertent arterial puncture.

Mode

The major modes available in bedside ultrasonography are two dimensional (2D), motion mode (M mode), and Doppler. Each mode provides a unique type of image and diagnostic information.

Two-Dimensional (2D) Mode

The most commonly known ultrasound is the 2D brightness mode, also known as the *2D* or *B-mode*. The piezoelectric crystals within the probe generate sound waves that travel through tissues until they encounter structures within the body that reflect signal back to the probe. Depending on the composition and echogenicity of the object encountered, the waves are transmitted through, accelerated, deflected, or reflected back to the probe. Depending on signal strength, angle, and depth, the computer processes these signals and creates a gray-scale image that is generated from the composition of the returning signal. Highly reflective structures such as bone cortex and diaphragm appear hyperechoic or bright white. Fluid-filled structures transmit the signal without attenuation and appear anechoic or hypoechoic, that is, dark. Other tissues and fluids have intermediate properties and appear as different degrees of gray, depending on the density of the structures being imaged (Figure 11-3).

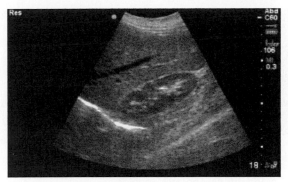

FIGURE 11-3 Example of variable echogenicity of tissues.

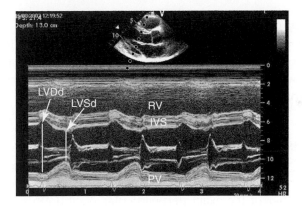

FIGURE 11-4 M-mode.

Motion Mode (M-Mode)

M-mode ultrasound is the original form of clinical ultrasound. This mode samples the anatomy along a single point of the ultrasound signal and reflects the information from that point graphically over time. M-mode provides a one-dimensional view of the structure of interest and is displayed as monochromic dots.[16] M-mode was initially used to image the heart, but its application has been expanded to multiple anatomic structures (Figure 11-4). M-mode is utilized in several diagnostic-imaging procedures to provide additional information useful in measuring changes in distance and indirectly measuring changes in volume and pressure.

Doppler (Spectral, Color, and Power)

The Doppler mode measures the velocity of fluid being examined and relies on a principle known as the "Doppler shift" caused by the change in frequency from the transmitting to the receiving object from motion toward or away from the receiving object. An everyday illustration of the increase in the audible sound—heard as a barking dog approaches along with the decrease in sound as the dog moves away—is an example of the Doppler shift. The three principal types of Doppler used in clinical sonography are Spectral Doppler, color-flow Doppler, and power Doppler.

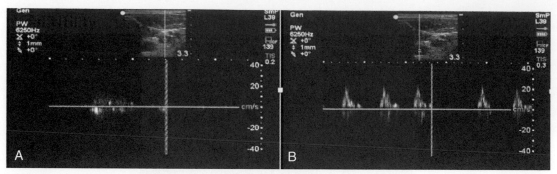

FIGURE 11-5 Venous and arterial spectral Doppler.

Spectral Doppler

Spectral Doppler is a graphic measurement of fluid flow with time on the X-axis and velocity of flow on the Y-axis. High-velocity flow results in a taller peak on the Y-axis. Spectral Doppler displays the obvious difference between arterial and venous spectral Doppler signals (Figure 11-5).

Color Doppler

Color Doppler allows the sonographer to determine whether fluid is flowing toward or away from the transducer; to obtain this view, the transducer must be angled to one side or the other of the exact perpendicular position in reference to the pathway of the fluid flow. A red signal represents flow toward the transducer, and a blue signal indicates flow away from the transducer, as opposed to the common misbelief that red is arterial and blue is venous. A common mnemonic device to remember which color Doppler represents which direction of flow is the acronym BART—Blue Away Red Toward. When colors other than red or blue are seen, it is often a sign of turbulent blood flow, as is seen with valve stenoses (Figure 11-6).

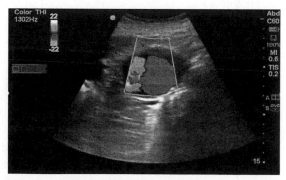

FIGURE 11-6 Representation of a Color Doppler Screen. Red (*here shown as light gray*) indicates flow toward the probe. Blue (*here shown as dark gray*) indicates flow away from the probe.

Power Doppler

A colored signal is also produced with power Doppler, but a single yellow-orange color identifies qualitative presence or absence of low velocity flow within tissues. This differs from the color Doppler that measures directionality of flow, as indicated by blue or red, and the spectral Doppler that measures quantitative velocities. The power Doppler mode would be used to identify vascular flow in low-flow states, to rule out testicular torsion, to identify small capillaries, or to image joints for signs of inflammation (Figure 11-7).

Care of the Ultrasound Machine

It is important that probes are treated carefully as broken crystals lead to suboptimal imaging with streak artifact. Additionally, a common error is improper attention to the care of the cords that connect the probes to the computer. Damage to the cords from kinking or being run over by the wheels of the ultrasound cart will lead to suboptimal imaging over time.

Cleaning the Ultrasound Machine

Care of the ultrasound probes and the machine is an overlooked, but critical, component of successful point-of-care ultrasonography. The probe and computer processor of an ultrasound machine require chemical solutions different from those used on the screen. For example, manufacturers recommend cleaning the screen with water or an alcohol-based cleaner and a cotton cloth. Use of bleach-based cleansers or similar harsh disinfectants may create a cloudy film on the screen, which would cause permanent damage and interfere with image quality and interpretation. It is imperative that the housing of the computer, keyboard, knobs, and transducers be cleaned before and after each use of the machine, even if a sterile probe cover and gloves were used during contact with the patient. A soft cloth with an approved germicidal solution is recommended when cleaning the machine and components. The equipment should be allowed to air-dry after cleaning to avoid prematurely removing disinfectant. If a

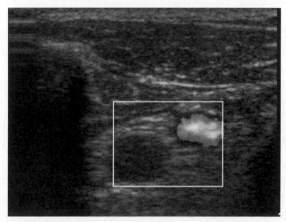

FIGURE 11-7 Representation of a Power Doppler Screen. A single yellow-orange color (*here shown as a solid gray cloud*) identifies qualitative presence or absence of low velocity flow within tissues.

patient is in isolation for drug-resistant pathogens, a manufacturer-approved disinfectant needs to be used to clean the entire ultrasound system, including the transducers prior to further use. Ultrasound machines have been implicated in the transmission of nosocomial infections; therefore, ensuring proper hygiene is critical.[17]

Inspection of the probes after each use is equally vital, as damaged probes may serve as vectors for transmission of infection and may also provide suboptimal images, thus potentially hampering patient care. Last, it is important not to forget to clean the ultrasound gel bottle as well after each patient to avoid cross-contamination. Specific protocols with regard to the most effective way to clean the ultrasound machine and probes are available from manufacturers and are a useful reference.

Patient Safety

Thorough cleaning of the ultrasound machine protects patients from nosocomial infections. Ensure that the probe and machine have been cleaned before and after every patient examination.

Cardiac Assessment

Cardiac evaluation is the most challenging aspect of point-of-care ultrasonography to teach and to learn. Despite this fact, studies support that basic critical care and emergency echocardiography can be successfully taught to health care providers other than cardiologists with excellent results in terms of quality and reproducibility of image acquisition and accuracy of interpretation, comprehension, and proper integration into patient care.[7,18] In a 2010 international expert statement regarding training for critical care ultrasonography, 29 experts and 12 professional critical care societies agreed that "basic level critical care echocardiography and general critical care ultrasound should be a required part of the training of every critical care unit physician."[19] The American College of Emergency Physicians (ACEP) has also recognized the indispensable nature of this diagnostic tool and routinely incorporates education on ultrasonography into its training pathways. In a consensus statement, the ACEP and the American Society of Echocardiography (ASE), state that "focused cardiac ultrasound has become a fundamental tool to expedite the diagnostic evaluation of the patient at the bedside and to initiate emergent treatment and triage decisions by emergency physicians."[6] The utility of this tool in the hands of the bedside clinicians has been clearly established, and its impact on patient care, decision making, and outcomes can be powerful.

Clinical Reasoning Pearl

Critical care societies now require all new trainees to learn point-of-care ultrasonography. Within a decade, one could reasonably expect bedside ultrasonography to be as common as the stethoscope and used as an extension of the physical examination. Familiarity with this modality is and will be an important part of taking care of critically ill patients.

Ultrasound Cardiac Windows

Three basic approaches or windows are taken to view the heart with the ultrasound. These include the subcostal, parasternal, and apical windows. Each view has its advantages and disadvantages. It is key to achieve competence in all windows, as many critically ill patients cannot be clearly imaged from every view because of multiple factors, including bowel gas, postsurgical changes, invasive tubes and lines, or inability to be repositioned because of hemodynamic instability. However, in one study that used a focused transthoracic echocardiographic protocol, usable images from at least one view were obtained in 97% of patients in the critical care unit. The information obtained from these examinations contributed positively to the assessment of patients in 97% of cases, provided new information in 35% of patients, and was decisive in enabling clear management in 25% of cases.[12]

Subcostal Window

The subcostal view of the heart takes advantage of the echogenicity of the liver to obtain a sonographic window of the heart, which sits on the opposite side of the diaphragm from where the probe comes into contact with the upper abdomen (Figure 11-8). For enough pressure and contact with the abdomen to obtain adequate images, this window is the only view of the heart that requires an overhand grip of the probe. As a result of the position of the probe that is relatively flat and almost parallel with the floor, this view may not be possible in patients with large abdomens as with pregnancy and massive ascites. It also may be a limited view after abdominal or cardiothoracic surgery because of overlying dressings, mediastinal tubes, or patient

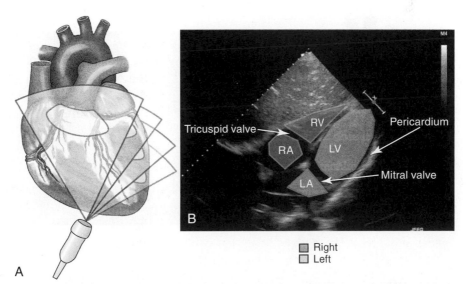

FIGURE 11-8 **Subcostal Window. A,** Position of the probe for subcostal view of the heart. **B,** Subcostal image of the heart.

discomfort. The subcostal window gives a long-axis view of the heart and all four chambers, and has utility in providing information about each cardiac chamber in terms of static and dynamic parameters. The pericardium, as well as any pericardial effusion that may be present, is well visualized from this view. In cardiac tamponade, this is the preferred approach for emergent ultrasound-guided pericardiocentesis. In addition, from the subcostal view, the probe can be rotated into the longitudinal plane of the body to obtain an image of the inferior vena cava as it courses into the right atrium. The utility of this view is to acquire information on volume status and likelihood of response to volume resuscitation. Finally, the subcostal view is the preferred window in certain populations, including patients with chronic obstructive pulmonary disease (COPD) and cardiac arrest, because of the difficulty of obtaining transthoracic views in these patient populations.

Apical Window

The apical views of the heart provide a long-axis, four-chamber view of the heart from the position of the apex of the heart where the point of maximal impulse is located (Figure 11-9). This view best shows the relative size and function of the right and left ventricles, evaluates for atrial enlargement, and is the optimal vantage point to assess mitral, tricuspid, and aortic insufficiency or stenosis with spectral Doppler because of the approximately parallel orientation with the flow of blood through these valves.

The aortic outflow tract is visualized via the apical window and is sometimes referred to as the fifth heart chamber. This view also enables evaluation of the pericardium and shows a portion of the pleural space as well as a cross-section of the

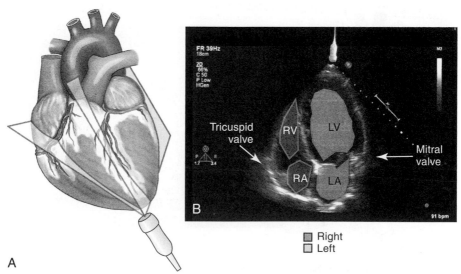

FIGURE 11-9 Apical Window. A, Position of the probe for apical view of the heart. **B,** Apical image of the heart.

descending aorta. This window is one of the key views needed to obtain velocity measurements across the aortic valve outflow tract, which are used in cardiac output calculations. Often, the patient must be positioned in the left lateral decubitus position with the left arm elevated above the head to achieve the apical images. This position serves to bring the heart close to the chest wall thereby displacing the poor acoustic medium of the lungs, and it also increases the space between ribs to reduce interference with the ultrasound beam. Again, this window may not be feasible in the critically ill or injured patient because of hemodynamic or spinal instability.

Parasternal View

The parasternal view of the heart is typically obtained in both parasternal long axis (PLAX) and parasternal short axis (PSAX), each with its own advantages (Figure 11-10). The PLAX view focuses the ultrasound vector along the long axis of the left ventricle and provides information regarding left ventricular (LV) size and function, interventricular septum size and function, left atrial size, mitral valve and aortic valve anatomy and function, aortic root size, ascending and descending aorta, pericardium, and pleural space. The descending aorta is a key landmark to differentiate pericardial fluid that lies between the heart and the descending aorta from pleural effusion that collects deep to this landmark. The long-axis view does not image the right ventricle in its entirety but, rather, only shows a portion of the right ventricular (RV) outflow tract (Figure 11-11). When the probe is rotated approximately 90 degrees clockwise from the long-axis position, the ultrasound beam divides the heart along its short axis. With proper angling, four levels of cross section can be imaged; these include the base with the aortic, tricuspid, and pulmonic valves, the mitral valve level, the papillary muscle level, and the apex.

The PSAX view highlights the relative size of the right ventricle and the left ventricle, can display LV wall motion abnormalities, and is an excellent view for determining volume status at the papillary level.

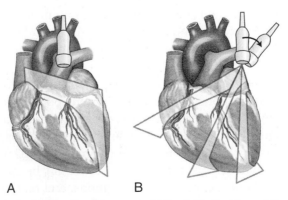

A   B

FIGURE 11-10 Positioning the Probe for Parasternal View. A, Position of the probe for parasternal short-axis view of the heart. **B,** Position of the probe for parasternal long-axis view of the heart.

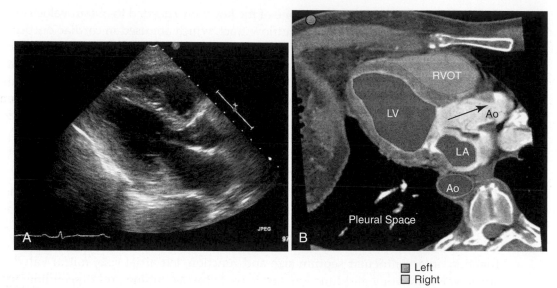

☐ Left
☐ Right

FIGURE 11-11 **Images of Parasternal View. A,** Parasternal long-axis image of the heart by ultrasonography. **B,** Parasternal long-axis image of the heart by computed tomography with structures labeled. *Ao,* Ascending and descending aorta; *LA,* left atrium; *LV,* left ventricle; *RVOT,* right ventricular outflow tract.

Fluid Volume Status Assessment

One of the most common questions in the management of seriously ill and unstable patients is whether the patient would benefit from intravenous fluid volume resuscitation. Cardiologists have long emphasized the evaluation of the jugular venous pulsation as a clue to underlying fluid status. Early goal-directed therapy (EGDT) and the Surviving Sepsis Campaign have given central venous pressure (CVP) measures a prominent role in the protocol for evaluation of patients with sepsis.[20,21] Reliance on CVP as a marker of central volume has been extrapolated to other areas such as trauma and burn surgery. However, CVP has consistently been shown to be unreliable in predicting volume status and fluid responsiveness except at the extremes.[22,23] In addition, CVP monitoring is invasive and carries with it risks of infection, hemorrhage, pneumothorax, and thrombosis. As an alternative or adjunct, it is possible to evaluate volume status and predict fluid responsiveness with the use of bedside ultrasonography by evaluating changes in preload, stroke volume, and aortic velocity during the respiratory cycle. This can be done fairly quickly in some populations of patients and without the risks of an invasive procedure such as a central venous catheter insertion. Fluid volume status evaluation should comprise several ultrasonographic and echocardiographic findings, as opposed to only one image or 2D view of the inferior vena cava, as the answer to this clinical question could be multifactorial and complex, depending on patient age, comorbid conditions, and real-time clinical acuity.

Volume status may, in part, be evaluated by measuring the size of the inferior vena cava and change in size of the inferior vena cava during the respiratory cycle; this change in vessel size is measured a few centimeters distal to the inferior vena cava and the right atrial junction. During the respiratory cycle, intrathoracic pressures vary; however, the interpretation of this depends on whether the patient is breathing spontaneously by using negative pressure generated by the diaphragm, or if the patient is being artificially ventilated via positive pressure from mechanical support. In spontaneously breathing patients, intrathoracic pressure is lowest at the end of inspiration, and in mechanically ventilated patients on positive pressure, intrathoracic pressures are lowest at end expiration. During the low intrathoracic pressure phase of the respiratory cycle, additional preload volume is drawn into the right side of the heart, and the inferior vena cava will collapse through a suction mechanism inversely proportional to the patient's volume status. In other words, the walls of the inferior vena cava of a volume-depleted patient are likely to collapse significantly when intrathoracic pressure drops.[24] A similar variability can also be observed in the superior vena cava (Figure 11-12).

The inferior vena cava collapsibility seen with normal breathing in spontaneously breathing patients has been correlated to CVP ranges. At the extreme low CVP equivalent, volume responsiveness is likely to occur (Table 11-3). Caution must be exercised to avoid overinterpretation of CVP in the middle or higher range of the scale because factors such as mechanical ventilation with positive end-expiratory pressure (PEEP), tricuspid regurgitation, and pulmonary hypertension may falsely elevate CVP. When the volume status of a patient places him or her on the steep part of the Frank-Starling curve (Figure 11-13), a change in preload will lead to a marked change in stroke volume. However, if a patient is fully volume repleted or fluid overloaded, changes in preload will not lead to changes in stroke volume or cardiac output. In addition, the respiratory variability of the inferior vena cava will be less marked when a patient is euvolemic or fluid overloaded. This phenomenon has been studied most often in mechanically ventilated patients. It has been shown that a stroke volume variation, as measured by differences in the velocity across the aortic valve of greater than 12% during the respiratory cycle, predicts an increase in cardiac output after an intravenous fluid bolus challenge. For spontaneously breathing patients who are not in respiratory distress, a greater than 12% variation in stroke volume with passive leg raise predicts a similar response to volume[25] (Figure 11-14). In summary, when patients are hypovolemic, pressure changes in the thorax may impact preload and ultimately change stroke volume. Markers of the change in stroke volume caused by changes in intrathoracic pressure are seen during bedside ultrasound evaluation, which can confirm a patient's hemodynamic position on the Starling curve and allow better understanding of management strategies.

Evaluation of the LV chamber size and contractility can also give clues to a patient's volume status. In the midparasternal short-axis view at the level of the papillary muscles, a small chamber size in systole or "kissing papillary sign" in addition to a small chamber size in diastole is a sign of a hyperdynamic heart likely caused by hypovolemia. This finding is predictive of volume responsiveness in patients who are displaying signs of hypoperfusion or hypotension.[26]

Even though inferior vena cava collapsibility, SV variations, and small LV dimensions may be noted on bedside ultrasonographic evaluation, it is imperative to put all of these findings in clinical context. For instance, if a patient has a normal mental status, normal lactate level, adequate urine output, normal kidney function, and is

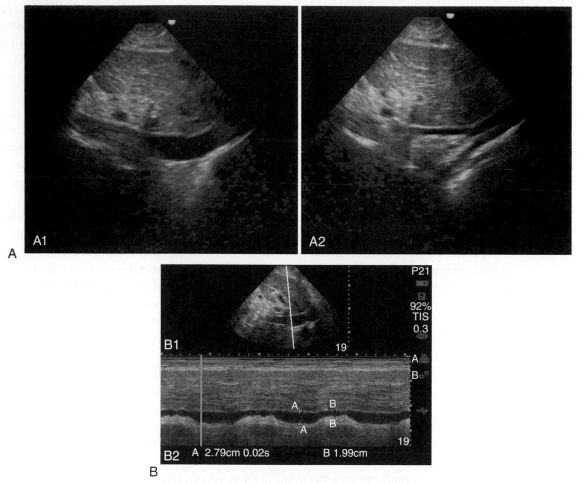

FIGURE 11-12 Consequences of Changes in Intrathoracic Pressure. A, Respiratory intrathoracic pressure changes impact inferior vena cava (IVC) diameter. When a spontaneously breathing patient takes a deep breath (inhalation) or sniffs, the blood in the IVC rapidly enters the right atrium and the IVC decreases in diameter—a collapsed IVC is a sign of hypovolemia. In contrast, when a patient performs a Valsalva maneuver, the IVC plumps out, with less blood going into the right atrium. **A1,** Exhalation (expiration): The IVC is at maximum diameter in a spontaneously breathing patient. **A2,** Inhalation (inspiration): The IVC has collapsed, indicating hypovolemia in a spontaneously breathing patient. **B,** Ultrasound in a spontaneously breathing patient. **B1,** 2-D ultrasound of IVC from the subxiphoid view. **B2,** M-Mode ultrasound showing changes in the IVC diameter with breathing: **A** indicates exhalation (expiration); **B** indicates inhalation (inspiration).

normotensive, then volume resuscitation may not be indicated. Additionally, some conditions dictate the need for a low CVP, and some patients such as athletes and young individuals may have a dilated inferior vena cava with normal CVP. The initial clinical question for each individual patient should always guide the response to the information uncovered during focused evaluation with sonography.

TABLE 11-3 Subcostal Inferior Vena Cava Assessment

INFERIOR VENA CAVA DIAMETER (CM)	% COLLAPSE	CENTRAL VENOUS PRESSURE (mm Hg)
<2 cm	>50%	0–5
>2 cm	>50%	5–10
>2 cm	<50%	10–15
>2 cm	Minimal	15–20
>2 cm	None + hepatic veins dilated	>20

Data from Lang RM, Bierig M, Devereux RB, et al.: Recommendations for Chamber Quantification: a report from the American Society of Echocardiography's Guidelines and Standards Committee and the Chamber Quantification Writing Group, developed in conjunction with the European Association of Echocardiography, a branch of the European Society of Cardiology, *J Am Soc Echocardiogr* 18(12):1440–1463, 2005.

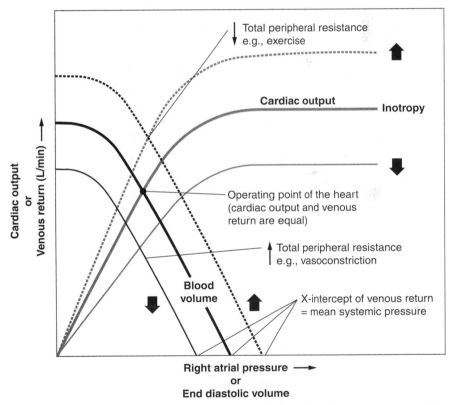

FIGURE 11-13 Cardiac output is dependent upon the interrelationship of venous return and cardiac function (Starling Curve) so that blood entering the right heart (venous return) will equal blood leaving the left heart (cardiac output). The intersection point of these curves will vary according to the quantity of venous return and cardiac output. For example, in hypovolemia, reduced venous return places the patient on the steep rising part of the Starling curve. In hypervolemia, a patient will be on the flatter part of the Starling Curve. Other factors such as vasodilation, change in contractility, and increased sympathetic stimulation or exercise will also shift the intersection point of the curves.

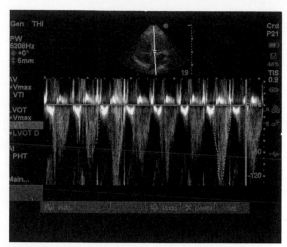

FIGURE 11-14 Stroke volume variation across the aortic valve indicative of a fluid responsive state.

Bedside Ultrasonography Protocols for Cardiac Assessment

Numerous protocols have been developed to guide systematic assessment with ultrasonography. The cardiac protocols include the FOCUS, FATE, and FEEL algorithms. These algorithms differ in minor ways and all seek to provide information about both static and dynamic features of cardiac function. Static parameters commonly evaluated include chamber size and wall thickness, whereas dynamic parameters include contractility, wall motion abnormalities, valvular insufficiency or stenosis, and evidence of tamponade physiology in the case of pericardial effusions.

The FATE examination is essentially the FOCUS examination with an added component of evaluation of the pleural space, as it is clear that significant pathology of the thoracic space such as large effusions or pneumothoraces can impact hemodynamic status.

The FEEL algorithm applies the expedited cardiac examination in the setting of cardiac arrest to evaluate for reversible etiologies. The FEEL protocol is an algorithm that is compliant with Advanced Cardiac Life Support (ACLS) and is similarly used to diagnose and treat reversible causes of cardiac arrest. The goal is to exclude pulmonary embolism, cardiac tamponade, severe LV dysfunction, and hypovolemia as causes of cardiac arrest. The protocol is unique in comparison with the FATE and FOCUS protocols in that it is integrated into the ACLS algorithm. The views used in the FEEL examination are subcostal, parasternal long axis, and apical. In one study, this protocol led to perceived changes in therapy in 89% of cases and at least one echocardiographic window was available in all patients.[10]

Pericardial Assessment and Cardiac Tamponade

The pericardial space is a potential space around the heart that usually contains trace serous fluid and fills appreciably with fluid only in pathologic conditions.[27] With an accumulation of fluid or other material in the pericardial space, the pressure within the space may rise and cause impaired return of blood to the heart, which, in turn,

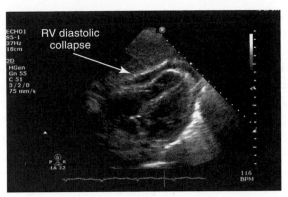

FIGURE 11-15 Diastolic collapse of the right ventricular free wall indicative of tamponade physiology.

could diminish cardiac output and cause severe hemodynamic compromise. This situation manifests clinically as cardiac tamponade, a rapidly progressing and potentially fatal condition. The amount of pericardial fluid that could lead to cardiac tamponade depends on how quickly this fluid accumulates. In an acute setting, less compliance exists in the pericardial space, and as such, a small amount of fluid accumulation in a short period may have significant hemodynamic implications. In the chronic setting, however, the stretch of the pericardium is progressive, and larger volumes of fluid are required to create hemodynamic compromise. Importantly, cardiac tamponade remains a clinical diagnosis, manifesting classically as hypotension, tachycardia, and jugular venous distention, as well as the more nuanced finding of pulsus paradoxus.

Echocardiography is the modality of choice for the diagnosis of pericardial effusion,[28] and such a finding could lend confidence to the diagnosis when the clinician is faced with clinical evidence of tamponade.[8,29,30] On careful inspection of all accessible cardiac windows, a pericardial effusion can be identified by a relatively anechoic space around the heart.[31] To detect tamponade, however, further pathophysiologic changes must be elicited. In its early phases, cardiac tamponade may lead to prominent changes in the blood flow and volume of either ventricle during normal breathing. This forms the basis of pulsus paradoxus and is quickly identifiable via Doppler by experienced ultrasonographers.[32] As the pathology progresses, echocardiographic evidence of right, and subsequently, left chamber collapse during diastole is seen (Figure 11-15). Intervention in these circumstances is lifesaving, and echocardiography is used to guide a therapeutic pericardiocentesis in a rapid and safe fashion when indicated.[33]

Pulmonary Edema or Fluid Overload Assessment

Ultrasonography of the lungs has proven utility in the evaluation of pneumothorax, pleural effusion, alveolar consolidation, and interstitial processes such as pulmonary edema or acute respiratory distress syndrome (ARDS).[34] The discovery of any of these findings factors heavily in the assessment of the hemodynamically unstable patient.

Traditionally, clinicians believed that lung ultrasonography did not have the same utility as solid organ ultrasonography. This stemmed from the knowledge that ultrasound waves are scattered by air and yield poorly discernible images. Once clinicians realized the diagnostic importance of lung ultrasound artifacts, the potential for lung ultrasonography became evident.[35] Consistent ultrasound findings are used to detect pulmonary pathologic conditions, and a clinically validated algorithm known as the BLUE protocol utilizes these findings in the setting of acute respiratory distress to make a diagnosis with reasonable accuracy[36] (Figure 11-16 and Table 11-4). In this algorithm, patients are examined at three points on the anterior, lateral, and posterior thorax bilaterally. The protocol also involves imaging of deep venous vasculature in the legs to rule out deep vein thrombosis. A low-frequency probe for the thorax examination is appropriate, and a high-frequency probe is used for the vascular examination. The BLUE protocol was originally performed in patients with acute respiratory failure of unknown etiology. The protocol enabled clinicians to categorize a patient's respiratory failure

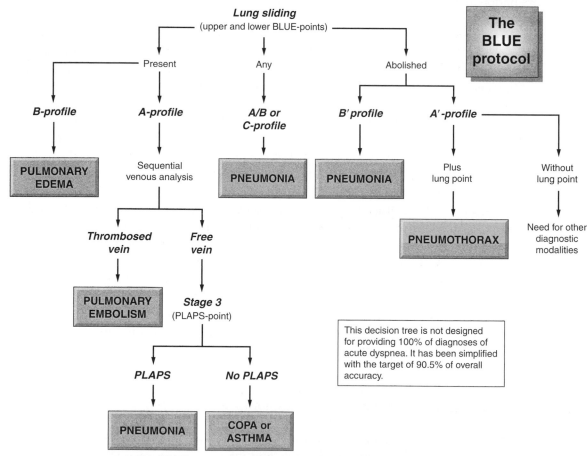

FIGURE 11-16 The BLUE protocol algorithm. (From Lichtenstein DA, Mezière GA: Relevance of lung ultrasound in the diagnosis of acute respiratory failure: the BLUE protocol, *Chest* 134 (1):117–125, 2008.) See Table 11-4 for definitions of the abbreviations used in the BLUE protocol.

TABLE 11-4	Categories of Lung Ultrasonography Artifacts for the BLUE Protocol
PROFILE	**DESCRIPTION**
A	Anterior predominant bilateral A-lines associated with lung sliding
A′	A profile with absent lung sliding and without a lung point
B	Anterior–predominant bilateral B-lines associated with lung sliding
B′	B-profile with abolished lung sliding
A/B	A-profile on one side and B-profile on the other
C	Anterior alveolar consolidation
PLAPS	Posterior and/or lateral alveolar and/or pleural syndrome, namely, the finding of consolidation or effusions in those dependent areas

Data from Lichtenstein DA, Mezière GA: Relevance of lung ultrasound in the diagnosis of acute respiratory failure: the BLUE protocol, *Chest* 134(1):117–125, 2008.

into specific disease processes, including pulmonary edema, pulmonary embolism, pneumonia, reactive airway disease, and pneumothorax. Without the use of any other clinical examination, the protocol provided the cause of patient's respiratory failure in 90.5% of patients.[37] The importance of these findings cannot be understated as the physical examination in critically ill patients has known limitations and computed tomography (CT) of the chest has significant radiation risks. Lung ultrasonography is now recommended over supine chest radiography to evaluate patients for pneumothorax,[38] and international recommendations with regard to the use of lung ultrasonography in the critically ill have now been created.[39]

> **Clinical Reasoning Pearl**
>
> Bedside ultrasonography is superior to plain-film radiography for many purposes such as evaluation of pneumothorax, evaluation of free fluid in the abdomen evaluation, and invasive procedure guidance and should be the go-to modality in these situations.

When a linear transducer is positioned on the chest wall at the midclavicular line across the second and third ribs, an image including two transected ribs with shadows behind and an interposed horizontal hyperechoic structure can be obtained (Figure 11-17).[40] The hyperechoic structure is the pleural interface and represents the meeting of the parietal and visceral pleura. The pleura glide against each other during respirations, a feature that is appreciated with real-time image acquisition and is referred to as "lung sliding." Normal lung tissue, which lies beyond the pleural interface, cannot be appreciated because of the presence of air deep to the pleura. In fact, much of the basis for clinically relevant ultrasound findings in the lung is not direct visualization of pathology but the presence of artifacts attributed to interactions between the air and the fluid-lined interfaces.

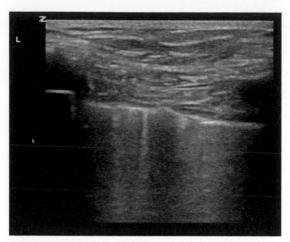

FIGURE 11-17 Ribs, rib shadows, and pleural line between ribs.

Two primary artifacts are useful for lung evaluation. These are known as *A-lines* and the *B-lines*. A-lines are horizontal reverberations of the pleural interface that occur at repeating intervals equivalent to the skin to pleural distance and are seen when the ultrasound beam encounters air (Figure 11-18). A-lines can be seen in normal lung as well as pathologic processes such as pneumothorax. B-lines are vertical, linear artifacts that spread in a comet tail fashion from the pleural interface to the edge of the screen, abolishing A-lines in the process. B-lines tend to occur as a result of localized physiologic or pathologic areas of fluid concentration in the interlobular septae that extend perpendicularly from the pleural surface. B-lines are typically few and faint in physiologic conditions and are referred to as *minor B-lines*. However, with a pathologic increase in extravascular lung water or with reduced aeration of lung tissue, an increased preponderance of major B-lines can be appreciated (Figure 11-19). The finding of multiple bilateral B-lines (>3 and in at least two regions per side) is significant and is typically referred to as the "interstitial syndrome."[41,42] In numerous studies, the interstitial syndrome correlated well to radiographic and clinical assessments

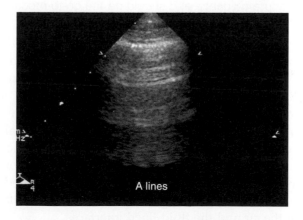

FIGURE 11-18 A-lines.

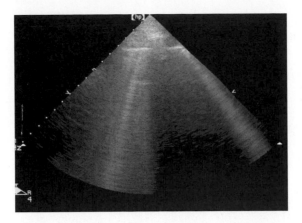

FIGURE 11-19 B-lines.

consistent with cardiogenic and non-cardiogenic pulmonary edema, pulmonary fibrosis, or interstitial pneumonia.[43] In addition, B-lines separated by approximately 7 millimeters (mm) are suggestive of interstitial edema, whereas B-lines attributed to alveolar edema tend to appear either 3 mm apart or confluent.

In the assessment for pleural effusions, a low-frequency probe is placed along the posterior diaphragm at the midclavicular line on an upright patient or midaxillary line in supine patients, with the primary aim of identifying the diaphragm as it abuts the spleen or the liver below[34,44,45] (Figure 11-20). In normally aerated lungs without pleural effusion, the diaphragm–air interface reflects the sound waves back to the probe and creates the appearance of the liver or the spleen as a mirror image artifact above the diaphragm (Figure 11-21). In the presence of a pleural effusion, a hypoechoic space without abdominal organ reflection will be evident (Figure 11-22). Ultrasound can help guide both therapeutic as well as diagnostic drainage of this space in a safe and rapid fashion when the need arises.[46]

Lung artifacts are particularly relevant in the ultrasound evaluation for pneumothorax, which is an important differential diagnosis in the evaluation of the hemodynamically unstable patient with respiratory distress. The three major structures to be identified in the ultrasound examination for pneumothorax are (1) absence or presence

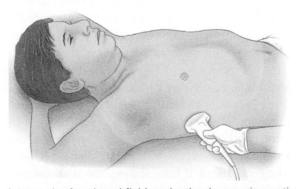

FIGURE 11-20 Position of the probe for pleural fluid evaluation in a supine patient.

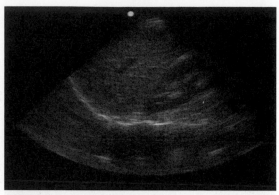

FIGURE 11-21 Mirror image artifact seen with normal lungs.

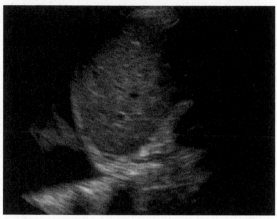

FIGURE 11-22 Pleural effusion.

of lung sliding on 2D mode and M-mode, (2) the absence or presence of A-lines, and (3) the existence or lack of B-lines. Lung sliding is the shimmering appearance of the visceral and parietal pleura as they slide together in the normally inflated lung. Sliding sign is absent in pneumothorax; instead, only the static parietal pleural line is seen. M-mode is paired with 2D ultrasound to verify the position of the lung relative to the chest wall. In pneumothorax, the M-mode appearance of the lung is distinct from that of the inflated lung. A pneumothorax appears like a classic bar code, and a normal lung that is adherent to the chest wall creates an image similar to waves coming into a sandy beach known as the "seashore sign" (Figure 11-23). The absence of lung sliding is a reasonable positive predictor for pneumothorax. However, absent lung sliding is well described in a variety of clinical conditions such as atelectasis, ARDS, and pneumonia and is therefore not specific enough alone to make the diagnosis. The constellation of absent lung sliding and the presence of A-lines without B-lines, however, are very sensitive for the presence of a pneumothorax. This paired with M-mode provides further evidence for a pneumothorax diagnosis. On the other hand, if lung sliding, the seashore sign, and B-lines are present, the presence of a pneumothorax is essentially ruled out, as these findings provide

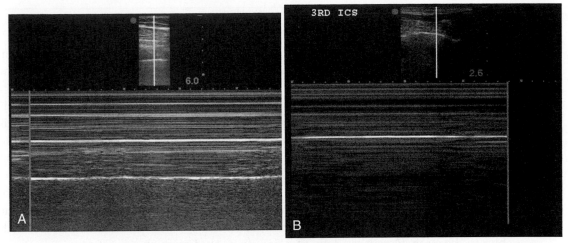

FIGURE 11-23 Normal Lung Compared with Pneumothorax. A, Seashore sign seen normally. **B,** Bar code sign seen with pneumothorax.

evidence of the intact visceral and parietal pleura interface. Finally, a very specific finding when assessing the possibility of a pneumothorax is the location of the "lung point." This finding describes the precise location where the visceral and parietal pleura separate. At this place, respiratory variation intermittently brings a partially collapsed lung up to the chest wall and allows visualization of findings that both support and refute a pneumothorax within the same rib space cyclically (Figure 11-24). This finding is 100% specific but often not visualized; however, its presence guarantees the diagnosis.[47,48]

In conclusion, diagnostic confidence for hemodynamically unstable patients is enhanced when lung ultrasonography is combined with cardiac or vascular ultrasonography. In the BLUE protocol, the presence of a normal lung profile with sonographic evidence for DVT raises the likelihood of a pulmonary embolism, and findings of right ventricular strain further support the bedside diagnosis of pulmonary embolism. In a similar fashion, the presence of diffuse B-lines, bilateral pleural effusions, and a noncollapsing inferior vena cava with poor ejection fraction raise the likelihood of cardiogenic pulmonary edema. Further case illustrations are provided at the end of this chapter.

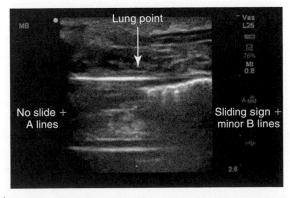

FIGURE 11-24 Lung point.

Vascular Assessment

Vascular ultrasonography is essential in many cases managed in the emergency department, critical care unit, and other acute care settings and is rapidly becoming the standard of care for central line placement.[49] In a similar fashion, the large veins of the lower extremities can be assessed for DVT. The presence or absence of DVT in a patient with clinical concern for pulmonary embolism is a valuable data point that factors significantly in the pretest probability of pulmonary embolism. However, standard full-leg evaluations of the lower extremities for DVT are time consuming and cumbersome and often not achievable in an unstable patient. Fortunately, mounting evidence indicates that a rapid two-point vascular examination of the lower extremities can reliably detect or rule out lower extremity DVT to a degree similar to formal ultrasound studies.[50–52] This is particularly helpful in the acute setting, where patients may be too unstable to be transferred to definitive imaging studies such as CT angiography or ventilation–perfusion (V/Q) scanning. Ultrasound evidence for hemodynamically significant pulmonary embolism can facilitate intervention more rapidly, when indicated.

For the two-point assessment, the high-frequency vascular probe is applied to bilateral common femoral veins as well as bilateral popliteal veins, and pressure is applied at each site in an attempt to fully compress the vessel. If it is difficult to compress the vein or evidence of echogenic thrombus within the vessel is seen at any site, the study is deemed positive (Figure 11-25). If each of the assessed sites is fully compressible without evidence of intraluminal clot, significant DVT can reliably be excluded.

FAST Examination

The oldest and best-known application for point-of-care ultrasonography is the FAST examination.[53,54] This examination was introduced in 1996 and is now an integral part of Advanced Trauma Life Support (ATLS). The FAST examination is performed after the initial primary survey of critically injured patients with blunt or penetrating trauma to the neck, chest, abdomen, or pelvis. The goal of the protocol is to quickly evaluate for injury that has resulted in internal bleeding, and the study is usually completed in less

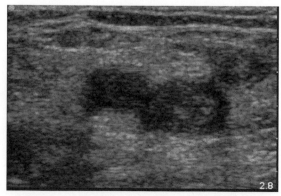

FIGURE 11-25 Poor compressibility and intraluminal opacity indicating deep vein thrombosis.

than 10 minutes. The protocol has essentially replaced the diagnostic peritoneal lavage for diagnosis of free fluid in the abdomen, as intraperitoneal free fluid volumes as little as 250 mL can be seen by the trained clinician. The sonographer focuses on four areas: the perihepatic, perisplenic, subxiphoid, and pelvic areas.

The perihepatic or right upper quadrant view looks at the hepatorenal interface known as Morison's pouch, subdiaphragmatic space, and the right chest. Typically, the area is viewed through the eighth through the eleventh intercostal spaces along the middle and posterior axillary lines. The low-frequency probe sweeps through the windows of the kidney, liver, paracolic gutter, diaphragm, and right lower costophrenic angle of the lung. During this sonography examination, the trained clinician can detect both small anechoic slivers of fluid as well as large volumes of occult fluid.

The perisplenic region is imaged next. The goals of this examination are very similar to those of the perihepatic examination except that in this window, the spleen and kidney are identified in the subdiaphragmatic space. The spleen is inherently more difficult to identify because of its homogeneous appearance; however, other components of the examination are similar.

A four-chamber view of the heart is obtained from the subcostal view and is used to rule out acute pericardial effusion and tamponade. The liver as a sonographic window, is used to obtain the four-chamber view of the heart.

The pelvic view evaluates for fluid between the bladder and rectum or the rectovesicular space; in women, fluid can collect posterior to the uterus, which is often referred to as the cul-de-sac of Douglas or the Douglas pouch. The target population for the FAST examination comprises trauma patients who have hypotension of unknown etiology and patients with any sort of blunt or penetrating thoracic or abdominal injury.

The FAST examination has a high specificity and is a screening tool for patients with traumatic injury. It is approximately 90% sensitive for detection of pathologic peritoneal fluid.[55] The original FAST protocol had significant limitations, including its minimal utility in detecting bowel injury and lung pathology. This led to the development of the extended FAST protocol (eFAST), which additionally addresses the possibility of pneumothorax in trauma patients. The eFAST requires examination of the four FAST protocol anatomic areas but adds the anterior of the thorax to assess for ultrasonographic signs of pneumothorax, including lung sliding, A-lines, B-lines, and the "seashore sign" along the anterior chest wall. The primary advantage of this technique is the avoidance of CT of the chest. Ultrasonography has superior sensitivity for detecting pneumothorax compared with chest radiography.[56]

Case Study #1

A 52-year-old man with history of dilated cardiomyopathy presents with difficulty breathing and hypotension. The emergency room physician performs bedside echocardiography and examination of the thorax.

Continued

Case Study #1—cont'd

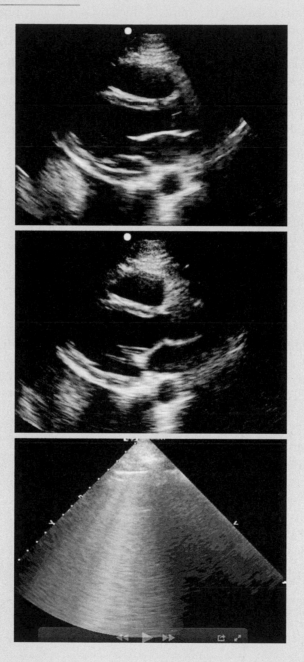

This picture shows a dilated heart with minimal change in LV size between diastole and systole and a pleural image consistent with B-lines seen in pulmonary edema. The patient was admitted with cardiogenic shock. ■

Case Study #2

A 33-year-old woman presents with symptoms of an upper respiratory viral illness that had progressed into gradually worsening dyspnea over the course of 5 days. An emergency room physician performs bedside echocardiography.

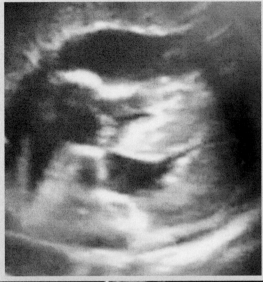

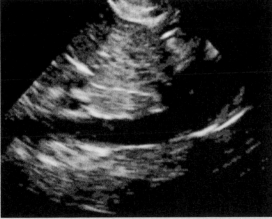

These images show a pericardial effusion that is causing clinical hemodynamic compromise as well as a dilated, noncollapsible inferior vena cava.

Case Study #3

A subclavian catheter is placed by a resident on a mechanically ventilated patient in the critical care unit. The patient develops hypoxia and hypotension within 1 hour of the procedure. An intensivist performs the RUSH examination.

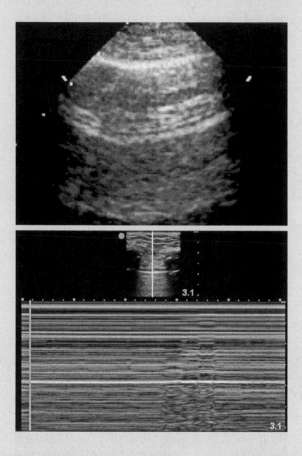

These images illustrate findings consistent with a pneumothorax with prominent A-lines and the loss of the "seashore" appearance of the pleura on M-mode. The clinical scenario leads to the diagnosis of a tension pneumothorax, and appropriate measures are taken immediately. ■

Case Study #4

A 62-year-old woman is in a car accident and is hypotensive when she is brought into the emergency room. A FAST examination is performed by a surgical resident.

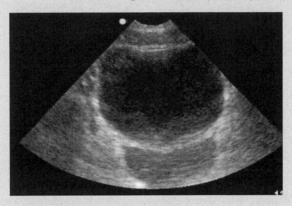

This picture demonstrates a positive FAST examination, with free fluid in the space posterior to the bladder and indicates the need for emergent laparotomy. ▪

Conclusion

In 2010, three major publications changed the landscape for critical care ultrasonography. Prior to that year, appreciation for the utility of bedside ultrasonography in the hands of noncardiologists and nonradiologists had been growing gradually, but at that time, a wide consensus did not exist regarding inclusion of point-of-care ultrasonography in the expected skill set of critical care and emergency clinicians. A consensus statement issued by the American Society of Echocardiography (ASE) and the Academy of Emergency Physicians (ACEP), delineated the roles of both formal and bedside ultrasonography and described the necessity of both in the care of emergency and critically ill patients.[6] This was one of the first formal acknowledgements of bedside ultrasonography by cardiologists, and the statement opened the door to greater acceptance of the practice of point-of-care ultrasonography. In addition, a Round Table Report on the role of critical care ultrasonography was created by 12 international critical care societies with unanimous consensus for the need for critical care ultrasonography as a requirement of practice.[19] As a result, training programs are now expected to include ultrasonography training for all critical care fellows as standard of care. Additionally, the RUSH protocol was introduced in 2010 and consolidated cardiac, abdominal, vascular, and pleural ultrasonography into a unified approach to the management of the patient in shock.[11] This has become the framework that emergency and critical care clinicians use to treat patients who are hemodynamically unstable, and the body of evidence for its utility is steadily growing.

References

1. Duncan DR, Morgenthaler TI, Ryu JH, Daniels CE: Reducing iatrogenic risk in thoracentesis: establishing best practice via experiential training in a zero-risk environment, *Chest* 135 (5):1315–1320, 2009.
2. Froehlich CD, Rigby MR, Rosenberg ES, et al.: Ultrasound-guided central venous catheter placement decreases complications and decreases placement attempts compared with the landmark technique in patients in a pediatric intensive care unit, *Crit Care Med* 37(3):1090–1096, 2009.
3. Karakitsos D, Labropoulos N, De Groot E, et al.: Real-time ultrasound-guided catheterisation of the internal jugular vein: a prospective comparison with the landmark technique in critical care patients, *Crit Care* 10(6):R162, 2006.
4. Via G, Hussain A, Wells M: International evidence-based recommendations for focused cardiac ultrasound, *J Am Soc Echocardiogr* 27(7):683.e1–e33, 2014.
5. Beaulieu Y: Specific skill set and goals of focused echocardiography for critical care clinicians, *Crit Care Med* 35(5 Suppl):S144–S149, 2007.
6. Labovitz AJ, Noble VE, Bierig M, et al.: Focused cardiac ultrasound in the emergent setting: a consensus statement of the American Society of Echocardiography and American College of Emergency Physicians, *J Am Soc Echocardiogr* 23(12):1225–1230, 2010.
7. Vignon P, Dugard A, Abraham J, et al.: Focused training for goal-oriented hand-held echocardiography performed by noncardiologist residents in the intensive care unit, *Intensive Care Med* 33(10):1795–1799, 2007.
8. Noritomi DT, Vieira ML, Mohovic T, et al.: Echocardiography for hemodynamic evaluation in the intensive care unit, *Shock* 34(Suppl 1):59–62, 2010.
9. Oren-Grinberg A, Talmor D, Brown SM: Focused critical care echocardiography, *Crit Care Med* 41(11):2618–2626, 2013.
9a. Howard ZD, Noble VE, Marill KA, et al.: Bedside ultrasound maximizes patient satisfaction, *J Emerg Med* 46(1):46–53, 2013.
10. Breitkreutz R, Walcher F, Seeger FH: Focused echocardiographic evaluation in resuscitation management: concept of an advanced life support-conformed algorithm, *Crit Care Med* 35 (5 Suppl):S150–S161, 2007.
11. Perera P, Mailhot T, Riley D, Mandavia D: The RUSH exam: Rapid Ultrasound in SHock in the evaluation of the critically ill, *Emerg Med Clin North Am* 28(1):29–56, 2010, vii.
12. Sloth E, Larsen KM, Schmidt MB, Jensen MB: Focused application of ultrasound in critical care medicine, *Crit Care Med* 36(2):653–654, 2008, author reply 654–655.
13. Lichtenstein DA, Mezière GM: The BLUE-points: three standardized points used in the BLUE-protocol for ultrasound assessment of the lung in acute respiratory failure, *Crit Ultrasound J* 3(2):109–110, 2011.
14. Frederiksen CA, Juhl-Olsen P, Sloth E: Perioperative use of focus assessed transthoracic echocardiography (FATE), *Anesth Analg* 115(5):1029–1032, 2012.
15. Aldrich JE: Basic physics of ultrasound imaging, *Crit Care Med* 35(5 Suppl):S131–S137, 2007.
16. Edler I, Lindstrom K: The history of echocardiography, *Ultrasound Med Biol* 30(12):1565–1644, 2004.

17. Schabrun S, Chipchase L, Rickard H: Are therapeutic ultrasound units a potential vector for nosocomial infection? *Physiother Res Int* 11(2):61–71, 2006.
18. Chalumeau-Lemoine L, Baudel JL, Das V, et al.: Results of short-term training of naïve physicians in focused general ultrasonography in an intensive-care unit, *Intensive Care Med* 35 (10):1767–1771, 2009.
19. International expert statement on training standards for critical care ultrasonography, *Intensive Care Med* 37(7):1077–1083, 2011.
20. Silva E, Akamine N, Salomao R, et al.: Surviving sepsis campaign: a project to change sepsis trajectory, *Endocr Metab Immune Disord Drug Targets* 6(2):217–222, 2006.
21. Rivers E, Nguyen B, Havstad S, et al.: Early goal-directed therapy in the treatment of severe sepsis and septic shock, *N Engl J Med* 345(19):1368–1377, 2001.
22. Janssens U, Graf J: [Volume status and central venous pressure], *Anaesthesist* 58(5):513–519, 2009.
23. Michard F, Teboul JL: Predicting fluid responsiveness in ICU patients: a critical analysis of the evidence, *Chest* 121(6):2000–2008, 2002.
24. Feissel M, Michard F, Faller JP, Teboul JL: The respiratory variation in inferior vena cava diameter as a guide to fluid therapy, *Intensive Care Med* 30(9):1834–1837, 2004.
25. Marx G, Cope T, McCrossan L: Assessing fluid responsiveness by stroke volume variation in mechanically ventilated patients with severe sepsis, *Eur J Anaesthesiol* 21(2):132–138, 2004.
26. Lamia B, Ochagavia A, Monnet X, et al.: Echocardiographic prediction of volume responsiveness in critically ill patients with spontaneously breathing activity, *Intensive Care Med* 33(7):1125–1132, 2007.
27. Spodick DH: Pathophysiology of cardiac tamponade, *Chest* 113(5):1372–1378, 1998.
28. Cheitlin MD, Armstrong WF, Aurigemma GP, et al.: ACC/AHA/ASE 2003 guideline update for the clinical application of echocardiography: a report of the American College of Cardiology/American Heart Association Task Force on Practice Guidelines (ACC/AHA/ASE Committee to Update the 1997 Guidelines for the Clinical Application of Echocardiography), *Circulation* 108(9):1146–1162, 2003.
29. Babic Z, Nikolic-Heitzler V, Bulj N, et al.: Hemodynamically unstable pericardial effusion in the Intensive Cardiac Unit: prospective study, *Acta Med Austriaca* 30(3):76–79, 2003.
30. Perera P, Lobo V, Williams SR, Gharahbaghian L: Cardiac Echocardiography, *Crit Care Clin* 30(1):47–92, 2014.
31. Mayo PH: Pericardial effusion and cardiac tamponade. In De Backer D, Cholley BP, Slama M, Vieillard-Baron A, Vignon P, editors: *Hemodynamic monitoring using echocardiography in the critically ill*, 2011, Springer-Verlag Berlin Heidelberg, pp 151–161, Springer.
32. Maisch B, Seferović PM, Ristić AD, et al.: Guidelines on the diagnosis and management of pericardial diseases executive summary: the task force on the diagnosis and management of pericardial diseases of the European society of cardiology, *Eur Heart J* 25(7):587–610, 2004.
33. Tsang TS, Enriquez-Sarano M, Freeman WK, et al.: Consecutive 1127 therapeutic echocardiographically guided pericardiocenteses: clinical profile, practice patterns, and outcomes spanning 21 years, *Mayo Clin Proc* 77(5):429–436, 2002.
34. Via G, Storti E, Gulati G, et al.: Lung ultrasound in the ICU: from diagnostic instrument to respiratory monitoring tool, *Minerva Anestesiol* 78(11):1282–1296, 2012.
35. Lichtenstein D, Mézière G, Biderman P, et al.: The comet-tail artifact. An ultrasound sign of alveolar-interstitial syndrome, *Am J Respir Crit Care Med* 156(5):1640–1646, 1997.
36. Lichtenstein D: Lung ultrasound in acute respiratory failure an introduction to the BLUE-protocol, *Minerva Anestesiol* 75(5):313–317, 2009.
37. Lichtenstein DA, Mezière GA: Relevance of lung ultrasound in the diagnosis of acute respiratory failure: the BLUE protocol, *Chest* 134(1):117–125, 2008.
38. Alrajhi K, Woo MY, Vaillancourt C: Test characteristics of ultrasonography for the detection of pneumothorax: a systematic review and meta-analysis, *Chest* 141(3):703–708, 2012.

39. Volpicelli G, Elbarbary M, Blaivas M, et al.: International evidence-based recommendations for point-of-care lung ultrasound, *Intensive Care Med* 38(4):577–591, 2012.
40. Piette E, Daoust R, Denault A: Basic concepts in the use of thoracic and lung ultrasound, *Curr Opin Anaesthesiol* 26(1):20–30, 2013.
41. Stefanidis K, Dimopoulos S, Kolofousi C, et al.: Sonographic lobe localization of alveolar-interstitial syndrome in the critically ill, *Crit Care Res Pract*, ID#179719, 7 pages, 2012.
42. Volpicelli G, et al.: Bedside lung ultrasound in the assessment of alveolar-interstitial syndrome, *Am J Emerg Med* 24(6):689–696, 2006.
43. Lichtenstein DA: Ultrasound examination of the lungs in the intensive care unit, *Pediatr Crit Care Med* 10(6):693–698, 2009.
44. Kocijančič I, Vidmar K, Ivanovi-Herceg Z: Chest sonography versus lateral decubitus radiography in the diagnosis of small pleural effusions, *J Clin Ultrasound* 31(2):69–74, 2003.
45. Lichtenstein D, Goldstein I, Mourgeon E, et al.: Comparative diagnostic performances of auscultation, chest radiography, and lung ultrasonography in acute respiratory distress syndrome, *Anesthesiology* 100(1):9–15, 2004.
46. Hibbert RM, Atwell TD, Lekah A, et al.: Safety of ultrasound-guided thoracentesis in patients with abnormal preprocedural coagulation parameters, *Chest* 144(2):456–463, 2013.
47. Lichtenstein D, Mezière G, Biderman P, Gepner A: The "lung point": an ultrasound sign specific to pneumothorax, *Intensive Care Med* 26(10):1434–1440, 2000.
48. Lichtenstein DA, Mezière G, Biderman P, Gepner A: Ultrasound diagnosis of occult pneumothorax, *Crit Care Med* 33(6):1231–1238, 2005.
49. Lewiss RE, Kaban NL, Saul T: Point-of-Care Ultrasound for a Deep Venous Thrombosis, *Global Heart* 8(4):329–333, 2013.
50. Theodoro D, Blaivas M, Duggal S, et al.: Real-time B-mode ultrasound in the ED saves time in the diagnosis of deep vein thrombosis (DVT), *Am J Emerg Med* 22(3):197–200, 2004.
51. Bernardi E, Camporese G, Büller HR, et al.: Serial 2-point ultrasonography plus D-dimer vs whole-leg color-coded Doppler ultrasonography for diagnosing suspected symptomatic deep vein thrombosis, *JAMA* 300(14):1653–1659, 2008.
52. Crisp JG, Lovato LM, Jang TB: Compression ultrasonography of the lower extremity with portable vascular ultrasonography can accurately detect deep venous thrombosis in the emergency department, *Ann Emerg Med* 56(6):601–610, 2010.
53. Rozycki GS, Shackford SR: Ultrasound, what every trauma surgeon should know, *J Trauma* 40 (1):1–4, 1996.
54. AIUM Practice Guideline for the Performance of the Focused Assessment With Sonography for Trauma (FAST) Examination, *J Ultrasound Med* 33(11):2047–2056, 2014.
55. Ma OJ, Mateer JR, Ogata M, et al.: Prospective analysis of a rapid trauma ultrasound examination performed by emergency physicians, *J Trauma* 38(6):879–885, 1995.
56. Blaivas M, Lyon M, Duggal S: A prospective comparison of supine chest radiography and bedside ultrasound for the diagnosis of traumatic pneumothorax, *Acad Emerg Med* 12 (9):844–849, 2005.

Arterial Waveform and Pressure-Based Hemodynamic Monitoring

12

Jan M. Headley

Monitoring cardiac output and other important cardiovascular variables is the cornerstone of hemodynamic assessment and management of the acutely ill. With recent advances in microprocessing and signal extraction, the use of arterial waveform and pressure-based technologies for determining flow parameters—stroke volume and cardiac output—and dynamic parameters—pulse pressure variation (PPV) and stroke volume variation (SVV)—is becoming more commonplace. Newer technologies provide improved reliability and accurate and precise measurements in a less invasive, to completely noninvasive, manner. By doing so, important patient hemodynamic parameters can be obtained in care areas where invasive monitoring is limited. More hemodynamically unstable patients can now be monitored in environments where less monitoring is available or for occasions when more invasive techniques are contraindicated.[1-3]

Historical Milestones

The concept of using the arterial pulse to assess pressure and flow to measure cardiac output has an interesting history. The two major coexisting theories for evaluating the arterial system are (1) measuring arterial pressure and (2) evaluating arterial blood flow. Pressure assessment requires an understanding of the relationships between vessel resistance and compliance. Arterial blood flow assessment is based on blood flow waves traveling both forward and backward in the vascular tree. Both theories have their strengths and weaknesses. Using the arterial pulse to assess flow or stroke volume is not new; however, the concept lost favor when quantitative blood pressure measuring devices became available. As measurement became more commonplace, it became accepted as the norm. It is interesting, from a historical perspective, how the two concepts of arterial pulsation and arterial pressure measurement emerged and then became nearly exclusive of each other.[4-7]

In the sixteenth century, William Harvey was the first to describe the circulation and that arteries and veins contained nothing but blood. In addition, he described quantitative hemodynamic measures such as stroke volume, cardiac output, and ejection fraction. In the mid-eighteenth century, Stephen Hales directly measured pressure by placing a hollow tube in the arteries of animal models to measure the "force of blood," or blood pressure. In the later 1800s and early 1900s, many other researchers developed tools that measured blood pressure more accurately and, more importantly, more easily. Key milestones were as follows: Riva-Rocci refined the use of the sphygmomanometer by adding a noninvasive bladder cuff in 1896. In 1901, Cushing modernized this approach by using a sphygmomanometer to measure arterial pressure. Korotkoff reported in 1905 that by placing a stethoscope to the brachial artery distal to the Riva-Rocci cuff, specific sounds caused by the blood flowing back into the artery could be heard. This practice is considered the standard for auscultatory blood pressure measurement even today.[4–7]

Other investigators were concurrently focusing on assessment of the arterial wave. In the nineteenth and early twentieth centuries, graphical recordings of the pulse wave were used to assess various conditions by waveform shape characteristics. During this time, the available technologies were cumbersome and obtaining recordings was time consuming.[4,7]

In the 1700s, Stephen Hales not only evaluated the arterial tree with his classic studies measuring intravascular pressures but also conceptualized the vascular tree as a compliant, elastic reservoir that dynamically impacted the flow of blood. Hales visualized the vessel expanding to hold more volume during ventricular systole and recoiling during diastole, and that the forward flow of blood would be more consistent. Hales used the air chamber model of the early fire engines as an analogy to describe this phenomenon, which has since been termed the *Windkessel effect*. Otto Frank published on the Windkessel concept in 1899 and used a mathematical model to describe it. The earliest description was a two-element model, which included vessel elasticity and distensibility. These combined concepts are now commonly referred to as *arterial compliance*.[4,7–10]

Windkessel Models

The Windkessel effect describes the interaction between left ventricular (LV) stroke volume, the aorta, and the larger arterial vessels. Depending on vessel compliance and elasticity, the ability of the artery to distend with additional blood volume added from ventricular systole varies. Vessel distension decreases from recoiling during diastole, which produces a more constant pressure downstream. The net effect causes dampening or cushioning of the forward wave to ensure blood flow is near constant at the capillary level.[9,11]

Larger arterial vessels are more compliant, that is, they have more elasticity, and can accommodate increases in blood volume, whereas the more distal peripheral vessels are more resistant to forward blood flow. These two components, compliance and resistance, comprised the two-element Windkessel model. Around the 1930s, various researchers were making physiologic models of the arterial system. A third component, namely impedance to forward blood flow from the aortic valve, was integrated. Wesseling et al.[12] subsequently developed a three-Windkessel-based approach, which included aortic impedance (cZ) assessment as well as factors that affect aortic compliance and peripheral resistance. He integrated Langewouters'[13] work, which incorporated age, gender, height, and weight as factors that influence aortic and large vessel compliance. This method, commonly termed *Modelflow*, is also a technique used to determine cardiac output from the arterial pulse.[4,9,12–14]

Physiology of Arterial Pressure and Pulse Contour

In 1904, Erlanger and Hooker suggested that the pulse pressure–related to stroke volume coupled with the pulse rate could provide an index of "circulation rate," or cardiac output. Deriving stroke volume from either the arterial waveform or the arterial pressure is the basic premise of arterial pulse– or arterial pressure–based technologies for determining cardiac output. This concept is further refined by two principles: (1) aortic pulse pressure, that is, the difference between systolic blood pressure and diastolic blood pressure, is proportional to stroke volume; and (2) an inverse proportionality to pulse pressure and aortic compliance exists. Once stroke volume is determined, arterial pulsations are counted to reflect heart rate. Cardiac output (CO) is expressed as pulse rate (PR) times stroke volume (SV) depicted in the following equations.[15,16]

$$CO = PR \times SV$$
$$HR \times SV = CO$$

Erlanger also noted that the relationship of pulse pressure to stroke volume is dependent on "systolic time and elasticity of the arteries."[17] Therefore, threats to stroke volume–pulse pressure proportionality assumptions are directly related to vessel compliance and peripheral vascular resistance changes. Both aortic and larger vessel compliance are impacted by factors such as age, gender, height, and weight, and their effects are relatively slow to change.[13,18] Peripheral vasculature is affected by factors such as peripheral vascular disease and causes of vasoconstriction or vasodilatation, which alter vessel stiffness. These changes are rather rapid and subsequently impact the arterial waveform and potentially arterial pressures. These complex interactions made it difficult for rudimentary arterial pressure cardiac output models to provide accurate results. For arterial pressures to be used in a reliable and accurate manner for determining stroke volume, compensation for changes in vascular tone was required; alternatively, the systems required external calibration.[4,6,8,15,16]

Pulse Waveform Contour, Pulse Power, and Arterial Pressure

Current technologies incorporate arterial pulse waveform contour, arterial pressures, or a combination of both to determine stroke volume. Each technology uses a proprietary algorithm for determination of stroke volume, and most require an invasive arterial line. Newer technologies are completely noninvasive and use a finger pressure cuff to obtain the arterial pulse. In addition, each technology requires the following components: a means to obtain the arterial signal such as a cuff or arterial line, a means to transfer the arterial signal such as a sensor or cable, and a special monitor or bedside module.[19–21] See Table 12-1 and Figure 12-1 for a comparison of current technologies.

TABLE 12-1 Arterial Pressure and Waveform Based Technologies

METHOD CATEGORY	PRODUCT-SYSTEM/ MANUFACTURER	PARAMETERS	METHOD OF CALIBRATION/ RECALIBRATION REQUIRED	SENSOR SITE LOCATION
LESS INVASIVE: CALIBRATED				
Less-Invasive Arterial Line-Calibrated	Volume View/ EV 1000; Edwards Lifesciences	SV/SVI/CO/CI/ SVV SVR/SVRI EVLW, GEDV, GEF, PVPI	Transpulmonary Thermodilution (TPTD)	Central venous catheter / specialized thermistor in femoral arterial line See Figure 12-1, A
Less-Invasive Arterial Line-Calibrated	PiCCO; Pulsion Medical Systems	SV/SVI/CO/CI/ SVV/PPV SVR/SVRI EVLW, GEDV, CFI, ITBI	Transpulmonary thermodilution (TPTD)	Central venous catheter / specialized thermistor in femoral or radial arterial line See Figure 12-1, A
Less-Invasive Arterial Line-Calibrated	LiDCO / PulseCO; LiDCO Ltd.	SV/SVI/CO/CI/ SVV/PPV SVR/SVRI	Lithium	Any venous catheter (central or peripheral) / any arterial line with lithium sampling device See Figure 12-1, A
LESS INVASIVE: NONCALIBRATED				
Less-Invasive Arterial Line-Noncalibrated	FloTrac/ Vigileo/ EV1000; Edwards Lifesciences	SV/SVI/CO/CI/ SVV SVR/SVRI when CVP input	Arterial pressure - Waveform analysis	Arterial line See Figure 12-1, B
Less-Invasive Arterial Line-Noncalibrated	LiDCOrapid; LiDCO Ltd.	SV/SVI/CO/CI/ SVV SVR/SVRI	Pulse power	Arterial line See Figure 12-1, B
Less-Invasive Arterial Line-Noncalibrated	PulsioFlex; Pulsion Medical Systems	SV/SVI/CO/ CI/SVV/PPV SVR/SVRI	Pulse contour	Arterial line See Figure 12-1, B
Less-Invasive Arterial Line-Noncalibrated	MOSTCARE/PRAM; Vytech * Not available in the United States	SV/SVI/CO/CI/ SVV/PPV/SPV SVR/SVRI	Pulse contour	Arterial line See Figure 12-1, B
NONINVASIVE				
Noninvasive finger cuff–Calibrated	CNAP; CN Systems	SV/SVI/CO/CI/ SVV SVR/SVRI	Incorporates Modelflow algorithm	Finger cuffs See Figure 12-1, C
Noninvasive finger cuff – Auto-Calibrated	ccNexfin/ Clearsight/ EV1000; Edwards Lifesciences	SV/SVI/CO/CI/ SVV SVR/SVRI	Incorporates Modelflow algorithm	Finger cuff(s) See Figure 12-1, C

The shaded arrow represents the progression of monitoring technologies from less invasive to noninvasive.
References: 1,4,6,8,15,26,27,35,42,43,92

CFI, Cardiac function index; *CI*, cardiac index; *CO*, cardiac output; *EVLW*, extravascular lung water; *GEDV*, global end-diastolic volume; *GEF*, global ejection fraction; *ITBI*, intrathoracic blood volume index; *PPV*, pulse pressure variation; *PVPI*, pulmonary vascular permeability index; *SPV*, systolic pulse variation; *SV*, stroke volume; *SVI*, stroke volume index; *SVR*, systemic vascular resistance; *SVRI*, systemic vascular resistance index; *SVV*, stroke volume variation; *TPTD*, transpulmonary thermodilution.

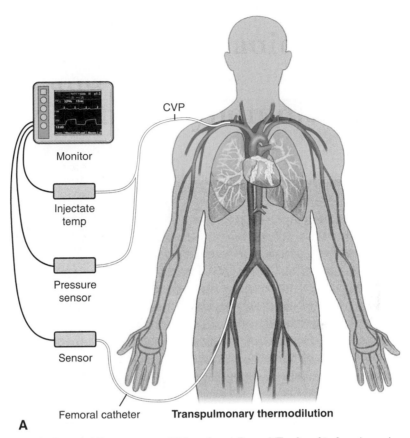

A

FIGURE 12-1 A, Arterial Pressure and Waveform Based Technologies. Less invasive transpulmonary thermodilution calibrated with normal saline: venous to arterial line: Volume View/ EV1000, Edwards Lifesciences; PiCCO, Pulsion Medical Systems.

The three basic technologies with unique attributes that use the arterial pressure or waveform for cardiac output determination are methods based on pulse contour, pulse power, and arterial pressure. All technologies are based on the simple concept that pulse pressure is proportional to stroke volume and inversely related to aortic compliance. However, each method includes different approaches to compensate for the fluctuating relationship caused by changes in vascular tone. *Arterial pulse contour analysis* is a near-generic term that describes the technique of measuring stroke volume on a beat-to-beat basis from the arterial waveform. The area under the systolic portion of the curve, from initial rise to the closure of the aortic valve, reflects the amount of blood ejected during systole and therefore stroke volume.[15,16,22] Pulse power analysis incorporates fluctuations in BP around a mean value caused by the volume of blood (stroke volume) forced into the arterial conduit by each systole. The magnitude of the change in pulse pressure is a function of the magnitude of the stroke volume and does not rely on pulse contour.[23] Aortic cross-section is

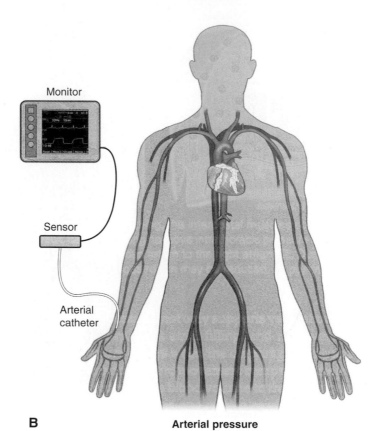

B   **Arterial pressure**

FIGURE 12-1 B, Arterial Pressure and Waveform Based Technologies. Less invasive calibrated with lithium chloride: venous to arterial line LiDCO/PulseCO, LiDCO Ltd. Less invasive non-calibrated: Arterial Pressure and Waveform analysis, FloTrac/Vigileo/EV1000, Edwards Lifesciences; Pulse power: LiDCOrapid, LiDCO Ltd; Pulse Contour: PulsioFlex, Pulsion Medical Systems; MOSTCARE/PRAM, Wytech Health.

accounted for by including equations for Langewouters' work.[6,13,22,23] Arterial pressure–based determination of cardiac output determines stroke volume by measuring the standard deviation of the full pulse wave over a given period and a robust waveform characteristic assessment. The algorithm incorporates the relationship of pressure measurements and flow by empiric formulas and compliance prediction models based on age, gender, height, and weight.[13,15,24,25] See Figure 12-2 for a comparison of various pulse-based methods.

Clinical Reasoning Pearl

Because arterial pressure–based methods incorporate the patient's age, gender, height, and weight for increased accuracy of values, it is imperative to obtain accurate weights and measure the patient's height rather than rely on estimates.

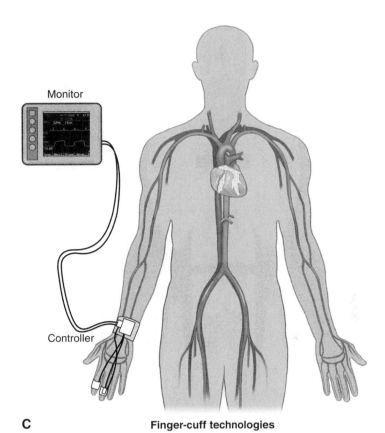

C **Finger-cuff technologies**

FIGURE 12-1 C, Arterial Pressure and Waveform Based Technologies. Noninvasive Finger cuff(s): CNAP, CN Systems; ccNexfin/Clearsight/EV1000, Edwards Lifesciences.

Physiologic Factors That Impact Measurement

The arterial waveform consists of two major components: (1) the forward flow wave, or incident wave, from the aorta and (2) the backward wave, or reflective wave, from the periphery. Waveform characteristics change from the aortic root to the more distal arterial branches. With increased age and decreased vascular tone, reflective waves may occur near the down-slope of the systolic wave and obscure the dicrotic notch. Therefore, when using a pulse contour analysis model to determine stroke volume, assumptions as to the location of actual aortic valve closure need to be considered on the basis of the location of the measured pulse wave. Various systems using this method attempt to account for waveform shape and vascular tone changes by including a correction factor into the algorithm.[15,16,26,27] See Figure 12-3 for the impact of reflective waves on dicrotic notch identification and Figure 12-4 for a description of the components of the arterial pulse arterial wave.

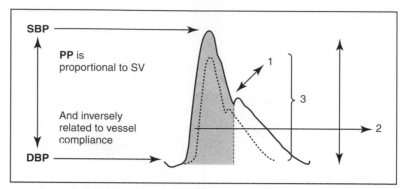

FIGURE 12-2 Various Arterial Pressure—Pulse Wave Technologies. All technologies are based on basic premise that pulse pressure is proportional to stroke volume and inversely related to aortic or large vessel compliance. Further stroke volume refinement is accomplished by various proprietary algorithms. The pulse amplitude reflects the heart rate, therefore, SV × HR = CO. 1: Pulse contour, requires identifying the dicrotic notch, considers upstroke to notch the systolic area (*shaded area*), and requires external calibration. 2: Pulse power, based on mean value to extrapolate the SV and not the waveform morphology, and requires external calibration. 3: Pulse pressure or flow, incorporates full wave in a mathematical standard deviation formula (*dotted lines*), is not dependent on dicrotic notch identification, and does not require external calibration. *CO,* Cardiac output; *DBP,* diastolic blood pressure; *PP,* pulse pressure; *SBP,* systolic blood pressure; *SV,* stroke volume.

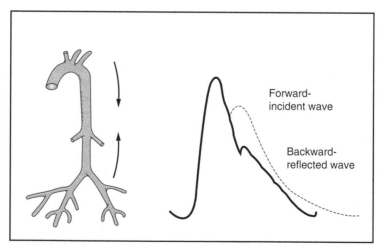

FIGURE 12-3 Impact of Reflective Wave on Dicrotic Notch Location. The arterial wave comprises a forward incident wave and a backward reflective wave. The solid line represents a normal arterial waveform. The dotted line reflects the potential impact of a reflective wave on identification of the dicrotic notch. Use of pulse contour in this situation makes the isolation of end of systole (closure of aortic valve as denoted by dicrotic notch) difficult.

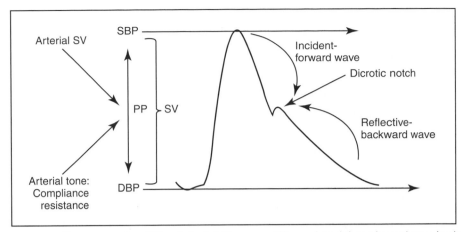

FIGURE 12-4 Components of the Arterial Pressure Wave. Arterial stroke volume is the forward blood volume from LV systole. This volume contributes to the systolic pressure in the arterial pulse. Arterial tone comprises larger vessel compliance and smaller vessel resistance. This component impacts the diastolic pressure more and adds to the PP. The difference between SBP and DBP is the PP. PP is best measured from the DBP to the next SBP. PP is proportional to SV. The actual arterial waveform contains the incident or forward wave and the reflective or backward wave from the periphery. Depending on the vessel compliance or resistance, the reflective wave can encroach anywhere on the arterial wave. In older adult patients with noncompliant vessels, the reflective wave may occur during systole and obscure the dicrotic notch or even the peak systolic portion of the waveform. *DBP*, Diastolic blood pressure; *LV*, left ventricle; *PP*, pulse pressure; *SBP*, systolic blood pressure; *SV*, stroke volume.

The pulse pressure analysis theory is not reliant on the contour of the pulse. This technology depends on obtaining an accurate value of the mean arterial pressure (MAP). A challenge to this concept is that since compliance and resistance are neither equal nor static, the pressure relationship changes. Use of a radial arterial line rather than a femoral site has been recommended, as reflective waves cause alterations in the pressures measured, altering MAP and subsequent stroke volume, cardiac output, and the cardiac index values, necessitating external calibration. However, after the initial calibration, the pulse pressure analysis method is used to determine the beat-to-beat stroke volume rather than a pulse contour approach.[6,23,26]

The arterial pressure–based determination of cardiac output technology includes factors such as age, gender, height, and weight that affect large vessel compliance. In addition, vascular tone changes the full waveform with a multi-modal algorithmic assessment of pressures and waveform characteristics. These are incorporated to compensate for these changes, so external calibration is not required.[25] In some situations, the normal relationship between central to peripheral pressures is reversed; instead of central pressures being lower than the periphery, they are higher. This may occur in extreme conditions of hyperdynamic and vasodilatory states such as severe sepsis, coming off cardiopulmonary bypass, and liver transplantation.[28–32] Earlier-generation algorithms could not compensate for this phenomenon. Newer algorithms have been shown to improve the accuracy and precision for stroke volume and cardiac output.[32–34]

Technologies That Require External Calibration

Current technologies that require external calibration use some form of an indicator dilution method. One system (LiDCO) uses lithium as the indicator, and two other systems (Edwards, Pulsion) use a large bolus of cold solution for transpulmonary thermodilution cardiac output determination. Once calibration is performed, the stroke volume and cardiac output values are updated by applying their respective pulse pressure analysis, pulse contour analysis, or arterial pressure–based determination of cardiac output algorithms.[35–37]

Required recalibration times vary according to manufacturer; some research has reported the need to recalibrate after any significant change in vascular tone, preload, afterload, and contractility or after administering vasoactive agents. Recalibration frequency has been reported from 1 to 24 hours.[35,38–41]

Technologies That Do Not Require External Calibration

Besides Edwards' EV1000/FloTrac arterial pressure–based determination of cardiac output system, LiDCO and Pulsion have released versions of their systems that do not require external calibration. Both have incorporated into their uncalibrated system a means to include patient characteristics, using a nomogram, to obtain an initial nominal stroke volume and cardiac output or cardiac index value. To increase accuracy, an external method of obtaining cardiac output is still recommended. Published data on each system vary, but overall trending for each shows promising results. The key to validating the various technologies is familiarity with the version of the algorithm being compared against the type of technology that is used as the reference.[1,19–21,26]

From the Arterial Line to Noninvasive Finger Cuff

Continuous noninvasive arterial blood pressure monitoring has been available for many years. Two devices with similar technology are commercially available. Each uses a finger cuff with infrared photoplethysmography to determine vessel size and volume of blood, and a pressure source that applies an intermittent "counterpressure" to obtain the patient's blood pressure. Depending on the technology used, a proprietary algorithm is incorporated to determine stroke volume and cardiac output or cardiac index as well as the dynamic parameters of PPV, SVV, or both. Both systems use a dedicated monitor to display the values.[21,35,42,43]

Technologies vary as to how they specifically adjust for the differences from the finger pressure to the brachial pressure, which is considered the clinical gold standard site to obtain blood pressure noninvasively. Continuous Noninvasive Arterial Pressure (CNAP) technology (http://www.cnsystems.at/cnsystems) is based on oscillometric principles and uses an algorithmic approach to eliminate the effects of rapid vascular tone changes. An initial brachial cuff pressure is required to calibrate the system, as the pressures in the finger are different from those in the brachial artery. In addition, a further mathematic analysis using a Modelflow approach is implemented to provide for estimation of cardiac output. The CNAP device uses repeated upper arm brachial cuff pressure measurements to compensate for effects of hydrostatic pressure changes.[21,42,44]

> ### Clinical Reasoning Pearl
>
> If employing a technology that requires calibration with a blood pressure cuff, ensure that the cuff is of appropriate size and placed in the correct location as it is used to obtain accurate calibration values.

After obtaining the pulse wave from the finger cuff, the ccNexfin device (www.edwards.com) transforms the finger waveform into a brachial blood pressure waveform. Cardiac output is then calculated from the systolic area under the brachial waveform, which is coupled with a three-element Windkessel model similar to Modelflow. Major vessel compliance is accounted for by including age–gender–height–weight data according to the Langewouters equations. To accommodate for peripheral vascular resistance changes, the monitor uses an autocalibration algorithm; therefore, no external calibration is required. In addition, a zeroing reference device is used to automatically correct for hydrostatic pressure changes.[21,35,43,45]

Being completely noninvasive, the new technologies have advantages in selected patient populations when more invasive monitoring is either not available or patient conditions preclude their use. Monitoring in a pre-emptive hemodynamic optimization strategy improves postoperative outcomes. However, since a certain level of monitoring is required, the noninvasive technologies fulfill that unmet need.[46,47] See Table 12-2 for technology development milestones.

Limitations

All of the technologies discussed above are dependent on obtaining either accurate arterial pressure or waveforms for optimal results. Accordingly, leveling of the sensor or air–fluid interface to the phlebostatic axis is required. Overdampened waveforms produce artificially low pressure measurements, which may lead to erroneously low values for stroke volume or cardiac output. Underdamped waveforms may lead to erroneously high pressure values, which may result in abnormally high values for stroke volume or cardiac output.[6,15,16,22] Because of the cyclic inflation of the finger cuff for the noninvasive technologies, use of the cuff for more than 8 hours is not recommended. In addition, conditions such as severe hypoperfusion, Reynaud syndrome, vasoconstriction, and edematous fingers may hamper signal acquisition.[43,45,48]

TABLE 12-2 Technology Development Milestones

DATE	AUTHOR	DEVELOPMENT
1899	Otto Frank	Developed Windkessel effect mathematical two-element model
1904	Erlanger and Hooker	Suggested stroke volume is proportional to pulse pressure
1948	Remington	Aortic compliance relationship evaluated in an animal model
1967	Penaz	Volume clamp invented to continuously measure pressure noninvasively
1970	Kouchoukos	Developed aortic systolic area–based pulse contour concepts
1974	Wesseling	Proposed cZ method; used a constant impedance (Z) to calculate stroke volume from pulsatile systolic area
1984	Langewouters	Measured thoracic and abdominal aortic compliance values in human cadavers
1993	Wesseling and Jansen	Developed Modelflow three-element Windkessel model for systolic area pulse contour and correction factors
1996	Band	Vascular compliance changes waveform correction incorporated in a "net" power algorithm approach
2005	Roteliuk and Hatib	Multi-modal signal processing algorithm for noncalibrated arterial pressure cardiac output technique
2005	Bogert and Van Lieshout	Noninvasive technology that incorporates three-element Windkessel model into an algorithm and reconstructs brachial waveform as substitute for aortic pressure

References: 4, 6, 7, 9, 12–14, 21–23, 25, and 42–44.

Arterial pressure–based technologies should be used with caution in patients with conditions that produce wide pulse pressures (e.g., severe aortic regurgitation) or conditions or interventions that produce abnormal arterial waveforms (e.g., intra-aortic balloon pumping or pulsus bisferiens).[1] Atrial fibrillation or other highly erratic cardiac rhythms while measuring stroke volume may produce varied values. Any condition that leads to a rapid and drastic change in vascular tone (e.g., severe sepsis, rapid bolus infusion, vasoconstrictors such as phenylephrine, or coming off cardiopulmonary bypass) may result in less reliable and reproducible values for cardiac output.[19,21,35,42,49,50] Caveats exist for all technologies; however, once understood, the values can be critically evaluated.[1,15]

Heart–Lung Interactions Affecting Arterial Pressures

Cardiac output and stroke volume assessment has historically been the mainstay for the determination of cardiac performance. Although both parameters are good indicators of blood flow, they are not good indicators for assessing if the patient will respond to fluid or not. Early work by Kussmaul in the late 1800s described pulsus paradoxus as an exaggeration of a normally occurring phenomenon; with spontaneous breathing during inspiration, systolic pressure decreases. Pulsus paradoxus occurs when the pressure decline becomes greater than 10 millimeters of mercury (mm Hg). The use of dynamic parameters for assessing the patient's volume status is based on heart–lung interactions caused by altered filling of the ventricles during the different phases of the respiratory cycle.[50-52]

Variations in stroke volume during the respiratory cycle are a normal phenomenon. During spontaneous breathing, the inspiratory phase causes a decreased (more negative) intrathoracic pressure thereby allowing more venous return to the right side of the heart. At the same time, the negative pressure effect is to allow more sequestering of blood volume in the pulmonary vasculature, which results in less returning to the left side of the heart, producing a smaller LV stroke volume and decrease in systolic blood pressure. This effect takes about three to five heartbeats to become apparent. On exhalation, the intrathoracic pressure is higher, and filling of the right ventricle from venous return is reduced. The sequestered blood volume in the pulmonary vascular bed is "squeezed" into the left side of the heart to augment LV filling. This increases LV pressure and stroke volume, and subsequently, systolic blood pressure increases after a few heartbeats in exhalation.[2,50,53-55]

On controlled positive pressure mechanical ventilation, the sequelae of the heart–lung interaction is reversed. The higher intrathoracic pressure during inspiration narrows the pressure gradient to fill the right ventricle. The volume of blood being held in the pulmonary vascular bed from the previous breath is now diverted to the left side of the heart, thereby increasing the systolic blood pressure. On exhalation, the opposite occurs, as the intrathoracic pressure is now lower. Venous return increases to fill the right side of the heart, and during expiration, blood volume is being held in the pulmonary vascular tree, causing a decrease in LV filling and subsequently lowering systolic blood pressure.[2,50,53-55] Figure 12-5 shows a comparison of spontaneous versus controlled ventilation.

The full respiratory cycle, whether on mechanical ventilation or spontaneous breathing, produces a normal variation in systolic blood pressure from inspiration to exhalation of about 5 to 10 mm Hg. When the difference is greater than 10 mm Hg, the phenomenon is called *pulsus paradoxus* or with controlled mechanical ventilation, termed *reverse pulsus paradoxus*. This exaggeration occurs when conditions of hypovolemia, conditions that restrict right ventricular (RV) filling (e.g., cardiac tamponade, restrictive pericardial disease), conditions of altered ventricular interdependence (e.g., RV and or LV failure), and conditions of severe respiratory restrictive diseases (e.g., acute asthma) exist.[2,19,50,53-56]

Clinical Reasoning Pearl

When arterial pressure waveform tracings are being observed on a bedside monitor, the term *respiratory swing* may be used to describe the variation in pressures noted. This is a somewhat subjective means to assess for pulsus paradoxus.

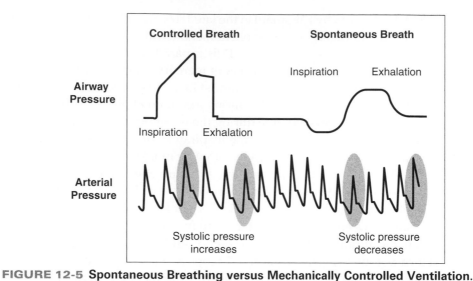

FIGURE 12-5 Spontaneous Breathing versus Mechanically Controlled Ventilation.
Changes in systolic blood pressure occur during the respiratory cycle. With a spontaneous breath, the systolic pressure will decrease after a few heartbeats during inspiration and the systolic pressure will increase during exhalation. With controlled breathing, the opposite occurs, during inspiration the systolic pressure increases and decreases during exhalation. The circled arterial waveforms identify the minimum and maximum values during a respiratory cycle. It is from the maximum and minimum values that the systolic pressure variation or pulse pressure variation is determined.

Dynamic Parameters to Assess Fluid Responsiveness

Fluid is often the first intervention for optimizing blood flow in the acutely ill patient. Typically, 50% of the patients who are given a fluid challenge respond with an increase in their stroke volume and cardiac output or cardiac index. Fluid or preload responsiveness is defined as an increase in stroke volume and cardiac output or cardiac index by 10% to 15% after a fluid challenge. Static or pressure-based indices such as right atrial pressure (central venous pressure [CVP]), pulmonary artery diastolic (PAD) pressure, or pulmonary artery occlusion pressure (PAOP) are used to evaluate the patient's volume status, with varying results. Volumetric parameters obtained either by a special pulmonary artery catheter (PAC) or by echocardiography are more useful than pressure-based parameters for preload assessment; however, these values are not sensitive predictors of preload responsiveness.[56–59] Dynamic parameters, or parameters termed *functional hemodynamic parameters*, can predict a positive increase in stroke volume and cardiac output or cardiac index to fluid (Table 12-3). They include SVV and its surrogates, PPV, and SPV and are more sensitive and specific compared with static parameters for predicting a response to fluid.[15,56,60–62] All dynamic parameters are calculated as either an absolute difference (in mm Hg) between the maximum and minimum SBP during a respiratory cycle or a ratio of the difference between the maximum

TABLE 12-3 Dynamic Parameters: Definitions, Normal Ranges, Responsive Indicator Range, Advantages, and Disadvantages

PARAMETER AND DEFINITION	NORMAL RANGE	FLUID RESPONSIVE RANGE	ADVANTAGE	DISADVANTAGE
Systolic pressure variation (SPV) Maximum–minimum systolic pressure over a respiratory cycle	<10 mm Hg	>10 mm Hg	Easy to calculate Can be assessed noninvasively with blood pressure cuff	Diastolic blood pressure can affect value Changes in pleural pressure can affect value On bedside monitor scaling may decrease visibility of "swing"
Delta Up (Δ Up) Systolic blood pressure increase at end-expiration compared to baseline Delta Down (Δ Down) Systolic blood pressure decrease at end-expiration from baseline	2–4 mm Hg	>5 mm Hg	Available on some bedside physiologic monitors Values combined affect SPV	Dependent on determining baseline value. Unable to continuously obtain value Accuracy requires end-expiratory pause Δ Up reflects intrathoracic pressure changes and is not a reliable marker of fluid responsiveness
Pulse pressure variation (PPV) Maximum PP – Minimum PP / Mean PP over a respiratory cycle (may be up to 32 sec when averaged on bedside monitor)	<13%–15%	>13%–15%	Available on some bedside physiologic monitors More precise than SPV or Δ Down	Difficult to obtain value related to respiratory phase
Stroke volume variation (SVV) Maximum SV – Minimum SV / Mean SV over a 20- to 30-sec period	<10%–15%	>10%–15%	More precise than SPV Measured by specific devices Proprietary algorithm provides increased accuracy with multiple ectopics	Cutoff values vary with different conditions (see text)

>, Greater than; <, less than.
References: 1, 6, 8, 15, 20, 22, 23, 26, 35, 55, and 92.

and minimum pulse pressure or stroke volume over approximately 20 seconds.[15,20,50,57]

Currently, focus on applying functional hemodynamic monitoring strategies in the acute care setting is increasing. The notion includes determining the effect a physiologic stressor has on the system or the value being monitored. An example of functional hemodynamic monitoring is using a fluid challenge as the stressor on stroke volume. The clinical importance of assessing the relationship between these two variables is to determine where the patient is on his or her individual Frank-Starling curve and to predict whether fluid therapy will produce a positive result or not.[19,36,50,54,62,63] Just as under-resuscitating a patient has detrimental effects, so does administering an excess amount of fluid.[2,56,57,62,63]

Dynamic parameters can be used to optimize the patient's Starling curve. The greater the variations in stroke volume, the greater is the patient's response to fluid, putting the data point for that patient on the steep portion of the Starling curve. The less the variation in stroke volume, the less responsive the patient is to fluid, putting the patient's data point near or on the plateau portion of the curve. Values greater than 10% to 15% have a high level of sensitivity and specificity for the need for fluid. However, a specific predetermined target value may not be optimal for the patient's condition. Implementing a "gray zone" approach is considered more clinically relevant. This approach determines the maximum value, wherein the likelihood of a positive response to fluid is identified, as well as the lowest value where the likelihood of a non-response to fluid lies. The area or values in-between is called the "gray zone," and further patient assessment and determination of cardiac performance is suggested. By assessing the dynamic parameter and the associated stroke volume, a fluid management strategy for optimizing (or maximizing) cardiac performance can be implemented.[1,2,19,36,62–64] See Figure 12-6 for a Starling curve showing stroke volume dynamic parameters and the physiologic challenge effect.

Dynamic Parameters: Caveats and Potential Limitations

Elevated dynamic parameters do not always reflect the need to administer volume, as neither decreased nor normal values indicate volume adequacy. The efficacy of the predictability of dynamic parameters relies not only on the preload status but also on the contractile state of the heart. In addition, patient assessment, baseline condition, and potential limitations affecting the accuracy of the value need to be considered.[50,57,63–65]

A significant change in intrathoracic pressure is required to result in a measurable heart–lung interaction to determine responsiveness. Caution with using dynamic parameters as indicators of fluid responsiveness relates to factors that affect intrathoracic pressure changes, for example, lower tidal volumes, high positive end-expiratory pressure (PEEP), and decreased lung compliance. The small variation in intrathoracic pressure may not be sufficient to cause a significant change in stroke volume, even in light of the patient being preload responsive. The cutoff values for responders are often higher. Also, factors that alter respiratory rates and inspiration-to-expiration (I:E) ratios impact the responsiveness accuracy such as high-frequency ventilation. A low

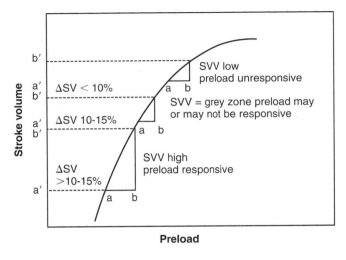

a – b = Physiologic challenge:
passive leg raise, fluid challenge

a′ – b′ = Response to challenge

FIGURE 12-6 **Starling curve.**

respiratory rate to heart rate ratio occurs when the respiratory rate is too fast to allow for cardiac cyclic changes in stroke volume. Most reports in the literature support the use of dynamic indices in patients who are on controlled mechanical ventilation, with a tidal volume greater than 6 to 8 milliliters per kilogram (mL/kg; some report up to 10 mL/kg), PEEP no greater than 10 centimeters of water (cm H_2O), and with fixed respiratory rates.[53,56,57,63,65] However, some reports show favorable results in spontaneously breathing patients or those on lower tidal volume ventilation, and support the use of synchronized intermittent mandatory ventilation (SIMV) modes.[8,62,66–73]

Factors that affect ventricular filling time such as HR and arrhythmias may impact dynamic parameters. Erratic arrhythmias produce erratic filling of the ventricles and therefore altered stroke volume and elevated SVV. The value then becomes nonspecific for predicting fluid responsiveness. One system, Edwards EV1000 FloTrac, has incorporated a newer algorithm that allows for a specific number of ectopics, or irregular beats per computation cycle (6 beats per one 20-second cycle). The newer version has a better sensitivity and specificity compared with the algorithm without this feature. In addition, the monitor alerts the clinicians when the rhythm is outside the filtering range and the value should be used with caution.[74] It is important to note, however, that even if the dynamic parameter of the system might be suspect, the stroke volume and cardiac output or cardiac index measurement remains valid.

An altered normal intrathoracic and juxtacardiac pressure relationship may also impact dynamic parameters. With increased intra-abdominal pressure, a higher cutoff value is noted for fluid responsiveness.[75–77] During open-chest surgery, changes in stroke volume produced by the heart–lung variation lose their predictive value.

The degree to which this occurs may depend on the type of surgery—if the pericardium is open or closed.[78,79] Also, certain patient positions such as the prone position alter the normal heart–lung relationships via abdominal and chest wall compression. These effects tend to induce a higher cutoff value for dynamic parameters.[80,81]

RV failure, LV failure, pulmonary hypertension, and cor pulmonale are conditions in which false-positive dynamic parameters may be misleading. The values are elevated, but the response to a fluid challenge does not improve stroke volume. The main reason is that the right ventricle has failed and is unable to deliver more volume to the left. Interestingly, conditions with elevated dynamic parameters unresponsive to volume alerts the clinicians to assess further for RV failure or acute cor pulmonale, especially in patients with acute respiratory distress syndrome (ARDS).[82–84]

Understanding the caveats with any technology or parameter in light of the patient's condition and underlying physiology can still make it a valuable tool in the clinician's hands. Specific strategies to determine if the patient will respond to fluid include incorporating another functional physiologic challenge in the care plan and then observe the change in stroke volume and cardiac output or cardiac index for a greater than 10% to 15% increase to determine responsiveness.[2,19,36,50,64,85] See Table 12-4 for dynamic parameters cautions and potential interventions.

Clinical Reasoning Pearl

Parameters should not be used in isolation but rather in conjunction with other variables and patient assessment.

Functional Physiologic Challenges

"Mini-Fluid" Boluses: When dynamic parameters are questioned, physiologic challenges can be performed to stress the system. The easiest way to challenge the system is to administer fluid and then observe the resulting stroke volume and cardiac output or cardiac index. A potential problem with this strategy is that if large bolus amounts such as 500 mL are used and administered frequently, the patient may develop fluid overload, and the result of fluid administration cannot be easily reversed. The use of a smaller "mini-challenge" of 50 to 100 mL administered over 5 to 10 minutes has been found to be specific for fluid responsiveness. By rapidly reassessing the patient after the small amount of fluid, potential overload is limited.[62]

Passive Leg Raise Maneuver: Another simple physiologic stressor is to perform a passive leg raise maneuver. Elevating the patient's legs 30 to 45 degrees in a passive manner diverts the blood volume from the lower extremities upward to the heart (see Figure 3-11 in Chapter 3). The amount of blood returning has been estimated to be between 150 and 500 mL, depending on leg raise technique and patient condition. A positive response to passive leg raise is an increase in stroke volume and cardiac output or cardiac index from baseline by 10% to 15%. Additionally, a decrease in the dynamic parameter may be noted. More importantly, passive leg raise can be used in patients with arrhythmias, in those who are spontaneously breathing or are on lower tidal volume ventilation, and when the dynamic parameter value is in question.

TABLE 12-4 Dynamic Parameters Cautions and Potential Interventions

POTENTIAL LIMITATION	TYPE OF ERROR/ VALUES SEEN	POTENTIAL ALTERNATIVE ACTIONS*
Spontaneous breathing	False positive/Elevated	Observe value during quiet, regular breathing. Perform physiologic challenge. Observe effect on stroke volume or the cardiac index.
Varied respiratory efforts	False positive/Elevated and/or false negative/ Lower	Observe values when breathing is quiet and regular. Perform physiologic challenge. Observe effect on stroke volume or cardiac index.
Tidal volume (Vt) <8–10 milliliters per kilogram (mL/kg)	False negative/Lower	Lower cutoff values for responders. Increase Vt for approximately a minute if patient can tolerate to assess parameters. Perform physiologic challenge. Observe effect on stroke volume or cardiac index.
Increased levels of positive end-expiratory pressure (PEEP)	False positive/Elevated	May have a higher cutoff value for fluid responsiveness. If patient can tolerate, lower PEEP for approximately 1 minute. Perform physiologic challenge. Observe effect on stroke volume or cardiac index.
Inverted inspiration-to-expiration (I:E) ratios	False positive/Elevated	May have a higher cutoff value for fluid responsiveness. If patient can tolerate, reverse I:E ratio for approximately 1 minute. Perform physiologic challenge. Observe effect on stroke volume or cardiac index.
Decreased chest wall compliance	False positive/Elevated	May occur with severe burns or chest wall edema, restrictive bandages, or morbid obesity. Attempt to correct underlying cause. Perform physiologic challenge. Observe effect on stroke volume or cardiac index.
Decreased lung compliance	False positive/Elevated	Dynamic parameters less accurate if lung compliance <30 milliliters per centimeters of water (mL/cm H_2O). Attempt to correct underlying cause. Perform physiologic challenge. Observe effect on stroke volume or cardiac index.
Cardiac arrhythmias	False positive/Elevated	Some monitors provide an alert (yellow heart icon) when SVV values should be questioned. Stroke volume and CO values are reflective of patient's condition. Perform physiologic challenge. Observe effect on stroke volume or cardiac index.

Continued

TABLE 12-4   Dynamic Parameters Cautions and Potential Interventions—cont'd

POTENTIAL LIMITATION	TYPE OF ERROR/VALUES SEEN	POTENTIAL ALTERNATIVE ACTIONS
Atrial fibrillation	False positive/Elevated	Some monitors provide an alert (yellow heart icon) when SVV values should be questioned. Stroke volume and cardiac output values remain valid and reflective of patient's condition. Perform a physiologic challenge or administer a small fluid challenge to verify fluid responsiveness. Observe effect on stroke volume or cardiac index.
Heart rate/Respiratory rate ratio <3.6	False negative/Lower	May have a lower cutoff value for fluid responsiveness. Perform physiologic challenge. Observe effect on stroke volume or cardiac index.
Respiratory rates <8 or >30	False negative/Lower	May have a lower cutoff value for fluid responsiveness. Perform physiologic challenge. Observe effect on stroke volume or cardiac index.
Open chest/Sternotomy	False negative/Lower	May have a lower cutoff value for fluid responsiveness. Perform physiologic challenge. Observe effect on stroke volume or cardiac index.
Increased intra-abdominal pressure	False positive/Elevated	May have a higher cutoff value for fluid responsiveness. Perform physiologic challenge. Observe effect on stroke volume or cardiac index.
Right ventricular failure (cor pulmonale)	False positive/Elevated	If SVV is high and stroke volume does not increase after administering fluid, suspect RV failure. Administering fluid may be detrimental to patient.
Pharmacologically induced vasodilatation	False positive/Elevated	Effectively a relative hypovolemia. Consider patient condition as to need for fluid.
Prone positioning	False positive/Elevated	Prone positioning increases dynamic values. Maintains ability to predict fluid responsiveness with a higher cutoff value.

*Delta stroke volume (SV) or delta cardiac output (CO) or cardiac index (CI) can be used to determine if the patient responded favorably to fluid. Typically an increase in SV, CO, or CI of 10% to 15% is considered a positive response. Maneuvers such as performing a passive leg raise can be implemented to determine if the patient is responsive or not. Alternatively, small fluid challenges may be tried.
References: 36, 50, 55–57, 62, 64–88, and 90.

Simply lowering the legs can also quickly reverse the effect of passive leg raise. Passive leg raise is a safe maneuver if the patient's physical condition can tolerate it, and this is true even when increasing the blood volume may be harmful, as in ARDS.[50,56,62,66,86,87]

Ventilator Manipulations: Ventilator maneuvers have also been proposed as means to providing a physiologic challenge to assess for responsiveness to fluid. A significant change in pleural pressure is needed to determine if this impacts the resultant stroke volume. Techniques suggested, with varied results, are placing a patient on an end-expiratory hold via the ventilator for a few seconds to evoke an increase in venous return and determine responsiveness to fluid.[66] Another suggestion, if the patient is on low tidal volume ventilation, is to increase the tidal volume to 8 mL/kg or greater for approximately 1 minute if the patient's condition does not prevent this.[88] For accurate assessment of the patient's response, a device that can rapidly measure the response is required.[2,87,89]

Performing a Valsalva maneuver is another strategy for assessing for responsiveness to fluid in the awake, spontaneously breathing, and cooperative patient. A physiologic challenge occurs when an inspiratory effort is made against a closed glottis, resulting in changes in intrathoracic pressure. A 20-second maneuver reliably predicts fluid responsiveness as measured with dynamic parameters in spontaneously breathing patients.[89]

The lack of precision in using a dynamic parameter because of potential limitations does not preclude the use of delta stroke volume and cardiac output or cardiac index to assess the patients' response to volume therapy. In certain conditions that render the dynamic parameters unusable or untrustworthy, stroke volume and cardiac output or cardiac index can be used. If the stroke volume and cardiac output or cardiac index values are unusable or cannot be depended on, dynamic parameters can be used. The most advantageous practice is to use both together to determine the optimal individual Starling curve position.[36,56,57,90] See Box 12-1 for determining true positives with elevated SVV.

BOX 12-1 Determining a True Positive with Elevated Stroke Volume Variation

- Elevated dynamics parameters signify need for fluid.
- Question an elevated stroke volume variation (SVV) % value.
- Assess the baseline stroke volume.
- Verify fluid responsiveness by:
  - Performing a passive leg raise or other physiologic challenge.
  - Administering a "mini-fluid challenge" 50 to 100 milliliters (mL) over 5 to 10 minutes.
  - Inducing a ventilator challenge, if patient can tolerate.

- Reassess stroke volume if greater than 10% to 15% increase = fluid responsive = true positive.
- If no change in stroke volume or less than 10% = not fluid responsive = false positive.
- If false positive, assess patient for signs of right ventricular failure, increased intra-abdominal pressure, or assess ventilatory status (e.g., respiratory rate, chest compliance, tidal volume).

Clinical Utility

Incorporating dynamic parameters into an algorithm for guiding fluid therapy as a means to optimize volume status has been shown to improve patients' outcomes. With the adoption of less invasive and noninvasive technologies, and the incorporation of a solid therapeutic algorithm, interventions may be made more rapidly, which may improve overall outcomes.[2,3,50,91] See Chapter 3 and Chapter 14 for a discussion on the use of dynamic parameters in an evidence-based approach to care.

Clinical Procedure and Technical Considerations

Arterial pulse cardiac output technologies are dependent on obtaining an accurate signal from either the arterial line or the finger cuff. See Chapter 3 for a discussion on arterial line considerations and Table 3-4 for troubleshooting tips. In addition to all of the techniques required for optimal arterial line placement and pressure monitoring, specific considerations relate to the proper input of patient-specific characteristics, if required, into the monitor for accurate values. These may include age, gender, height, and weight. Leveling or placing the zero reference devices at the heart or phlebostatic axis is paramount for optimal readings. Always be sure to check the manufacturer's operations manuals and instructions for use for full operation guidelines and specific cautions related to the individual device.[92]

Caring for the patient by using these technologies is also similar to caring for a patient with an invasive arterial line. Line patency must be maintained for accurate values and patient safety. Aseptic technique is used to eliminate or decrease the opportunity for line infection.[92]

For noninvasive cuff technology, it is important to evaluate the patient's finger where the cuff is applied to assess for decreased perfusion to the finger. It is not uncommon to see a bluish tint related to venous stasis. However, if a question of compromised perfusion to the digit arises, the device has to be cycled down. It is recommended to cycle down the device or change to another finger at least every 8 hours or sooner if perfusion is in doubt and if another digit that the cuff fits appropriately can be used.[48,93]

Troubleshooting techniques are similar to all invasive and noninvasive monitoring devices. Specific actions include ensuring that the input signal from the arterial line is free of artifact and is properly damped, not underdamped or overdampened. With the arterial line–based methods, the flush system must be free of air bubbles. Performing a square wave test helps confirm optimal damping and provides determination of potential cause of altered signals. The zero reference port needs to be level with the heart or the phlebostatic axis. For the noninvasive method, the heart reference system should be zeroed at the level of the finger prior to instituting monitoring.[48,92]

Patient Care Considerations

As with all forms of hemodynamic or patient monitoring, an evaluation consisting of physical assessment, general vital signs, and obtaining current and past histories, as well as advanced hemodynamics parameters, provides the clinician with a sound baseline for assessing any change in the patient's condition. Absolute changes in values are important, as are trends. It is important to evaluate the parameters obtained in context of the whole picture rather than in isolation.[50] What may be a normal value for one patient may not be for another. Assessing the overall balance between oxygen delivery and oxygen demand is paramount.[8]

Monitoring, no matter how accurate, does not improve outcomes unless coupled with a therapy that has been proven to improve outcomes.[8] Incorporating functional hemodynamics in a therapeutic approach has been proven to improve outcomes. Targets include administering fluid if the dynamic parameters are elevated and if the resultant change in stroke volume and cardiac output or cardiac index is more than a 10% to 15% increase (delta stroke volume). The combined parameters identify where the patient is on his or her individual Starling curve and help determine if the patient is hypovolemic, euvolemic, or hypervolemic. Improved outcomes with the incorporation of this strategy in the perioperative patient has been well established by research; however, it needs to be further explored in other populations.[2,3,8,50,64,91]

Conclusion

Adding flow-based and dynamic parameters to patient assessment strategies, coupled with a proven therapeutic approach, provides an opportunity to improve both patient and economic outcomes. The advent of less to noninvasive tools to monitor these variables expands the care areas in which these strategies can be applied. As more experience with the various new technologies is gained and algorithm improvements continue, newer applications will continue to be increasingly used.

Case Study: Applying Dynamic Parameters

Mr. S, a 64-year-old male, height 72 inches, weight 79 kg, BSA 2.01 postoperative on-pump coronary artery bypass graft to right coronary artery (RCA), left anterior descending (LAD) artery, and Circumflex artery, was admitted to the cardiac surgical critical care unit. He was intubated and on controlled ventilation: tidal volume (Vt) 8 mL/kg; fraction of inspired oxygen (FiO_2) 0.30; temperature 36.8°C. ∎

Continued

Case Study:
Applying Dynamic Parameters—cont'd

TIMES	16:05	16:10	16:15	16:20	16:25	16:30	16:35	16:40	16:45
Stroke volume mL/beat	30	38	48	68	40	37	44	49	67
Stroke volume variation (SVV) %	30	24	18	10	29	35	38	18	11
Cardiac index (CI) mL/min/m^2	1.7	2.0	2.2	2.6	2.0	2.0	2.2	2.1	2.5
Central venous pressure (CVP) mm Hg	6	6	7	6	5	5	6	6	7
Heart rate, beats per minute	113	105	91	76	100	108	100	85	75
Systolic/Diastolic Mean arterial pressure (MAP) mm Hg	98/62 73	102/64 77	112/66 81	118/68 85	104/66 78	100/64 76	110/68 82	118/68 84	122/70 87
Heart rhythm	Sinus tachycardia (S Tach)	S Tach	Sinus rhythm (NSR)	NSR	Atrial fibrillation (Afib)	Afib	Afib	NSR	NSR
Interventions	250 mL crystalloid	250 mL crystalloid	250 mL colloid	_____	_____	Passive leg raise (PLR)	250 mL colloid	_____	_____

TIMES COMMENTS

16:05 — Arrival into unit. Patient was warmed. Heart rhythm sinus tachycardia with rate of 113. Blood pressure within acceptable range with SBP 98, DBP 62 and mean arterial pressure (MAP) of 73. Stroke volume and cardiac index were low with an elevated SVV. CVP unremarkable at 6. Because of the low flow parameters and higher-than-normal dynamic parameter SVV, the patient was determined to be hypovolemic. 250 mL crystalloid was administered over 5 minutes.

16:10 — Repeat assessment after the fluid challenge shows a slight increase in blood pressure and decrease in heart rate. The stroke volume change (delta ΔSV) was 27% from 30 to 38 mL with SVV decrease of 20% from 30 to 24. Since the values were still indicative of a need for fluid, another 250 mL of crystalloid was administered over a few minutes.

16:15 — A colloid was administered with the intent of inducing a more sustainable fluid loading.

16:20 — Target SVV of 10% achieved. The ΔSV was 42%, and cardiac index reached 2.6.

16:25 — Heart rhythm spontaneously converted to atrial fibrillation with a slightly elevated response of 100. Note the stroke volume has decreased—68 to 40—partially as a result of loss of atrial contribution resulting in a decreased cardiac index. SVV had greatly increased—10% to 29%. Atrial fibrillation causes an irregular R-to-R interval which produces an irregular filling of the ventricles. This, in turn, results in an irregular stroke volume value and therefore elevated SVV. The question then becomes: Is the elevated SVV caused by the cardiac activity or the need for fluid, or potentially both? Performing a physiologic challenge such as a passive leg raise maneuver is a quick way to provide an autologous fluid challenge.

16:30 — After passive leg raise, SVV decreased and stroke volume increased. This was determined to be a positive response to volume, so a fluid bolus was begun.

16:35 — A 250-mL fluid bolus of colloid was administered.

16:40 — Converted spontaneously back into a regular sinus rhythm at a rate of 85 beats/minute.

16:45 — After the colloid, the patient's hemodynamics became stable. Note that during the course of interventions, CVP rarely changed with or without fluid, nor was CVP indicative that the patient would respond to fluid.

References

1. Chamos C, Vele L, Hamilton M, Cecconi M: Less invasive methods of advanced hemodynamic monitoring: principles, devices, and their role in the perioperative hemodynamic optimization, *Perioperat Med* 2:19, 2013.
2. Cannesson M: Arterial pressure variation and goal-directed fluid therapy, *J Cardiothorac Vasc Anesth* 24:487–497, 2010.
3. Gruenwald M, Bein B: Goal directed therapy. In Vincent JL, editor: *Annual update in intensive care and emergency medicine*, New York, 2013, Springer-Verlag, pp 249–259.
4. Thiele RH, Durieux ME: Arterial waveform analysis for the anesthesiologist: past, present, and future concepts, *Anesth Analg* 113:766–776, 2011.
5. Booth J: A short history of blood pressure measurement, *Proc Roy Soc Med* 70:792–799, 1977.
6. Cecconi M, Rhodes A, Della Rocca G: From arterial pressure to cardiac output. In Vincent JL, editor: *Yearbook of intensive care and emergency medicine*, New York, 2008, Springer-Verlag, pp 591–601.
7. Ghasemzadeh N, Maziar Zafari A: A brief journey into the history of the arterial pulse. *Cardiol Res Pract* Volume 2011, Article ID 164832, doi:10.4061/2011/164832
8. Cove ME, Pinsky MR: Perioperative hemodynamic monitoring, *Best Pract Res Clin Anaesthesiol* 26:453–462, 2012.
9. Westerhof N, Lankhaar JW, Westerhof BE: The arterial Windkessel, *Med Biol Eng Comput* 47(2):131–141, 2009.
10. Smith IB: The impact of Stephen Hales on medicine, *J Roy Soc Med* 86:349–352, 1993.
11. Mackenzie IS, Wilkinson IB, Cockcroft JR: Assessment of arterial stiffness in clinical practice, *Q J Med* 95:67–74, 2002.
12. Wesseling KH, Jansen JRC, Settels JJ, Schreuder JJ: Computation of aortic flow from pressure in humans using a nonlinear, three-element model, *Model Physiol* 2566–2573, 1993.
13. Langewouters GJ: The static elastic properties of 45 human thoracic and 20 abdominal aortas in vitro and the parameters of a new model, *J Biomech* 17:425–435, 1984.
14. Vermeersch SJ, Rietzschel ER, De Buyzere ML, et al.: The reservoir pressure concept: the 3-element Windkessel model revisited? Application to the Asklepios population study, *J Eng Math* 64(4):417–428, 2009.
15. Headley JM: Arterial pressure-based technologies: a new trend in cardiac output monitoring, *Crit Care Nurs Clin North Am* 18:179–187, 2006.
16. Romano SM, Pistolesi M: Assessment of cardiac output from systemic arterial pressure in humans, *Crit Care Med* 30(8):1834–1841, 2002.
17. Rosen IT, White HL: The relation of pulse pressure to stroke volume, *Exp Biol Med* 23 (8):746–748, 1926.
18. Hamilton WF, Remington JW: The measurement of the stroke volume from the pressure pulse, *Am J Physiol* 148:14–23, 1947.
19. Ramsingh D, Brenton A, Cannesson M: Clinical review: does it matter which hemodynamic monitoring system is used? *Crit Care* 17:208, 2013.
20. Alhashemi JA, Cecconi M, Hofer CK: Cardiac output monitoring: an integrative perspective, *Crit Care* 15:214, 2011.
21. Truijen J, Lieshout JJ, Wesselink WA, Westerhof BE: Noninvasive continuous hemodynamic monitoring, *J Clin Monit Comput* 26:267–278, 2012.
22. Jansen JRC, van den Berg PCM: Cardiac output by thermodilution and arterial pulse contour techniques. In Pinsky MR, editor: *Functional hemodynamic monitoring*, 2005, Springer-Verlag Berlin Heidelberg.
23. Payen D: Update in intensive care and emergency medicine, 42, New York, 2005, Springer-Verlag, pp. 135–152.

24. Linton N, Linton R: Estimation of changes in cardiac output from the arterial blood pressure waveform in the upper limb, *Br J Anaesth* 86:486–496, 2001.

25. McGee WT, Horswell JL, Calderon J, et al.: Validation of a continuous, arterial pressure-based cardiac output measurement: a multicenter, prospective clinical trial, *Crit Care* 11(5):R105, 2007.

26. Pratt B, Roteliuk L, Hatib F, et al.: Calculating arterial pressure-based cardiac output using a novel measurement and analysis method, *Biomed Instrum Tech* 41(5):403–411, 2007.

27. Marik PE: Noninvasive cardiac output monitors: a state-of-the-art review, *J Cardiothorac Vasc Anesth* 27(1):121–134, 2012.

28. Oren-Grinberg A: *The PiCCO Monitor International Anesthesia Clinics,* Philadelphia, 2010, Lippincott Williams & Wilkins.

29. Dorman T, Breslow MJ, Lipsett PA, et al.: Radial artery pressure monitoring underestimates central arterial pressure during vasopressor therapy in critically ill surgical patients, *Crit Care Med* 26:1646–1649, 1998.

30. Hynson JM, Katz JA, Mangano DT: On the accuracy of intra-arterial pressure measurement: the pressure gradient effect, *Crit Care Med* 26:1623–1624, 1998.

31. Smith J, Camporota L, Beale R: Monitoring arterial blood pressure and cardiac output using central or peripheral arterial pressure waveforms. In Vincent JL, editor: *Yearbook of intensive care and emergency medicine*, Heidelberg, 2009, Springer, pp 285–296.

32. Biais M, Nouette-Gaulain K, Cottenceau V, et al.: Cardiac output measurement in patients undergoing liver transplantation: pulmonary artery catheter versus uncalibrated arterial pressure waveform analysis, *Anesth Analg* 106:1480–1486, 2008.

33. Monnet X, Anguel N, Naudin B, et al.: Arterial pressure-based cardiac output in septic patients: different accuracy of pulse contour and uncalibrated pressure waveform devices, *Crit Care* 14(R109), 2010.

34. DeBacker D, Marx G, Tan G, et al.: Arterial pressure-based cardiac output monitoring: a multicenter validation of the third-generation software in septic patients, *Intens Care Med* 37:233–240, 2011.

35. Vasdev S, Chauhan S, Choudhury M, et al.: Arterial pressure waveform derived cardiac output FloTrac/Vigileo system (third generation software): comparison of two monitoring sites with the thermodilution cardiac output, *J Clin Monit Comput* 26(2):115–120, 2012.

36. Geisen M, Rhodes A, Cecconi M: Less-invasive approaches to perioperative haemodynamic optimization, *Curr Opin Crit Care* 18:377–384, 2012.

37. Biais M, Ouattara A, Janvier G, Sztark F: Case scenario: respiratory variations in arterial pressure for guiding fluid management in mechanically ventilated patients, *Anesthesia* 116:1354–1361, 2012.

38. Bendjelid K, Marx G, Kiefer N, et al.: Performance of a new pulse contour method for continuous cardiac output monitoring: validation in critically ill patients, *Br J Anaesth* 111 (4):573–579, 2013.

39. Cecconi M, Fawcett J, Grounds RM, Rhodes A: A prospective study to evaluate the accuracy of pulse power analysis to monitor cardiac output in critically ill patients, *BMC Anesthesiol* 8:3, 2008.

40. Bein B, Meybohm P, Cavus E, et al.: The reliability of pulse contour-derived cardiac output during hemorrhage and after vasopressor administration, *Anesth Analg* 105(1):107–113, 2007.

41. Cooper ES, Muir WW: Continuous cardiac output monitoring via arterial pressure waveform analysis following severe hemorrhagic shock in dogs, *Crit Care Med* 35:1724–1729, 2007.

42. Hamzaoui O, Monnet X, Richard C, et al.: Effects of changes in vascular tone on the agreement between pulse contour and transpulmonary thermodilution cardiac

output measurements within an up to 6-hour calibration-free period, *Crit Care Med* 36 (2):434–440, 2008.

43. Bogert LWJ, Wesseling KH, Schraa O, et al.: Pulse contour cardiac output derived from non-invasive arterial pressure in cardiovascular disease, *Anaesthesia* 112(6):1392–1402, 2010.

44. Perel A, Settels JJ: Totally non-invasive continuous cardiac output measurement with the Nexfin CO-Trek. In Vincent J-L, editor: *Annual Update in Intensive Care and Emergency Medicine*, Berlin/Heidelberg, 2011, Springer-Verlag, pp 434–442.

45. Biais M, Stecken L, Ottolenghi L, et al.: The ability of pulse pressure variations obtained with CNAP™ device to predict fluid responsiveness in the operating room, *Anesth Analg* 113(3):523–528, 2011.

46. Chen G, Meng L, Alexander B, et al.: Comparison of noninvasive cardiac output measurements using the Nexfin monitoring device and the esophageal Doppler, *J Clin Anesth* 24:275–283, 2012.

47. Maguire S, Rinehart J, Vakharia S, Cannesson M: Technical communication: respiratory variation in pulse pressure and plethysmographic waveforms: intraoperative applicability in a North American academic center, *Anesth Analg* 112(1):94–96, 2011.

48. Hamilton M, Cecconi M, Rhodes A: A systematic review and meta-analysis on the use of pre-emptive hemodynamic intervention to improve postoperative outcomes in moderate and high-risk surgical patients, *Anesth Analg* 112(6):1392–1402, 2011.

49. Imholz BPM, Wieling W, van Montfrans GA, et al.: Fifteen years' experience with finger arterial pressure monitoring: assessment of the technology, *Cardiovasc Res* 38:605–616, 1998.

50. Meng L, Tran NP, Alexander BS, et al.: The impact of phenylephrine, ephedrine, and increased preload on third-generation Vigileo-FloTrac and esophageal Doppler cardiac output measurements, *Anesth Analg* 113(4):751–757, 2011.

51. Perel A, Habicher M, Sander M: Bench-to-bedside review: functional hemodynamics during surgery—should it be used for all high-risk cases? *Crit Care* 17:203, 2013.

52. Johnson SK, Naidu RK, Ostopowicz RC, et al.: Adolf Kussmaul: distinguished clinician and medical pioneer, *Clin Med Res* 7(3):107–112, 2009.

53. Hamzaoui O, Monnet X, Teboul JL: Pulsus paradoxus, *Eur Respir J* 42(6):1696–1705, 2013.

54. Michard F: Changes in arterial pressure during mechanical ventilation, *Anesthesia* 103:419–428, 2005.

55. Bridges EJ: Arterial pressure-based stroke volume and functional hemodynamic monitoring, *JCVN* 23(2):105–112, 2008.

56. da Silva Ramos FJ, Costa ELV, Amato MBP: Bedside monitoring of heart-lung interactions. In Vincent JL, editor: *Annual Update in Intensive Care and Emergency Medicine*, Berlin Heidelberg, 2013, Springer-Verlag, pp 373–384.

57. Marik PE, Monnet X, Teboul J-L: Hemodynamic parameters to guide fluid therapy, *Ann Intens Care* 1(1), 2011.

58. Enomoto TM, Harder L: Dynamic indices of preload, *Crit Care Clin* 26:307–321, 2010.

59. Kumar A, Anel R, Bunnell E, et al.: Pulmonary artery occlusion pressure and central venous pressure fail to predict ventricular filling volume, cardiac performance, or the response to volume infusion in normal subjects, *Crit Care Med* 32:691–699, 2004.

60. Osman D, Ridel C, Ray P, et al.: Cardiac filling pressures are not appropriate to predict hemodynamic response to volume challenge, *Care Med* 35:64–68, 2007.

61. Marik PE, Baram M, Vahid B: Does central venous pressure predict fluid responsiveness? A systematic review of the literature and the tale of seven mares, *Chest* 134:172–178, 2008.

62. Marik PE, Cavallazzi R: Does the central venous pressure predict fluid responsiveness? An updated meta-analysis and a plea for some common sense, *Crit Care Med* 41:1774–1781, 2013.

63. Monnet X, Teboul J-L: Assessment of volume responsiveness during mechanical ventilation: recent advances. In Vincent JL, editor: *Annual Update in Intensive Care and Emergency Medicine*, Berlin, 2013, Springer-Verlag, pp 385–396.

64. McGee WT, Raghunathan K: Physiologic goal-directed therapy in the perioperative period: the volume prescription for high-risk patients, *J Cardiothorac Vasc Anesth* 27(6):1079–1086, 2013.

65. Zhang J, Chen CQ, Lei XZ, Zhu SM: Goal-directed fluid optimization based on stroke volume variation and cardiac index during one-lung ventilation in patients undergoing thoracoscopy lobectomy operations: a pilot study, *Clinics* 68(7):1065–1070, 2013.

66. Cannesson M, Le Manach Y, Hofer CK, et al.: Assessing the diagnostic accuracy of pulse pressure variations for the prediction of fluid responsiveness. A "gray zone" approach, *Anesthesia* 115(2):231–241, 2011.

67. Monnet X, Bleibtreu A, Ferre A, et al.: Passive leg raising and end-expiratory occlusion tests perform better than pulse pressure variation in patients with low respiratory system compliance, *Crit Care Med* 40:152–157, 2012.

68. De Backer D, Heenen S, Piagnerelli M, et al.: Pulse pressure variations to predict fluid responsiveness: influence of tidal volumes, *Int Care Med* 31:517–523, 2005.

69. De Backer D, Taccone FS, Holsten R, et al.: Influence of respiratory rate on stroke volume variation in mechanically ventilated patients, *Anesthesia* 110:1092–1097, 2009.

70. Huang CC, Fu JY, Hu HC, et al.: Prediction of fluids responsiveness in acute respiratory distress syndrome patients ventilated with low tidal volume and high positive end-expiratory pressure, *Crit Care Med* 36(10):2810–2816, 2008.

71. Soubrier S, Saulnier F, Hubert H, et al.: Can dynamic indicators help the prediction of fluid responsiveness in spontaneously breathing critically ill patients? *Intens Care Med* 33:1117–1124, 2007.

72. De Backer D, Pinsky MR: Can one predict fluid responsiveness in spontaneously breathing patients? *Intens Care Med* 33:1111–1113, 2007.

73. Zaniboni M, Formenti P, Umbrello M, et al.: Pulse and systolic pressure variation assessment in partially assisted ventilatory support, *J Clin Monit Comput* 22:355–359, 2008.

74. Muller L, Louart G, Bousquet PJ, et al.: The influence of the airway driving pressure on pulsed pressure variation as a predictor of fluid responsiveness, *Intens Care Med* 36:496–503, 2010.

75. Cannesson M, Tran NP, Cho M, et al.: Predicting fluid responsiveness with stroke volume variations despite multiple extrasystoles, *Crit Care Med* 40:193–198, 2012.

76. Malbrain M, Inneke DL: Functional hemodynamics and increased intra-abdominal pressure: same thresholds for different conditions? *Crit Care Med* 37(2):781–783, 2009.

77. Bendjelid K, Duperret S, Colling J, et al.: Pulse pressure variation and stroke volume variation during increased intra-abdominal pressure: an experimental study, *Crit Care* 15 (R33), 2011.

78. Jacques D, Bendjelid K, Duperret S, et al.: Pulse pressure variation and stroke volume variation during increased intra-abdominal pressure: an experimental study, *Crit Care* 15(R33), 2011.

79. De Waal EEC, Rex S, Kruitwagen CLJJ, et al.: Dynamic preload indicators fail to predict fluid responsiveness in open-chest conditions, *Crit Care Med* 37:510–515, 2009.

80. Reuter DA, Goepfert MSG, Goresch T, et al.: Assessing fluid responsiveness during open chest conditions, *Br J Anesth* 94(3):318–323, 2005.

81. Biais M, Bernard O, Ha JC, et al.: Abilities of pulse pressure variations and stroke volume variations to predict fluid responsiveness in prone position during scoliosis surgery, *Br J Anaesth* 104:407–413, 2010.

82. Marks R, Silverman R, Fernandez R, et al.: Does the systolic pressure variation change in the prone position? *J Clin Monit Comput* 23:279–282, 2009.

83. Daudel F, Tuller D, Krahenbuhl S, et al.: Pulse pressure variation and volume responsiveness during acutely increased pulmonary artery pressure: an experimental study, *Crit Care* 14:R122, 2010.

84. Mesquida J, Kim HK, Pinsky MR: Effect of tidal volume, intrathoracic pressure, and cardiac contractility on variations in pulse pressure, stroke volume, and intrathoracic blood volume, *Intens Care Med* 37:1672–1679, 2011.

85. Sondergaard S: Pavane for a pulse pressure variation defunct, *Crit Care* 17(327), 2013.

86. Benes J, Zatloukal J, Kletecka J, Simanova A: Respiratory induced dynamic variations of stroke volume and its surrogates as predictors of fluid responsiveness: applicability in the early stages of specific critical states, *J Clin Monit Comput* 28(3):225–231, 2013.

87. Biais M, Vidil L, Sarrabay P, et al.: Changes in stroke volume induced by passive leg raising in spontaneously breathing patients: comparison between echocardiography and Vigileo/FloTrac device, *Crit Care* 13(R195), 2009.

88. Cavallaro F, Sandroni C, Marano C, et al.: Diagnostic accuracy of passive leg raising for prediction of fluid responsiveness in adults: systematic review and meta-analysis of clinical studies, *Intens Care Med* 36:1475–1483, 2010.

89. García MIM, Cano AG, Monrove JCD: Arterial pressure changes during the Valsalva maneuver to predict fluid responsiveness in spontaneously breathing patients, *Intens Care Med* 35:77–84, 2009.

90. Shujaat A, Bajwa AA: Optimization of preload in severe sepsis and septic shock, *Crit Care Res Pract* 2012, 761051, http://dx.doi.org/10.1155/2012/761051.

91. Lanspa MJ, Grissom CK, Hirshberg EL, et al.: Applying dynamic parameters to predict hemodynamic response to volume expansion in spontaneously breathing patients with septic shock, *Shock* 39(2):155–160, 2013.

92. Ramsingh DS, Sanghvi C, Gamboa J, et al.: Outcome impact of goal directed fluid therapy during high risk abdominal surgery in low to moderate risk patients: a randomized controlled trial, *J Clin Monit Comput* 27(3):249–257, 2013.

93. Kern ME: Arterial pressure based cardiac output monitoring. In Wiegand , Lynn-McHale D, editors: *AACN procedure manual for critical care*, 6 ed., St. Louis, MO, 2011, Saunders, pp 548–554.

94. Gravenstein JS, Paulus DA, Feldman J, McLaughlin G: Tissue hypoxia distal to a Pefiaz finger blood pressure cuff, *J Clin Monit Comput* 1:120–125, 1985.

Implantable Hemodynamic Monitoring

Nancy M. Albert

13

Four predominant themes are related to the current management of heart failure support and implantable hemodynamic monitoring: (1) Pulmonary artery thermodilution catheter, also known as internal or invasive hemodynamic monitoring, is used less often in the management of acute heart failure decompensation; (2) The numerous signs and symptoms of heart failure identified during a physical examination are insensitive markers of acute decompensation and elevated left ventricular filling pressures; (3) Impedance assessment obtained with a noninvasive impedance cardiography device does not have good accuracy as a surrogate of pulmonary arterial occlusion pressure (PAOP), also described as a wedge pressure; (4) Noninvasive telemonitoring has not been useful in reducing death and rehospitalization. Each of these four themes will be briefly reviewed to provide a foundation for the value of implantable hemodynamic monitoring.

Historical Milestones in Internal Hemodynamic Monitoring

Internal hemodynamic monitoring, with placement of invasive catheters for patients with heart failure, was a very common practice in the 1970s after development of the pulmonary artery thermodilution catheter, also known as the Swan-Ganz catheter. In the early days of heart failure treatment, when only digoxin and diuretics were available for outpatient management, patients received an indwelling pulmonary artery catheter to normalize the hemodynamic profile in two scenarios: (1) an acute decompensated heart failure episode consistent with cardiogenic shock after myocardial infarction[1] and (2) when symptoms were refractory after receiving optimal outpatient heart failure care, necessitating hospitalization.[2] Internal hemodynamic monitoring became more important in the late 1970s, when intravenous vasodilator therapies were introduced to treat cardiogenic shock and in the 1980s, when intravenous inotropic therapies were prominent adjuncts to the treatment of low cardiac output states. These medications were also used to improve kidney function, especially in patients being treated in a critical care environment or having a cardiac surgical procedure.[3,4]

In the 1990s, internal hemodynamic monitoring with an invasive pulmonary artery catheter (PAC) lost favor as a means of assessing hemodynamic function and managing therapies in intensive care environments. Researchers were unable to find evidence of decreased mortality[5,6] or improvements in other clinical outcomes.[7,8] Further, known risks and patient safety issues related to pulmonary artery rupture, bleeding at the insertion site, infection, and prolonged balloon occlusion of a pulmonary arterial segment were highlighted.

The Evaluation Study of Congestive Heart Failure and Pulmonary Artery Catheterization Effectiveness (ESCAPE) trial was designed in 2000 to determine the safety and clinical outcomes in hospitalized patients with reduced ejection fraction (rEF) and acutely decompensated chronic heart failure, or with severe symptoms.[9] Patients were randomized to either clinical assessment alone, or clinical assessment with a pulmonary artery catheter.[9]

From a hemodynamic monitoring perspective, no differences were observed in the signs and symptoms of volume overload (used as a marker for elevated cardiac filling pressures) in patients monitored with or without a PAC. Further, the use of a PAC increased anticipated in-hospital adverse events.[9] Results of the ESCAPE trial were followed by a meta-analysis of 13 randomized controlled trials of PAC use in critically ill patients. The odds ratios for death and number of days hospitalized were similar between those who received and those who did not receive a PAC to guide care; however, use of inotropic and vasodilator therapies were higher among patients who received a PAC.[10] More recently, a retrospective cohort design of adult admissions from 2001 to 2008 was used to create a better understanding of the use of the PAC in critically ill patients. Usage decreased from 10.8% during the first 3-year period to 6.2% in the 3-year period ending in 2008. Noticeably, usage was higher in teaching hospitals, among surgical critical care units, and in unit settings with the leadership of a surgeon.[11]

Heart Failure Management

Heart Failure Management Guided by Pulmonary Artery Catheter

In patients with heart failure, the value of internal hemodynamic monitoring may not be apparent during hospitalization when most people are being aggressively treated to alleviate congestion. It may be more important to record PAOP readings after receiving heart failure medications so that evidence-based decisions about the breadth and depth of post-discharge care requirements can be made. In clinical research, long-term outcomes varied, depending on the hemodynamic monitoring values obtained after heart failure stabilization. For example, in patients hospitalized for decompensated heart failure, a PAOP of 16 mm Hg (millimeters of mercury) or less after treatment with intravenous diuretics and vasodilators was associated with 2-year survival, but cardiac index levels were not associated with survival.[12] In the ESCAPE trial, researchers also demonstrated that PAOP less than or equal to 22 mm Hg had value in predicting 6-month post-discharge survival, and similar to previous research, cardiac output was not a prognostic factor.[9] In addition to high PAOP readings, congestion was also a marker of 2-year survival. When researchers assessed patients 4 to 6 weeks after hospital discharge, those with moderate symptoms of congestion (orthopnea, peripheral edema, weight gain, need to increase baseline diuretic dose, and jugular venous distension) had significantly worse 2-year survival rates.[13] Thus, high left ventricular filling pressures, whether measured as PAOP or as a factor known to be associated with congestion, have prognostic importance.

Heart Failure Management Guided by Physical Assessment

It would seem easy to draw a conclusion that if congestion can be determined via physical examination, internal or implantable hemodynamic monitoring is not a necessity. However, many caveats exist as to identifying markers of congestion on physical examination. In an emergency department setting, the overall sensitivity of signs and symptoms in those who actually had heart failure diagnoses was low.[14] Further, in the ESCAPE trial, the sensitivity of physical examination findings in detecting a PAOP greater than 22 mm Hg was surprisingly poor. Pulmonary crackles (rales), ascites, edema, hepatomegaly, jugular venous pressure greater than 11 cm (centimeters), and presence of an S3 heart sound all had sensitivities at or below 65%. Only orthopnea (two or more pillows) and positive hepatojugular reflux had sensitivities of 86% and 83%, respectively.[15] Another problem is the reliance of health care providers (nurses and physicians) to accurately determine prognostic risks following an episode of acute heart failure decompensation. In patients with advanced heart failure enrolled in the ESCAPE trial, nurses had significantly higher predictive accuracy in determining death, even though for both groups it was not overly strong, and both nurses and physicians had weak accuracy in predicting rehospitalization.[16] Ultimately, if accurate assessment of congestion cannot be determined with enough precision by a health care provider on the basis of general assessment and physical examination findings during an episode of decompensation, implantable hemodynamic monitoring may be a necessity in both acute care and ambulatory settings.

Heart Failure Management Guided by Noninvasive Monitoring

As an alternative to implantable hemodynamic monitoring, noninvasive impedance cardiography technology became available in the early 2000s. It used a change in impedance across the thorax to assess hemodynamic values. Researchers found fairly accurate correlations between stroke volumes and cardiac outputs in noninvasive impedance cardiography and PAC readings; however, intrathoracic impedance values, measured in kilo-ohms (kOhms), were not associated with left ventricular filling pressures.[17–19] Thus, impedance values obtained with noninvasive impedance cardiography systems should not be used as a surrogate for PAOP obtained from internal hemodynamic monitoring.

Without validated noninvasive systems that can provide an accurate surrogate of left-sided filling pressures, direct assessment of hemodynamic values from implantable hemodynamic monitoring systems are warranted and may gain increasingly greater importance in determining prognostic risk, as the pressure to reduce heart failure hospitalization and mortality increases with health care reform.

Heart Failure Management Guided by Telemonitoring

Finally, clinicians and researchers had great hope that noninvasive telemonitoring would provide surrogate information of high left-sided filling pressures and impending heart failure decompensation that would lead to proactive heart failure treatments and improved clinical outcomes. Unfortunately, randomized controlled trials of telemonitoring of hemodynamic and nonhemodynamic data such as weight, blood pressure, oxygenation, heart rate, worsening dyspnea and orthopnea, and other markers of worsening heart failure failed to improve the primary endpoints of death or hospitalization.[20-22] In clinical trial reports, researchers hypothesized why telemonitoring failed. The reasons included too many gadgets; too much support from the telemonitoring vendor; good support from cardiologists and primary care providers (making telemonitoring a non-necessity); and inability of telemonitoring to reconcile medications, provide caregiver support, or develop or maintain heart failure self-care lifestyle recommendations.[20-22] Another issue was the patients' willingness to use telemonitoring. In one trial, nearly one third of eligible candidates declined to participate in the trial. Of those who received telemonitoring, 14% never used the system, and in the final week of the study intervention, 45% of study participants had stopped using the system.[20] Therefore, telemonitoring may have issues with initial desirability and durability over time. In a qualitative report of patients who declined or withdrew from telemonitoring programs, three barriers to telemonitoring emerged: (1) technical competence issues related to feeling alienated from technology, having misperceptions about how to use technology, and having difficulty dealing with alarms or slow response from experts when issues occurred; (2) threats to identity, independence, and self-care; and (3) expectations and experiences of disruption to usual-care medical services.[23]

Implantable Hemodynamic Monitoring

The ideal implantable hemodynamic monitoring system would have the following qualities. First, implantable hemodynamic monitoring should provide intermittent or continuous hemodynamic data to health care providers in a way that negates or minimizes "data collection" actions by patients. Second, implantable hemodynamic data should be available to health care providers (assuming optimal technology capabilities are available), even when patients are nonadherent to self-care expectations or are traveling. Third, implantable hemodynamic data should be used by health care providers in a way that minimizes patient congestion, maintains homeostasis, reduces heart failure–related hospitalization, and improves heart failure–related quality of life and survival. Finally, implantable hemodynamic data must be highly accurate and automatically downloadable to help health care providers with quick, easy retrieval and trusted findings. The last expectation is especially important to health care providers who manage large populations.

Evolution of Management of Heart Failure

In 1997, a paper was published by Steimle et al. describing clinical and hemodynamic responses after 8 or more months of delivery of chronic heart failure therapies (diuretics, angiotensin-converting enzyme inhibitors, and nitrates) based on early hemodynamic monitoring responses in 25 patients with advanced heart failure who had been referred for cardiac transplantation.[24] For the cohort, early reductions in PAOP and systemic vascular resistance (SVR) were maintained and were accompanied by an increase in stroke volume, improvement in functional class, and freedom from resting symptoms.[24] Study results provided new evidence that early hemodynamic responses to treatments were sustained over time and led to further improvement in stroke volume.

Implantable Stand-Alone Devices

At or near the same time, researchers were establishing the feasibility of using implantable sensor technology to monitor hemodynamic measurements for long-term use in ambulatory patients.[25–29] By implanting a sensor in the right ventricle, researchers hypothesized that a reasonable estimate of pulmonary arterial diastolic pressure could be obtained, since pressure in the pulmonary artery was equal to pressure in the right ventricle when the pulmonic valve opened.[25]

Accuracy and stability of sensors were reported in 2001 on the basis of data from a multicenter study of 21 patients who maintained an implantable hemodynamic monitor for 1 year. Researchers were able to demonstrate reproducibility and stability of data, even though slight variations existed in right ventricular systolic and diastolic pressures and mixed venous oxygen saturation compared with data obtained from right heart catheterization. Researchers also learned more about oxygen sensor and pressure sensor failures, both of which occurred during the study period.[28]

In 2002, researchers reported the accuracy of an implantable hemodynamic monitor for measuring right heart pressures in 32 patients with heart failure: at baseline; at 3, 6, and 12 months; and in various physiologic conditions (rest, exercise, and with Valsalva maneuver). Right ventricular systolic and diastolic pressures and pulmonary artery diastolic pressures were correlated to PAC measurements initially and over time, demonstrating reproducibility of monitoring patients' hemodynamic conditions.[30] On the basis that an implantable hemodynamic monitor might improve day-to-day management of patients with chronic heart failure, data from the 12-month study were also assessed for changes during volume overload events. Researchers learned that right ventricular pressure increased in most patients about 4+ days before the exacerbation leading to hospitalization.[31] Learning that pressure elevations occurred days before clinical symptoms were recognized was an important finding. Also, learning that stable estimated pulmonary artery diastolic pressures were associated with clinical stability and lack of hospitalization provided more evidence of the value of monitoring intracardiac pressures.[32] Conceivably, health care providers could use hemodynamic data to alter treatment plans and possibly avoid or reduce hospitalization events.

Heart Failure Management Guided by Implantable Devices

Three implantable hemodynamic monitoring devices have been studied in patients with heart failure.

Chronicle

The first device, called the *Chronicle* (Medtronic Inc., Minneapolis, MN), was never approved by the U.S. Food and Drug Administration (FDA) and is no longer available. The implantable right ventricular pressure sensor was studied in 274 patients with advanced heart failure and New York Heart Association (NYHA) functional classes of III or IV. The study was named the Chronicle Offers Management to Patients with Advanced Signs and Symptoms of Heart Failure (COMPASS-HF) trial.[33] Patients were randomized to receive a *Chronicle* device or were control subjects. Hemodynamic data, specifically right ventricular systolic pressure and right ventricular diastolic pressure, provided estimates of pulmonary artery diastolic pressure and were used to guide patient management in the device group, with all patients receiving optimal medical therapies for 6 months. The primary efficacy endpoint was not met; a 21% nonsignificant reduction was seen in all heart failure–related events in those who received the device compared with control subjects. However, in a retrospective analysis, time to first hospitalization was prolonged in the Chronicle device group.[33] In the COMPASS-HF study, 70 patients had advanced heart failure with preserved ejection fraction (HFpEF). Results were similar to the primary efficacy endpoint in that a 20% nonsignificant reduction occurred in all heart failure events in participants with HFpEF, and no difference existed in the relative risk of heart failure hospitalization between the two groups.[34] The COMPASS-HF trial provided new knowledge about hemodynamic monitoring of ambulatory patients with advanced heart failure. One important factor was learning the estimated pulmonary artery diastolic pressure, that was associated with event risk. Participants with estimated pulmonary artery diastolic pressures of 25 mm Hg or higher, were at higher risk. Additionally, patients whose pressures did not decline below 25 mm Hg over time were at higher risk.[35]

HeartPOD

The second implantable device used a left atrial pressure sensor to measure left atrial pressure, obtain an intracardiac electrocardiogram, and record the core temperature. The sensor is placed transapically, and a coil antenna was implanted in the subpectoral area.[36] The sensor lead was attached to an implantable communications module. The system was called *HeartPOD* (developed by Savacor Co, Los Angeles, CA and sold to St. Jude Medical, St. Paul, MN in 2005). This device was never submitted to the FDA for approval and devices are no longer being implanted (Figure 13-1). The HeartPOD system used an external component, a patient advisory module that powered the HeartPOD by inductive radiofrequency (Figure 13-2). The patient advisory module was a hand-held device that monitored left atrial pressure, stored data, alerted patients to monitor left atrial pressure and instructed patients regarding medications, activity, and when to contact their physician. In real time, patients downloaded their

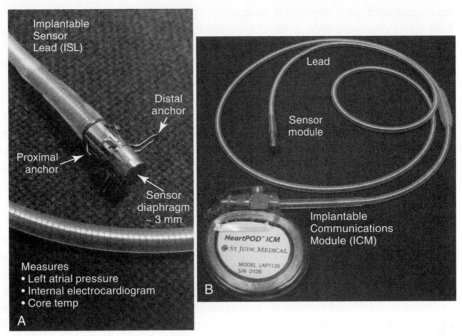

FIGURE 13-1 The HeartPOD implantable sensor lead (**A**) and implantable communication module (**B**). (Photos provided courtesy of St. Jude Medical.)

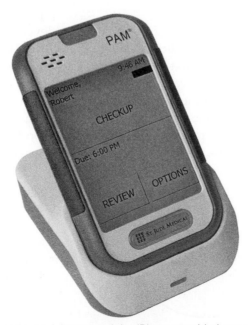

FIGURE 13-2 The HeartPOD patient advisory module. (Photo provided courtesy of St. Jude Medical.)

measurements and used their data to titrate their treatment in a very precise manner. Left atrial pressure data were also uploaded to the health care provider's office computer, allowing for changes in the plan of care. The first report of this monitoring technology was published in 2010.[36] Researchers implanted devices in 40 patients with advanced HFrEF or HFpEF and NYHA functional class III-IV. During the first 3 months, patients and clinicians were blinded to the twice-a-day readings. Then, therapies were guided by left atrial pressure readings and data were disclosed to patients. In the first 3 months of pressure-guided therapy mean daily left atrial pressures were reduced, heart failure–related vasodilator and beta-blocker therapies were uptitrated, and doses of loop diuretics were reduced.[36] Although it was a small study, researchers learned about the potential to improve hemodynamics, symptoms, and clinical outcomes in patients with advanced heart failure.

The left atrial pressure sensor and the HeartPOD system were being studied in a randomized controlled study titled the Left Atrial Pressure Monitoring to Optimize Heart Failure Therapy (LAPTOP-HF) trial, however, patient enrollment was stopped. The purpose of LAPTOP-HF was to evaluate the safety and clinical effectiveness of using left atrial pressure measurements and a management system that was physician directed and patient managed. The system guided adjustments in heart failure medications (similar to insulin therapy being guided by blood sugar levels). Clinical effectiveness may be measured by episodes of worsening heart failure and hospitalizations, and patients will be compared on the basis of being managed with the left atrial pressure system or usual care.[37]

CardioMEMS HF System

The third device is the *CardioMEMS HF System* (developed by CardioMEMS, Atlanta, GA and sold to St. Jude Medical, St. Paul, MN, in 2014), a fully implantable, wireless pulmonary artery device that monitors pulmonary artery systolic, mean, and diastolic pressures.[38] This device was approved for clinical use by the FDA in May 2014. CardioMEMS uses a lead-less sensor that is placed in a distal branch of the pulmonary artery (Figure 13-3), home electronics that allow for daily pressure readings to be transmitted to health care providers, and a trend report of pressure information and individual waveforms. The sensor itself is a very small capsule covered by silicone

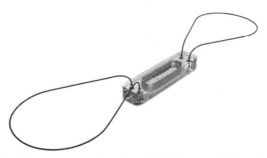

FIGURE 13-3 CardioMEMS lead-less sensor placed in a distal branch of the pulmonary artery. (Photo provided courtesy of St. Jude Medical.)

(15 millimeters [mm] in length, 3.4 mm in width, and 2 mm in thickness) that contains a coil and pressure-sensitive capacitor. [38] Two nitrol loops, one on each end of the sensor, maintain the sensor in place in the pulmonary artery. No batteries need to be placed in the sensor, as an external antenna from the home electronics is held against the patient's body to create electromagnetic coupling and power the device. The antenna continuously measures resonate frequencies, which are converted into pressure waveforms, based on an electrical circuit that is created by the coil and capacitor. [38]

In 2011, the outcomes of the CardioMEMS Heart Sensor Allows Monitoring of Pressure to Improve Outcomes in NYHA Class III Heart Failure Patients (CHAMPION) trial were reported. [39] The trial involved implantation of a CardioMEMS sensor in 550 patients, a one-night hospital stay, and training of patients to use the home electronics. All patients were told to take daily pressure readings, which were uploaded to a secure patient database. Data from the sensor was only available to patients randomized to the treatment group. Company-sponsored nurse communication was also available to the treatment group. When the pulmonary artery pressures exceeded the protocol-defined treatment goals and when signs and symptoms of worsening heart failure were identified on the basis of standard of care practices, physicians were expected to use neurohormonal, diuretic, and vasodilator heart failure therapies to reduce pressures and alleviate symptoms. [39] The usual care group received alterations in heart failure therapies based on standards of care. At 6 months and during the entire randomization period, patients in the treatment group had significant reductions in heart failure–related hospitalizations, and compared with the usual care group, the treatment group had a significant reduction in mean pulmonary artery pressure and more days alive outside of the hospital. [39]

Because of concerns regarding the effects of nurse communication to enhance protocol adherence in the treatment group of the CHAMPION trial, a 13-month open access assessment period (part 2) followed the 17.6-month randomized access data collection period (part 1, described above). In part 2, both the former usual care and the treatment groups received standard heart failure management and both had physician knowledge of pulmonary artery pressures. Moreover, neither group received nurse communications, thereby addressing issues that were raised during the initial FDA review. [40] In part 2, 177 former treatment patients and 170 former usual care patients participated with 119 and 127, respectively, completing the open access assessment period. Data were analyzed for heart failure hospitalization rates. [40]

In part 2 analysis, physician access to pulmonary artery pressure measurements led to a significant reduction in the annualized heart failure hospitalization rate among patients in the open access control group compared with the rates from part 1, reflecting the benefit of physician access to hemodynamic data. [40] Of the treatment group patients, no differences in annualized heart failure hospitalization rates existed between part 1 and part 2 groups, reflecting that the part 1 nurse communication component may not have had a large influence on physician treatment decisions.

Alternatively, physicians could have learned new management options to reduce pulmonary artery pressures during the randomized access period, then used these strategies during the open access period. Additionally, patient gains in part 1 associated with stabilization of hemodynamic status may have been maintained in part 2.

When the magnitude of change in annualized hazard ratios for heart failure hospitalization was assessed between part 1 and 2 of the control and treatment groups, a significant change (improvement) was seen in the control group (from 0.68 to 0.36) and no change in the treatment group (from 0.48 to 0.45), reflecting the benefit of access to pulmonary artery pressure monitoring in the former control group. Analysis also revealed that hemodynamic monitoring created early gains but that prolonged monitoring did not lead to a continued reduction in the annualized heart failure hospitalization hazard rate.[40] Features of devices with hemodynamic monitoring features are provided in Table 13-1.

TABLE 13-1   Devices with Hemodynamic Monitoring Features

DEVICE NAME (TRIAL NAME)	HEMODYNAMIC MONITORING FEATURES	NON-HEMODYNAMIC MONITORING FEATURES	DATA TRANSMISSION	COMMENTS
Stand-Alone				
HeartPOD St. Jude Medical (LAPTOP-HF)	• Measures and stores IEGMs • Measures and stores LAP, mm Hg	• Measures and stores core temperature • Feedback loop for medication adjustments • Implantable communications module that contains a telemetry coil • Patient advisor module that stores medications, symptoms, BP, weight; provides a reminder to take medications a minimum of twice per day	• Patient advisor module • Patient self-management	• Goal is to minimize abnormal LAP readings • Sensing and communication technology for both health care providers and patients or caregivers • Three systems were available: HeartPOD, the Auricle System (which provides left atrial pressure monitoring as part of CRT-D), and the Promote left atrial pressure system (which provided left atrial pressure monitoring, impedance monitoring, and CRT-D)

TABLE 13-1   Devices with Hemodynamic Monitoring Features—cont'd

DEVICE NAME (TRIAL NAME)	HEMODYNAMIC MONITORING FEATURES	NON-HEMODYNAMIC MONITORING FEATURES	DATA TRANSMISSION	COMMENTS
CardioMEMs HF System St. Jude Medical (CHAMPION)	• PAS, mm Hg • Mean PA, mm Hg • PAD, mm Hg	• None	• Directly to a secure website for physician assessment	• Goal is to control PA pressures in the normal range • Wireless sensing and communication technology for health care providers
With CRT-D				
Biotronics	• Mean HR, beats per minute • HR variability	• Arrhythmia detection via IEGM • Real-time 30-second EGM strip • Activity • AF burden • Percent of CRT pacing • VES/hour	• Automatic, wireless cellular phone (global system for mobile communications) or landline-based patient monitor transmits patient data to a home monitoring center • Immediate detection of clinical events • Internet alerts via simple messaging service, electronic mail, and fax	• 5 of 7 parameters (see the "features" column; all but activity and HR variability) may trigger an alert if programmed and are customizable • Intuitive, color-coded, web-based system of classification of patient status • Cannot integrate external sensors (blood pressure, weight scale) • Easy to travel with system
Boston Scientific	• Mean HR, beats per minute • HR variability	• Activity • Arrhythmia detection and documentation • Weekly patient symptom self-report using questions that require Likert-type or fill-in-the-blank responses	• Manual and automatic communicator transmits patient data • Uses telephone line to transfer data and Internet for health care providers	• External sensors (weight scale and blood pressure) can be integrated and use Bluetooth technology to send results to the communicator • Communicator options when interrogating the device include push button, wireless; touch screen, wireless and wanded

Continued

TABLE 13-1	**Devices with Hemodynamic Monitoring Features—cont'd**			
DEVICE NAME (TRIAL NAME)	**HEMODYNAMIC MONITORING FEATURES**	**NON-HEMODYNAMIC MONITORING FEATURES**	**DATA TRANSMISSION**	**COMMENTS**
Medtronic	• Intrathoracic impedance fluid status monitoring • Average ventricular rate (beats per minute) • HR variability, milliseconds	• Activity; hours/day • Burden and rate of AT/AF, hours per day • Atrial and ventricular pacing, percent	• Portable home monitor reader to transmit patient data; requires telephone or a cellular accessory; report can be faxed to the office • Password protected Internet service for automatic monitoring (health care providers) available 24/7; shows trended values	• System network can provide data that matches an in-office device check • In addition to a full parameter summary, data are provided on percent pacing; battery voltage and longevity; A-V conduction histograms and dysrhythmia summary
St. Jude Medical	• Congestion duration exceeded programmed thresholds • Mean HR, beats per minute	• Arrhythmia detection and documentation (burden and duration greater than threshold) • Atrial and ventricular pacing, percent	• Radiofrequency (wireless) daily transfer of data to Internet server via a telephone; alerts communicated via simple messaging services, electronic mail, and fax	• Data from Internet server can be linked to an electronic medical record • Allows for prerecorded messages from clinic to patient to remind them of office visits and missed follow-up or to confirm transmitted data • Direct alert patient notifier feature • Online scheduling tools

AF, Atrial fibrillation; *AT*, atrial tachycardia; *BP*, blood pressure; *CRT-D*, cardiac resynchronization therapy-defibrillator; *D*, diastole; *HR*, heart rate; *IEGM*, intracardiac electrogram; *LAP*, left atrial pressure; *PA*, pulmonary artery; *S*, systole; *VES*, ventricular episodes; *VT/VF*, ventricular tachycardia/ventricular fibrillation.

Monitoring Features of Implanted Cardiac Resynchronization Therapy-Defibrillator (CRT-D) Devices

In the early 2000s, two of the four major pacemaker device companies developed internal monitoring features for some models of cardiac resynchronization therapy (CRT) devices. Currently, internal monitoring features are available in all implantable CRT-defibrillator (CRT-D) devices, although the features offered by each company vary (see Table 13-1).

Most internal monitoring features of CRT-D devices are not hemodynamic monitoring specific; for example, recording patient activity level and percent of atrial and ventricular pacing. Other CRT-D devices record intrathoracic impedance, average ventricular day and night heart rate, and heart rate variability. The intrathoracic impedance feature provides a lung volume impedance measurement that reflects thoracic fluid, which is usually a surrogate for lung edema. High intrathoracic impedance and low fluid index values reflect a dry lung state. Thoracic fluid status can be monitored from the patient's home as a stand-alone data point or with other CRT-D internal monitoring data and may be used by health care providers to facilitate outpatient management of heart failure.[41,42] Data points or data trends could provide early warning that could facilitate treatment changes that prevent hospitalization.

The literature contains many case studies and research reports of health care providers' use of internal monitoring data from internal cardiac devices. Clinicians described a decrease in intrathoracic impedance and a subsequent rise in fluid index that were associated with a decrease in patient activity, a rise in night-time heart rate, and a decrease in heart rate variability over time, which matched patients' reports of worsening symptoms of heart failure. Further, trends were reversed once diuretics were administered.[43,44] In 23 patients who had intrathoracic impedance validated by PAOP obtained by the echocardiography–Doppler method, the kappa-coefficient was 0.70 (standard error, 0.113), reflecting strong accuracy. Further, the impedance alert detected clinical heart failure deterioration with 92% sensitivity and 67% positive predictive value.[45] Since the positive predictive value was only 67%, it must be remembered that not all changes in intrathoracic impedance were caused by lung edema.

Internal monitoring data was used in a multi-center, retrospective, cohort study, of impedance-monitoring capabilities via a CRT-D, where 326 patients were monitored for fluid index levels that rose above the threshold level (labeled as an "event"). Patients with more than three threshold crossings of fluid index values per year had a significantly higher likelihood of a heart failure hospitalization during the study period.[46] Thus, serial decreases in intrathoracic impedance leading to high fluid index levels that cross established thresholds provide opportunities for health care providers to reassess current management strategies and ensure that guideline-directed medical therapies are optimized. Of note, a modified CRT-D algorithm was developed to detect a reference impedance and fluid index level. In a study of 81 subjects, the modified algorithm decreased unexplained fluid index threshold crossings.[47] To date, the modified algorithm is not available clinically; a multi-center, randomized controlled study would be required prior to FDA approval.

Intrathoracic impedance values were also associated with hemodynamic and physiologic values. Researchers found strong correlations between stroke impedance and both stroke volume and pulse pressure.[48] In another report of CRT internal monitoring features, persistent atrial fibrillation burden, for longer than 24 hours, worsened heart rate variability and activity level and increased night-time heart rate.[49] Also, it took approximately 30 days after the atrial fibrillation episode ended before activity and heart rate variability levels returned to preatrial fibrillation values.[49]

In a study of patients who were monitored for 8.6 months, atrial tachycardia events preceded a fluid index event (reflecting a drop in intrathoracic impedance and presence of lung edema) in 43% of cases. Atrial tachycardia events followed a fluid index event in 29% of cases, and was simultaneous or intermediate in 22% of cases.[50] Thus, patients with heart failure had increased susceptibility to temporary atrial tachycardia with worsening pulmonary congestion. In another study, researchers learned that ventricular tachydysrhythmic events occurred within 30 days of a fluid index threshold crossing event.[51] This knowledge may lead to a better understanding of the interplay between atrial or ventricular tachyarrhythmias and neurohormonal and cardiac remodeling events in heart failure.

Using Implantable Hemodynamic Monitoring

Implantable hemodynamic monitoring may offer many benefits, but some potential issues have to be considered as well. In the case of both stand-alone devices and the internal monitoring features of CRT-D, no new knowledge is available that suggests that the device data can be used in isolation from other history and physical examination findings. Therefore, current benefits are relative in that device data must be coupled with other patient data before treatment plans are finalized, to ensure patient safety and minimization of adverse outcomes. In the following section, both benefits and potential issues are discussed.

Benefits

Thus far, pulmonary artery sensor technologies have been reasonably safe, accurate, and seemingly durable, although more research is warranted. An implantable hemodynamic monitor that wirelessly transmits pulmonary artery pressures to patients and health care providers allows for distant, ambulatory control of moderate to severe heart failure. In the case of internal monitoring features that are part of CRT-D, electrophysiology cardiologists have a long history of placing devices in patients. The technology is safe, and benefits of the core device (CRT, implantable cardioverter-defibrillator or CRT-D) are well known to outweigh risks. Both pulmonary artery catheter stand-alone devices and hemodynamic monitoring features that are part of CRT-D devices offer quick, timely and ongoing access to data that could effectively decrease heart failure events and acute decompensation requiring hospitalization. Freedom from heart failure events may improve heart failure–related pharmacologic profiles, quality of life, and clinical outcomes.

Potential benefits of implantable hemodynamic monitoring are associated with electronic data capture. If hemodynamic data can be downloaded to multiple health care providers, as needed, problem identification and optimal treatment planning might be maximized. Multi-disciplinary collaboration among health care providers might increase, creating uniformity in the plan of care revisions, and consistent messaging to patients and families.

Potential Issues

Potential issues with stand-alone hemodynamic monitoring involve the comfort and ease of health care providers in making decisions that impact patient outcomes. In the CHAMPION trial, the CardioMEMS system was not initially approved for use by the FDA because decision makers were unable to determine the effectiveness of the data in changing clinical practice.[40] During the trial, company representatives advised physicians in dealing with abnormal hemodynamic values. Thus, the impressive reduction in hospitalization could have been caused by external support that would not be available once the device was approved for use in clinical practice. Considering that many patients with heart failure are managed by primary care providers, and not cardiac specialists, outcomes may be hard to replicate in clinical practice. When hemodynamic data are provided as stand-alone data, treatment decisions involving aggressive diuretic or vasodilator therapies could lead to hypotension, dizziness, or neurohormonal stimulation that worsens heart failure.[52] If, indeed, the CHAMPION trial health care providers used other diagnostic and symptom measures such as B-type natriuretic peptide to make decisions, a need for transparency exists to learn how treatment decisions were really made so that the value of implantable hemodynamic monitoring can be accurately determined.

If a hemodynamic monitoring system has accurate, reliable, and safe medication management algorithms, both the potential issues of failing to act when pressures increase above present thresholds and overreacting to too-high pressures could be avoided, that is, assuming the algorithm was complete and health care providers followed the actions as determined. However, the problem with algorithm use is that many health care providers believe that the art of managing heart failure is just as important as the science of heart failure management. With an algorithm, specific circumstances that could have preceded the changes in hemodynamic pressures may not have been considered. Further, if medication management decisions are made without knowledge of special circumstances, changes in medication prescriptions may be incomplete or suboptimal.

Implantable hemodynamic monitoring is a new era in patient management that allows for data generation with simple patient actions or without patient interface. Since traditional history and physical examination data are not used to determine the cause of deterioration or improvement, patients may feel distanced from health care providers, especially when only red flags are acted upon. Patients may believe that heart failure self-care expectations are not necessary, or they may believe that they will be contacted only when a significant change in status requires attention, whether or not health care providers are really paying attention to incoming data. The patient may feel like a "patient," rather than a person with heart failure, and resent expectations of daily activity associated with monitoring. Patients may have fears related to home electronics alarms. Thus, barriers to using telemonitoring may also be barriers to implantable hemodynamic monitoring.

Electronic data capture is a potential benefit of hemodynamic monitoring; however, it could also be a burden. Often, a large portion of downloaded data cannot be acted on. If episodic office-based follow-up is going to change to continuous or frequent device assessment, system changes will need to occur. Health care personnel will need to allocate time to be able to triage data and identify data abnormalities that require action. The downloaded implantable hemodynamic monitoring data will need to be reliable and trusted to result in economic and patient benefits. In one study of remote monitoring, some measurements did not correlate with others; for example, blood pressure did not correlate with weight, activity, or the difference between mean and resting heart rates.[53] Measurements that are not associated with others and do not offer additional value need to be identified and isolated.

Management Considerations

Implantable hemodynamic monitoring requires specific nursing and physician considerations that relate to time, education, and systems to enhance teamwork and communication. Table 13-2 provides details of each consideration. To have a successful program, all areas must be addressed. Currently, most acute care and ambulatory nurses do not have the available time to download data from a company server, and to save data to an electronic medical record. Further, even though only a specific percentage of data might require a health care provider's review and response, if the goal is to assess for trends of worsening hemodynamics before an impending emergency care visit or hospitalization, it might be necessary to build time into the work plan, especially if there is a need to download device data during an office visit or hospitalization.

From an education standpoint, clinicians will require new or renewed knowledge about hemodynamic waveform interpretation. Factors such as mitral regurgitation and chronic pulmonary disease could influence hemodynamic monitor values provided in devices; it may become necessary to assess waveforms. Most nonsurgical critical care areas have reduced the usage of PACs, and noncritical care nurses may not be familiar with waveform interpretation at all. Further, because of the underlying heart failure diagnosis, some hemodynamic waveforms are abnormal compared with waveforms presented in textbooks. Clinicians will need to recognize abnormal hemodynamic waveforms and understand differing treatment expectations based on both waveforms and values.

Development of systems that enhance teamwork and communication are essential when implantable hemodynamic monitoring is used, especially when primary care or family practice physicians and nurses are the medical providers of care. When assessed

TABLE 13-2   Management Considerations Specific to Implantable Hemodynamic Monitoring

CLINICAL CONSIDERATIONS	ACTIONS NEEDED TO INITIATE AND MAINTAIN IMPLANTABLE HEMODYNAMIC MONITORING	RATIONALE
Time	• To access hemodynamic monitoring device waveforms, values, and ancillary data available through system • To assess patient's adherence to HF self-care activities • To download and store data in office systems (file or EHR)	• Some systems require multiple steps to retrieve data • Having context for changes in hemodynamic data may enhance decision making • To maintain evidence of hemodynamics
Education	• Of normal and abnormal hemodynamic waveforms (waves and descents) • Of normal and abnormal hemodynamic values • Of clinical presentations when hemodynamic waveforms should be used rather than values	• To ensure correct interpretation of waveforms • To ensure correct interpretation of values • To ensure that the right data is used in making clinical decisions
Systems for enhanced teamwork and communication	• A system that provides coverage for off-shift, weekend and holiday data retrieval and interpretation • An algorithm of specialty personnel names and contact information to provide guidance in care planning decisions, based on hemodynamics • Develop a system for automatic download of data into the EHR • Develop and assess outcomes of a distance-care system or program for patients that includes implantable hemodynamic monitoring	• To ensure an appropriate response to data received when primary caregivers are away from the workplace • To facilitate communication among ancillary providers of care so that patient follow-up is based on full disclosure of current status and actions • Saves time and enhances multidisciplinary communication • Allow patients to receive hemodynamic monitoring–related care without leaving home

EHR, Electronic health record; *HF*, heart failure.

through survey research, cardiology-based care was associated with more investigative and diagnostic requests and improved use of evidence-based medications.[54] As an example, in the CHAMPION trial, nurses employed by the company communicated with heart failure specialists to facilitate a more aggressive approach to managing pulmonary artery pressures above threshold levels. Ultimately, device technology provides information, but health care providers must act upon abnormal data for patients to have improved outcomes.

Conclusion

Implantable hemodynamic monitoring provides an objective assessment of low intrathoracic impedance and elevated pulmonary artery pressures, as abnormal values may represent lung edema and heart failure decompensation. Physical examination and signs and symptoms of heart failure are not sensitive enough to identify patients who require medication and self-care changes. Additionally, some implantable hemodynamic devices provide patients with data that can be used to manage heart failure, achieve euvolemia, improve quality of life, reduce morbidity, and improve survival. As implantable hemodynamic monitoring systems are approved for use and systems become more commonplace, distance care will most likely increase, saving patients time and energy associated with receiving health care at an office or hospital. However, clinicians must have dedicated time to assess and analyze hemodynamic waveforms and values, make knowledgeable decisions about changes in pharmacologic and nonpharmacologic care requirements, and ensure ideal communication with all health care providers and patients to facilitate evidence-based care delivery and optimal follow-up.

Finally, implantable hemodynamic monitoring devices are expensive to insert and use and may not be needed by all patients. It will be important to determine the predictors of normal and abnormal hemodynamic values and realistic outcomes when hemodynamic monitoring is used. In part 2 of the CHAMPION study, long-term hemodynamic monitoring did not lead to further incremental reductions in heart failure hospitalization. Thus, hemodynamic monitoring may be a short-term solution or an acute care solution to optimal treatment of fluid overload and may be unnecessary after the initial period of monitoring and pharmacologic and nonpharmacologic alterations. As the technology matures and develops, future research will answer questions about ideal patients, ideal clinical presentations, and ideal treatment strategies to facilitate and maintain hemodynamic homeostasis.

References

1. Rutherford BD, McCann WD, O'Donovan TP: The value of monitoring pulmonary artery pressure for early detection of left ventricular failure following myocardial infarction, *Circulation* 43(5):655–666, 1971.
2. Russell Jr RO, Hunt D, Potanin C, Rackley CE: Hemodynamic monitoring in a coronary intensive care unit: clinical application, *Arch Intern Med* 130(3):370–376, 1972.
3. Armstrong PW: Contributions of hemodynamic monitoring to the treatment of chronic congestive heart failure, *Can Med Assoc J* 121(7):913–918, 1979.
4. Russell Jr RO, Mantle JA, Rogers WJ, Rackley CE: Current status of hemodynamic monitoring: indication, diagnoses, complications, *Cardiovasc Clin* 11(3):1–13, 1981.
5. Harvey S, Harrison DA, Singer M, et al.: PAC-Man study collaboration: assessment of the clinical effectiveness of pulmonary artery catheters in management of patients in intensive care (PAC-Man): a randomised controlled trial, *Lancet* 366(9484):472–477, 2005.
6. Richard C, Warszawski J, Anguel N, et al.: French Pulmonary Artery Catheter Study Group: early use of the pulmonary artery catheter and outcomes in patients with shock and acute respiratory distress syndrome: a randomized controlled trial, *JAMA* 290(20):2713–2720, 2003.
7. Connors Jr AF, Speroff T, Dawson NV, et al.: The effectiveness of right heart catheterization in the initial care of critically ill patients. SUPPORT Investigators, *JAMA* 276(11):889–897, 1996.

8. Sandham JD, Hull RD, Brant RF, et al.: Canadian Critical Care Clinical Trials Group: a randomized, controlled trial of the use of pulmonary-artery catheters in high-risk surgical patients, *N Engl J Med* 348(1):5–14, 2003.

9. Binanay C, Califf RM, Hasselblad V, et al.: ESCAPE Investigators and ESCAPE Study Coordinators: Evaluation study of congestive heart failure and pulmonary artery catheterization effectiveness: the ESCAPE trial, *JAMA* 294(13):1625–1633, 2005.

10. Shah MR, Hasselblad V, Stevenson LW, et al.: Impact of the pulmonary artery catheter in critically ill patients: meta-analysis of randomized clinical trials, *JAMA* 294(13):1664–1670, 2005.

11. Gershengorn HB, Wunsch H: Understanding changes in established practice: pulmonary after catheter use in critically ill patients, *Crit Care Med* 41(12):2667–2676, 2013.

12. Fonarow GC: The treatment targets in acute decompensated heart failure. *Rev Cardiovasc Med* 2 (Suppl 2):S7–S12.

13. Lucas C, Johnson W, Hamilton MA, et al.: Freedom from congestion predicts good survival despite previous class IV symptoms of heart failure, *Am Heart J* 140:840–847, 2000.

14. Mueller C, Frana B, Rodriguez D, et al.: Emergency diagnosis of congestive heart failure: impact of signs and symptoms, *Can J Cardiol* 21:921–924, 2005.

15. Drazner MH, Hellkamp AS, Leier CV, et al.: Value of clinician assessment of hemodynamics in advanced heart failure: the ESCAPE trial, *Circ Heart Fail* 1(3):170–177, 2008.

16. Yamokoski LM, Hasselblad V, Moser DK, et al.: Prediction of rehospitalization and death in severe heart failure by physicians and nurses of the ESCAPE trial, *J Card Fail* 13(1):8–13, 2007.

17. Drazner MH, Thompson B, Rosenberg PB, et al.: Comparison of impedance cardiography with invasive hemodynamic measurements in patients with heart failure secondary to ischemic or nonischemic cardiomyopathy, *Am J Cardiol* 89(8):993–995, 2002.

18. Albert NM, Hail MD, Li J, Young JB: Equivalence of the bioimpedance and thermodilution methods in measuring cardiac output in hospitalized patients with advanced, decompensated chronic heart failure, *Am J Crit Care* 13(6):469–479, 2004.

19. Kamath SA, Drazner MH, Tasissa G, et al.: Correlation of impedance cardiography with invasive hemodynamic measurements in patients with advanced heart failure: the BioImpedance CardioGraphy (BIG) substudy of the Evaluation Study of Congestive Heart Failure and Pulmonary Artery Catheterization Effectiveness (ESCAPE) Trial, *Am Heart J* 158 (2):217–223, 2009.

20. Chaudhry SI, Mattera JA, Curtis JP, et al.: Telemonitoring in patients with heart failure, *N Engl J Med* 363(24):2301–2309, 2010.

21. Boyne JJ, Vrijhoef HJ, Crijns HJ, et al.: TEHAF investigators: tailored telemonitoring in patients with heart failure: results of a multicentre randomized controlled trial, *Eur J Heart Fail* 14 (7):791–801, 2012.

22. Takahashi PY, Pecina JL, Upatising B, et al.: A randomized controlled trial of telemonitoring in older adults with multiple health issues to prevent hospitalizations and emergency department visits, *Arch Intern Med* 172(10):773–779, 2012.

23. Sanders C, Rogers A, Bowen R: Exploring barriers to participation and adoption of telehealth and telecare within the Whole System Demonstrator trial: a qualitative study, *BMC Health Serv Res* 12(220), 2012.

24. Steimle AE, Stevenson LW, Chelimsky-Fallick C, et al.: Sustained hemodynamic efficacy of therapy tailored to reduce filling pressures in survivors with advanced heart failure, *Circulation* 96(4):1165–1172, 1997.

25. Ohlsson A, Bennett T, Nordlander R, et al.: Monitoring of pulmonary arterial diastolic pressure through a right ventricular pressure transducer, *J Card Fail* 1:161–168, 1995.

26. Ohlsson A, Bennett T, Ottenhoff C, et al.: Long-term recording of cardiac output via an implantable hemodynamic monitoring device, *Eur Heart J* 17:1902–1910, 1996.

27. Ohlsson A, Nordlander R, Bennett T, et al.: Continuous ambulatory hemodynamic monitoring with an implantable system, *Eur Heart J* 19:174–184, 1998.

28. Ohlsson A, Kubo S, Steinhaus D, et al.: Continuous ambulatory monitoring of absolute right ventricular pressure and mixed venous oxygen saturation in patients with heart failure using an implantable hemodynamic monitor: one-year multi-center feasibility study, *Eur Heart J* 11:942–954, 2001.

29. Steinhaus DM, Lemery R, Bresnahan Jr DR, , et al.: Initial experience with an implantable hemodynamic monitor, *Circulation* 93:745–752, 1996.

30. Magalski A, Adamson P, Gadler F, et al.: Continuous ambulatory right heart pressure measurements with an implantable hemodynamic monitor: a multicenter, 12-month follow-up study of patients with chronic heart failure, *J Card Fail* 8(2):63–70, 2002.

31. Adamson PB, Magalski A, Braunschweig F, et al.: Ongoing right ventricular hemodynamics in heart failure: clinical value of measurements derived from an implantable monitoring system, *J Am Coll Cardiol* 41(4):565–571, 2003.

32. Zile MR, Bennett TD: St. John Sutton M, et al.: Transition from chronic compensated to acute decompensated heart failure: pathophysiological insights obtained from continuous monitoring of intracardiac pressures, *Circulation* 118(14):1433–1441, 2008.

33. Bourge RC, Abraham WT, Adamson PB, et al.: COMPASS-HF Study Group. Randomized controlled trial of an implantable continuous hemodynamic monitor in patients with advanced heart failure: the COMPASS-HF study, *J Am Coll Cardiol* 51(11):1073–1079, 2008.

34. Zile MR, Bourge RC, Bennett TD, et al.: Application of implantable hemodynamic monitoring in the management of patients with diastolic heart failure: a subgroup analysis of the COMPASS-HF trial, *J Card Fail* 14(10):816–823, 2008.

35. Stevenson LW, Zile M, Bennett TD, et al.: Chronic ambulatory intracardiac pressures and future heart failure events, *Circ Heart Fail* 3(5):580–587, 2010.

36. Ritzema J, Troughton R, Melton I, et al.: Physician-directed patient self-management of left atrial pressure in advanced chronic heart failure, *Circulation* 121(9):1086–1095, 2010.

37. ClinicalTrials.gov. *Left atrial pressure monitoring to optimize heart failure therapy (LAPTOP-HF).* http://clinicaltrials.gov/ct2/show/NCT01121107?term=HeartPOD&rank=3. Accessed December 12, 2013.

38. Adamson PB, Abraham WT, Aaron M, et al.: CHAMPION trial rationale and design: the long-term safety and clinical efficacy of a wireless pulmonary artery pressure monitoring system, *J Card Fail* 17(1):3–10, 2011.

39. Abraham WT, Adamson PB, Bourge RC, et al.: CHAMPION Trial Study Group: Wireless pulmonary artery hemodynamic monitoring in chronic heart failure: a randomised controlled trial, *Lancet* 377(9766):658–666, 2011.

40. Food and Drug Administration and CaridoMEMS. *CardioMEMS Champion HF Monitoring System PMA Amendment P100045.* http://www.fda.gov/downloads/AdvisoryCommittees/CommitteesMeetingMaterials/MedicalDevices/MedicalDevicesAdvisoryCommittee/CirculatorySystemDevicesPanel/UCM370692.pdf. Accessed December 9, 2013.

41. Lüthje L, Vollmann D, Drescher T, et al.: Intrathoracic impedance monitoring to detect chronic heart failure deterioration: relationship to changes in NT-proBNP, *Eur J Heart Fail* 9 (6–7):716–722, 2007.

42. Wang L: Fundamentals of intrathoracic impedance monitoring in heart failure, *Am J Cardiol* 99 (10A):3G–10G, 2007.

43. Santine M, Ricci RP, Lunati M, et al.: Remote monitoring of patients with biventricular defibrillators through the CareLink system improves clinical management of arrhythmias and heart failure episodes, *J Interv Card Electrophysiol* 24(1):53–61, 2009.

44. Guéguin M, Roux E, Hernández AI, et al.: Exploring time series retrieved from cardiac implantable devices for optimizing patient follow-up, *IEEE Trans Biomed Eng* 55(10):2343–2352, 2008.

45. Maines M, Catanzariti D, Cirrincione C, et al.: Intrathoracic impedance and pulmonary wedge pressure for the detection of heart failure deterioration, *Europace* 12(5):680–685, 2010.

46. Small RS, Wickemeyer W, Germany R, et al.: Changes in intrathoracic impedance are associated with subsequent risk of hospitalizations for acute decompensated heart failure: clinical utility of implanted device monitoring without a patient alert, *J Card Fail* 15(6):475–481, 2009.

47. Sarkar S, Hettrick DA, Koehler J, et al.: Improved algorithm to detect fluid accumulation via intrathoracic impedance monitoring in heart failure patients with implantable devices, *J Card Fail* 17(7):569–576, 2011.

48. Bocchiardo M, Meyer zu Vilsendorf D, Militello C, et al.: Intracardiac impedance monitors stroke volume in resynchronization therapy patients, *Europace* 12(5):702–707, 2010.

49. Puglisi A, Gasparini M, Lunati M, et al.: Persistent atrial fibrillation worsens heart rate variability, activity and heart rate, as shown by a continuous monitoring by implantable biventricular pacemakers in heart failure patients, *J Cardiovasc Electrophysiol* 19(7):693–701, 2008.

50. Jhanjee R, Templeton GA, Sattiraju S, et al.: Relationship of paroxysmal atrial tachyarrhythmias to volume overload: assessment by implanted transpulmonary impedance monitoring, *Circ Heart Fail* 2(5):488–494, 2009.

51. Sekiguchi Y, Tada H, Yoshida K, et al.: Significant increase in the incidence of ventricular arrhythmic events after an intrathoracic impedance change measured with a cardiac resynchronization therapy defibrillator, *Circ J* 75(11):2614–2620, 2011.

52. Krum H: Telemonitoring of fluid status in heart failure: CHAMPION, *Lancet* 377(9776):616–618, 2011.

53. Lieback A, Proff J, Wessel K, Fleck E, Götze S: Remote monitoring of heart failure patients using implantable cardiac pacing devices and external sensors: results of the Insight-HF study, *Clin Res Cardiol* 101(2):101–107, 2012.

54. Rutten FH, Grobbee DE, Hoes AW: Differences between general practitioners and cardiologists in diagnosis and management of heart failure: a survey in every-day practice, *Eur J Heart Fail* 5(3):337–344, 2003.

Hemodynamics of Mechanical Ventilation and Acute Respiratory Distress Syndrome

14

John J. Gallagher

Positive pressure mechanical ventilation is a common intervention used to support patients with respiratory failure resulting from a variety of causes. Although ventilators have increased in complexity and capability over the last 60 years, the main function is largely unchanged. Positive pressure ventilators generate a positive flow of gas into the lungs through a cuffed tube to achieve a predetermined target of either volume (volume control) or pressure (pressure control) to ventilate the patient. It is difficult to imagine providing modern critical care without this essential tool, but positive pressure ventilation is unnatural and has the potential to interfere with normal cardiopulmonary physiology. This is further complicated by the ventilation mode strategy, as well as underlying cardiopulmonary pathophysiology such as heart failure and acute respiratory distress syndrome (ARDS). In this chapter, we will explore the effects of positive pressure mechanical ventilation and ARDS on hemodynamic function in the critically ill patient.

Physiologic Breathing

The normal breathing process supports cardiovascular function. Unlike positive pressure ventilation, natural breathing is a negative pressure process within the thoracic cavity. During a natural breath, the intercostal muscles and diaphragm contract to expand the chest cavity. The lungs expand with the chest cavity because of the adherence of the visceral and parietal pleural layers. The inspiratory effort of a normal breath creates a negative intrathoracic pressure relative to the atmosphere, drawing air into the trachea, large and small airways and eventually expanding the alveoli. Peripheral alveoli expand first, followed by more central alveoli (Figure 14-1).[1]

Patient Comfort

- Assess for pain by using patient self-report or nonverbal pain assessment scales.
- Administer analgesic agents based on assessment findings and prior to anticipated painful events such as turning, suctioning, or repositioning the artificial airway.
- Utilize continuous lateral rotation sleep surfaces to improve gas exchange, as indicated.

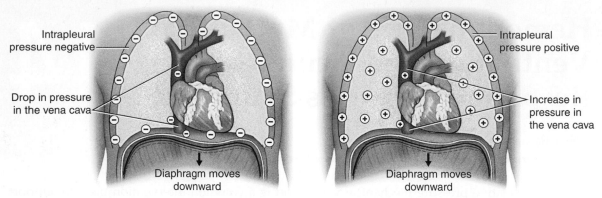

Intrapleural
pressure negative

Drop in pressure
in the vena cava

Diaphragm moves
downward

Intrapleural
pressure positive

Increase in
pressure in
the vena cava

Diaphragm moves
downward

FIGURE 14-1 A, During spontaneous breathing, the intercostal muscles contract, and the diaphragm expands the thoracic cavity, creating negative intrathoracic pressure drawing air into the lungs. This negative pressure supports venous return to the right atrium. **B,** During the inspiratory phase of positive pressure ventilation, venous return may be reduced, as positive pressure is exerted on the vena cava and right atrium.

The negative intrathoracic pressure not only supports ventilation of the lung but also promotes central venous return, right atrial filling, and right ventricular preload.[2–7] Augmentation of venous return occurs when the diaphragm contracts pressing down on the abdominal cavity. This downward movement compresses the mesenteric venous complex, thus promoting return of this blood volume to the central venous circulation. Known as the "thoracic pump," this is one of two mechanisms supporting venous return to the right side of the heart. The second mechanism, the "skeletal pump," promotes venous return through contraction of muscles around the peripheral veins (Figure 14-2).[3,4,7,8] Contraction of the skeletal muscles compresses the veins, propelling venous blood volume from the capacitance vessels to the central venous system, further augmenting right ventricular preload.[8] The combined function of the thoracic pump and skeletal pump mechanism is essential for normal circulatory function.

Venous Return

Key to appreciating the effects of ventilation and disease states on clinical hemodynamics is an understanding of venous return. The venous (capacitance) system comprises highly distensible vessels that hold approximately 70% of the body's blood volume (Figure 14-3). This volume can be classified as either "unstressed" volume or "stressed" volume. Unstressed volume represents the largest volume of blood in the venous reservoir that is under minimal pressure.[4] The stressed volume accounts for 30% of the total blood volume and is the venous volume under pressure resulting from increase in vascular tone or pressure surrounding the venous system.[3,4,9–11] Unstressed volume can be converted to stressed volume as vascular tone or pressure surrounding the venous system increases. Vascular tone may be increased through the effects of endogenous catecholamines or the administration of exogenous (vasopressor) agents.[2,3,12]

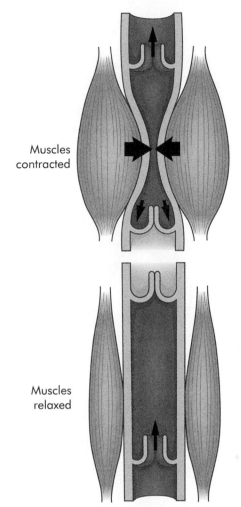

FIGURE 14-2 Contraction of the skeletal muscles compresses the veins converting unstressed blood volume to stressed volume thereby supporting venous return to the heart. (From Huether SE, McCance KL: *Understanding pathophysiology*, ed 5, St. Louis, 2012, Mosby.)

The mean systemic filling pressure (also called the mean circulatory filling pressure) is generated from the stressed volume and it largely determines the blood flow to the right side of the heart, specifically the right atrium. This concept was illustrated by Magder (Figure 14-4) as a reservoir with a drain in the side. The volume above the drain represented stressed volume, and the volume under the opening of the drain represented unstressed volume. In this model, the stressed volume (mean systemic filling pressure), combined with right atrial pressure and resistance to venous return, determines blood flow back to the heart.[4]

Right atrial pressure can impact venous return relative to the mean systemic filling pressure. This is the pressure of the venous blood volume that returns to the right heart. Normally, right atrial pressure is the lower value, allowing for forward flow from the venous circulation into the right atrium. The normal gradient from the venous system

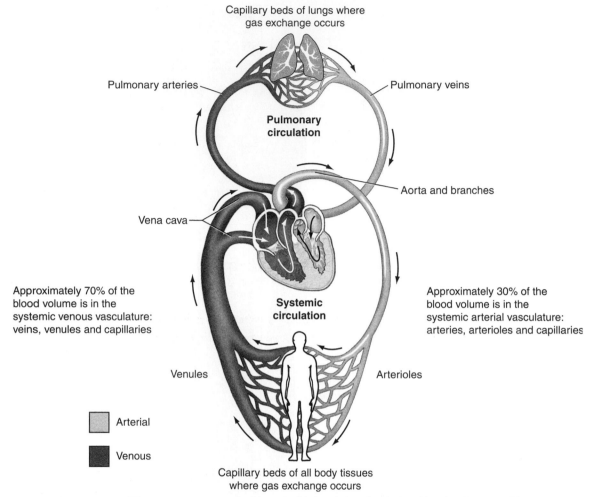

Capillary beds of lungs where
gas exchange occurs

Pulmonary arteries

Pulmonary veins

**Pulmonary
circulation**

Aorta and branches

Vena cava

Approximately 70% of the
blood volume is in the
systemic venous vasculature:
veins, venules and capillaries

Approximately 30% of the
blood volume is in the
systemic arterial vasculature:
arteries, arterioles and capillaries

**Systemic
circulation**

Venules

Arterioles

Arterial

Venous

Capillary beds of all body tissues
where gas exchange occurs

FIGURE 14-3 The venous system holds two thirds of the circulating blood volume and is described as a capacitance system, where the flow of blood that returns to the right side of the heart can be increased or decreased, as needed. Volume that exerts pressure on vessel walls is described as *stressed volume*, defined as a transmural pressure above zero. Venous volume in a non–pressure state is referred to as the *unstressed volume*, defined as a transmural pressure of zero. Veins are over 20 times more compliant than similar arteries and can thus hold the additional volume. The sum of the stressed and unstressed volume represents the total volume in the system. See Figure 14-4 for a further explanation of this concept.

to the right atrium is approximately 4 to 8 millimeters of mercury (mm Hg). Venous return is maximal when right atrial pressure equals zero.[2-4,7,13] Conditions that improve venous return include those that increase the stressed volume and decrease venous compliance, resistance, and right atrial pressure. Conditions that increase right heart afterload such as positive pressure ventilation, positive end-expiratory pressure (PEEP), or right ventricular heart failure will increase right atrial pressure relative to mean systemic filling pressure, thus reducing venous return.[13]

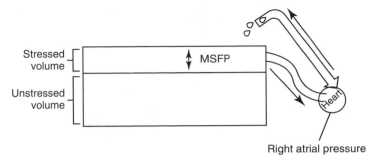

FIGURE 14-4 The "bathtub" reservoir represents the total volume that can potentially return to the right heart. The volume above the drain represents stressed volume, whereas the volume under the opening of the outflow drain represents unstressed volume. Stressed volume, generates the mean systemic filling pressure (MSFP), and combined with right atrial pressure and resistance to venous return, determines the volume of blood that flows back to the right atrium and the right ventricle. The unstressed volume represents a reserve volume that can be mobilized when physiologically required. See Figure 14-3 for a further explanation of this concept. (Adapted from Magder S: Point: Counterpoint: The classical Guyton view that mean systemic pressure, right arterial pressure, and venous resistance govern venous return is/is not correct, *J Appl Physiol* 101 (5): 1523–1525, 2006.)

The skeletal pump described above may contribute to the conversion of unstressed volume to stressed volume. Patients who are immobile lose the skeletal pump contribution, resulting in venous or lymphatic stasis and edema. Early mobility in the critically ill ventilated patient may help limit the effects of immobility through restoration of the skeletal pump mechanism.[8]

Circulating Blood Volume

Conditions that alter vascular volume may also impact venous return. Hypovolemia, regardless of cause, reduces circulating vascular volume, venous return, and, eventually, cardiac output. Compensatory mechanisms for decreased preload, for example, tachycardia and vasoconstriction, have time-limited effectiveness.[3,7,14] Conversely, hypervolemia may increase venous return. Hypervolemia may occur as a result of overzealous fluid resuscitation. Although usually well tolerated with normal cardiac function, it will be detrimental with left ventricular failure.[3,7,14–18]

Guyton described the interaction of venous return and cardiac function through the illustration of a venous return curve combined with the cardiac function curve, or Starling curve (Figure 14-5).[9–11,16] The venous return curve represents venous flow (stressed volume) from the reservoir to the right heart (atrium). In this relationship, the Starling curve represents cardiac function and is plotted against right atrial pressure. The intersection of these curves provides the working or optimal value for this relationship (see Figure 14-5, point A).[4,10,11,16] This relationship can change, depending on increases or decreases in venous return or subsequent shifts in cardiac function. Conditions such as hypovolemia or venodilation may reduce venous return (stressed volume) shifting the curve to the left (see Figure 14-5, from point A to point B

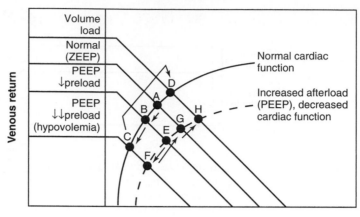

Right atrial pressure

FIGURE 14-5 The normal relationship between venous return and the cardiac function curve is illustrated by the intersection at point A. The application of positive end-expiratory pressure (PEEP) may reduce venous return and preload from point A to point B. In hypovolemia, the addition of PEEP may markedly reduce preload (point A/B to C). Volume administration can increase preload and restore the normal relationship back to point A or to supra-normal levels (D). PEEP may also shift the cardiac output curve to the right as a result of increased afterload. This combination of preload reduction and afterload increase, would reduce overall cardiac output and change the intersection of the venous return and cardiac function (point E). In the face of hypovolemia, venous return and subsequent cardiac function may become markedly depressed (point F). However, PEEP may also increase the mean systemic filling pressure (MSFP) by increasing stressed volume through activation of the sympathoadrenal response. This would increase venous return and maintain the venous return/cardiac function relationship to near normal (point G). Administration of fluid volume may further augment venous return (point H).

or C),[2–4,7,13] whereas increases in stressed volume (vasoconstriction) or fluid administration may increase venous return shifting the curve to the right (see Figure 14-5, point C or B back to A). These shifts can have subsequent effects on cardiac performance as well.[2,3,7,9] Although combinations of these volume and pressure interactions are many, this chapter will focus on hemodynamic interactions associated with positive pressure ventilation and PEEP.

Positive Pressure Ventilation

Patient Education

- Explain the indications for ventilator support.
- Explain the reason for any changes to ventilator settings or strategies and the expected outcomes.
- Review any hemodynamic monitoring devices and describe their purpose in monitoring changes associated with mechanical ventilation and management.

- Explain any changes in hemodynamic variables, and address concerns as they arise.
- Describe the procedure for ventilator liberation and assessment strategies during the process.
- Explain that the patient will be doing more of the work of breathing as ventilator support is reduced.

The implementation of positive pressure mechanical ventilation alters the complementary physiologic balance between normal breathing and hemodynamic function (see Figure 14-1). During a positive pressure breath, gas flow enters the trachea, bronchi, bronchioles, and alveoli filling from the central airways to the peripheral alveoli.[1,3,19] This sequence is opposite to that of physiologic breathing, as described above. Because of this, peripheral alveoli may be under-filled, depending on the tidal volume used in relation to the patient's lung capacity.

The hemodynamic effects of positive pressure ventilation result from alteration in the normal relationship between physiologic ventilation and cardiovascular function. These changes may affect venous return as well as cardiac function.[1–3,6,18,20] Additionally, they may be further determined by underlying cardiopulmonary pathophysiology. Each of these factors will be discussed further.

Venous Return and Positive Pressure Ventilation

Venous return is determined primarily by the gradient between mean systemic filling pressure and the right atrial pressure.[4,10] Both positive pressure ventilation and PEEP have the potential to reduce venous return by increasing pressure on the superior and inferior vena cava in the thoracic cavity thereby reducing flow to the right atrium (see Figure 14-1).[2,13,21–24] Increases in venous return through an increase in mean systemic filling pressure may occur as a result of neurohumoral responsiveness, vasopressor administration, or volume administration.[1–3,7,19,25]

The degree to which venous return is impacted by positive pressure ventilation is dependent on various factors. Such factors may include intravascular volume status, right heart function, and positive pressure increases in intrathoracic pressure transmitted to the heart and vascular structures. Intrathoracic pressure influence is complex because it is determined by chest wall and lung mechanics, as well as the ventilation mode parameters. Pulmonary mechanics include airway resistance, compliance, and elastance.[18,26,27] Ventilation parameters include tidal volume, PEEP level, and use of inverse ratio ventilation, or spontaneous breathing modes such as pressure-support and biphasic ventilation. Each of these factors, individually or in combination, will affect patients differently. When possible, this impact should be anticipated to prevent hemodynamic compromise. Each of these factors will be discussed further.

Positive Pressure Ventilation and Effect on the Right Heart

Right Heart Preload

Alterations in right heart hemodynamics associated with positive pressure ventilation primarily include reduction in preload and increase in afterload. Preload is impacted through reduction of venous return by mechanisms already discussed. Although reduction in preload as a result of decreased venous return is often cited as the cause of diminished right heart output, other evidence suggests that increased afterload on the right ventricle plays a more significant role.[2,12,13,28–30]

Ventilation and Perfusion Ratio

From a physiologic standpoint, total lung ventilation (V) and perfusion (Q) are equally matched with the V/Q ratio equal to 0.8 to 1. In reality, the V/Q ratio varies, depending on the lung region, patient position, mechanical ventilation, and pathophysiologic alterations in ventilation, perfusion, or both.

Lung Zone Pressures

In 1964, West described the relationship between alveolar, arterial, and venous pressures in the lung, progressing from the apex to base when a person is in an upright position (Figure 14-6, *A*).[31] In this model, Zone 1 is the upper third of the lung, where ventilation is greater than perfusion. Zone 2 is the middle portion of the lung, where ventilation and perfusion are more equally matched. Zone 3 is the bottom portion of the lung, where perfusion is greater than ventilation.[31] Although often described as progressing from the apices to the base of the lung, these zones progress from the anterior to the posterior lung when the patient is lying in the supine position.

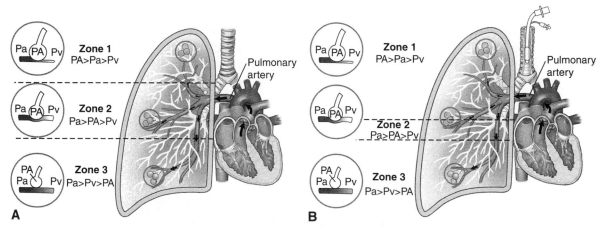

FIGURE 14-6 A, Lung Model developed by John West demonstrating ventilation and perfusion relationships: **Zone I**: Alveolar ventilation pressure (PA) predominates, followed by arterial pressure (Pa) and venous pressure (Pv) in the circulation, written as PA > Pa > Pv. **Zone II**: Pulmonary arterial pressure predominates (Pa) followed by alveolar pressure (PA) and venous pressure (Pv), written as Pa > PA > Pv. **Zone III**: Pulmonary arterial pressure predominates (Pa), followed by venous pressure (Pv) and alveolar (PA) pressure, written as Pa > Pv > PA. **B,** When applying alveolar recruitment strategies and positive pressure ventilation, Zone 1 may significantly impact Zone 2.

Even though physiologic variations in the V/Q ratio may occur as described above, pathophysiologic changes in the V/Q ratio also occur. Ventilation in excess of perfusion, or perfusion in excess of ventilation, results in a V/Q mismatch. When these imbalances occur to the extreme, they result in dead space or shunt conditions. Dead space ventilation conditions occur when the alveoli are ventilated, but there is no perfusion through the associated alveolar capillaries. Pulmonary embolism is a classic example of dead space ventilation (see Chapter 8, Figure 8-7). A shunt condition results when alveoli are not ventilated (fluid filled or collapsed), but perfusion to the alveoli is relatively normal. Pulmonary edema, pneumonia, or ARDS may result in shunt conditions. Clinically, both dead space and shunt conditions may co-exist simultaneously. Patients with ARDS have alveolar collapse (shunt) as well as perfusion abnormalities that result in dead space conditions. This is further complicated by the application of positive pressure ventilation.

The normal ventilation perfusion relationships described above can be altered by positive pressure ventilation and PEEP as alveolar overdistention may increase Zone 1 conditions into Zone 2 as shown in Figure 14-6, *B*. In addition to causing alveolar damage, overdistention may compress adjacent pulmonary capillaries, limiting blood flow to overdistended alveoli and resulting in V/Q mismatch or dead space conditions. This compression also redirects capillary blood flow in the direction of least resistance toward underventilated or collapsed alveoli. Perfusion will increase to these derecruited alveolar areas without the benefit of matched ventilation, resulting in worsening shunt (Figure 14-7).[13,24,32–35]

Pulmonary Pitfalls of PEEP

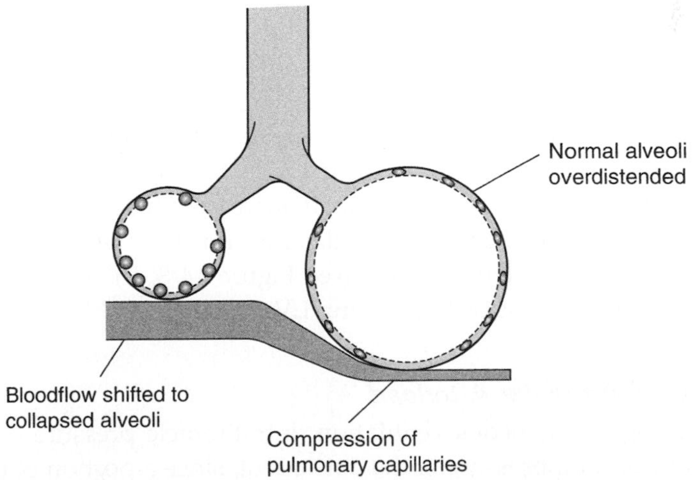

Normal alveoli overdistended

Bloodflow shifted to collapsed alveoli

Compression of pulmonary capillaries

FIGURE 14-7 Overdistention of normal functioning alveoli will compress adjacent capillaries, moving blood flow toward the collapsed alveoli and potentially increasing shunt.

Right Ventricular Afterload

In addition to mechanical vasoconstriction associated with alveolar overdistention, hypoxic vasoconstriction in the lung may further increase pulmonary vascular resistance and right ventricular afterload. Hypoxic vasoconstriction, mediator-induced vasoconstriction, and microvascular clots in the pulmonary circulation contribute to the right ventricular (RV) dysfunction often seen in ARDS.[36-38] These concepts will be discussed later in this chapter.

RV dilation may also negatively impact coronary artery blood flow, as high wall tension compresses the right coronary artery reducing blood flow to the myocardium. Increased RV afterload associated with vasoconstriction and positive pressure ventilation may further increase myocardial oxygen demand, leading to ischemia and infarction.[2,4,28,29,39-42]

Therapeutic strategies to reduce right heart afterload include the use of recruitment strategies to open collapsed alveoli to improve ventilation or oxygenation and reverse hypoxic vasoconstriction. Also, pulmonary vasodilators such as inhaled prostacyclin and nitric oxide may be used to reduce pulmonary vascular resistance and decrease afterload.[13,30,43-45] These inhaled agents are distributed to the best-ventilated regions of the lung. They cross the alveolar capillary membrane into the adjacent capillaries, causing vasodilation and improved perfusion to the ventilated alveoli. This, in turn, improves the V/Q matching of these units, allowing for better gas exchange.[46,47] Although these changes may be beneficial from a physiologic standpoint, reductions in mortality have not been demonstrated, even with severe hypoxemia.[48]

Positive Pressure Ventilation and Effect on the Left Heart

Left Heart Preload

The impact of positive pressure ventilation and PEEP on the left heart is caused by the downstream effects of intrathoracic pressure on the right heart. Left ventricular (LV) preload is reduced as a result of reduced RV output. Though positive pressure ventilation may expel some blood from the pulmonary circulation into the left atrium contributing to LV preload, this does not fully compensate for the reductions in left heart preload associated with the reduction in RV output to the left side of the heart.[1,2,4,15,17,18,29,39,49]

Similarly, ventricular interdependence (Figure 14-8, *A*) contributes to reduction of LV preload. As RV afterload increases, the right ventricle becomes distended, displacing the shared ventricular septum into the left ventricle, reducing the filling capacity of the left ventricle (see Figure 14-8, *B*). This decreases the diastolic filling capacity, subsequently reducing LV output.[2,3,13,39,50]

Left Ventricular Afterload

During spontaneous ventilation, intrathoracic pressure decreases more so than the intraluminal pressure of the aortic root, since a portion of the aorta is located outside of the thoracic cavity. LV afterload is greater during spontaneous inspiration than

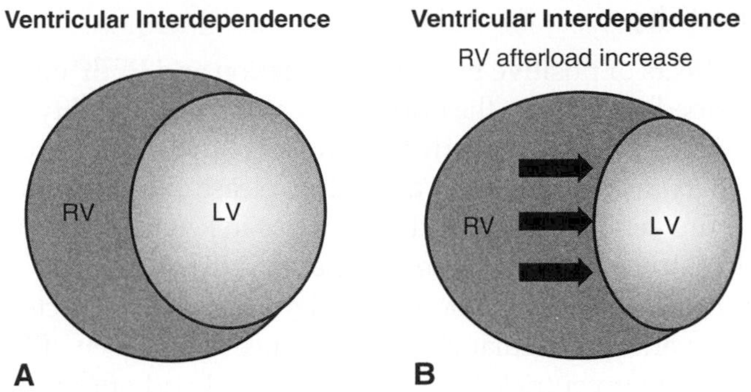

Ventricular Interdependence

Ventricular Interdependence

RV afterload increase

A

B

FIGURE 14-8 A, The shared intraventricular septum between the right and left ventricles gives rise to the concept of ventricular interdependence. Changes in the size of one ventricle may impact the size of the other because of the shared septal wall. **B,** Increases in right ventricular afterload as a result of positive pressure may result in right ventricular dilation and a shift of the intraventricular septum to the left.

during spontaneous expiration. Additionally, RV filling during spontaneous inspiration results in transient displacement of the ventricular septum into the left ventricle, reducing LV size, compliance, and preload.[2,4,13] This does not negatively impact cardiac output in those with normal LV function, but in patients with LV failure, increased work of spontaneous breathing may further increase myocardial oxygen demand, which results in ischemia.[1,19,51] This factor should be considered during ventilator liberation as the patient transitions from positive pressure ventilator support to spontaneous breathing. In patients with impaired ventricular function, transition from full support to spontaneous breathing may increase LV workload. Spontaneous breathing augments venous return to the right heart (RV preload), which results in an increase in left heart preload as well as in LV afterload. Increased work of breathing may also increase myocardial oxygen demand.[1,3,17-19]

During positive pressure ventilation, the transient increase in pressure during the inspiratory phase results in higher intrathoracic pressure relative to the extrathoracic pressure. Higher intrathoracic pressure applied to the mediastinum and intrathoracic aorta results in an elevated extramural pressure relative to the intraluminal pressure of the aorta and the circulatory system outside of the thorax at atmospheric pressure. This pressure gradient transiently reduces LV afterload and improves LV output.[2,4,13,52-54] With the application of PEEP, intrathoracic pressure remains elevated during the expiratory phase as well, sustaining the benefit of some afterload reduction during the exhalation phase of the positive pressure ventilation breath. Although this application of PEEP should theoretically improve cardiac output in the normal heart, it does not result in appreciable improvements. This may be due to co-existing reductions in RV preload, increased RV afterload and subsequent decrease in LV preload.[3] In LV failure, however, there is an increased sensitivity to preload reduction. PEEP may, therefore, have a beneficial effect in improving LV function by reducing LV preload and LV afterload in a similar fashion to vasodilators in heart failure.[1,2,4,13,29]

Cardiac Contractility

The effects of positive pressure ventilation and PEEP on preload and afterload are well described. However, the impact on cardiac contractility, the third component of stroke volume is less clear. Inotropic function may be indirectly affected by reduction in coronary artery blood flow as well as release of humoral mediators as a result of positive pressure ventilation and PEEP. Increase in RV afterload may reduce RV ejection fraction and worsen cor pulmonale associated with ARDS.[13,29,30,42,55] LV contractility may be reduced as overdistention of the right ventricle impacts the left ventricle through the septum and ventricular interdependence. Conversely, PEEP may improve contractility in the failing ventricle by reducing preload and afterload as described above.[13]

Heart Rate

Reductions in stroke volume are normally compensated by an increase in heart rate to maintain physiologic cardiac output. This is primarily mediated through the carotid baroreceptors (see Chapter 1, Figure 1-16). With positive pressure ventilation and PEEP, this chronotropic compensatory response appears to be blunted.[13] Despite reduction in stroke volume, some patients maintain normal or even reduced heart rates. Activation of pulmonary stretch receptors may be implicated in this response. The classic Hering-Breur reflex results in a transient increase in heart rate during inspiration. This is often the underlying cause of sinus arrhythmia. Inflation with higher pressures, however, may result in lower heart rate or bradycardia. Such may be the case with positive pressure ventilation and PEEP. This is clinically important, since the expected tachycardic response traditionally associated with reduced stroke volume may be blunted and not be a reliable hemodynamic finding in these patients.

Positive End-Expiratory Pressure

PEEP is a positive pressure applied through the ventilator, maintained during the expiratory phase of the ventilator breath to prevent alveolar collapse. Under normal physiologic conditions, alveolar collapse is prevented during exhalation by the volume of air remaining within the lungs; this is known as the functional residual capacity or FRC. Surfactant secreted by the type II alveolar cells reduces alveolar surface tension, resisting alveolar collapse associated with normal elasticity. Certain disease conditions such as ARDS may disrupt this normal function resulting in alveolar collapse.[36,37,56]

Atelectasis may result in alveolar collapse from hypoventilation. Resolution may be achieved in spontaneously breathing patients with deep breathing exercises or incentive spirometry. During mechanical ventilation, adding PEEP may resolve or prevent atelectasis. The level of PEEP required to achieve this goal is patient-specific; however, PEEP levels up to 5 centimeters of water (cm H_2O) are often employed empirically in the intubated patient to prevent atelectasis.[57] In more severe conditions such as ARDS, the alveoli fill with proteinaceous fluid resulting from immune-mediated injury to the alveolar capillary membrane.[36,56,58,59] This alteration in permeability leads to pulmonary edema that reduces alveolar gas exchange and inactivates surfactant, resulting in both fluid filled and collapsed alveoli.[36,56,59] Edema is most prominent in dependent regions of the lung, with the edema pattern shifting, depending on patient position.[56,58] Further, the weight of the fluid-filled lung tissue may compress the regions below them, thus worsening the alveolar collapse. This collapse may range in severity and result in varying degrees of shunt.

In these conditions, PEEP may be used to prevent end-expiratory alveolar collapse after delivery of the ventilator breath or, at higher levels, used to assist in the lung recruitment. Many patients are placed on low levels of physiologic PEEP (5 cm H_2O) as a standard setting on mechanical ventilation. This level does not impact hemodynamics but may prevent or improve atelectasis.[57] At higher levels, PEEP may affect hemodynamics in a similar fashion to positive pressure ventilation as discussed above. The terms "low" PEEP and "high" PEEP are not defined consistently in the literature. A recent Cochrane review compared high versus low PEEP in mechanically ventilated adult patients with acute lung injury and ARDS and included seven studies in the meta-analysis. Across all studies, the definition of low versus high PEEP differed.[60] In most cases, low PEEP was less that 10 cm H_2O, and high PEEP was greater than 10 cm H_2O. The absolute PEEP value is less likely to predict the hemodynamic effect. Rather, it is the combination of PEEP, lung mechanics, and vascular volume status that determine how a patient will respond to the set PEEP. It is important to remember that unlike the episodic pressure changes associated with the inspiratory and expiratory phases of the positive pressure ventilation breath, PEEP is maintained during exhalation as well.[23,32,61,62] Therefore, hemodynamic changes will be sustained or altered, depending on the level of PEEP and for any increases or decreases in the PEEP settings.

Positive End-Expiratory Pressure and Venous Return

When PEEP is not applied, a condition of zero PEEP (ZEEP) is assumed. The relationship of venous return to cardiac output (see Figure 14-5, point A) is maintained.

PEEP and Low Preload: With the addition of PEEP, the venous return curve may be shifted to the left (see Figure 14-5, point B) reducing preload. In the face of pre-existing hypovolemia, the addition of PEEP may markedly reduce preload (see Figure 14-5, point C). Volume administration can restore the normal relationship (back to point A) or to above normal levels (see Figure 14-5, point D).

PEEP and Increased Afterload: However, PEEP may also shift the cardiac output curve to the right as a result of increased afterload.[3,4,13,33] PEEP has combination hemodynamic effects of both RV preload reduction and increased RV afterload, thus PEEP can reduce overall cardiac output (see Figure 14-5, point E).

PEEP and Mean Systemic Filling Pressure: In the face of hypovolemia, venous return may decrease and subsequent cardiac function may become markedly depressed (see Figure 14-5, point F). However, PEEP may also increase the mean systemic filling pressure of the venous return by increasing stressed volume through activation of the sympathoadrenal response.[2,3,7,13] This would increase venous return and maintain the venous return–cardiac function relationship to near normal (see Figure 14-5, point G).

Administration of fluid volume may further augment venous return (see Figure 14-5, point H). The concepts of mean systemic filling pressure and stressed volume are illustrated in Figures 14-3 and 14-4.

Reductions in venous return related to PEEP seems to be effected by vascular volume status. For patients who are hypovolemic, increases in PEEP may result in compression of the superior vena cava as demonstrated by echocardiography.[28,40,63] Patients who are euvolemic or hypervolemic may not experience reduction in venous return, even at PEEP level of up to 20 cm H_2O.[2,3,13,33,42,64,65] Conversely, those who have underlying hypovolemia may experience hypotension resulting from reduced cardiac preload and increased afterload, as previously discussed.

Positive End-Expiratory Pressure and Right Heart Function

Reductions in RV preload from PEEP are the result of reduced venous return. However, PEEP may also impact RV afterload by decreasing or increasing pulmonary vascular resistance. In the collapsed regions of the lung, pulmonary vascular resistance is increased because of hypoxic vasoconstriction as well as compression of alveolar capillaries by fluid-filled alveoli.[2,4,13,30,54,66] When positive pressure is applied to re-expand the collapsed regions, it improves gas exchange and oxygenation, thus reversing hypoxic vasoconstriction and reducing pulmonary vascular resistance. Additionally, PEEP reduces pulmonary vascular resistance by inflating the collapsed regions, restoring the functional residual capacity (FRC) and opening small pulmonary capillaries.[13,38,43,67,68] At lung volumes below the FRC, vascular resistance is high. As alveoli are re-expanded to normal FRC from residual volume, the expansion of the alveoli opens capillaries, improving alveolar capillary blood flow and reducing pulmonary vascular resistance. These two mechanisms highlight the beneficial impact of PEEP in improving RV function through afterload reduction.[2,3] It is important to note however that overinflation of alveoli toward total lung capacity will cause capillary compression increasing pulmonary vascular resistance and RV afterload. This is an important consideration, as increased RV afterload combined with decreased preload will reduce overall cardiac output.[2–4,29,33]

Although some studies have shown that RV function is preserved with PEEP levels up to 20 cm H_2O or greater, others have noted reduction of RV function and the development of cor pulmonale with the use of PEEP. This may be even more prominent in patients with ARDS, when ARDS is associated with RV afterload elevation from alveolar collapse, pulmonary vasoconstriction, and pulmonary capillary microthrombosis. Lung-protective strategies aimed at reducing overdistention (low stretch) and recruitment are desirable to reduce RV afterload and improve cardiac output.[30,33,42,55,69–71]

Positive End-Expiratory Pressure and Left Heart Function

Left heart preload may be reduced by PEEP because of reduction in RV output from the mechanism described above. Additionally, ventricular interdependence associated with a shared ventricular septum results in decreased LV preload resulting from displacement of the septum into the left ventricle from RV dilation (Figure 14-8, *B*). For patients with failing LV function, PEEP, similar to venodilators, may improve function by reducing LV preload and by reducing afterload through an increase in juxtacardiac pressure in relation to extrathoracic pressure. This gradient improves the ejection of blood from the left ventricle.[4,7,13,29,53,72]

Patient Safety

Onset of hypotension in the ventilated patient should cause immediate suspicion of tension pneumothorax. This often manifests as hypotension that progresses to pulseless electrical activity (PEA). Diminished breath sounds on the affected side as well as subcutaneous emphysema and jugular vein distension may be present. Immediate treatment involves needle decompression of the affected side and insertion of a chest tube.

Hemodynamic Alterations in Acute Respiratory Distress Syndrome

Acute respiratory distress syndrome (ARDS) is a condition that results from an alveolar permeability defect that leads to pulmonary edema, causing refractory hypoxemia and respiratory failure. The 2012 Berlin Definition of ARDS provides updated criteria for the identification and severity classification of ARDS (Table 14-1) and may be helpful

TABLE 14-1 Comparison of ARDSnet and Berlin Criteria for Acute Respiratory Distress Syndrome (ARDS)

CRITERIA	ARDSnet[72a]	BERLIN[58]
Onset	Acute	Acute within 1 week of clinical insult
PEEP	Not included in definition	Incorporated into categories
Chest radiograph CT (Berlin only)	Diffuse or homogenous Patchy infiltrates	Bilateral opacities not explained by effusions, lung collapse or nodules
Classification with P/F ratio		
P/F <300 on 0.4 FiO_2	ALI (Acute Lung Injury)	Mild ARDS: PEEP or CPAP ≥5 cm H_2O
P/F <200 on 0.4 FiO_2	ARDS regardless of PEEP	Moderate ARDS: PEEP or CPAP ≥5 cm H_2O
P/F <100	–	Severe ARDS: PEEP or CPAP ≥5 cm H_2O
Left heart dysfunction	PAOP <18 mm Hg	Respiratory failure not explained by heart failure, overload or history. Echocardiography for objective assessment

cm H_2O, Centimeters of water; *CPAP*, continuous positive airway pressure; *CT*, computed tomography; *FiO_2*, fraction of inspired oxygen; *mm Hg*, millimeters of mercury; *PAOP*, pulmonary artery occlusion pressure; *PEEP*, positive end-expiratory pressure; *P/F*, PaO_2/FiO_2 ratio.

in distinguishing ARDS from other conditions. Alveolar capillary membrane damage with fluid-filled and collapsed alveoli is a hallmark finding. This damage results in a decrease in lung compliance (high elastance) and other pathophysiologic changes that may impact normal cardiopulmonary function.[58,59,73] Vasoconstriction with microvascular thrombi formation, bronchoconstriction, and alterations in normal oxygen delivery and consumption associated from inflammatory cytokines are also evident. The combination of these factors results in increased RV afterload and disease-associated RV failure or cor pulmonale. Mortality associated with ARDS has remained largely unchanged since its description in 1967.[59] Improvements in outcome have been attributed to support strategies rather than to treatment of the condition itself. Key to this support has been improvements in ventilator technology, our understanding of lung ventilator interactions in ARDS, and modifications in ventilation strategy based on this knowledge.[69,74–77]

Ventilation and Acute Respiratory Distress Syndrome

Although mechanical ventilation is a mainstay of support in ARDS, the use of large tidal volumes relative to the size of the injured lung have been implicated in the development of ventilator-induced lung injury and worsening RV failure. The Acute Respiratory Distress Syndrome Network (ARDSnet) trial compared a traditional tidal volume of 12 milliliters per kilogram (mL/kg) predicted body weight, to a low tidal volume of 6 mL/kg predicted body weight, in patients with ARDS, and demonstrated a 22% lower mortality rate in patients ventilated with the low tidal volume strategy.[77] This led to the recommendation that low tidal volumes between 4 to 8 mL/kg of predicted body weight be used as a lung protective strategy. Although the survival benefit may have been based on the reduction in ventilator-induced lung injury, emerging evidence suggests that the use of low tidal volume has also reduced the incidence of RV failure in this population.[28,30,33,40,78]

In the face of reduced lung compliance, larger tidal volumes result in higher inflation pressures in the lung. This has potential to increase RV afterload significantly, in addition to those factors associated with the disease state itself. Using a smaller tidal volume and targeting a plateau pressure of less than 30 cm H_2O would reduce inspiratory pressure and afterload.[13,28,30,40,55,75,78–81] This strategy, along with recruitment tactics (described below) to improve alveolar ventilation and reverse hypoxic vasoconstriction, may be responsible for the lower incidence of RV failure than was observed in the past.[55]

Recruitment Strategies and Hemodynamic Impact

Recruitment strategies are employed to reverse alveolar collapse and improve gas exchange. This practice is part of an "open lung" approach aimed not only at re-expanding collapsed alveoli, but preventing repeated end-expiratory alveolar collapse and atelectatic trauma. Recruitment strategies may be carried out in several ways. Two general approaches include the intermittent or episodic recruitment maneuver and transition to a recruitment mode of ventilation.[23,34,35,50,61,65,68,82]

Intermittent recruitment maneuvers involve the application of a brief 30 to 40-second sustained inflation of the lungs with the use of continuous positive airway pressure (CPAP) at a level of 30 to 40 cm H_2O to open collapsed alveoli. After the maneuver, it is essential to set the PEEP higher than the premaneuver level to sustain the gained alveolar recruitment.[32,35,41,50,68] During the recruitment maneuver, patients may experience hypotension related to reduced cardiac output resulting from increased intrathoracic pressure. Whether this occurs, or the degree to which this occurs, is, in part, dependent on the patient's intravascular volume status and the degree to which inflation pressures are transmitted to the cardiovascular structures.[24,32,50,65,66,83–85]

Another approach to lung recruitment is the conversion to a ventilation mode that facilitates alveolar recruitment by the style of ventilator breath delivery. Common modes in this category include pressure control ventilation (PCV), with or without inverse ratio, as well as dual control modes; biphasic airway pressure release ventilation (APRV); and high-frequency oscillation ventilation (HFOV). While each of these modes is different, they are similar in that they promote recruitment of the collapsed lung regions through a sustained increase in mean airway pressure (Paw). This may improve both oxygenation and ventilation over time.

With the exception of HFOV, the other modes listed above are pressure modes of ventilation with similar breath delivery styles as described below.

Clinical Reasoning Pearl

Patients on PEEP greater than 10 cm H_2O or on nontraditional ventilation modes such as APRV should be maintained on the ventilator rather than manually ventilated with bag–valve mask during transport. These parameters are challenging to maintain and duplicate with manual ventilation and may result in alveolar derecruitment, hypoxia, and hemodynamic instability. If converting to manual ventilation or another mode of ventilation for transport, a brief trial period on the new strategy should be undertaken before transport to ensure that it will support the patient adequately.

Pressure control ventilation (PCV), with or without inverse ratio, provides some advantages over conventional volume control ventilation in the way the breath is delivered and the impact on Paw.[85,86] In volume control ventilation, a positive pressure flow of gas is delivered to the lungs until the set tidal volume is reached. The peak inspiratory pressure (PIP) is reached when the full tidal volume is delivered. This corresponds with the highest inspiratory pressure generated in the lungs (Figure 14-9). For any delivered tidal volume, the pressure generated to deliver that volume will vary, depending on airway resistance and lung compliance. Although the delivered volume

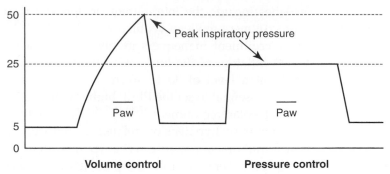

FIGURE 14-9 Comparison of a volume-control versus a pressure-control ventilator waveform. The peak inspiratory pressure of the volume control breath is brief, occurring at the end of breath when the full volume is delivered. The pressure of the pressure-controlled breath is delivered throughout the duration of the breath. Pressure control allows for better distribution of gas over time with potential recruitment of collapsed alveoli.

is consistent breath to breath, the pressure generated to deliver the volume may vary. In patients with reduced lung compliance, alveolar pressures may exceed 30 cm H_2O. This may result in ventilator induced lung injury; this is best avoided through implementation of strategies to keep alveolar pressures below this threshold. Because alveolar pressure cannot be directly measured clinically, plateau pressure is measured as a surrogate for alveolar pressure. Plateau pressure may be measured by performing an inspiratory hold maneuver on the ventilator in the volume control mode. The maneuver will display the plateau pressure, which is less than the peak inspiratory pressure, as well as the static lung compliance. On current mechanical ventilators, these measurements are displayed automatically on the screen when the inspiratory hold maneuver is completed.

In pressure control ventilation, a positive pressure flow of gas is delivered until the set inspiratory pressure is reached. This target pressure is maintained for the duration of the set inspiratory time. This allows for control of the peak inspiratory pressure, but the tidal volume will vary, depending on patient airway resistance and lung compliance. Pressure control ventilation produces a square pressure waveform. The advantage of the square pressure waveform is sustained time for alveolar inflation and recruitment. When combined with inverse ratio ventilation, the physiologic inspiration-to-expiration ratio (I:E) of 1:2 is reversed to 2:1. This shortens the expiratory time before the next breath, preventing full exhalation.[66,86–88] This technique results in a condition called auto-PEEP whereby PEEP is generated in the respiratory system without being set on the machine (Figure 14-10). The clinical benefit of the phenomena is sustained end-expiratory pressure, alveolar recruitment, and prevention of alveolar derecruitment. The negative effects hemodynamically are related to reduced RV preload and increased afterload from sustained positive pressure in the thorax. This, again, is dependent on intravascular volume and ventricular function in the particular patient.[7,33]

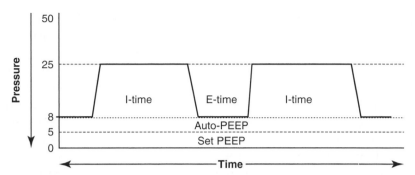

FIGURE 14-10 Pressure-controlled ventilation with inverse ratio results in a shortened expiratory time and generation of auto-PEEP (positive end-expiratory pressure). Auto-PEEP may assist in alveolar recruitment but may also result in reduction of right ventricular preload and increased afterload.

Patient Safety

Routine disconnection of the ventilator circuit from the airway in patients on high PEEP or on modes such as PCV and APRV should be avoided to prevent alveolar derecruitment. If disconnection of the circuit must be done (i.e., ventilator circuit change), clamping the endotracheal tube at end-inspiration prior to disconnection may preserve PEEP and prevent alveolar collapse.

Dynamic Hyperinflation

Dynamic hyperinflation is a condition in which the lungs become hyperinflated from insufficient emptying. This may occur with the use of short expiratory times as part of the ventilation strategy (inverse ratio) or as a result of lung pathology such as bronchoconstriction with impaired lung elasticity.[13,89–91]

The purpose of inverse ratio ventilation is to increase the mean airway pressure to improve oxygenation and ventilation through alveolar recruitment. The risk in doing this is that the lungs may become hyperinflated, especially when extremely short expiratory times are used (3:1). Inverse ratios may also be achieved unintentionally when high respiratory rates are set on the ventilator or when the patient becomes tachypneic. In either condition, a higher respiratory rate will reduce the expiratory time, creating auto-PEEP and some degree of hyperinflation.[61,68,92–94]

The above condition associated with ventilator settings may be further complicated by bronchoconstriction and reduced elastic recoil of the lungs. Bronchoconstriction occurs in many disease states associated with the need for mechanical ventilation. In asthma, histamine-mediated bronchoconstriction, airway swelling, and increased mucous production impede expiratory gas flow, which results in lung hyperinflation.[36,37,56,59] In emphysema, expiratory small airway collapse and loss of lung elasticity result in air trapping and hyperinflation.[90,95] Patients with ARDS may develop bronchoconstriction from leukocyte-released mediators known as leukotrienes.

Regardless of cause, dynamic hyperinflation results in sustained positive pressure in the chest, reducing cardiac output by mechanisms previously described. Tactics to prevent dynamic hyperinflation and hemodynamic sequelae include reducing airway resistance and increasing expiratory time. Airway resistance may be reduced by using the largest appropriate endotracheal tube and by administering bronchodilators and mucolytic agents to improve expiratory flow.[95–97] Expiratory time may be increased by reducing the breath frequency, which increases the inspiratory flow rate.[90,96–98] Reducing the degree of inverse ratio ventilation to 1.5:1 or equal I:E may be necessary if hyperinflation is adversely impacting hemodynamic stability. This must be weighed against any potential therapeutic benefit dynamic hyperinflation ventilation may have in improving gas exchange.

Although controversial, immediate treatment for hemodynamic instability indicated by dynamic hyperinflation may require disconnecting the ventilator circuit from the airway to allow the patient to fully, passively exhale.[91,97,99] This will usually result in improvement in blood pressure but may result in derecruitment of the lung with deoxygenation. The immediate issue will be resolved, but clinicians should be prepared to address the sequelae of resulting hypoxia such as bradycardia or other arrhythmias.[97]

Ventilation Mode and Hemodynamic Impact

In the previous sections, the global effects of positive pressure ventilation and PEEP, as well at the two main categories of ventilation, volume control (targeted) and pressure control (targeted) ventilation, were described. Volume control and pressure control describe the endpoint to which gas flow is delivered—set volume with variable pressure or set pressure with variable volume, respectively. The other consideration that may impact hemodynamic performance is the mode of ventilation, or the way the breath is delivered. These include full-support modes such as assist control, mixed modes such as synchronous intermittent mandatory ventilation (SIMV), and spontaneous breathing modes such as pressure support.[100–102] Newer modes, including biphasic pressure modes (bilevel and APRV), allow spontaneous breaths to occur in tandem with ventilator-delivered breaths. Spontaneous breathing modes provide some advantage over control modes, as they allow for more natural breathing that supports venous return and optimal V/Q matching.[71,93,94,103]

Clinical Reasoning Pearl

Modes such as biphasic and APRV allow the patient to take spontaneous breaths along with machine-delivered breaths. This use of the diaphragm during spontaneous breathing improves ventilation in the lung bases and posterior regions thereby improving V/Q matching and gas exchange in these regions. Additionally, spontaneous breathing improves venous return and decreases right heart afterload.

During spontaneous breathing, use of the diaphragm improves ventilation to the posterior and basilar lung regions that are not well ventilated during positive pressure ventilation. Physiologically, regions along the dorsal portion of the lung are also the best perfused, so this improves V/Q matching as well.[94,103–105] Spontaneous ventilation also benefits venous return compared with traditional positive pressure ventilation. Sedation can be reduced, and no neuromuscular blockade (generally) is required when using these modes, as spontaneous ventilation further improves venous return.[5,103,105–107]

Hemodynamic Monitoring and Mechanical Ventilation

Modern hemodynamic monitoring technology is broad in capability and application. Traditional pressure-based parameters such as central venous pressure (CVP), pulmonary artery pressure and pulmonary artery occlusion pressure (PAOP), also known as "wedge" pressure, have been used to estimate vascular volume status. The limitation of using these static pressure-based endpoints as surrogates for volume is well described in the literature. Broadly, this includes an inability to accurately measure and track true changes in vascular volume.[4,12,18,25,44,108–112] These limitations are often magnified in patients on positive pressure ventilation and PEEP because of the associated intravascular pressure changes. Because of the limitations in pressure-based endpoints, newer hemodynamic endpoints such as dynamic stroke volume indices are increasingly used. These dynamic measures include: stroke volume variation (SVV), pulse pressure variation (PPV), and echocardiographic measures of vascular volume and heart chamber visualization.[18,25,108,111,113,114] These dynamic indices are better predictors of vascular volume and cardiac chamber function. The technology used to obtain the measurements varies in degree of invasiveness, capability, and clinician proficiency to utilize and interpret the clinical information provided. Many of these devices are discussed in detail elsewhere in this text. It is important, however, to understand how the above hemodynamic endpoints are altered by mechanical ventilation.

Pressure-Based Parameters

Pressure-based endpoints such as CVP and PAOP reflect the intravascular pressure and are often used as surrogates for vascular volume. Rise in intrathoracic pressure with positive pressure ventilation and PEEP may falsely indicate an increase in measured vascular pressure as ventilation pressure is transmitted to the cardiac chambers and venous system. The degree to which this will happen is patient dependent and is related to multiple factors, including respiratory system compliance (lung and chest wall compliance) in addition to other limitations such as ventricular afterload, valvular dysfunction, and pulmonary vascular resistance.[4,12,18,20,25,108,115] These factors will influence pressure-based hemodynamic measurements in the ventilated patient.

One proposed formula used to correct the measured vascular pressure with the application of PEEP involves subtracting half the PEEP value from the CVP or PAOP after converting the PEEP value to mm Hg from cm H_2O.[13] This formula may be helpful in correcting CVP and PAOP for applied PEEP only when lung and chest wall compliance is normal. When lung compliance is decreased, the transmitted pressure may be less to the cardiovascular structure, and this formula will not hold true.[22,116] Such is the case in patients with ARDS and intra-abdominal hypertension.[13,21,38,117–120]

Clinical Reasoning Pearl

Increases in intrathoracic pressure from positive pressure ventilation and PEEP cause elevation in pulmonary capillary pressure that may elevate PAOP and CVP. This makes these parameters less reliable as endpoints for patient management. Non–pressure-based endpoints such as dynamic change in stroke volume or pulse pressure should be considered as volume resuscitation endpoints.

Dynamic changes in stroke volume or measures of PPV and SVV are valuable hemodynamic endpoints for volume resuscitation. Changes in stroke volume and evaluation of PPV and SVV may be helpful when assessing the hemodynamic impact of ventilator setting or mode changes and can help guide decisions in fluid administration.[18,20,25,111,113,114,121]

Determining the need to administer volume may be assisted through application of the passive leg raise maneuver or the administration of a fluid challenge to determine the effect on improving stroke volume or reducing the percentage of PPV and SVV.[25,122,123] Passive leg raise is a reversible volume-challenge maneuver, in which the patient's own blood volume from the lower extremities is utilized. The patient is transitioned from an elevated head of bed position, such as 45 degrees, to a flat supine position, with elevation of the legs to 45 degrees (See Figure 3-11 in Chapter 3). This results in a reversible auto-transfusion of blood from the legs. If the patient is volume responsive, this maneuver should result in an increase in measured stroke volume. This evaluation requires a dynamic monitoring system to detect these changes before and after the challenge.[25,111,113,113,114,121] Baseline and post-intervention evaluation of cardiac output and surrogates for vascular volume such as great vessel diameter and end-diastolic area through echocardiography are also useful in guiding volume administration.[4,55,124,125] This is especially important in patients with limited cardiac reserve and ARDS, in whom euvolemia is desirable and consistent with better outcomes.[126–132]

The diagnostic value and accuracy of PPV and SVV rely on the heart–lung interactions resulting from positive pressure ventilation. The inspiratory increase in intrathoracic pressure results in cyclic changes in blood flow, reducing right ventricular preload and stroke volume, and subsequently reducing LV stroke volume.[18,25,111] The changes in intrathoracic pressure result in respiratory variation in blood flow observed in both PPV and SVV. The degree of variance is determined by the degree of cyclic changes in blood flow.[20,80] Hence, a high degree or percentage of variance means that the heart is operating on the steep portion of the Starling curve and may be volume responsive, whereas lower variation indicates adequate volume with the heart operating on the flat portion of the curve.[6,9,16,80] Normal PPV is less than 13%, whereas normal SVV is less than 10%.[20,25,110,111,113,120] Higher degrees of variation may signal the need for intravascular volume.

Although PPV and SVV are helpful, these parameters have some limitations related to their use in the mechanically ventilated patient. Clinical conditions that may influence the reliability of these parameters include tidal volumes under 8 mL/kg, open chest conditions, spontaneous breathing efforts, elevated intra-abdominal pressure and PEEP.[27,113,117,119,133–136]

Several investigators have shown that the predictive value of PPV and SVV is reduced with tidal volumes less than 8 mL/kg. Lower tidal volumes may result in less change in intrathoracic pressure and a lower degree of cyclic changes in stroke volume.[27,133,134] Given the accepted use of low-tidal volume ventilation to protect the lungs, this must be considered when interpreting these values in patients on low-tidal volume ventilation. In patients with restrictive lung conditions such as ARDS, lower tidal volumes (less than 8 mL/kg) may still be sufficient to influence dynamic changes in PPV and SVV.[133,134,137–140]

In addition to low tidal volumes, spontaneous breathing efforts will affect the measurement of PPV and SVV and reliability of data observed. These endpoints require positive pressure ventilation to create the cyclic changes in volume and pressure. Spontaneous breathing will create negative intrathoracic pressure conditions and may falsely elevate or reduce PPV and SVV. Clinically, this is significant, since many patients may be supported by spontaneous breathing modes such as pressure support or biphasic ventilation.[27,133]

The open chest is another condition that will reduce the reliability of PPV and SVV. When the chest is open, the cyclic changes created by positive pressure ventilation are reduced and the degree of variation is compromised. Clinically, it is not recommended that PPV and SVV are used in patients with an open chest.[80,136]

Intra-abdominal hypertension results in elevations in intra-abdominal pressure, potentially reducing venous return from the inferior vena cava, increasing LV afterload, and increasing the intrathoracic pressure from upward compression of the diaphragm. These changes may create false variation in PPV and SVV, which would fail to predict true fluid responsiveness due to the degree of intra-abdominal pressure elevation. Because of these limitations, use of PPV and SVV are not recommended in the presence of intra-abdominal hypertension.[21,117,121,135]

PEEP increases intrathoracic pressure by distending the lungs and both reducing preload and increasing afterload. Both PPV and SVV are noted to increase in the presence of PEEP in both open-chest and closed-chest conditions. This elevation may not be truly reflective of a hemodynamic response to volume. Caution must be taken when interpreting these values in light of these limitations.[4,13,44,113,137,141–143]

Echocardiography

Echocardiography, either transthoracic or transesophageal, may be beneficial to assess volume status and cardiac function in patients who are mechanically ventilated.[124,125] Echocardiography requires skill in performance and interpretation but provides concurrent information to guide treatment decisions related to fluid administration, pharmacotherapy, or mechanical support of the heart.[124,125]

Hemodynamic Changes with Ventilator Liberation

The method and timing of ventilator liberation are points of considerable debate. Although many approaches exist, it is generally agreed that the patient should be hemodynamically stable with resolution of the clinical reason for initiation of ventilator support.[144–148]

As positive pressure ventilator support is withdrawn, the work of breathing increases and may result in alterations in gas exchange and hemodynamic function.[1,19,149] This is dependent on a number of factors, including the method of weaning and the patient's underlying cardiopulmonary function.[144,145,150–153]

Withdrawal of ventilator support may be rapid or gradual and is dependent on patient condition and duration of ventilation. Following a spontaneous awakening trial, a spontaneous breathing trial (SBT) is employed to determine readiness to wean and is extended if the patient tolerates the trial.[144–146,146,154–157] This method moves the patient from full ventilator support to minimal support or spontaneous breathing. Other liberation methods may include pressure support ventilation with gradual tapering of the level of support. Although this may extend the weaning process, it may be necessary for patients who are deconditioned. In either case, transition from supported breathing to unsupported spontaneous breathing results in an increase in work of breathing as well as cardiac workload.[144,145,150,157–161]

For patients with normal cardiac function, the transition to spontaneous breathing is less acute or uneventful. Patients may have an increase in stroke volume and heart rate (cardiac output) without any clinical consequences. However, patients with unresolved hypoxia and limited cardiac reserve may develop more severe hypoxia and hemodynamic instability during the transition, indicating the need for a slower, more supportive weaning plan.[1,19,51,151,153,162,163]

The change from positive pressure ventilation to spontaneous breathing may result in alveolar collapse and hypoxic vasoconstriction.[1,26,38,41,44,45,164] This, in turn, would increase pulmonary vascular resistance and RV afterload. Venous return may also increase as positive pressure effects on preload are eliminated. The combined effect may be RV dilation with subsequent impact on LV function. In the case of marginal LV function, increase in LV afterload may further reduce LV function as PEEP and positive pressure give way to spontaneous breathing. These effects on both ventricles may result in increased oxygen demand and decreased coronary artery perfusion from ventricular dilation. The combined effects may cause myocardial ischemia and infarction.[1,19,51,144,152,153,158,162]

Pre-weaning parameters should include assessment of underlying cardiac disease, resolution of conditions requiring initiation of ventilation, and hemodynamic stability.

Patient Safety

Reduction of PEEP and transition from full ventilator support to spontaneous breathing may increase myocardial workload, especially in LV dysfunction. Increase or decrease in heart rate or rhythm, nonvariability in heart rate, tachypnea, or other changes in vital signs may signal intolerance of ventilator liberation.

During the weaning trial, assessment should continue beyond the initial spontaneous breathing trial period. Clinically, patients that are less able to hemodynamically compensate during weaning may be unsuccessful, since they cannot meet the required pulmonary and cardiovascular demands of spontaneous breathing.[1,19] Re-establishment of ventilator support may be necessary until the underlying issues are corrected. A more gradual approach to weaning may then be undertaken.

Mechanical Ventilation Case Study

Mr. S, a 45-year-old male, was involved in a motor vehicle crash. He had not been wearing his seat belt and had sustained severe chest and abdominal injuries that required immediate surgery and massive transfusion of blood products. Postoperatively, he was admitted to the critical care unit and required mechanical ventilation and ongoing resuscitation. His initial ventilator settings were: Volume control (VC) assist control (A/C) mode on a rate of 12 breaths per minute; tidal volume (Vt): 550 mL, fraction of inspired oxygen (FiO$_2$): 1.0, and positive end-expiratory pressure (PEEP): 5 cm H$_2$O.

PARAMETER	ADMISSION	12 HOURS	16 HOURS	20 HOURS	96 HOURS
Heart rate	120	128	124	118	116
Blood pressure in mm Hg	100/68	88/50	100/76	112/66	120/76
Central venous pressure in mm Hg	6	10	12	10	8
Stroke volume	Unknown	55 mL	50 mL	62 mL	75 mL
Ventilation mode	VC-A/C	VC-A/C	APRV	APRV	PSV
Tidal volume (mL) in VC-A/C mode	550 mL	550 mL			15 cm H$_2$O (350 mL Vt)
Inspiratory pressure (cm H$_2$O) and Tidal volume (Vt) in mL in APRV mode			28 cm H$_2$O (450 mL Vt)	28 cm H$_2$O (450 mL Vt)	
Set rate/ Spontaneous	12/0	12/4	13 /22	13 /22	0/22

Continued

Mechanical Ventilation Case Study—cont'd

Set inspiratory time in seconds (sec)	N/A	N/A	4 sec	4 sec	N/A
Set expiratory time in seconds (sec)	N/A	N/A	0.6 sec	0.6 sec	N/A
PEEP (cm H_2O)	5	10	0	0	5
FiO_2	0.7	1.0	1.0	1.0	0.45
Peak inspiratory pressure (cm H_2O)	26	38	28	28	18
Plateau pressure (cm H_2O)	12	33	N/A	N/A	
Static compliance (mL/cm H_2O)	0.046	0.017	N/A	N/A	0.055

Over the next 12 hours, his oxygen requirements were increasing. The decision was made to increase his PEEP to 10 cm H_2O, which quickly resulted in hypotension (88/55 mm Hg), tachycardia, and minimal improvement in oxygenation. He was given a fluid bolus of 500 mL, based on his hemodynamic changes. Additionally, the intensivist used echocardiography to examine the heart and major vessels, and initiated a minimally invasive cardiac output monitor to measure dynamic changes in stroke volume and cardiac output. Chest radiography revealed bilateral infiltrates. His arterial blood gas was not improving with these measures. His measured plateau pressure was rising (33 cm H_2O), and static lung compliance was decreasing (0.17 mL/cm H_2O). Echocardiography showed a dilated right atrium with reduced ejection fraction, but no evidence of LV dysfunction. His hemodynamic measurements after increasing PEEP and fluid bolus are listed in the table (12 hours column).

The intensivist diagnosed moderate ARDS, per the Berlin definition (see Table 14-4), since the patient had a P/F ratio of 160 as shown by the following calculation:

Partial pressure of arterial oxygen (PaO_2): 160 mm Hg/ FiO_2: 1.0 = 160.

Chest radiography revealed bilateral infiltrates, and no evidence that LV failure was contributing to the pulmonary condition. Additionally, the patient had several insults that might have triggered the ARDS (injury, shock, massive transfusion). Because of worsening oxygenation, worsening lung compliance, and elevated plateau pressure, the patient was transitioned to a lung-protective ventilation strategy. The ventilation mode was changed to Airway Pressure Release Ventilation (APRV). Initial settings included inspiratory pressure of 28 cm H_2O (resultant tidal volume dropped to 450 mL), inspiratory time of 4 seconds

Mechanical Ventilation Case Study—cont'd

(ventilator rate of approximately13 breaths per minute), PEEP of 0 cm H_2O with an expiratory time of 0.6 second, and FiO_2 of 1.0 (16 hours column).

Inhaled prostacyclin (Epoprostenol) was initiated to improve oxygenation and reduce RV afterload. Additionally, the patient was placed in continuous lateral rotation to 40 degrees bilaterally. Oxygenation began to improve, although the partial pressure of arterial carbon dioxide ($PaCO_2$) rose as minute ventilation had been decreased to protect the lungs (permissive hypercapnea). Hemodynamic data revealed elevation of CVP, but stroke volume decreased with institution of APRV. Echocardiography revealed a flattened vena cava and underfilled right ventricle. The decision was made to give a fluid bolus, but because the patient's hemoglobin was 8 milligrams per deciliter (mg/dL), a unit of packed red blood cells was administered instead to increase stroke volume and oxygen-carrying capacity. Stroke volume increased by 20%, and repeat echocardiography showed improved RV filling and improved cardiac function (20 hours column).

Over the next 72 hours, the patient was hemodynamically stable. Chest radiography revealed resolution of infiltrates, and the patient was weaned off Epoprostenol. FiO_2 was reduced to 0.45 (45%), and the ventilation mode was changed to volume-control ventilation with A/C rate of 14, Vt: 500 mL, and FiO_2: 0.45 with PEEP: 5 cm H_2O. The next day, he progressed to pressure support ventilation (PSV) at 15 cm H_2O (spontaneous Vt of 350 mL and rate of 22 breaths per minute). Over the next 12 hours, PSV was reduced to 7 cm H_2O (96 hours column).

Mr. S was successfully extubated to a high flow, high-humidity nasal cannula. ▪

Conclusion

Mechanical ventilation is an essential tool in the management of the critically ill patient. The hemodynamic side effects that result from disruption of the physiologic heart–lung interactions that support normal function are often underappreciated. Thorough understanding of the hemodynamic impact of positive pressure ventilation, PEEP, and interactions in clinical conditions such as ARDS are essential in managing the mechanically ventilated patient.

References

1. Frazier SK: Cardiovascular effects of mechanical ventilation and weaning, *Nurs Clin North Am* 43(1):1–15, 2008.
2. Feihl F, Broccard AF: Interactions between respiration and systemic hemodynamics. part II: practical implications in critical care, *Intensive Care Med* 35(2):198–205, 2009.
3. Feihl F, Broccard AF: Interactions between respiration and systemic hemodynamics. part I: basic concepts, *Intensive Care Med* 35(1):45–54, 2009.
4. Magder S: Hemodynamic monitoring in the mechanically ventilated patient, *Curr Opin Crit Care* 17(1):36–42, 2011.

5. Neumann P, Schubert A, Heuer J, et al.: Hemodynamic effects of spontaneous breathing in the post-operative period, *Acta Anaesthesiol Scand* 49(10):1443–1448, 2005.

6. Fessler HE: The cycles of heart, lungs, and science, *Crit Care Med* 37(5):1816–1817, 2009.

7. Funk DJ, Jacobsohn E, Kumar A: The role of venous return in critical illness and shock-part I: physiology, *Crit Care Med* 41(1):255–262, 2013.

8. Miller JD, Pegelow DF, Jacques AJ, Dempsey JA: Skeletal muscle pump versus respiratory muscle pump: modulation of venous return from the locomotor limb in humans, *J Physiol (Lond)* 563(Pt 3):925–943, 2005.

9. Guyton AC, Lindsey AW, Kaufmann BN: Effect of mean circulatory filling pressure and other peripheral circulatory factors on cardiac output, *Am J Physiol* 180(3):463–468, 1955.

10. Guyton AC, Lindsey AW, Abernathy B, Richardson T: Venous return at various right atrial pressures and the normal venous return curve, *Am J Physiol* 189(3):609–615, 1957.

11. Guyton AC: The venous system and its role in the circulation, *Mod Concepts Cardiovasc Dis* 27 (10):483–487, 1958.

12. Magder S: Invasive intravascular hemodynamic monitoring: technical issues, *Crit Care Clin* 23 (3):401–414, 2007.

13. Luecke T, Pelosi P: Clinical review: positive end-expiratory pressure and cardiac output, *Crit Care* 9(6):607–621, 2005.

14. Lopes MR, Auler Jr JO, Michard F: Volume management in critically ill patients: new insights, *Clinics* 61(4):345–350, 2006.

15. Chen Y, Chen P, Hanaoka M, et al.: Mechanical ventilation in patients with hypoxemia due to refractory heart failure, *Intern Med* 47(5):367–373, 2008.

16. Guyton AC: Determination of cardiac output by equating venous return curves with cardiac response curves, *Physiol Rev* 35(1):123–129, 1955.

17. Maestroni A, Aliberti S, Amir O, et al.: Acute effects of positive end-expiratory pressure on left ventricle diastolic function in healthy subjects, *Intern Emerg Med* 4(3):249–254, 2009.

18. Pinsky MR: Heart-lung interactions, *Curr Opin Crit Care* 13(5):528–531, 2007.

19. Frazier SK, Stone KS, Moser D, et al.: Hemodynamic changes during discontinuation of mechanical ventilation in medical intensive care unit patients, *Am J Crit Care* 15(6):580–593, 2006.

20. Michard F: Changes in arterial pressure during mechanical ventilation, *Anesthesiology* 103 (2):419–428, 2005.

21. Krebs J, Pelosi P, Tsagogiorgas C, et al.: Effects of positive end-expiratory pressure on respiratory function and hemodynamics in patients with acute respiratory failure with and without intra-abdominal hypertension: a pilot study, *Crit Care* 13(5):R160, 2009.

22. deBoisblanc BP, Girod-Espinoza A, Welsh DA, Taylor DE: Hemodynamic monitoring in acute lung injury and acute respiratory distress syndrome, *Respir Care Clin N Am* 9(4):457–479, 2003.

23. Di Marco F, Devaquet J, Lyazidi A, et al.: Positive end-expiratory pressure-induced functional recruitment in patients with acute respiratory distress syndrome, *Crit Care Med* 38 (1):127–132, 2010.

24. Gernoth C, Wagner G, Pelosi P, Luecke T: Respiratory and haemodynamic changes during decremental open lung positive end-expiratory pressure titration in patients with acute respiratory distress syndrome, *Crit Care* 13(2):R59, 2009.

25. Marik PE, Cavallazzi R, Vasu T, Hirani A: Dynamic changes in arterial waveform derived variables and fluid responsiveness in mechanically ventilated patients: a systematic review of the literature, *Crit Care Med* 37(9):2642–2647, 2009.

26. Glenny RW: Determinants of regional ventilation and blood flow in the lung, *Intensive Care Med* 35(11):1833–1842, 2009.

27. De Backer D, Taccone FS, Holsten R, et al.: Influence of respiratory rate on stroke volume variation in mechanically ventilated patients, *Anesthesiology* 110(5):1092–1097, 2009.

28. Jardin F, Vieillard-Baron A: Monitoring of right-sided heart function, *Curr Opin Crit Care* 11 (3):271–279, 2005.
29. Wallis TW, Robotham JL, Compean R, Kindred MK: Mechanical heart-lung interaction with positive end-expiratory pressure, *J Appl Physiol* 54(4):1039–1047, 1983.
30. Vieillard-Baron A, Schmitt JM, Augarde R, et al.: Acute cor pulmonale in acute respiratory distress syndrome submitted to protective ventilation: incidence, clinical implications, and prognosis, *Crit Care Med* 29(8):1551–1555, 2001.
31. West JB, Dollery CT, Naimark A: Distribution of blood flow in isolated lung; relation to vascular and alveolar pressures, *J Appl Physiol* 19:713–724, 1964.
32. Gattinoni L, Caironi P, Cressoni M, et al.: Lung recruitment in patients with the acute respiratory distress syndrome, *N Engl J Med* 354(17):1775–1786, 2006.
33. Fougeres E, Teboul JL, Richard C, et al.: Hemodynamic impact of a positive end-expiratory pressure setting in acute respiratory distress syndrome: importance of the volume status, *Crit Care Med* 38(3):802–807, 2010.
34. Dellaca RL, Andersson Olerud M, Zannin E, et al.: Lung recruitment assessed by total respiratory system input reactance, *Intensive Care Med* 35(12):2164–2172, 2009.
35. Kacmarek RM, Villar J: Lung recruitment maneuvers during acute respiratory distress syndrome: is it useful? *Minerva Anestesiol* 77(1):85–89, 2011.
36. Cortes I, Penuelas O, Esteban A: Acute respiratory distress syndrome: evaluation and management, *Minerva Anestesiol* 78(3):343–357, 2012.
37. Derdak S: Acute respiratory distress syndrome in trauma patients, *J Trauma* 62(6 Suppl):S58, 2012.
38. McCann 2nd UG, Schiller HJ, Gatto LA, et al.: Alveolar mechanics alter hypoxic pulmonary vasoconstriction, *Crit Care Med* 30(6):1315–1321, 2002.
39. Jardin F: Acute leftward septal shift by lung recruitment maneuver, *Intensive Care Med* 31 (9):1148–1149, 2005.
40. Jardin F, Vieillard-Baron A: Right ventricular function and positive pressure ventilation in clinical practice: from hemodynamic subsets to respirator settings, *Intensive Care Med* 29 (9):1426–1434, 2003.
41. Meade MO, Cook DJ, Griffith LE, et al.: A study of the physiologic responses to a lung recruitment maneuver in acute lung injury and acute respiratory distress syndrome, *Respir Care* 53(11):1441–1449, 2008.
42. Mitchell JR, Whitelaw WA, Sas R, et al.: RV filling modulates LV function by direct ventricular interaction during mechanical ventilation, *Am J Physiol Heart Circ Physiol* 289(2):H549–H557, 2005.
43. Namendys-Silva SA, Dominguez-Cherit G: Mechanical ventilation can cause changes in pulmonary circulation, *Crit Care Med* 38(8):1759–1760, 2010.
44. Her C, Mandy S, Bairamian M: Increased pulmonary venous resistance contributes to increased pulmonary artery diastolic-pulmonary wedge pressure gradient in acute respiratory distress syndrome, *Anesthesiology* 102(3):574–580, 2005.
45. Huh JW, Hong SB, Lim CM, Koh Y: Effect of the alveolar recruitment manoeuvre on haemodynamic parameters in patients with acute respiratory distress syndrome: relationship with oxygenation, *Respirology* 15(8):1220–1225, 2010.
46. Khan M, Frankel H: Adjuncts to ventilatory support part 1: nitric oxide, surfactants, prostacyclin, steroids, sedation, and neuromuscular blockade, *Curr Probl Surg* 50(10):424–433, 2013.
47. Allan PF, Codispoti CA, Womble SG, et al.: Inhaled prostacyclin in combination with high-frequency percussive ventilation, *J Burn Care Res* 31(2):347–352, 2010.
48. Adhikari NK, Dellinger RP, Lundin S, et al.: Inhaled nitric oxide does not reduce mortality in patients with acute respiratory distress syndrome regardless of severity: systematic review and meta-analysis, *Crit Care Med* 42(2):404–412, 2014.

49. David M, von Bardeleben RS, Weiler N, et al.: Cardiac function and haemodynamics during transition to high-frequency oscillatory ventilation, *Eur J Anaesthesiol* 21(12):944–952, 2004.
50. Iannuzzi M, De Sio A, De Robertis E, et al.: Different patterns of lung recruitment maneuvers in primary acute respiratory distress syndrome: effects on oxygenation and central hemodynamics, *Minerva Anestesiol* 76(9):692–698, 2010.
51. Zapata L, Vera P, Roglan A, et al.: B-type natriuretic peptides for prediction and diagnosis of weaning failure from cardiac origin, *Intensive Care Med* 37(3):477–485, 2011.
52. van den Berg PC, Jansen JR, Pinsky MR: Effect of positive pressure on venous return in volume-loaded cardiac surgical patients, *J Appl Physiol* 92(3):1223–1231, 2002.
53. van den Berg PC, Grimbergen CA, Spaan JA, Pinsky MR: Positive pressure inspiration differentially affects right and left ventricular outputs in postoperative cardiac surgery patients, *J Crit Care* 12(2):56–65, 1997.
54. Van de Louw A, Medigue C, Papelier Y, Cottin F: Positive end-expiratory pressure may alter breathing cardiovascular variability and baroreflex gain in mechanically ventilated patients, *Respir Res* 11:38, 2010.
55. Osman D, Monnet X, Castelain V, et al.: Incidence and prognostic value of right ventricular failure in acute respiratory distress syndrome, *Intensive Care Med* 35(1):69–76, 2009.
56. Caironi P, Langer T, Gattinoni L: Acute lung injury/acute respiratory distress syndrome pathophysiology: what we have learned from computed tomography scanning, *Curr Opin Crit Care* 14(1):64–69, 2008.
57. Futier E, Constantin JM, Petit A, et al.: Positive end-expiratory pressure improves end-expiratory lung volume but not oxygenation after induction of anaesthesia, *Eur J Anaesthesiol* 27(6):508–513, 2010.
58. ARDS Definition Task F, Ranieri VM, Rubenfeld GD, et al.: Acute respiratory distress syndrome: the Berlin definition, *JAMA* 307(23):2526–2533, 2012.
59. Ashbaugh DG, Bigelow DB, Petty TL, Levine BE: Acute respiratory distress in adults, *Lancet* 2(7511):319–323, 1967.
60. Santa Cruz R, Rojas JI, Nervi R, et al.: High versus low positive end-expiratory pressure (PEEP) levels for mechanically ventilated adult patients with acute lung injury and acute respiratory distress syndrome, *Cochrane Database Syst Rev* 6:009098, 2013.
61. Albert SP, DiRocco J, Allen GB, et al.: The role of time and pressure on alveolar recruitment, *J Appl Physiol* 106(3):757–765, 2009.
62. Borges JB, Okamoto VN, Matos GF, et al.: Reversibility of lung collapse and hypoxemia in early acute respiratory distress syndrome, *Am J Respir Crit Care Med* 174(3):268–278, 2006.
63. Vieillard-Baron A, Augarde R, Prin S, et al.: Influence of superior vena caval zone condition on cyclic changes in right ventricular outflow during respiratory support, *Anesthesiology* 95(5):1083–1088, 2001.
64. Bindels AJ, van der Hoeven JG, Graafland AD, et al.: Relationships between volume and pressure measurements and stroke volume in critically ill patients, *Crit Care* 4(3):193–199, 2000.
65. Bohm SH, Thamm OC, von Sandersleben A, et al.: Alveolar recruitment strategy and high positive end-expiratory pressure levels do not affect hemodynamics in morbidly obese intravascular volume-loaded patients, *Anesth Analg* 109(1):160–163, 2009.
66. Toth I, Leiner T, Mikor A, et al.: Hemodynamic and respiratory changes during lung recruitment and descending optimal positive end-expiratory pressure titration in patients with acute respiratory distress syndrome, *Crit Care Med* 35(3):787–793, 2007.
67. Petersson J, Ax M, Frey J, et al.: Positive end-expiratory pressure redistributes regional blood flow and ventilation differently in supine and prone humans, *Anesthesiology* 113(6):1361–1369, 2010.
68. Fan E, Wilcox ME, Brower RG, et al.: Recruitment maneuvers for acute lung injury: a systematic review, *Am J Respir Crit Care Med* 178(11):1156–1163, 2008.

69. MacIntyre N: Ventilatory management of ALI/ARDS, *Semin Respir Crit Care Med* 27 (4):396–403, 2006.

70. Grasso S, Stripoli T, De Michele M, et al.: ARDSnet ventilatory protocol and alveolar hyperinflation: role of positive end-expiratory pressure, *Am J Respir Crit Care Med* 176 (8):761–767, 2007.

71. Putensen C, Theuerkauf N, Zinserling J, et al.: Meta-analysis: ventilation strategies and outcomes of the acute respiratory distress syndrome and acute lung injury, *Ann Intern Med* 151 (8):566–576, 2009.

72. Steiner S, Schannwell CM, Strauer BE: Left ventricular response to continuous positive airway pressure: role of left ventricular geometry, *Respiration* 76(4):393–397, 2008.

72a. The Acute Respiratory Distress Syndrome Network: Ventilation with lower tidal volumes as compared with traditional tidal volumes for acute lung injury and the acute respiratory distress syndrome, *N Engl J Med* 342(18):1301–1308, 2000.

73. Maniatis NA, Orfanos SE: The endothelium in acute lung injury/acute respiratory distress syndrome, *Curr Opin Crit Care* 14(1):22–30, 2008.

74. Chatburn RL: Understanding mechanical ventilators, *Expert Rev Respir Med* 4(6):809–819, 2010.

75. Haas CF: Mechanical ventilation with lung protective strategies: what works? *Crit Care Clin* 27 (3):469–486, 2011.

76. Keszler M: State of the art in conventional mechanical ventilation, *J Perinatol* 29(4):262–275, 2009.

77. The Acute Respiratory Distress Syndrome Network: Ventilation with lower tidal volumes as compared with traditional tidal volumes for acute lung injury and the acute respiratory distress syndrome, *N Engl J Med* 342(18):1301–1308, 2000.

78. Schultz MJ, Haitsma JJ, Slutsky AS, Gajic O: What tidal volumes should be used in patients without acute lung injury? *Anesthesiology* 106(6):1226–1231, 2007.

79. Reis Miranda D, Klompe L, Mekel J, et al.: Open lung ventilation does not increase right ventricular outflow impedance: an echo-Doppler study, *Crit Care Med* 34(10):2555–2560, 2006.

80. Pinsky MR: Heart-lung interactions, *Curr Opin Crit Care* 13(5):528–531, 2007.

81. Jellinek H, Krafft P, Fitzgerald RD, et al.: Right atrial pressure predicts hemodynamic response to apneic positive airway pressure, *Crit Care Med* 28(3):672–678, 2000.

82. Kacmarek RM, Kallet RH: Respiratory controversies in the critical care setting. Should recruitment maneuvers be used in the management of ALI and ARDS? *Respir Care* 52 (5):622–631, 2007.

83. Costa EL, Amato M: Hemodynamic and respiratory changes during lung recruitment and descending optimal positive end-expiratory pressure titration with acute respiratory distress syndrome, *Crit Care Med* 35(8):1998–1999, 2007.

84. Park KJ, Oh YJ, Chang HJ, et al.: Acute hemodynamic effects of recruitment maneuvers in patients with acute respiratory distress syndrome, *J Intensive Care Med* 24(6):376–382, 2009.

85. Nielsen J, Ostergaard M, Kjaergaard J, et al.: Lung recruitment maneuver depresses central hemodynamics in patients following cardiac surgery, *Intensive Care Med* 31(9):1189–1194, 2005.

86. Nichols D, Haranath S: Pressure control ventilation, *Crit Care Clin* 23(2):183–199, 2007.

87. Kallet RH, Campbell AR, Dicker RA, et al.: Work of breathing during lung-protective ventilation in patients with acute lung injury and acute respiratory distress syndrome: a comparison between volume and pressure-regulated breathing modes, *Respir Care* 50 (12):1623–1631, 2005.

88. Katsaragakis S, Stamou KM, Androulakis G: Independent lung ventilation for asymmetrical chest trauma: effect on ventilatory and haemodynamic parameters, *Injury* 36(4):501–504, 2005.

89. Caramez MP, Borges JB, Tucci MR, et al.: Paradoxical responses to positive end-expiratory pressure in patients with airway obstruction during controlled ventilation, *Crit Care Med* 33 (7):1519–1528, 2005.

90. Oddo M, Feihl F, Schaller MD, Perret C: Management of mechanical ventilation in acute severe asthma: practical aspects, *Intensive Care Med* 32(4):501–510, 2006.

91. Marini JJ: Dynamic hyperinflation and auto-positive end-expiratory pressure: lessons learned over 30 years, *Am J Respir Crit Care Med* 184(7):756–762, 2011.

92. Kallet RH: Patient-ventilator interaction during acute lung injury, and the role of spontaneous breathing: part 2: airway pressure release ventilation, *Respir Care* 56(2):190–203, 2011.

93. Maung AA, Kaplan LJ: Airway pressure release ventilation in acute respiratory distress syndrome, *Crit Care Clin* 27(3):501–509, 2011.

94. Putensen C, Wrigge H: Clinical review: biphasic positive airway pressure and airway pressure release ventilation, *Crit Care* 8(6):492–497, 2004.

95. Ward NS, Dushay KM: Clinical concise review: mechanical ventilation of patients with chronic obstructive pulmonary disease, *Crit Care Med* 36(5):1614–1619, 2008.

96. Brenner B, Corbridge T, Kazzi A: Intubation and mechanical ventilation of the asthmatic patient in respiratory failure, *J Emerg Med* 37(2 Suppl):S23–S34, 2009.

97. Koh Y: Ventilatory management in patients with chronic airflow obstruction, *Crit Care Clin* 23 (2):169–181, 2007.

98. Burns SM: Ventilating patients with acute severe asthma: what do we really know? *AACN Adv Crit Care* 17(2):186–193, 2006.

99. Calverley PM, Koulouris NG: Flow limitation and dynamic hyperinflation: key concepts in modern respiratory physiology, *Eur Respir J* 25(1):186–199, 2005.

100. Pertab D: Principles of mechanical ventilation—a critical review, *Br J Nurs* 18(15):915–918, 2009.

101. Richard JC, Lefebvre JC, Tassaux D, Brochard L: Update in mechanical ventilation 2010, *Am J Respir Crit Care Med* 184(1):32–36, 2011.

102. Singer BD, Corbridge TC: Pressure modes of invasive mechanical ventilation, *South Med J* 104 (10):701–709, 2011.

103. Kuhlen R, Rossaint R: The role of spontaneous breathing during mechanical ventilation, *Respir Care* 47(3):296–303, 2002.

104. Putensen C, Hering R, Muders T, Wrigge H: Assisted breathing is better in acute respiratory failure, *Curr Opin Crit Care* 11(1):63–68, 2005.

105. Yoshida T, Rinka H, Kaji A, et al.: The impact of spontaneous ventilation on distribution of lung aeration in patients with acute respiratory distress syndrome: airway pressure release ventilation versus pressure support ventilation, *Anesth Analg* 109(6):1892–1900, 2009.

106. Kamath SS, Super DM, Mhanna MJ: Effects of airway pressure release ventilation on blood pressure and urine output in children, *Pediatr Pulmonol* 45(1):48–54, 2010.

107. Marik PE, Young A, Sibole S, Levitov A: The effect of APRV ventilation on ICP and cerebral hemodynamics, *Neurocrit Care* 17(2):219–223, 2012.

108. Marik PE, Cavallazzi R: Does the central venous pressure predict fluid responsiveness? An updated meta-analysis and a plea for some common sense, *Crit Care Med* 41(7):1774–1781, 2013.

109. Heresi GA, Arroliga AC, Wiedemann HP, Matthay MA: Pulmonary artery catheter and fluid management in acute lung injury and the acute respiratory distress syndrome, *Clin Chest Med* 27(4):627–635, 2006.

110. Pinsky MR, Payen D: Functional hemodynamic monitoring, *Crit Care* 9(6):566–572, 2005.

111. Pinsky MR: Hemodynamic evaluation and monitoring in the ICU, *Chest* 132(6):2020–2029, 2007.

112. Barnett CF, Vaduganathan M, Lan G, et al.: Critical reappraisal of pulmonary artery catheterization and invasive hemodynamic assessment in acute heart failure, *Expert Rev Cardiovasc Ther* 11(4):417–424, 2013.

113. Renner J, Scholz J, Bein B: Monitoring fluid therapy, *Best Pract Res Clin Anaesthesiol* 23 (2):159–171, 2009.

114. Marik PE: Noninvasive cardiac output monitors: a state-of the-art review, *J Cardiothorac Vasc Anesth* 27(1):121–134, 2013.

115. Kardos A, Vereczkey G, Szentirmai C: Haemodynamic changes during positive-pressure ventilation in children, *Acta Anaesthesiol Scand* 49(5):649–653, 2005.

116. Ferguson ND, Meade MO, Hallett DC, Stewart TE: High values of the pulmonary artery wedge pressure in patients with acute lung injury and acute respiratory distress syndrome, *Intensive Care Med* 28(8):1073–1077, 2002.

117. Malbrain ML, Ameloot K, Gillebert C, Cheatham ML: Cardiopulmonary monitoring in intra-abdominal hypertension, *Am Surg* 77(Suppl 1):S23–S30, 2011.

118. Ameloot K, Gillebert C, Desie N, Malbrain ML: Hypoperfusion, shock states, and abdominal compartment syndrome (ACS), *Surg Clin North Am* 92(2):207–220, 2012.

119. Torquato JA, Lucato JJ, Antunes T, Barbas CV: Interaction between intra-abdominal pressure and positive-end expiratory pressure, *Clinics* 64(2):105–112, 2009.

120. Pinsky MR: Cardiovascular issues in respiratory care, *Chest* 128(5 Suppl 2):592S–597S, 2005.

121. Renner J, Gruenewald M, Quaden R, et al.: Influence of increased intra-abdominal pressure on fluid responsiveness predicted by pulse pressure variation and stroke volume variation in a porcine model, *Crit Care Med* 37(2):650–658, 2009.

122. Monnet X, Bleibtreu A, Ferre A, et al.: Passive leg-raising and end-expiratory occlusion tests perform better than pulse pressure variation in patients with low respiratory system compliance, *Crit Care Med* 40(1):152–157, 2012.

123. Monnet X, Rienzo M, Osman D, et al.: Passive leg raising predicts fluid responsiveness in the critically ill, *Crit Care Med* 34(5):1402–1407, 2006.

124. Noritomi DT, Vieira ML, Mohovic T, et al.: Echocardiography for hemodynamic evaluation in the intensive care unit, *Shock* 34(Suppl 1):59–62, 2010.

125. Vignon P, AitHssain A, Francois B, et al.: Echocardiographic assessment of pulmonary artery occlusion pressure in ventilated patients: a transoesophageal study, *Crit Care* 12(1):R18, 2008.

126. Levitt JE, Matthay MA: Treatment of acute lung injury: historical perspective and potential future therapies, *Semin Respir Crit Care Med* 27(4):426–437, 2006.

127. Pino-Sanchez F, Lara-Rosales R, Guerrero-Lopez F, et al.: Influence of extravascular lung water determination in fluid and vasoactive therapy, *J Trauma* 67(6):1220–1224, 2009.

128. Heresi GA, Arroliga AC, Wiedemann HP, Matthay MA: Pulmonary artery catheter and fluid management in acute lung injury and the acute respiratory distress syndrome, *Clin Chest Med* 27(4):627–635, 2006.

129. Neamu RF, Martin GS: Fluid management in acute respiratory distress syndrome, *Curr Opin Crit Care* 19(1):24–30, 2013.

130. Tinti M, Gracias V, Kaplan LJ: Adjuncts to ventilation part II: monitoring, fluid management, bundles, and positioning, *Curr Probl Surg* 50(10):433–437, 2013.

131. van der Heijden M, Verheij J, van Nieuw Amerongen GP, Groeneveld AB: Crystalloid or colloid fluid loading and pulmonary permeability, edema, and injury in septic and nonseptic critically ill patients with hypovolemia, *Crit Care Med* 37(4):1275–1281, 2009.

132. National Heart, Lung, and Blood Institute Acute Respiratory Distress Syndrome (ARDS) Clinical Trials Network, Wiedemann HP, Wheeler AP, Bernard GR, et al.: Comparison of two fluid-management strategies in acute lung injury, *N Engl J Med* 354(24):2564–2575, 2006.

133. De Backer D, Heenen S, Piagnerelli M, et al.: Pulse pressure variations to predict fluid responsiveness: influence of tidal volume, *Intensive Care Med* 31(4):517–523, 2005.

134. De Backer D, Scolletta S: Why do pulse pressure variations fail to predict the response to fluids in acute respiratory distress syndrome patients ventilated with low tidal volume? *Crit Care* 15 (2):150, 2011.

135. Malbrain ML, De Laet I: Functional haemodynamics during intra-abdominal hypertension: what to use and what not use, *Acta Anaesthesiol Scand* 52(4):576–577, 2008.

136. Wyffels PA, Sergeant P, Wouters PF: The value of pulse pressure and stroke volume variation as predictors of fluid responsiveness during open chest surgery, *Anaesthesia* 65(7):704–709, 2010.

137. Huang CC, Fu JY, Hu HC, et al.: Prediction of fluid responsiveness in acute respiratory distress syndrome patients ventilated with low tidal volume and high positive end-expiratory pressure, *Crit Care Med* 36(10):2810–2816, 2008.

138. Michard F, Descorps-Declere A, Lopes MR: Using pulse pressure variation in patients with acute respiratory distress syndrome, *Crit Care Med* 36(10):2946–2948, 2008.

139. Payen D, Vallee F, Mari A, et al.: Can pulse pressure variations really better predict fluid responsiveness than static indices of preload in patients with acute respiratory distress syndrome? *Crit Care Med* 37(3):1178, 2009.

140. Teboul JL, Monnet X: Pulse pressure variation and ARDS, *Minerva Anestesiol* 79(4):398–407, 2013.

141. Nunes S, Valta P, Takala J: Changes in respiratory mechanics and gas exchange during the acute respiratory distress syndrome, *Acta Anaesthesiol Scand* 50(1):80–91, 2006.

142. Sundaresan A, Chase JG, Hann CE, Shaw GM: Cardiac output estimation using pulmonary mechanics in mechanically ventilated patients, *Biomed Eng Online* 9(1):80, 2010.

143. Cavallaro F, Sandroni C, Antonelli M: Functional hemodynamic monitoring and dynamic indices of fluid responsiveness, *Minerva Anestesiol* 74(4):123–135, 2008.

144. Branson RD: Modes to facilitate ventilator weaning, *Respir Care* 57(10):1635–1648, 2012.

145. Burns SM: Weaning from mechanical ventilation: where were we then, and where are we now? *Crit Care Nurs Clin North Am* 24(3):457–468, 2012.

146. Cappati KR, Tonella RM, Damascena AS, et al.: Interobserver agreement rate of the spontaneous breathing trial, *J Crit Care* 28(1):62–68, 2013.

147. Hess DR: The role of noninvasive ventilation in the ventilator discontinuation process, *Respir Care* 57(10):1619–1625, 2012.

148. Macintyre NR: Evidence-based assessments in the ventilator discontinuation process, *Respir Care* 57(10):1611–1618, 2012.

149. Teixeira C, Teixeira PJ, de Leon PP, Oliveira ES: Work of breathing during successful spontaneous breathing trial, *J Crit Care* 24(4):508–514, 2009.

150. Thille AW, Cortes-Puch I, Esteban A: Weaning from the ventilator and extubation in ICU, *Curr Opin Crit Care* 19(1):57–64, 2013.

151. Mekontso Dessap A, Roche-Campo F, Kouatchet A, et al.: Natriuretic peptide-driven fluid management during ventilator weaning: a randomized controlled trial, *Am J Respir Crit Care Med* 186(12):1256–1263, 2012.

152. Mongodi S, Via G, Bouhemad B, et al.: Usefulness of combined bedside lung ultrasound and echocardiography to assess weaning failure from mechanical ventilation: a suggestive case, *Crit Care Med* 41(8):e182–e185, 2013.

153. Caille V, Amiel JB, Charron C, et al.: Echocardiography: a help in the weaning process, *Crit Care* 14(3):R120, 2010.

154. Girard TD, Kress JP, Fuchs BD, et al.: Efficacy and safety of a paired sedation and ventilator weaning protocol for mechanically ventilated patients in intensive care (awakening and breathing controlled trial): a randomised controlled trial, *Lancet* 371(9607):126–134, 2008.

155. Hooper MH, Girard TD: Sedation and weaning from mechanical ventilation: linking spontaneous awakening trials and spontaneous breathing trials to improve patient outcomes, *Crit Care Clin* 25(3):515–525, 2009.

156. Teixeira C, Teixeira PJ, de Leon PP, Oliveira ES: Work of breathing during successful spontaneous breathing trial, *J Crit Care* 24(4):508–514, 2009.

157. Verceles AC, Diaz-Abad M, Geiger-Brown J, Scharf SM: Testing the prognostic value of the rapid shallow breathing index in predicting successful weaning in patients requiring prolonged mechanical ventilation, *Heart Lung* 41(6):546–552, 2012.

158. Ambrosino N, Gabbrielli L: The difficult-to-wean patient, *Expert Rev Respir Med* 4(5):685–692, 2010.

159. Haas CF, Loik PS: Ventilator discontinuation protocols, *Respir Care* 57(10):1649–1662, 2012.

160. Jubran A, Grant BJ, Duffner LA, et al.: Effect of pressure support vs unassisted breathing through a tracheostomy collar on weaning duration in patients requiring prolonged mechanical ventilation: a randomized trial, *JAMA* 309(7):671–677, 2013.

161. Kaplan LJ, Toevs CC: Weaning from mechanical ventilation, *Curr Probl Surg* 50(10):489–494, 2013.

162. Lara TM, Hajjar LA, de Almeida JP, et al.: High levels of B-type natriuretic peptide predict weaning failure from mechanical ventilation in adult patients after cardiac surgery, *Clinics* 68(1):33–38, 2013.

163. Russell JA: Biomarker (BNP)-guided weaning from mechanical ventilation: time for a paradigm shift? *Am J Respir Crit Care Med* 186(12):1202–1204, 2012.

164. Girgis K, Hamed H, Khater Y, Kacmarek RM: A decremental PEEP trial identifies the PEEP level that maintains oxygenation after lung recruitment, *Respir Care* 51(10):1132–1139, 2006.

Hemodynamics of Mechanical Circulatory Support

15

Julie A. Shinn

Mechanical circulatory support (MCS) has evolved to become a routine therapy for patients with advanced heart failure and is provided at most major medical centers worldwide.

Historical Milestones

Intra-aortic balloon pump (IABP) counterpulsation therapy emerged in the late 1960s as the first invasive device to treat inability to wean from cardiopulmonary bypass following heart surgery or as a treatment for cardiogenic shock following acute myocardial infarction. IABP therapy augments cardiac function by increasing coronary perfusion and unloading the left ventricle. Because it has no direct ability to maintain blood pressure and systemic circulation, the ability of the device to resuscitate patients is severely limited. Timing of therapy and initial application was reserved for patients with dismal prognoses, which, not unexpectedly led to poor outcomes. Since that time, a better understanding of IABP application, timing, and refinement of technology has led to widespread application with excellent outcomes.

The evolution and application for MCS therapy in the early years was similar to that of the IABP. Some milestones of MCS therapy are listed in Table 15-1. The MCS field has seen great advancements in the last two decades to include a variety of devices for short-term and long-term support of patients with advanced heart failure. Unlike IABP therapy, these devices are capable of supporting the systemic circulation. They have evolved to the point of being capable of supporting patients as destination therapy in lieu of heart transplantation. Many major medical centers have at least two or three forms of MCS support that can be utilized for management of advanced heart failure. Examples of the more commonly used devices are outlined in this chapter and provide an insight into how the various designs impact and support cardiovascular hemodynamics.

TABLE 15-1   Milestones of Mechanical Circulatory Support Therapy

YEAR	INVESTIGATORS AND CLINICAL TRIALS	DEVELOPMENT
1953	John H. Gibbon	First intracardiac repair with cardiopulmonary bypass
1966	Michael A. DeBakey	First successful postcardiotomy left ventricular assist device (LVAD) for bridge to recovery
1967	Adrian Kantrowitz	First clinical use of the intra-aortic balloon pump (IABP)
1969	Denton Cooley and Domingo Liotta	First human total artificial heart (TAH) implantation for bridge to transplantation
1882	William DeVries	First TAH destination therapy implantation—Jarvik 7
1984	Philip Oyer	First successful LVAD bridge to transplantation—Novacor
2001	Rose, et al.*	REMATCH trial—destination therapy with HeartMate XVE
2003		FDA approval of HeartMate XVE for destination therapy
2004		FDA approval of the SynCardia TAH for bridge to transplantation
2007	Miller, et al.†	HeartMate II bridge to transplantation trial
2008		FDA approval of HeartMate II for bridge to Transplantation
2009	Slaughter, et al.‡	HeartMate II destination therapy trial
2010		FDA approval of HeartMate II for destination therapy
2012	Aaronson, et al.‖	HeartWare bridge to transplantation trial
2012		FDA approval of HeartWare for bridge to transplantation

FDA, United States Food and Drug Administration.
*Rose EA, Gelijns AC, Moskowitz AJ, et al.: Long-term use of a left ventricular assist device for end-stage heart failure, *N Engl J Med* 345(20):1435–1443, 2001.
†Miller LW, Pagani FD, Russell SD, et al.: Use of a continuous-flow device in patients awaiting heart transplantation, *N Engl J Med* 357(9):885–896, 2007.
‡Slaughter MS, Rogers JG, Milano CA, et al.: Advanced heart failure treated with continuous-flow left ventricular assist device, *N Engl J Med* 361(23):2241–2251, 2009.
‖Aaronson KD, Slaughter MS, Miller LW, et al.: Use of an intrapericardial, continuous-flow, centrifugal pump in patients awaiting heart transplantation, *Circulation* 125(25):3191–3200, 2012.

Categories of Mechanical Circulatory Support

Short-Term Mechanical Circulatory Support Devices

These devices are designed to be used in conjunction with the native heart and are used as a temporary measure to augment the function of the failing heart. Their capability ranges from augmentation to fully supporting the circulation for a limited amount of time. The intent of this therapy is to allow time for myocardial recovery and return of heart function or provide time to evaluate whether the patient is a suitable candidate for a long-term MCS device. Examples of commonly used devices in this category are the IABP, the Tandem Heart (Cardiac Assist, Pittsburgh, PA), the Impella device (Abiomed Inc., Danvers, MA), Centrimag (Thoratec Corp., Pleasanton, CA), and extracorporeal membrane oxygenation (ECMO). These devices are limited to cardiovascular systemic support for a period of days to weeks until ventricular recovery occurs or until the patient is bridged to either heart transplantation or to a more durable device.

Intermediate-Term Mechanical Circulatory Support Devices

Intermediate-term MCS devices are designed to fully support a patient's circulation for weeks to months during myocardial recovery or while waiting for cardiac transplantation. These devices are typically left ventricular assist devices (LVADs) and can also be used to support the right ventricle (RVAD). Blood enters these pumps from a patient's circulation through an inflow cannula placed in the atrium or the ventricle. Blood is returned to the patient's circulation through an outflow cannula, which is anastomosed to the ascending aorta (LVAD) or to the pulmonary artery (RVAD). These pumps are capable of providing flows of 3 to 10 liters per minute (L/min).

Intermediate-term devises are pulsatile and typically are placed outside of the body (extracorporeal), although they can also be placed inside the body (intracorporeal). Alternating compressed air and vacuum from an external source (driver) are necessary for these devices to run. This feature makes them more cumbersome for patients to use and limits their use for long-term support outside of the hospital. Two commonly used intermediate-term pulsatile pumps are the Thoratec PVAD and IVAD (Thoratec Corporation, Pleasanton, CA), and the Abiomed AB5000 (Abiomed Inc., Danvers, MA).

Long-Term Mechanical Circulatory Support Devices

Long-term MCS devices have evolved into small, nonpulsatile, continuous flow pumps that are implanted inside the patient's pericardial space or in a surgically created "pocket" just below the patient's diaphragm. They have a small driveline that is tunneled through the skin and exits the body to be connected to a monitor and an electrical power source. They are quiet and require minimal external equipment, which makes it easy for the patient to live with these devices outside the hospital. As a result, these devices are capable of supporting patients for an extended period while waiting for heart transplantation or as long-term treatment for advanced heart failure, which is described as destination therapy. Two commonly used continuous flow pumps are the HeartMate II (Thoratec Corporation, Pleasanton, CA), and HeartWare Left Ventricular Assist System (LVAS) (HeartWare Inc., Framingham, MA).

Total Artificial Heart Device

An alternative for patients with biventricular heart failure is complete ventricular replacement with the total artificial heart (TAH). The TAH is used in cases of severe biventricular failure when an LVAD alone would not provide adequate support.

A failing right ventricle may not be able to maintain adequate filling of the left heart with only an LVAD. The TAH is actually composed of two pumps that attach to the two atria and completely replace all native ventricular function. Clinical issues that might impair TAH pump function include hypovolemia, tamponade, right heart failure, thrombus formation in the pump, and inflow or outflow cannula obstruction.

Short-Term Mechanical Circulatory Support Therapy

Intra-aortic Balloon Pump Counterpulsation Therapy

IABP counterpulsation is the most widely used form of MCS and has become a mainstay in the management of hemodynamic instability in patients with ischemic and dysfunctional myocardium. The hemodynamic effects and benefits of IABP counterpulsation therapy result from the alternating addition and displacement of volume to and from the aorta in a manner opposite to, or counter to, the cardiac cycle.[1] A percutaneously inserted catheter-mounted balloon is advanced into the descending aorta from the femoral artery. Figure 15-1 depicts the correct position of the catheter in the aorta. The balloon capacities range from 30- to 50-milliliter (mL) volume in adult patients.

Hemodynamic and Physiologic Effects of Intra-aortic Balloon Pump Therapy

Intra-aortic Balloon Pump Inflation. At the beginning of diastole, the balloon is inflated with helium gas, which efficiently displaces the aortic blood volume and pushes blood toward the aortic root. The increase in aortic root pressure increases flow into the coronary arteries. As a result, myocardial oxygen supply is increased. Distal perfusion pressure is also enhanced as balloon inflation improves renal and mesenteric arterial blood flow. These are two vascular beds that are frequently underperfused with myocardial dysfunction and advanced heart failure.

Intra-aortic Balloon Pump Deflation. Deflation is timed to occur just prior to the next systolic ejection of the heart. The displacement of blood from the aorta reduces impedance to left ventricular (LV) ejection resulting in a larger stroke volume with lower ventricular wall tension (Figure 15-2). The clinical outcome is decreased afterload and reduced myocardial oxygen demand. Indirectly, this will improve contractility. Greater stroke volume per beat results in decreased preload and decreased pulmonary congestion, which are two prevalent features of myocardial dysfunction and advanced heart failure.

The hemodynamic and physiologic effects of IABP counterpulsation therapy are summarized in Table 15-2. The degree to which the desired hemodynamic effects are achieved will, in part, depend on the size or volume of the balloon, the degree to which the balloon occludes the aorta during diastole, correct positioning of the balloon in the aorta, and how well timed the balloon inflation and deflation are relative to the patient's cardiac cycle.[2]

To achieve ideal counterpulsation, the balloon must have adequate volume relative to the size of the patient. Ideally, the inflated balloon should occlude 95% of the aorta to increase coronary blood flow during inflation and achieve optimal afterload reduction

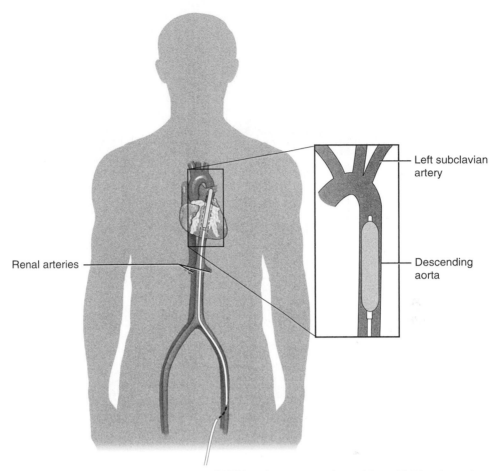

FIGURE 15-1 Intra-aortic balloon pump (IABP) catheter correctly positioned in the thoracic aorta just below the left subclavian artery and above the renal arteries.

during deflation. The degree to which this is achieved depends on how well the balloon size fits the diameter of the aorta. Balloon sizes range from 30 to 50 mL in volume in adult patients. A person with a height less than 5 feet and 2 inches would most likely require the 30-mL size because the larger balloon will extend too far down into the abdominal aorta potentially inflating against a calcified aorta, thus increasing the risk of balloon rupture. A lower position may also interfere with renal artery blood flow. A person taller than 6 feet and 2 inches would most likely require a 50-mL balloon to ensure adequate blood volume displacement during balloon inflation. For all other individuals, the 40-mL balloon is adequate.

The correct position of the balloon in the aorta is just below the left subclavian artery and above the renal arteries. This position can be visualized on the chest radiograph. The catheter tip should be located 2 centimeters (cm) below the origin of the left subclavian artery at the second to third intercostal space. A position too high in the aorta

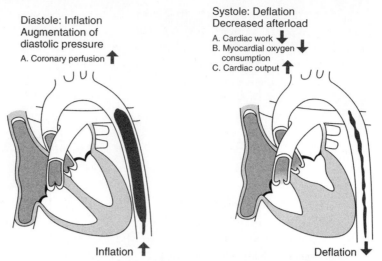

FIGURE 15-2 Effects of Intra-aortic balloon pump (IABP) catheter inflation and deflation. Augmentation of coronary blood flow and distal perfusion occurs during balloon inflation. Deflation of the balloon during systole enhances forward flow of blood from the ventricle and decreases impedance to ejection resulting in afterload reduction. (Courtesy of Maquet Cardiac Assist (Datascope Corp.), Inc.)

TABLE 15-2 **Physiologic and Hemodynamic Effects of IABP Inflation and Deflation**

CLINICAL OR HEMODYNAMIC INDICATOR	INFLATION	DEFLATION
↑ Coronary blood flow	+++	None
↓ Symptoms and signs of ischemia Angina ST segment changes Arrhythmias	+++	+++
↓ Afterload	None	+++
↓ Preload (PAOP)	+ - ++	+++
↓ Heart rate (indirect effect)	++	++
↑ Cardiac index	+ - +	+++
↑ Urine output (indirect effect)	+ - ++	+++
↓ MVO$_2$	+ - ++	+++

+ = mild
++ = moderate
+++ = major
IABP, Intra-aortic balloon pump; *MVO$_2$,* myocardial oxygen demand; *PAOP,* pulmonary artery occlusion pressure (wedge).

may interfere with blood flow to the left subclavian artery. A position too low in the aorta may interfere with renal artery blood flow. Routine assessment of the patient with an IABP includes assessment for the presence of the left radial pulse. A change in radial pulse character might be an indication that the balloon is too high in the aorta and limiting left subclavian arterial blood flow. Any unexpected decrease in urine output in the patient should be investigated, as it may result from a low balloon position limiting renal artery blood flow.

Timing of balloon inflation and deflation to the patient's cardiac cycle is critical for achieving optimal coronary perfusion and afterload reduction. The hemodynamic consequences of balloon mistiming are listed below:

- **Early inflation:** A balloon that inflates too early might abruptly force closure of the aortic valve before the end of systole due to the increased pressure in the aorta.
- **Late inflation:** When inflation is too late, it does not take advantage of the total time in diastole to increase coronary perfusion.
- **Early deflation:** Balloon deflation that is too early may not result in significant afterload reduction just before the next systolic contraction. Aortic pressure may have time to rise to baseline after an early deflation resulting in no afterload reduction effect.
- **Late deflation:** Balloon deflation that is too late may result in higher afterload as the impedance to ejection is increased at the beginning of systole because of the still inflated balloon. This inflation error is the most harmful to the patient because it actually causes increased myocardial oxygen demand; defeating a primary purpose of IABP therapy.

The accurate timing of balloon inflation and deflation is illustrated in Figure 15-3. Present-day IABP consoles use computer or automatic timing. The most accurate IABP timing is achieved with newer fiberoptic catheters.[1]

Indications and Contraindications of Intra-aortic Balloon Pump Therapy

IABP therapy is indicated and effective for a variety of cardiac conditions. A frequent application is for the support of low cardiac output following cardiopulmonary bypass. The duration of support is rarely more than 72 hours, by which time the myocardium has recovered from any stunning, edema, or other transient effects of the surgery. Common medical indications include cardiogenic shock from LV failure or following myocardial infarction. IABP therapy can be helpful in supporting patients who have incurred acute mitral regurgitation from papillary muscle injury, or ventricular septal rupture with left-to-right shunting following myocardial infarction. The decreased afterload and increased stroke volume helps decrease the amount of regurgitation and left-to-right shunt from these two mechanical problems until surgical repair. Other indications are intractable angina or myocardial ischemia, refractory heart failure, intractable arrhythmias, and as a bridge to further therapy such as LVAD, heart transplantation, or cardiac surgery.[3] IABP therapy is used in some centers as adjunctive therapy for high-risk patients undergoing interventional procedures in the cardiac catheterization laboratory.

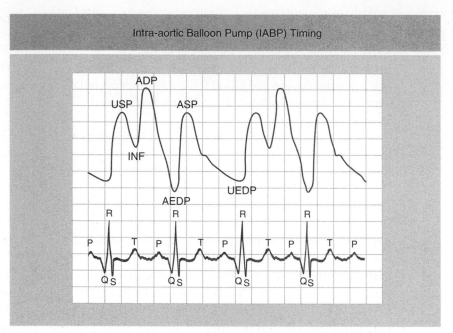

FIGURE 15-3 Arterial waveform shows balloon inflation during diastole and balloon deflation during systole. Diastolic augmentation results from balloon inflation, which causes a rise in diastolic blood pressure during diastole. The augmentation of blood pressure is the source of increased coronary artery perfusion pressure. The evacuation of volume from the balloon just prior to the assisted systole cause a drop in aortic pressure which decrease impedance to the next systolic ejection and afterload is effectively reduced. Evidence of afterload reduction is demonstrated by the assisted end-diastolic pressure being lower than the unassisted end-diastolic pressure and by the assisted systolic pressure being lower than the unassisted systole. *ADP*, Assisted diastolic pressure; *AEDP*, assisted end-diastolic pressure; *ASP*, assisted systolic pressure; *INF*, inflation; *UEDP*, unassisted end-diastolic pressure; *USP*, unassisted systole. (From Crawford MH, DiMarco JP, Paulus WJ, editors: *Cardiology*, ed 2, Philadelphia, 2004, Mosby.)

Contraindications to IABP therapy are few. Severe peripheral vascular disease is a contraindication because of the risk of the catheter compromising blood flow distal to the cannulated femoral artery. This condition could potentially lead to limb ischemia or compartment syndrome. Other contraindications include the presence of an aortic aneurysm, as well as aortic dissection, since dissection may further increase with higher pressures during diastole. Aortic insufficiency is also a contraindication because the increased pressure during diastole would serve to create greater valve regurgitation. Because patients must be anticoagulated while receiving IABP therapy, any uncontrolled bleeding disorder may be a contraindication for insertion.

Potential Complications of Intra-aortic Balloon Pump Therapy

Complications associated with IABP therapy are well established and primarily vascular in nature, especially in the presence of peripheral arterial disease.[2] Common complications are listed in Box 15-1.[4-6] In keeping with the theme of this chapter, only those

---

BOX 15-1   Complications of Intra-aortic Balloon Pump Therapy[4-6]

Limb ischemia
Compartment syndrome
Visceral ischemia
Aortic dissection
Vascular injury
Retroperitoneal bleeding
Balloon rupture

Balloon entrapment resulting from thrombus
    formation inside the balloon after rupture
Cerebral emboli from dislodged thrombus on
    the catheter tip
Plaque dislodgement causing embolization
Thrombocytopenia

---

complications that affect hemodynamic effectiveness are discussed. The clinical issues that might impair IABP effectiveness other than what has previously been discussed include hypovolemia and right heart failure. In the cardiothoracic surgery patient, bleeding from extensive surgical dissection, trauma to platelets from cardiopulmonary bypass, and residual effects from anticoagulation may cause hypovolemia, which must be treated with volume replacement before the benefits of improved cardiac index from IABP therapy can be appreciated. A second issue that may preclude hemodynamic improvement from IABP therapy is the presence of significant right heart failure. Increased coronary perfusion may help to a certain extent, but if the clinical problem is primary right heart failure, improved cardiac index cannot be achieved. Left heart afterload reduction might be attained but inadequate filling of the left heart will still result in low output and cardiac index.

Hemodynamic Effectiveness and Limitations in Intra-aortic Balloon Pump Therapy

For decades, IABP counterpulsation therapy has been the first-line MCS for patients with acute myocardial infarction undergoing percutaneous revascularization intervention because of its widespread availability, ease of use, low cost, and relatively low rates of serious complications. However, the utility of IABP therapy has recently been challenged.[7] The results of two large randomized controlled trials have called into question the effectiveness of IABP therapy in acute myocardial infarction.

The Counterpulsation to Reduce Infarct Size Pre-PCI Acute Myocardial Infarction (CRISP-AMI) trial compared IABP support before percutaneous coronary intervention (PCI), with standard PCI care in 337 patients with acute myocardial infarction *without* cardiogenic shock. No difference was observed in infarct size reduction between the two groups.[8]

The Intra-aortic Balloon Pump in Cardiogenic Shock II (IABP- SHOCK II) trial compared 30-day mortality rates in 595 patients between those with acute myocardial infarction *and* cardiogenic shock undergoing early PCI revascularization and those with primary PCI alone.[9] Pre-PCI insertion of the IABP did not lower mortality at 30 days[9] or at 12 months.[10] These results can be interpreted in several ways. Perhaps

IABP does not have added benefit in acute myocardial infarction *without* cardiogenic shock as long as the time to coronary revascularization is short;[11] or it may be that the SHOCK II trial results indicate that more substantial MCS support is required for myocardial infarction patients *with* cardiogenic shock. The mortality risk of acute myocardial infarction with cardiogenic shock is about 40%.[9] Therefore, it is important to escalate MCS support in patients with refractory cardiogenic shock, as IABP therapy may not provide adequate support.[12]

Impella Ventricular Assist Device

Microaxial continuous flow pumps provide the next level of temporary MCS support. An example of this type of pump is the Impella device. The two commonly used sizes are the Impella 2.5, and the Impella 5.0. The pump is inserted through the femoral artery and passed in a retrograde manner up the aorta, across the aortic valve, and into the left ventricle under fluoroscopic or echocardiographic guidance. The pump directly off-loads the left ventricle by pulling blood from the LV inflow cannula and propelling it through the outflow into the ascending aorta (Figure 15-4). The pump is mounted on a 9-French (Fr) catheter, which houses a motor driveline and purge line system.

The Impella 2.5 has a pump diameter of 12 Fr and can usually be placed without a surgical cut down. The Impella 5.0 has a pump diameter of 21 Fr that necessitates a femoral arterial cut-down for placement.[13] The Impella pumps can also be placed directly into the aorta in patients with cardiogenic shock or low cardiac output syndrome following cardiothoracic surgery. This direct approach utilizes a vascular graft that is sewn directly to the ascending aorta. The pump-mounted catheter is then passed

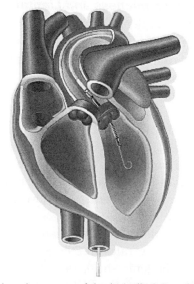

FIGURE 15-4 Transaortic valve placement of the Impella 2.5 and 5.0 pumps. (Courtesy Abiomed Inc., Danvers, MA.)

through the graft and directed in a retrograde manner across the aortic valve into the left ventricle. With this approach, only the skin of the chest wound is closed until the pump is removed. The rationale for this chest approach is the rapid initiation of circulatory support in an emergency situation with catastrophic hemodynamic deterioration.[14] A newer pump design created for transaortic placement is the Impella LD. It is shorter than the 2.5 and 5.0 pumps and does not have a pigtail at the tip. The catheter provides flows up to 5 L/min. The Impella 2.5 pump is capable of generating up to 2.5 L/min blood flow, and the Impella 5.0 is capable of 5.0 L/min. Another new pump is the Impella CP, which is built on the Impella 2.5 platform but with a larger diameter (14 Fr versus 12 Fr) so that it can provide flows of 3.5 to 4.0 L/min.

Each of these pumps has been used to support patients for periods up to 7 or more days allowing time to develop a more definitive treatment strategy or for recovery to occur.[14,15] Despite the large size of these pumps, the incidence of limb ischemia or vascular repair has been similar to that associated with IABP therapy.[16,17] The patient must receive anticoagulation therapy. Intraoperative activated clotting times are typically maintained between 160 and 180 seconds to prevent clot formation in the motor.[13,15] Postoperatively, partial thromboplastin times are maintained between 40 to 50 seconds with a continuous infusion of heparin.[14,15]

Hemodynamic and Physiologic Effects of Impella Device Therapy

The propulsion of blood ejected from the left ventricle results in an increase in mean arterial pressure (MAP) and an increase in the cardiac index. Coronary artery perfusion pressure should improve, thus increasing myocardial oxygen supply. Improved forward flow will lower the pulmonary artery occlusion pressure (PAOP). This mechanical unloading of the ventricle reduces LV workload and myocardial oxygen demand.[13] As with IABP therapy, improved distal flow and a higher cardiac index should enhance renal and mesenteric arterial blood flow.

Indications and Contraindications of Impella Device Therapy

Current indications for use of the Impella pump include hemodynamic support for high-risk percutaneous interventions, acute ST-elevation myocardial infarction with cardiogenic shock and low output syndrome, or cardiogenic shock following cardiothoracic surgery. Contraindications include severe peripheral vascular disease that would make peripheral insertion difficult and compromise blood flow distal to the insertion site with great risk of limb ischemia. The presence of LV thrombus precludes intraventricular placement of the pump because of the high risk of embolization to the cerebrovascular circulation causing a stroke. The presence of a mechanical aortic valve, moderate to severe aortic valve insufficiency, or aortic valve stenosis are also contraindications.

Potential Complications of Impella Device Therapy

The vascular injury potential of this pump is similar to IABP therapy because of the peripheral cannulation of the femoral artery. Limb ischemia and bleeding complications also have a reported incidence that is similar to IABP therapy.[17] Mild hemolysis may occur with the use of any mechanical pump and has been reported in up to 20% of patients.[18] Patients receiving higher flows with faster motor revolutions may be at greater risk for hemolysis.

Impaired Hemodynamic Effectiveness and Limitations of Impella Device Therapy

Hypovolemia following cardiothoracic surgery presents a threat to the optimal performance of the pump and can easily be addressed with volume replacement. A greater threat is the development of cardiac tamponade, which would impair LV filling (pump preload) and therefore impair pump output. Relief of cardiac tamponade is a surgical emergency. This event is more likely to occur with transaortic placement of the device.

As with all devices that support the left ventricle, the coexistence of right heart failure will inhibit the ability of the pump to provide optimal output. If the right ventricle has difficulty filling the left heart, there is less volume to support pump flow and a reduced contribution by the left ventricle to overall blood pressure. In this situation, inotropic support would be indicated to support right ventricular (RV) function. Care must be taken during insertion to position the pump away from the papillary muscles and the mitral subvalvular apparatus to avoid damage to those structures (see Figure 15-4). The suction effect generated by the pump might result in inflow obstruction from adjacent tissue. It is also important to maintain adequate anticoagulation to prevent thrombus formation within the pump that would impair function and might even necessitate removal or exchange.

TandemHeart

The TandemHeart is another example of a percutaneous continuous flow MCS system. TandemHeart support is indicated in patients with refractory cardiogenic shock following myocardial infarction, in decompensated heart failure as temporary support until there is ventricular recovery, as a bridge to a more permanent device, or as a bridge to heart transplantation. The TandemHeart circuit includes a venous cannula, a trans-septal left atrium to femoral artery cannula, and an external, nonpulsatile centrifugal pump (see Figure 15-5). Contained within the pump is a six-blade rotating impeller that spins at speeds between 3000 and 7500 revolutions per minute (RPM), generating flows of up to 5 L/min. Placement of the pump is performed in the cardiac catheterization laboratory under fluoroscopic guidance or by direct vision in the case of a cardiothoracic surgery patient.

The inflow to the pump is via a 21-Fr femoral venous cannula that is advanced up the inferior vena cava to the right atrium. The cannula is then advanced across the atrial septum into the left atrium via septotomy. The end of the cannula has 14 side holes that allow oxygenated blood to be pulled from the left atrium to the extracorporeal centrifugal pump.[13] It is important to maintain the cannula in the correct position with 3 cm traversing the septum. The pump returns blood to the femoral or iliac arterial systemic circulation. A 14-Fr to 19-Fr cannula is used for this purpose. The position of the pump

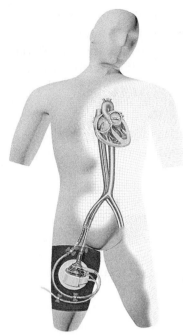

FIGURE 15-5 TandemHeart pVAD. (Courtesy CardiacAssist, Inc.)

and the transseptal cannulation of the left atrium is shown in Figure 15-5. It is critical not to jeopardize the position of the left atrial cannula. For that reason, patients are relatively immobile during TandemHeart support.

Patient positioning concerns with regard to this pump include recommendations that patients be tilted rather than turned, that the cannulated extremity not be flexed, and that the head of the bed not be elevated more than 20 degrees. Cooperative patients require only light sedation, but some patients may require extended sedation to limit mobility for their safety. These are reasons this therapy has a limited duration of only several days. Anticoagulation is required when this pump is in use. Activated clotting times are maintained between 180 and 220 seconds with anticoagulation. Anticoagulation is titrated to maintain partial thromboplastin times between 65 and 85 seconds in the post-insertion period.

Hemodynamic and Physiologic Effects of TandemHeart Therapy

The TandemHeart is capable of significant pressure and volume unloading of the left ventricle. It can relieve LV distention and decrease ventricular wall strain, which are important components of myocardial oxygen demand. The LV unloading will also unload the right ventricle, improving right heart function, as evidenced by a decrease in the central venous pressure. The improved cardiac index will enhance the support of end-organ function with increased tissue perfusion. These effects have been reported in patients with cardiogenic shock, high-risk interventional cardiology patients, and cardiothoracic surgery patients.[19–21]

As stated, it is critical to prevent dislodgement of the left atrial cannula. A sudden drop in peripheral oxygen saturation is a first indication of cannula malposition, which can be confirmed with an arterial blood gas (ABG) measurement. This event is an emergency. If the catheter has slipped back into the right atrium, deoxygenated blood will be pulled from the right atrium and returned to the systemic circulation. In addition, the acute left-to-right shunt from the left atrium to the right atrium will volume-overload the right ventricle. Resuscitation with chest compressions may dislodge the left atrial cannula and also pose a risk of left atrial perforation; if needed, such resuscitation should be performed under the supervision of a physician.

Indications and Contraindications for the TandemHeart

Indications for the use of the TandemHeart include refractory cardiogenic shock in ST-segment elevation myocardial infarction, as a bridge to recovery, or a bridge to decision, allowing time to determine whether to offer a more durable form of support for longer-term therapy.

Contraindications to the use of this pump include severe peripheral vascular disease, as is the case for the other peripherally inserted therapies previously discussed. Left atrial thrombosis can be a source of systemic emboli. The degree of anticoagulation required for this pump is greater than the Impella or the IABP, so any coagulopathy might be a contraindication. Since the pump primarily addresses LV function, severe right heart failure is a contraindication if the right ventricle is not capable of adequately filling the left side of the heart.

Potential Complications of TandemHeart Therapy

The placement of a large cannula in the femoral artery creates a risk of lower limb ischemia. Cannulation of the femoral artery brings a risk of artery dissection. Other complications reported in the TandemHeart Registry include groin hematomas, bleeding around the cannula sites, sepsis, gastrointestinal bleeding, coagulopathy, and stroke.[22] Given the larger bore of the TandemHeart catheters, infection at the insertion site is a much greater risk than with the previously described devices. These patients are also much more likely to require blood transfusions compared with patients receiving IABP or Impella support.

Impaired Hemodynamic Effectiveness and Limitations of TandemHeart Therapy

As with other devices, hypovolemia will impair pump performance, so it is important to assess the patient's fluid volume status regularly. This assessment is critical to all assist devices. Tamponade may occur if the left atrial wall is perforated. Randomized controlled trials of the TandemHeart with mortality as an outcome are not available, possibly because the TandemHeart is rarely inserted as an elective procedure.[12]

CentriMag

Like the TandemHeart, the CentriMag device is an extracorporeal, electrically driven, continuous-flow, centrifugal pump designed for short-term use in patients in cardiogenic shock. The CentriMag can be used in patients with acute cardiogenic shock of any etiology, but its initial reported use was frequently in postcardiotomy patients because a median sternotomy is required for placement.[23,24] No specific cannulas are required, so cardiopulmonary bypass cannulas can easily be used with this pump, which makes it relatively quick and easy to place a patient on support in situations where rapid deterioration occurred following attempts to wean from cardiopulmonary bypass.[25,26] A typical placement of cannulas would be inflow from the right atrium with return to the pulmonary artery for an RVAD and left atrial inflow with return to the ascending aorta for an LVAD.[23,24,27] The unique feature of this device is an impeller that floats and rotates in a magnetic field, so there is no mechanical contact with any other part of the pump (see Figure 15-6).

Put simply, the magnetic field is created by the electrical energy powering the pump. The impeller is uniformly washed by blood flow to minimize areas of blood stagnation and turbulence that can be sources of thrombus formation.[28] This feature also minimizes hemolysis. Unlike the TandemHeart, patients with CentriMag can become mobile once their condition has stabilized because of the central cannulation. The pump battery system can provide up to 120 minutes of untethered support at a speed of 3500 RPM. The CentriMag device has been used for periods of up to 30 days to support patients as a bridge to decision, bridge to recovery, or bridge to transplantation.[23,24,28] It can be used as an LVAD, RVAD, or biventricular assist device (BI-VAD).

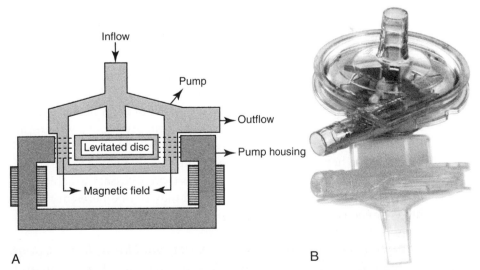

FIGURE 15-6 A, Schematic of CentriMag pump with the floating impeller being maintained by a magnetic field (inside view). **B,** Outer housing of CentriMag Pump. (**A,** From Salaunkey K et al.: Mechanical support for heart failure, *Journal of the Intensive Care Society* 14(3): 220–225, 2013; **B,** Courtesy Thoratec Corporation, Pleasanton, CA.)

If needed, the CentriMag pump can be combined with an oxygenator to deliver what is traditionally thought of as ECMO support.[26] The device is capable of providing flows of up to 10 L/min. Usual pump flows are between 4 and 5 L/min at speeds of 3000 to 4000 RPM.

Hemodynamic and Physiologic Effects of CentriMag Therapy

The hemodynamic and physiologic effects of the CentriMag device are similar to what one expects to see with the TandemHeart. Those are pressure and volume unloading of the left ventricle and, in the case of the CentriMag, pressure and volume unloading of the right ventricle if used as an RVAD or BI-VAD. The resultant decrease in myocardial oxygen demand will support the heart and allow time for potential recovery or for a bridge to re-evaluating the plan of care for the patient. Early initiation of support should have the effect of minimizing the damage to end-organ function and enhance organ recovery from cardiogenic shock.

Contraindications to Use of the CentriMag Device

The primary contraindication to the use of this device is any contraindication to anti-coagulation. This contraindication would primarily apply to the evaluation of medical patients because surgical patients have already been screened and anticoagulated for cardiopulmonary bypass. If heparin-induced thrombocytopenia (HIT) should occur, patients can be converted to a direct thrombin inhibitor such as argatroban.

Potential Complications of CentriMag Therapy

As would be expected with a surgically implanted device, bleeding is the most commonly reported complication of device placement. The incidence of bleeding has been reported to be between 21% and 44%.[23,24,28] The presence of cardiac tamponade should always be investigated when low flows occur in the presence of optimized volume loading. Thrombus may be less likely to occur within the pump but can develop in the atria, in the ventricle, or at the cannula connector sites, so a stroke as a result of thromboembolism is still possible.[24] Low flows will increase the risk of thrombus. Low flows should also prompt an evaluation of right heart function in a patient with an LVAD. Right heart failure is a common source of poor LV filling and low preload for the pump. Hemolysis incidence has been reported to be low (5%) and not clinically relevant.[23,28] When hemolysis does occur, it is likely related to the speed of the pump. The pump should not be run at higher speeds than necessary to achieve adequate flows. For example, flows of greater than 5 L/min may not be necessary and may only serve to increase the risk of hemolysis.

Impaired Hemodynamic Effectiveness and Limitations of CentriMag Therapy

The common theme for all devices is maintaining adequate pump filling, decreasing resistance to pump flow by active management of any systemic or pulmonary hypertension, and inotropic support of right heart function as required in patients with an LVAD. If these issues are not addressed, pump outflow can be affected, and this will impair effectiveness. A disadvantage of the CentriMag device is the requirement of a median sternotomy for cannula placement often in a hemodynamically unstable patient. Placement using a mini-thoracotomy has been reported and may be preferred in patients who have had a previous median sternotomy because of the greater risk of bleeding and the need for more complicated surgery.[29]

Peripheral Extracorporeal Membrane Oxygenation System

ECMO has been successfully used to treat refractory cardiogenic shock and failure to wean patients from cardiopulmonary bypass. Survival rates have been reported to be over 60% for non-postcardiotomy patients and 45% for postcardiotomy patients.[30,31] The survival rate of over 60% in medical patients is similar to that achieved for acute respiratory failure indications. Acute respiratory failure is a longstanding indication for the use of this technology.[32] Survival is about half that in patients resuscitated from cardiac arrest.[33]

The advent of centrifugal pumps has made the idea of ECMO following cardiopulmonary bypass more appealing. It is actually an extension of cardiopulmonary bypass with or without oxygenation support. Centrifugal pumps cause much less trauma to blood than the traditional roller pumps associated with cardiopulmonary bypass and can provide support to patients for days. Advantages of ECMO are that it can provide both cardiac and pulmonary support and it can be inserted percutaneously using the femoral artery and vein. Insertion is simple and rapid and can be achieved during cardiopulmonary resuscitation. The speed of application is the major appeal, as ECMO can be accomplished at the bedside.[31] It is also one of the least costly forms of MCS therapy. As mentioned, the system consists of venous-to-arterial cannulation for the support of cardiac failure. In case of failure to wean from cardiopulmonary bypass, the previously opened chest allows for direct right atrial cannulation with return to the ascending aorta. In this application, the chest is left open until the cannulas are removed. Many companies have centrifugal pumps that can be set up with membrane oxygenators. Figure 15-7 is a schematic illustration of a venous-to-arterial central and peripheral ECMO circuit.

Indications and Contraindications of Extracorporeal Membrane Oxygenation Therapy

Virtually all situations where ECMO is considered are emergencies where time is of the essence. The patient may be too unstable for complex device insertion or too unstable to move to the cardiac catheterization laboratory or operating room. Indications include cardiogenic shock refractory to inotropic or IABP therapy, cardiac arrest, cardiogenic shock after cardiothoracic surgery with failure to wean from cardiopulmonary bypass, and post–heart transplantation graft failure. Patients may also be bridged to decision when the transplantation status is unknown, for example, following cardiac arrest when the patient's neurologic status and comorbidities are unknown. For the majority of cardiothoracic surgery patients, the goal is bridge to

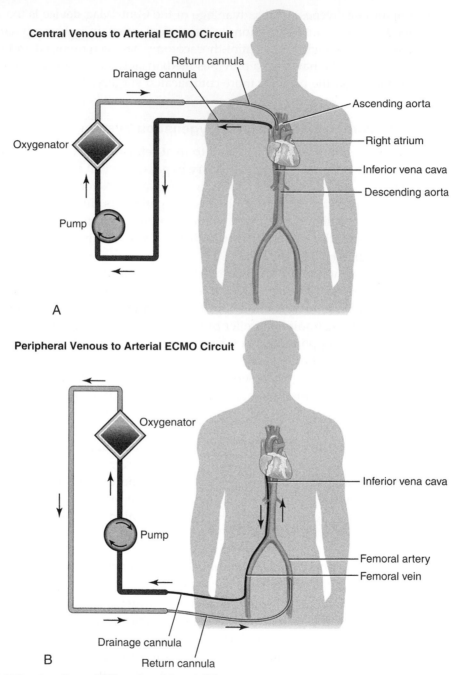

FIGURE 15-7 Central **(A)** and peripheral **(B)** placement of an extracorporeal membrane oxygenation (ECMO) circuit. (Modified from Hung M et al.: Extracorporeal membrane oxygenation: coming to an ICU near you, *Journal of the Intensive Care Society* 13(1): 31–38, 2012.)

recovery. Unfortunately, the duration of ECMO support is limited to usually no more than 7 to 9 days because of bleeding complications.[30,31] In many areas of the United States, finding a heart donor in this short period is an unrealistic expectation, so, in this case, a longer-term device should be considered as a continued bridge-to-heart transplantation.

Absolute contraindications to ECMO include known neurologic dysfunction (e.g., dementia), pre-existing kidney failure, pre-existing liver failure, and significant aortic valve insufficiency. Prolonged shock with acidosis, oliguria, and prolonged hypotension will often be associated with poor outcomes, but consideration will be given to patient age and the degree to which kidney and liver functions have been affected. Relative contraindications include compromised pre-existing functional status and lack of social support if transplantation were to be considered an option. Advanced age is also a risk factor for poor outcomes.[34] Given the emergent situation, it is left to individual physicians to make the best decisions about a patient's likelihood for survival, as data to predict outcomes are limited.

Potential Complications of Extracorporeal Membrane Oxygenation Therapy

Bleeding is the most common complication with virtually all patients requiring transfusion after placement.[30,31] Initial activated clotting time guidelines are initially targeted for 210 to 230 seconds, which might have to be reduced in a patient who is bleeding. Any bleeding is further complicated by the requirement for systemic anticoagulation to prevent the circuit from clotting off. Cerebral bleeding resulting in brain death is another devastating complication. Cardiac tamponade may be seen in postcardiotomy patients. Multi-organ failure occurs in approximately one third of patients.[31] Other complications include sepsis, leg ischemia, pulmonary complications, and thrombus formation in the ECMO circuit. Large or mobile clots require an immediate change out of the pump circuit. It is important to have nurses or other experts who will continually monitor for the presence of clots and are capable of changing out the circuit. The greatest risk occurs when the activated clotting time is reduced in the presence of bleeding. Use of heparin carries a risk of heparin induced thrombocytopenia (HIT, which will require switching the patient to a direct thrombin inhibitor such as argatroban.

Impaired Hemodynamic Effectiveness and Limitations of Extracorporeal Membrane Oxygenation Therapy

Hemodynamic effectiveness of ECMO therapy will primarily be limited by problems with the pump circuit, for example, clotting and limitations of cannula size. Another consideration is not allowing blood returning from the bronchial circulation to distend the left ventricle. Afterload reduction for the left ventricle—through concomitant IABP therapy and optimal coronary perfusion—helps minimize this. Volume optimization will help with maintenance of optimal circuit flows, thus minimizing the risk of clotting. The ECMO circuit continuously monitors hemoglobin and hematocrit. Continuous monitoring of venous oxygen saturation (SvO_2) is used to assess the adequacy of tissue perfusion. SvO_2 assessment also serves as a marker for weaning tolerance from

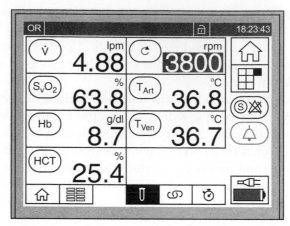

FIGURE 15-8 Extracorporeal membrane oxygenation (ECMO) monitoring parameters.

ECMO. Other monitoring indicators include esophageal echocardiographic determination of ejection fraction and right heart contractile performance.

Core temperature is monitored continuously. The long length of the cannulas, from the patient to the bedside ECMO pump, increases the risk of heat loss through the cannulas. Some circuits are capable of either warming or cooling. After cardiac arrest, patients are actively cooled to 32° C to 34° C for periods of up to 36 hours. Otherwise the patients are maintained at normothermia.[31] Figure 15-8 shows the ECMO monitor screen, where flow, pump RPM, temperature, and other parameters are continuously displayed.

Intermediate-Term Mechanical Circulatory Support Therapy

Thoratec Paracorporeal Ventricular Assist Device and Abiomed AB5000

Emergency situations arise where there is an immediate need for circulatory support in cases of acute cardiogenic shock or failure to wean from cardiopulmonary bypass, and the patient outcome is unknown. A decision must be made in spite of not knowing if cardiac recovery will occur, whether the patient is a heart transplantation candidate, and if the patient's neurologic status will be normal.[35] The emergent nature of the situation calls for a device that is easy to implant and one that has the potential to totally support the circulation and support the patient for longer periods than all of the previously discussed devices. The ideal device should also allow patients to become mobile in recovery.

The two first-generation devices that serve this purpose are paracorporeal pulsatile pumps. The term *paracorporeal* means that the pumps are positioned outside the body, with only inflow and outflow cannulas contained within the chest. The two pumps described here are the Thoratec paracorporeal ventricular assist device (PVAD) and the Abiomed AB5000. Thoratec also makes an implantable version of the PVAD that is intracorporeal or implanted in the body (Thoratec IVAD). The surgical implantation procedure is more complex than just placing cannulas in the chest, so it may not be the first choice of procedure in an emergency situation. Pulsatile devices were originally thought to have the advantage of being more physiologic with regard to end-organ function, so they became widely used before the advent of the third-generation, continuous flow pumps. See Figures 15-9 and 15-10 for an illustration of the Thoratec PVAD and the Abiomed AB5000 pumps.

Increasingly, larger medical centers are using the continuous flow devices for intermediate-term support. The pneumatic devices currently still have a role in biventricular support in centers that do not have access to the artificial heart or other devices that can be used for longer-term RV support. They may also still have a place in centers without access to another longer-term, but simpler-to-implant, LVAD when a patient is critically ill.

Both the Thoratec PVAD and Abiomed AB5000 devices are pneumatic systems that are driven by alternating pressure and vacuum, to compress a blood-filled bladder creating pump ejection and fill during systole, with the assist of vacuum during pump diastole. The bladders are housed in a rigid outer shell allowing for the flow of compressed air in and out of the chamber. They both run asynchronous to the native heart in a "fill to empty" mode. The pumps are triggered to eject when they reach full fill. Each pump contains inflow and outflow valves to maintain unidirectional blood flow. The Thoratec PVAD incorporates mechanical tilting disk valves, whereas the AB5000 utilizes synthetic tri-leaflet valves.

An advantage of the Thoratec PVAD and Abiomed AB5000 pumps is that they are housed outside the body, so space is available in the chest to accommodate two sets of inflow and outflow cannulas for biventricular support. Figure 15-11 illustrates the

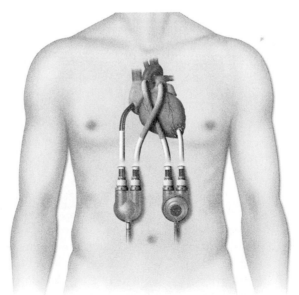

FIGURE 15-9 Thoratec PVAD with bi-ventricular support. (Courtesy Thoratec Corporation, Pleasanton, CA.)

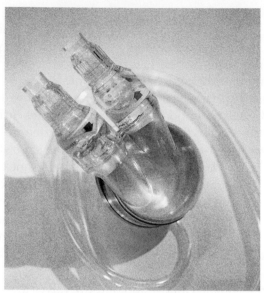

FIGURE 15-10 Abiomed AB5000 pump shows inflow and outflow synthetic valves. (Courtesy Abiomed Inc., Danvers, MA.)

Biventricular support cannulation

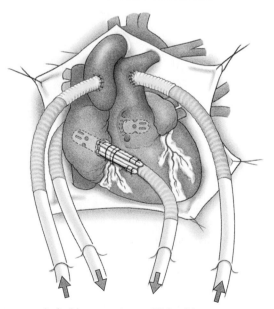

Left side support   Right side support

FIGURE 15-11 Biventricular support, illustrating a technique avoiding left ventricular cannulation. (Courtesy Abiomed Inc., Danvers, MA.)

cannula configuration for biventricular support. In many instances, LVAD therapy alone is sufficient. Patients who have signs of RV failure, as indicated by elevated right atrial pressures of more than 15 mm Hg, RV ejection fraction of less than 20%, pulmonary vascular resistance of more than 4 Wood units, or severe tricuspid regurgitation, most likely also need an RVAD.[36] It is important to institute biventricular support early, as earlier support is associated with improved survival, reduced need for re-operation, improved end-organ perfusion and the best opportunity to reverse multi-organ failure.

When used for biventricular support, the right atrium houses the inflow cannula, bringing blood to the paracorporeal pump subcostally. The return cannula from the pump is placed in the main pulmonary artery. Left-sided flow is captured in either the left atrium or the left ventricle. Left atrial cannulation is employed in any patient expected to recover. A disadvantage of left atrial cannulation is an expected smaller flow rate than can be achieved with LV cannulation. In the past, it was thought that it was less optimal to cannulate the ventricle if recovery was expected. However, ventricular cannulation is now common for any application because of the better flows that can be achieved. Left atrial cannulas exit the body subcostally to the external pump. Blood is returned to the systemic circulation via a cannula anastomosed to the ascending aorta. Figure 15-11 illustrates biventricular cannulation avoiding the left ventricle. Situations where recovery might be anticipated to occur include myocarditis, postpartum cardiomyopathies, and postcardiotomy failure.[37] Median sternotomy with cardiopulmonary bypass is required to place the Thoratec PVAD and Abiomed AB5000 pumps. Each of these pumps is capable of generating flow greater than 5 to 6 L/min. Both will respond to increased venous return by filling faster, generating a faster beat rate, and thereby increasing flow with increased activity.

Indications and Contraindications of Paracorporeal Devices

The overarching indication for implantation of one of these devices is cardiogenic shock when a longer-term device operation is considered too high risk and where heart transplantation candidacy is unknown. Paracorporeal devices are typically used for bridge to recovery, bridge to decision when the neurologic status is unclear, or potential bridge to transplantation when candidacy has been determined.

The major contraindications for these devices would be any situation where transplantation is not an option, when recovery is not expected, and the prognosis for any neurologic recovery is poor, for example, prolonged unconsciousness following cardiopulmonary arrest. Severe right heart failure would be considered a contraindication for left heart assist alone because of the considerable risk of mortality. In these patients, biventricular support should be considered. The minimum size requirement for the cannulas is a body surface area of 1.3 square meters (m^2), which accommodates most adolescents and small adults.

Potential Complications of Paracorporeal Devices

The Thoratec PVAD and Abiomed AB5000 devices are volume dependent, so hypovolemia will decrease pump preload and impair pump performance. Aggressive volume replacement is therefore indicated. Inadequate volume replacement will be evidenced by low pump output. The sternum is closed after pump placement, so tamponade is a concern. The atria have to be well filled to provide flow to support adequate pump output. If used only for LV support, particular attention must be paid to how the right ventricle responds. Patients may need inotropic support for several days after the implant to assist with the maintenance of adequate filling of the left ventricle. A unique feature of biventricular support is the importance of balancing the right-sided flow and the left-sided flow. It is important not to allow the right-sided flow to exceed the left-sided flow, which could precipitate pulmonary edema.

Anticoagulation is required for both the Thoratec PVAD and Abiomed AB5000 pumps. Anticoagulation is started within the first 24 hours after chest tube output has decreased. Intravenous anticoagulation is maintained until the patient achieves a therapeutic international normalized ratio (INR) on warfarin therapy. The INR goal range will vary somewhat at different centers but will be targeted to reach a level of 2.0 to 2.5. Daily aspirin is also used to prevent platelet aggregation on mechanical surfaces. Pump thrombosis and thromboembolic events are both potential complications with use of these pumps. Operating the pumps in a "fill to empty" mode and maintaining optimal pump stroke volume will promote good washing of blood through the pumps and help minimize the formation of pump thrombi. Pumps should be visually inspected often for the presence of early clot formation. A thrombus will necessitate changing of the pump, which can be accomplished fairly easily in the operating room. Biventricular support is associated with more hemolysis compared with implanted continuous-flow pumps, which are discussed in the next section, and this can contribute to lower hemoglobin levels over time.[38]

Impaired Hemodynamic Effectiveness and Limitations of Paracorporeal Devices

As with other devices discussed, inflow or outflow obstruction will impair the hemodynamic performance of the pumps. Partial obstruction is less likely the result of thrombus. The more common culprit of reduced inflow is a kink in the cannula or the angulation of cannula placement. Kinking may occur externally and is easily rectified by a change in patient position. Internal placement problems may require surgical correction, if severe. External cannula assessment and care also include meticulous wound care at the entrance and exit sites to prevent infection.

Patient Safety

Anticoagulation

- Wait to initiate anticoagulation until chest tube drainage has stopped.
    - It is usually safe to wait until patients can take oral medication.
    - Some centers will start heparin or another thrombin inhibitor after 24 to 48 hours and maintain until warfarin is therapeutic.

Patient Safety—cont'd

- Warfarin is titrated to an INR of 1.8 to 2.5, depending on the specifications of a particular device.

- Antiplatelet therapy with aspirin is titrated according to thromboelastography with doses, usually ranging from 81 milligrams (mg) to 325 mg.

- Hypertension should be prevented, as it may increase risk of bleeding.

- Patients on warfarin who have a fall in INR below 1.8 should be considered for heparin therapy to prevent thrombus formation in the pump.

- Provide patient education about foods that interact with warfarin and how eating inconsistent amounts of foods high in vitamin K may increase the risk of subtherapeutic INR levels.

- Patients need to recognize the following signs of a potential bleeding emergency:

  - Vomiting blood

  - Bright red blood in sputum or stool

  - Severe or unusual headache

  - Headache with confusion, weakness, or numbness

Long-Term Mechanical Circulatory Support Therapy

Continuous-Flow Pumps

The newer, continuous-flow pumps have several advantages over their predecessors. They are much smaller, which makes them suitable for smaller men, most women, adolescents, and some children. Continuous-flow pumps are quiet, which helps patients have a more normal life outside of the hospital. They have been engineered to have fewer moving parts, thus improving durability, reducing mechanical problems, and decreasing the risk of thrombogenicity compared with other pumps previously described; all desirable attributes of a long term pump. The percutaneous driveline for the delivery of power to the implanted pump is smaller and easier to care for than the first generation implanted pumps. All of these features have contributed to the ease of living with these pumps on a long-term basis. They are becoming acceptable alternatives to heart transplantation for many people.

More than 95% of all device implants reported to the Interagency Registry for Mechanically Assisted Circulatory Support (INTERMACS) database are now continuous flow devices.[39] Patients receive these durable pumps as bridge to heart transplantation, as destination therapy, or as bridge to decision. Patients with advanced systolic heart failure, severely reduced LV function, functional limitations from their heart failure, and frequent heart failure related hospital admissions are appropriate candidates for elective bridge to heart transplantation.[40] These include patients who may be hospitalized with decompensated heart failure and are deemed too sick to wait any longer for a heart transplant because of declining end-organ function. Patients who have contraindications to transplantation, for example, advanced age, comorbid conditions, or recent malignancy, may be candidates for destination therapy. Destination therapy now represents 40% of all MCS implants reported to the IMTERMACS database.[41] Bridge to decision includes patients who may have conditions that contraindicate heart transplantation but these conditions are potentially transient or temporary, for example, pulmonary hypertension, obesity, medication adherence issues, smoking, recent drug use, acute kidney injury, and liver dysfunction with the possibility of improvement.[40]

Contraindications are primarily related to anticoagulation therapy. Size limitations for adults are minimal. Patients must also be deemed competent for self-care and the ability to learn the management and response to alarms. They must also have the linguistic ability to read alarm conditions displayed on monitors and controllers. Caregiver support and social support are important requirements if a patient is to be considered for discharge from the hospital on a continuous-flow pump, on a long-term basis.

Currently, only two continuous-flow circulatory assist LVAD devices are available: (1) the HeartMate II and (2) the HeartWare LVAS. The HeartMate II was approved by the U.S. Food and Drug Administration (FDA) for bridge to transplantation in 2008 and as destination therapy in 2010. The HeartWare LVAS was FDA approved for bridge to transplantation in 2012 and is pending approval as destination therapy. Its current use as destination therapy is limited to centers participating in clinical trials. The HeartMate II and HeartWare LVAS are examples of the newer-generation of continuous flow pumps that are LVADs.

A third FDA-approved bridge-to-transplantation device is the SynCardia TAH (SynCardia Systems, Inc., Tucson, AZ), which is discussed separately. The SynCardia TAH is a volume-displacement pneumatic pump, which is used for patients with pulmonary hypertension when LVAD therapy alone is insufficient. Patients can be discharged from the hospital with any of these devices for long-term support. The categories of long-term MCS support and appropriate devices per category are listed in Figure 15-12.

HeartMate II

The HeartMate II device is an axial flow pump that is implanted in parallel or in circuit with the native heart and can generate flows of up to 10 L/min. Axial flow, which can be likened to an Archimedes screw effect, is created by the continual rotation of an impeller or rotating blade within the pump. This action results in continuous propulsion of blood through the pump. The HeartMate II pump has only one moving part, the impeller or rotor assembly, which spins on bearings located at either end of the pump assembly. The system uses electromagnetic energy to produce axial motion. The speed range of the pump is 8000 to 12,000 RPM. Since the pump is a nonpulsatile, continuous-flow pump, it is not necessary for the valves to maintain unidirectional flow. This feature

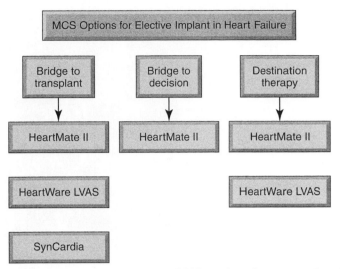

FIGURE 15-12 Mechanical circulatory support (MCS) options for greater than 30 days' support for patients with heart failure.

dramatically decreases the thrombogenicity of this pump compared with first-generation pumps. However, thrombosis is, unfortunately, still a troubling problem.

Inflow to the pump is achieved through cannulation of the LV apex with a rigid inflow cannula, which directs blood flow from the left ventricle to the pump generally placed within a surgically created pre-peritoneal pocket. Blood is returned from the pump to the ascending aorta through an outflow graft. Ventricular cannulation achieves better flows through larger diameter cannulas.

Attached to the pump is a percutaneous lead that houses wiring for the pump to receive external electrical energy and to deliver data on power use and the impeller's revolutions per minute (pump speed) from the pump to an external controller and monitor. From these data, the system controller calculates the pump flow rate and pulsatility index. See Figure 15-13. This connection is also used to change the speed settings as required.

The percutaneous lead is tunneled subcutaneously to exit the body in the right or sometimes the left upper abdominal quadrant. The lead is covered by polyester velour, which allows for endothelial cell in-growth into the material, effectively sealing the track to prevent infection along the percutaneous lead. It is critical during the first 10 to 14 days to ensure this lead is kept immobile so that the initial cell in-growth is not disrupted. Any interference with this process such as intermittent pulling or tension on the lead may disrupt cell in-growth, leading to a separation between the tissues and the lead. This disruption may lead to the development of a tract allowing bacteria on the skin to migrate toward the pump along the driveline. This disruption may occur at any time after implantation, so it is always important to keep the lead immobile. However, after the first 10 to 14 days, scarring and adhesions along the percutaneous lead will aid in protecting cell in-growth by limiting movement. Once a patient has a

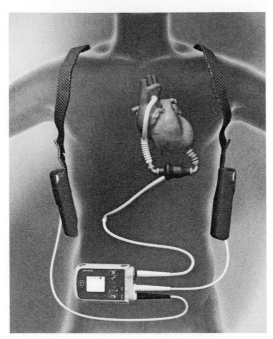

FIGURE 15-13 HeartMate II implant showing the pump, percutaneous driveline and controller connected to batteries. (Courtesy Thoratec Corporation, Pleasanton, CA.)

driveline infection, antibiotics may be required for an extended amount of time or indefinitely through the duration of pump support. Sometimes, the only definitive way to treat this type of infection is the removal of the foreign object by either redirecting the path of the driveline or removal of the pump and driveline, which would occur at the time of transplantation. The real danger is that the driveline infection eventually reaches the pump pocket or worse, the mediastinum.

HeartMate II Controller. The percutaneous lead from the pump is attached to a controller, which is actually the "brains" of the pump. Two versions of the HeartMate II controller exist. The newer version depicted in Figure 15-13 has only been available to patients since 2013, so many destination therapy patients are currently living with an older design that can only generate alarms and has no visual display.

The controller is programmed to monitor for alarm conditions such as low flow, pump disconnection, controller failure, or limited battery time. The controller then generates an alarm for the clinician or the patient. If the patient is attached to the bedside display or has the newest-generation controller, the alarm is accompanied by displayed text message instructions. The controller can be queried to continuously displays pump flow, speed, pulse index, and power.

HeartMate II Battery Support. The HeartMate II pump can operate on alternating current (AC) or battery power. A monitor continually displays the data from the pump and logs any alarm conditions. The patient is connected to the AC base unit with a 20-foot cable, which provides the patient with some mobility in the proximity of the base unit. This pump has been designed for active patients with the idea that they will not be constantly tethered to AC power, allowing the patients to live as normal a life as possible outside of the hospital. The HeartMate II has portable lithium ion batteries, each with the capability of 8 to 10 hours of support. The patient wears two batteries together, which easily allows the patient a full day of activity before a battery change or a re-connection to AC power is needed.

Pump Power Usage. Another parameter that is monitored besides the pump speed and alarm conditions is the pump power usage. Power usage should not vary by more than plus or minus 2 watts in a 24-hour period. A sudden, unsustained increase in the power requirement indicates that something is interfering with the usual rotation of the impeller. This is an indicator of the presence of a thrombus in the pump or a thrombus passing through the pump. A steady and consistent rise in the power requirement over time is an indication that interference with impeller movement is increasing, which is likely the result of a growing thrombus. This indicator is important to monitor closely because as with a paracorporeal pump, visual inspection is not possible.

HeartMate II Pulse Index. The pulse index is a calculated number that is an indication initially of the volume surge through the pump with LV contraction. Once ventricular contractility is stable, it becomes more reflective of the status of ventricular filling. As the ventricle contracts, an increase in ventricular pressure increases flow through the pump. These flow surges are measured, averaged, and translated into a pulse index calculation. The greater the surge with contractions, the higher the number will be. Initially, the number is low, given the impaired ventricular contractility after surgery. Lower ventricular filling will also result in a lower pulse index. As the ventricular contractile effect eventually stabilizes, the number remains fairly constant, and the rise and fall of the pulse surge or index is usually a reflection of the patient's ventricular filling. The more optimized the preload, the stronger is the pulse surge and the higher is the pulse index. If the preload diminishes, the volume in the left ventricle is less, and a smaller surge in blood flow occurs through the pump with each ventricular contraction. That translates into a lower displayed pulse index. If the pulse index significantly drops in an otherwise stable patient, this decrease may indicate a decrease in circulating blood volume. Pulse indexes that become elevated may be an indication of problems with percutaneous lead wear or fatigue.

HeartWare Left Ventricular Assist System

HeartWare Pump. The HeartWare left ventricular assist system (LVAS) device is also a continuous-flow pump. However, its design is different from that of the HeartMate II because it is a centrifugal pump. It has an impeller inside the pump housing that floats in blood and spins according to the revolution speed set by the clinician. It is the only moving part in the pump and has no contact with other pump surfaces. The impeller blades push blood from the left ventricle through the pump by using hydrodynamic and centrifugal forces. The energy to rotate the impeller is provided through electromagnetic coupling between permanent magnets enclosed within the impeller and the base of the pump. Like the HeartMate II, this pump is valveless, so it relies on adequate volume (preload) and decreased systemic vascular resistance to keep blood

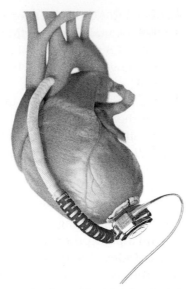

FIGURE 15-14 HeartWare pump implanted in the left ventricle with the outflow graft anastomosed to the ascending aorta. (Courtesy HeartWare Inc., Framingham, MA.)

flow moving forward. The speed range of the pump is 1800 to 4000 RPM. It can generate flows up to 10 L/min. The pump has a displaced volume of 50 mL and weighs 160 grams.

The system consists of a centrifugal blood pump with an integrated inflow cannula that is placed directly in the LV apex and secured with a sewing ring attached to the myocardium. A polyester outflow graft returns blood from the pump to the ascending aorta. Because of the small size of the pump, it is totally contained within the pericardial space. Placement of the HeartWare pump is shown in Figure 15-14.

HeartWare Left Ventricular Assist System Percutaneous Lead and Controller. The HeartWare pump has a percutaneous driveline, which is covered with a woven polyester fabric that encourages cellular in growth to protect the patient from infection similar to the HeartMate II. The driveline connects the pump to a controller, which is the microprocessor unit that controls and manages the pump. It sends power and operating signals to the pump and retrieves data. The controller continuously displays pump flow, pump speed, and power. The HeartWare LVAD controller will display any alarms with instructions as to what action must be taken to resolve the alarm conditions. The power indication should not vary by more than plus or minus 2 watts. An increase in power for any given speed setting has the same implications of possible pump thrombosis as described for the HeartMate II (Box 15-2).

HeartWare Left Ventricular Assist System Flow Waveform. As with the HeartMate II, the HeartWare LVAD monitor displays a flow waveform, which illustrates the surge in flow through the pump during LV systole. The greater the peak of this waveform, the greater is LV contractility; therefore, it essentially provides similar information to that provided by the pulse index of the HeartMate II. The monitor also provides a continuous graph of power usage in addition to the numerical indicators.

BOX 15-2 Percutaneous Lead Care

- Daily sterile dressing changes
- Cleansing site with chlorhexidine
- Assessment for signs of infection
- Immobilization of lead
  - Securing with a locking device over lead that secures to the skin (as with a urinary catheter)

- Use of abdominal binders or a stabilization belt supplied by companies for abdominal leads
- Assessment of skin for pressure points at any lead securing device—rotation of site, as needed

---

HeartWare Left Ventricular Assist System Battery. The controller has two power ports, which are connected to a battery and AC power or two battery sources. Each lithium ion battery lasts 4 to 6 hours, so a patient on battery support alone has approximately 8 hours less than does the HeartMate II patient before batteries are totally depleted. The HeartWare LVAS depletes one battery at a time and automatically switches to the second battery when the first is depleted. An alarm alerts the patient when the first battery is becoming low on power.

Potential Complications and Impaired Hemodynamic Effectiveness of Continuous-Flow Pumps

Continuous-flow pumps have many potential complications in common with other MCS devices previously discussed. Of note are bleeding complications associated with anticoagulation and infection. Potential complications are listed in Box 15-3. The complications discussed here are limited to those that impair the hemodynamic effectiveness of the pumps.

Right Heart Failure. Right heart failure is a potential complication early after implantation. It is critical that RV contractility and output be adequate to maintain LV preload. Without this, the MCS device will not be able to generate adequate flow

---

BOX 15-3 Potential Complications Associated with Left Ventricular Assist Device (LVAD) Therapy

Bleeding
Death
Device malfunction
Driveline infection
Liver dysfunction
Multi-organ failure
Neurologic dysfunction

Peripheral thromboembolism
Kidney failure
Respiratory failure
Right heart failure
Sepsis
Stroke

because of inadequate pump preload. Assessment of RV function is both imperative and difficult. Transesophageal echocardiography as well as right heart catheterization can help determine the degree of dysfunction. RV failure will be more likely to be seen in patients who have elevated pulmonary pressures and elevated central venous pressures preoperatively. The LVAD depends on the right ventricle to provide preload for the left ventricle and the pump, and a hallmark of RV failure is low pump output. Given time and adequate inotropic support, the right ventricle will likely recover from the insult of surgery.

To assist with afterload reduction for the right ventricle, treatment with pulmonary vasodilators is helpful. One mechanism is the delivery of nitric oxide through the ventilator circuit, although this is a very expensive therapy. An effective alternative is inhaled epoprostenol.[42] Patients can eventually be converted to oral sildenafil citrate to support afterload reduction of the right ventricle until pulmonary pressures decrease, which may happen over time. It is important to determine the degree of RV dysfunction and pulmonary hypertension preoperatively. If a patient is at excessively high risk, RVAD implantation may be reconsidered. Prolonged right heart failure will eventually affect liver function and may cause death. An alternative for the bridge to transplantation would be a TAH.

RV function and overall hemodynamics may be affected by inappropriate pump speed settings. Too high a speed may cause a leftward septal shift that creates abnormal RV geometry and can adversely affect RV function.[43,44] High speed can also collapse the left ventricle and obstruct inflow into the pump from the ventricle. This occurrence is called a *suction event*. Too low a speed results in inadequate unloading of the left ventricle and may result in increased mitral valve regurgitation, which may impair RV function. The optimal speed is often determined for each individual patient using a ramped speed study with transesophageal echocardiography and hemodynamic assessment. Optimal speed is that which results in no right shift or in left shift of the septum with an optimally filled left ventricle. The speed study assesses ventricular volume, size, septal position, blood pressure, and aortic valve opening at different speeds to identify the best speed setting for an individual patient.[45] Some centers reserve these studies for use when there are problems with clinically determining the optimal speed or when thrombus is suspected. How often the aortic valve should open is still debated. Higher pump speeds will pull blood through the ventricle quickly so that ventricular pressure decreases enough to cause the aortic valve not to open at all. A static valve is not desirable because of the risk of thrombus formation on the immobile aortic leaflets. Common practice is to adjust the pump speed to a setting that results in aortic valve opening every two to three beats, which is a frequency sufficient to reduce risk of thrombosis of the aortic valve.[43] That frequency also is an indication that the ventricle is reasonably filled, protecting the patient from suction events. The HeartWare pump has a suction alarm that will alert the clinician as well as a flow waveform on the monitor display that will illustrate the suction event. The HeartMate II device will protect the patient from suction by slowing down to a preset low speed limit when suction is detected. Slowing of the pump will allow the ventricle more time to fill. When suction is no longer detected, the pump will slowly increase the speed back to the presuction event setting. The maintenance of a fuller ventricle may have the advantage of being able to generate some pulsatile flow, depending on the patient's native ventricular function.

Pump Thrombosis. The primary cause of pump thrombosis is inadequate anti-coagulation. However, inadequate flows and low volumes can contribute to thrombus formation. Low flow rates are an indication to possibly increase the level of anticoagulation. Monitoring of anticoagulation is critical and patients may initially require frequent adjustments to their warfarin and aspirin therapy until they are stable and within therapeutic range. The target INR for these pumps varies, depending on the manufacturer's recommendations. It is typically kept between 1.5 and 2.5, depending on the particular device and the preference of the MCS team.[43] The risk of thrombotic events increases when the INR drops below 1.5 but the risk of hemorrhagic events is present at all INR ranges, especially when the INR is greater than 2.5.[46] Thromboelastography may be utilized to titrate the optimal dose of aspirin that should be administered to achieve adequate anti-platelet effect. This ability to customize each patient's aspirin therapy is an important adjunct to anticoagulation therapy.

Pump thrombosis is suspected with a gradual increase in the pump power requirement over time with no change in pump speed. Abrupt but nonsustained increases in power may also indicate that thrombosis is present in the pump. Thrombus accumulation will impair the movement of the impellers, requiring more power to maintain the set speed. A ramp echocardiography study will help identify the presence of pump thrombosis.[45]

Hemolysis has been identified as a marker of pump thrombosis, and the presence of hemolysis is associated with higher mortality.[47,48] Hemolysis likely occurs because of increased shear stress on the red blood cells as they pass through the pumps. Hemolysis may also occur in advance of the obvious power elevation associated with pump thrombosis. Hemolysis should be suspected in the setting of new anemia with no evidence of bleeding, elevation of lactate dehydrogenase (LDH), elevated plasma-free hemoglobin (Hgb) and undetectable haptoglobin (<8 grams per deciliter [g/dL]).[47] Early detection of hemolysis may allow for increased anticoagulation that may prevent the need for pump replacement.

Left Ventricular Assist Device (LVAD) Case Study

A 62-year-old man is admitted to the cardiovascular critical care unit (status: post–HeartMate II LVAD implantation) for destination therapy. He is not a candidate for heart transplantation because of pulmonary hypertension and diabetes. His preoperative pulmonary artery pressures were 62/28 mm Hg.

At 0900, he is in his fourth postoperative hour. The chest tube drainage has been 150 mL in the past 2 hours. Tachycardia and hypertension are concerns, and the resident elects to decrease the epinephrine infusion to 0.03 microgram per kilogram per minute (mcg/kg/min).

Continued

Left Ventricular Assist Device (LVAD) Case Study—cont'd

At 1000, there has been a definite change in the patient's hemodynamics. The nurse has turned off the nitroprusside because of concerns about hypotension. The resident is worried about the hypotension, continued tachycardia, and decreased urine output and orders an infusion of 1 liter of lactated Ringer solution.

At 1100, the situation is decidedly worse. Arterial blood gas (ABG) reveals metabolic acidosis, with a pH of 7.3 and bicarbonate (HCO_3^-) of 17, providing evidence of poor tissue perfusion. The partial pressure of arterial carbon dioxide ($PaCO_2$) is 40 and the partial pressure of arterial oxygen (PaO_2) is 150. Bedside transthoracic echocardiography reveals severely depressed RV function and decreased LV volume.

Explanation: This patient started to develop a progressive decrease in RV function when the epinephrine infusion was decreased. The loss of inotropic support in the face of high RV afterload from elevated pulmonary pressures resulted in decreased LV filling, hypotension, low urine output, and low LVAD flow. The 1-liter fluid challenge made the RV failure even more evident. The correct initial approach would have been to increase medications to reduce RV afterload, to address the pulmonary hypertension, and to leave the inotropic support with epinephrine unchanged. Clearly, his right ventricle was not yet ready to have inotropic support decreased.

At 1200, the epinephrine was increased back to 0.07 mcg/kg/min, and a nitroprusside infusion was restarted, which resulted in a dramatic improvement in blood pressure and LVAD flow. This case study illustrates the importance of RV function in achieving optimal LVAD flows and support of systemic circulation. ▪

TIME	0900	1000	1100	1200
Heart rate (beats/min)	120 Sinus rhythm	114 Sinus rhythm	100 Sinus rhythm with PVCs	100 Sinus rhythm
Blood pressure (systolic/diastolic) (mm Hg)	130/85	110/50	70/43	104/70
Mean arterial pressure (MAP) mm Hg	100	70	52	81
Right atrial pressure/central venous pressure (RAP/CVP) (mm Hg)	15	18	20	14
Pulmonary artery pressure (PAP) (mm Hg)	54/28	48/22	52/26	48/20
Pulmonary artery occlusion pressure (PAOP) (mm Hg)	24	20	20	18
Urine output (U/O) (mL/hour)	75	30	<30	60
LVAD flow (L/min)	4.6	4.0	3.4	4.8

Dopamine (mcg/kg/min)	5.0	5.0	5.0	5.0
Epinephrine (mcg/kg/min)	0.07	0.03	0.03	0.07
Sodium nitroprusside (mcg/kg/min)	0.2	Off	Off	0.25

Preload and Afterload Sensitivity

Both these MCS pumps are very sensitive to preload and afterload. Frequent volume shifts occur in the early postoperative period. Neurohormonal changes that occur when the patient is on cardiopulmonary bypass result in fluid accumulation caused by the release of antidiuretic hormone and aldosterone. Volume changes also occur because of bleeding, intravascular volume depletion, and active diuresis. Frequent echocardiographic assessment is advised to determine the volume status and size of the left ventricle. It is important to maintain afterload reduction, as a significant rise in the patient's systemic blood pressure may adversely affect pump output. Elevated blood pressure is also a risk factor for pump thrombosis.[49] Continuous flow results in an elevation of diastolic blood pressure and a narrowing of the pulse pressure to a degree that often makes it difficult or impossible to accurately determine blood pressure or palpate a pulse. Early in the postoperative period, blood pressure is continuously monitored by arterial catheter. Blood pressure is actively managed with vasoactive and inotropic medications. It is recommended that MAP be maintained below 80 mm Hg in patients with continuous-flow devices.[50] Many patients will require an oral antihypertensive regime to maintain blood pressure within that range. When the arterial line is removed, blood pressure is obtained by Doppler assessment. Clinical assessment of blood pressure and LVAS flow are the usual indicators in any patient; warm extremities, brisk capillary refill, good urine output, and clear mentation.

Clinical Reasoning Pearl

- It is important to find the optimal continuous-flow pump speed.
  - A speed that is too low will result in less than optimal pump flows.
  - A speed that is too fast may cause ventricular collapse or inflow obstruction and precipitate arrhythmias.
- The most optimal method of determining the safe operating speed for individual patients is with a ramped speed study by echocardiography.
- Ramped speed studies are helpful to determine the presence of pump thrombosis.
- A continuous-flow LVAD does not have valves. If the pump were to stop, blood flow could reverse creating acute aortic regurgitation and acute hemodynamic compromise. It is important to prevent inadvertent power interruption at all times.[43]

SynCardia Total Artificial Heart

Patients with biventricular failure may need to be bridged to transplantation with a TAH. The ventricles in this device are implanted in the chest. The currently available TAH system is a volume-displacement, pulsatile pump, although research on the use of more durable centrifugal and axial flow pump designs that could support both ventricles is in progress. A TAH is indicated as a bridge to transplantation for patients with severe biventricular failure, ventricular or septal rupture following myocardial infarction, calcified LV aneurysms, failed cardiac transplantation, prior mechanical valve replacement, infiltrative or restricted cardiomyopathy, complex congenital heart disease, and intractable arrhythmias.[51–54]

Two total artificial hearts developed in the United States are the Abiocor (Abiomed, Inc., Danvers, MA) and the CardioWest TAH (SynCardia Systems, Inc., Tucson, AZ). The Abiocor is no longer in production. It is mentioned here because of one unique aspect of the Abiocor system. It utilized transcutaneous electrical energy transfer, so a percutaneous driveline was not needed, which reduced infection risk.[51,54] This feature of MCS support is continuing to be pursued in other devices that are in research and development.

With the CardioWest TAH, now referred to as the SynCardia TAH, much greater experience has been gained in more centers. The SynCardia has multi-national (United States, Canada, European Union) approval for use as a bridge to transplantation device, and greater than 900 implants have been performed worldwide.[53,55]

SynCardia Pump

The SynCardia TAH is a pneumatically driven system that is placed in the orthotopic position; that is, it replaces the normal heart and has a volume displacement of 70 milliliters (mL). Patients require a body surface area of 1.7 m^2 and ample mediastinal enlargement to accommodate the large device size. The anteroposterior dimension of the chest has to be at least 10 cm at the 10th thoracic vertebrae, as determined by computed tomography (CT).[55] Both native ventricles and all four native valves are removed and replaced by two separate blood pumps that attach to the cuffs of the remaining atria after native ventricular excision. The blood pumps are adjustable in the chest to allow for optimal orientation, and they can be attached to each other with a Velcro patch present on both pumps (Figure 15-15).

Each pump is constructed with a rigid outer shell, which contains two mechanical disk valves and a four-layer polyurethane diaphragm that separates the blood from the air space. Blood flows from the atria across the mechanical valve into the blood sac of each artificial ventricle. Alternating pressure and vacuum is used to move the diaphragm (see Figure 15-15). The rate of the pump, (beats per minute), and the amount of time allowed for filling, is determined by the clinician. Each ventricle is run at the same rate. The rate is determined by the need to not allow the pump to fill completely. At the end of diastole, pressurized air fills the air space, pushing up on the diaphragm causing ejection to occur. When complete ejection has been achieved, vacuum is

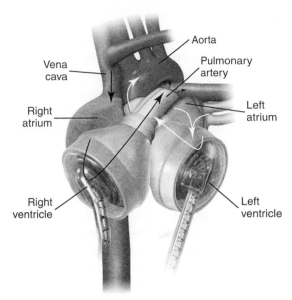

FIGURE 15-15 SynCardia total artificial heart. (Courtesy of SynCardia Systems Inc.)

applied to the air space and to the diaphragm to assist with pump filling. Pressure and vacuum are set separately for each ventricle but vacuum assist is essentially the same for both sides. Wire-reinforced drivelines attached to each pump are directed out of the body through subcostal incisions that supply alternating pressure and vacuum (Figure 15-16). Each pump has a volume capacity of 70 mL, with an output capacity for each pump of 9.5 L/min.

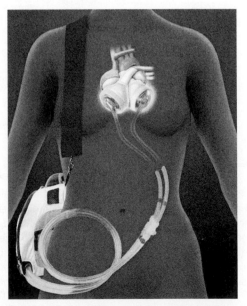

FIGURE 15-16 Total Artificial Heart showing ventricles, percutaneous drivelines and attachment to a portable Freedom Driver. (Courtesy of SynCardia Systems Inc.)

SynCardia Monitoring

A computer screen on the SynCardia monitor displays a continuous reading of the beat rate, which is usually set between 125 and 140 beats/min. Faster rates are usually only needed in the early postoperative period when more hemodynamic and volume instability is present. The preset driveline pressure and vacuum are displayed. The clinician can adjust the rate, pressure, and vacuum to attain optimal outputs from the pumps. The fill volume and pump output from each ventricle are continuously displayed. A key tenet of the system is that the fill volume of each pump should never reach full capacity, so the device can compensate appropriately for any increased venous return that occurs with activity. If venous return increases when the pumps are at full fill, flash pulmonary edema could occur because the left pump is not able to accommodate the increased flow from the right side. Fill volumes are generally maintained at 50 to 60 mL to prevent this complication. The lower fill volumes are the reason for the high beat rate. Another key tenet is to ensure that complete ejection occurs with each beat. This function ensures effective washing of blood out of the pump and minimizes the risk of thrombus formation. The clinician must monitor the air pressure waveform and the filling air flow waveform to make sure that complete ejection occurs and only partial filling occurs with each cardiac cycle (Figure 15-17).

Compared with the HeartMate II and the HeartWare LVAD, the SynCardia is not as sensitive to afterload because it has valves as components of the system and because systole is driven by pressurized air flow. It is, however, sensitive to preload. The system

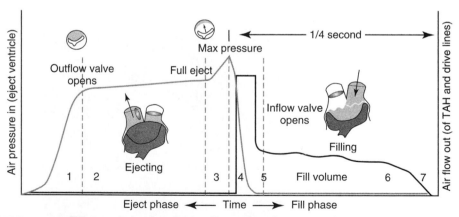

FIGURE 15-17 Filling and ejection phases illustrating air pressure into the ventricle air sac with systole and air flow moving out of the pump with diastole. The illustration during the fill phase shows all air leaving the pump that would mean the blood sac had fully filled. In practice, the blood sac would never be allowed to fill fully. 1, Beginning of eject phase; 2, outflow valve opens—start of upward diaphragm movement; 3, full ejection with diaphragms at maxim upward position; 4, end of eject phase—start of fill phase; 5, inflow valve opens—diaphragms begin to move down due to pressure from blood volume; 6, normal end of fill phase without full fill; 7, full fill. (Courtesy of SynCardia Systems Inc.)

has a portable driver that is available to centers participating in a clinical trial (see Figure 15-16). The SynCardia TAH received FDA approval in July 2014. Patients can be discharged to home on this device, as it can be operated with AC power or battery.

Potential Complications and Impaired Hemodynamic Effectiveness

A lot of the issues encountered with LVADs are eliminated with the SynCardia TAH. Because both native ventricles are removed, problems such as potential ventricular septal defects, LV thrombus, right heart failure, or arrhythmias are not present. The patient does not have detectable electrical activity, so electrocardiography (ECG) is not required. No concern exists about an aortic valve that does not open often, as the mechanical valve or outflow in the SynCardia TAH opens with every systolic ejection. Inotropic support is not needed because the ventricles are now mechanical. A vasopressor such as neosynephrine or vasopressin may be required in the early postoperative period to maintain vascular tone and increase blood pressure. The SynCardia pump is sensitive to preload, and venous tone must be supported to ensure adequate venous return and filling of the right ventricle. The CVP is usually maintained below 10 mm Hg.

One problem seen after TAH replacement is low levels of natriuretic peptide following removal of the native ventricles. Patients with heart failure typically have increased levels of plasma natriuretic peptides with downregulation of natriuretic receptors. At times, patients may have acute kidney injury after implantation that is not reversible with increased cardiac output alone.[51] It may take some time for neurohormonal receptors to recover, so natriuretic peptide infusion may be required in the short term to assist with recovery from acute kidney injury and to promote urine output.

Because of the size of the two ventricles, it is important to monitor the pump output response at chest closure. Any compression of the vena cava will impair filling of the right atrium and thus pump output. A drop in output from the ventricles is a possible indication to leave the chest open for 24 to 48 hours. This occurs in approximately 45% of cases (personal communication, Jack Copeland MD) Mechanical ventilation with high levels of positive end-expiratory pressure (PEEP) may have the same effect by compressing the vena cava and pulmonary veins. Patients should be extubated as soon as possible. Another important aspect of post-implantation care is to make sure that central lines do not enter the right atrium. If the distal end of the line is close to the mechanical valve, it may become entrapped in the valve, which would likely be fatal. All central lines should be placed under fluoroscopic guidance, including any peripherally inserted central catheter (PICC). If the patient has any cardiovascular emergency, clinicians need to be aware that chest compressions will have no effect because of the rigid housing of the pumps and the typical advanced cardiac life support (ACLS) medication protocols will be ineffective. The use of an epinephrine bolus may be deleterious, as increased venous return from vasoconstriction may cause the ventricles to reach full fill and precipitate pulmonary edema.

The major complications associated with the SynCardia TAH include bleeding, tamponade, stroke, and infection. Anticoagulation should be managed by prothrombin times, thromboelastography, and platelet aggregation studies as with other pumps. It is important to manage platelet aggregation and prevent thrombus. As with LVADs, patients with the SynCardia TAH are prone to the von Willebrand phenomenon and associated platelet dysfunction, which may manifest as gastrointestinal bleeding. Patients with this device also tend to have chronic anemia related to chronic hemolysis, inflammation, and abnormal erythropoiesis.[56] It has been postulated that since the heart participates in many neurohormonal signaling pathways, the ventricles may have a yet unidentified role in a cardiac-specific signaling pathway that modulates bone marrow function and is disrupted by removal of the ventricles.[56]

Because patients with the SynCardia TAH are candidates for bridge to transplantation, they generally do not receive a transfusion, unless symptoms of anemia occur, to avoid exposure to additional foreign antigens. Cardiac tamponade is an emergency condition as with any other cardiothoracic surgery patient. In the presence of pressure on the vena cava and pulmonary veins, the mechanical ventricles will not receive adequate volume inflow, and output from the ventricles will be compromised. Similar to the other devices described in this chapter, inadequate anticoagulation may result in thromboembolic events because of increased thrombogenicity of blood contacting the surfaces of the pump. Conversely, excessive anticoagulation puts the patient at risk for cerebrovascular bleeding as well as bleeding in other locations. Optimal anticoagulation management is, therefore, critical.

Patient Education

Critical Patient Education Prior to Discharge for Patients on Mechanical Circulatory Support

- Percutaneous driveline care
  - Dressing changes
  - Immobilization
- Switching back and forth from alternating current (AC) to battery power
- Switching to backup controllers or drivers
- How to call for help
- Care of the equipment
- Understanding the displayed data on monitors and controllers—"normal numbers"
- The importance of anticoagulation monitoring and taking medication as prescribed
- Signs of possible thrombus formation in pumps

> **Patient Education—cont'd**
>
> - How to shower safely
> - Signs and symptoms of infection
> - Signs and symptoms of bleeding
> - Signs and symptoms of stroke
> - See Table 15-3 for a summary of the features of each device described in this chapter.

TABLE 15-3 Ventricular Assist Device Overview

DEVICE	CONFIGURATION	PLACEMENT	FLOW TYPE	FLOW CAPABILITY	USE
Impella 2.5	LVAD	Intracorporeal	Axial continuous flow	2.5 L/min	BTR, BTT, BTV
Impella 5.0	LVAD	Intracorporeal	Axial continuous flow	5.0 L/min	BTR, BTT, BTV
Tandem Heart	LVAD	Extracorporeal	Centrifugal continuous flow	5.0 L/min	BTR, BTT, BTV
ECMO	BVAD	Extracorporeal	Centrifugal continuous flow	5.0 L/min	BTR, BTT, BTV
Centrimag	LVAD, RVAD, BVAD	Extracorporeal	Centrifugal continuous flow	5.0 L/min	BTR, BTT, BTV
Thoratec PVAD	LVAD, RVAD, BVAD	Extracorporeal	Pulsatile	5-6 L/min	BTT
Thoratec IVAD	LVAD, RVAD, BVAD	Extracorporeal	Pulsatile	5-6 L/min	BTT
Abiomed AB5000	LVAD, RVAD, BVAD	Intracorporeal	Pulsatile	5-6 L/min	BTT
HeartMate II	LVAD	Intracorporeal	Axial continuous flow	10 L/min	BTT, DT
HeartWare	LVAD	Intracorporeal	Centrifugal continuous flow	10 L/min	BTT
Syncardia	TAH	Orthotopic	Pulsatile	9.5 L/min	BTT

BTR, Bridge to recovery; *BTT*, bridge to transplant; *BTV*, bridge to a longer-term ventricular assist device; *BVAD*, bi-ventricular assist device; *DT*, destination therapy; *L/min*, liters per minute; *LVAD*, left ventricular assist device; *RVAD*, right ventricular assist device; *TAH*, total artificial heart.

Future Direction

For destination therapy to truly be a replacement for heart transplantation, the ideal long-term MCS device should be able to support the systemic circulation for years without mechanical malfunction. Devices have to demonstrate complication frequencies or adverse event profiles similar to those of transplantation to meet this benchmark. Ideal MCS devices should be nonthrombogenic, require minimal anticoagulation, cause minimal damage to blood cells, be fully implantable, be small and quiet, have a low risk of infection, be cost effective, and result in good to excellent quality of life compared with baseline.

Much has been learned about pump design that minimizes thrombogenicity, but the incidence of stroke and cerebral bleeding that occurs with MCS therapy is still unacceptable. Anticoagulation, to some degree, will remain a requirement of long-term MCS support for the near future. Newer designs presently in development are incorporating the knowledge gained from Abiocor and similar pumps related to the effective use of transcutaneous energy transfer systems, which would eliminate the driveline and, thus, driveline infections. That would give patients the freedom to enjoy swimming or other water sports and eliminate daily dressing changes of the driveline site. It would also eliminate the most common source of infection. Present-day LVADs are smaller and quieter, but it is conceivable that at some point in the future, they will be similar in size to an implanted defibrillator. Presently, considerable financial burden is associated with the placement of these devices. That will likely always be true for patients in cardiogenic shock. However, with earlier referral of patients with heart failure for destination therapy, outcomes will continue to improve, with fewer adverse events and decreased costs. If these outcomes are sustainable for several years, they will approach the gold standard outcomes of heart transplantation. Currently, 1-year survival on destination therapy is 80%.[41] MCS would then be available to many patients who cannot currently benefit from heart transplantation because of limited donor availability and other contraindications.

References

1. Hanlon-Pena PM, Quaal SJ: Resource document: evidence supporting current practice in timing assessment, *AJCC* 20(4):323–333, 2011.
2. Santa-Cruz RA, Cohen MG, Ohman EM: Aortic counterpulsation: a review of the hemodynamic effects and indications for use, *Catheter Cardiovasc Interv* 67(1):68–77, 2006.
3. Kapelios CJ, Terrovitis JV, Nanas JN: Current and future applications of the intra-aortic balloon pump, *Curr Opin Cardiol* 29(3):258–265, 2014.
4. Funk M, Ford CF, Foell DW, et al.: Frequency of long-term lower limb ischemia associated with intraaortic balloon pump use, *Am J Cardiol* 70(13):1195–1199, 1992.
5. Barnett MG, Swartz MT, Peterson GJ, et al.: Vascular complications from intraaortic balloons: risk analysis, *J Vasc Surg* 19(1):81–87, 1994.
6. Tatar H, Çiçek S, Demirkilic U, et al.: Vascular complications of intraaortic balloon pumping; unsheathed versus sheathed insertion, *Ann Thorac Surg* 55(6):1518–1521, 1993.

7. Unverzagt S, Machemer MT, Solms A, et al.: Intra-aortic balloon pump counterpulsation (IABP) for myocardial infarction complicated by cardiogenic shock, *Chochrane Database Syst Rev* 7:2011, CD007398.
8. Patel MR, Smalling RW, Thiele H, et al.: Intra-aortic balloon counterpulsation and infarct size in patients with acute anterior infarction without shock: the CRISP-AMI randomized trial, *JAMA* 306(12):1329–1337, 2011.
9. Thiele H, Zeymer U, Neumann FJ, et al.: IABP SHOCK II trial Investigators Intra-aortic balloon support for myocardial infarction with cardiogenic shock, *N Engl J Med* 367 (14):1287–1296, 2012.
10. Thiele H, Zeymer U, Neumann FJ, et al.: Intra-aortic balloon counterpulsation in acute myocardial infarction complicated by cardiogenic shock (IABP-Shock II): final 12 month results of a randomized, open label trial, *Lancet* 382(9905):1638–1645, 2013.
11. Vermulapalli S, Zhou Y, Gutberlet M, et al.: Importance of total ischemic time and preprocedural infarct-related artery blood flow in predicting infarct size in patients with anterior wall infarction (from the CRISP-AMI Trial), *Am J Cardiol* 112(7): 911–917, 2013.
12. Werdan K, Gielen S, Henning E, et al.: Mechanical circulatory support in cardiogenic shock, *Eur Heart J* 35(3):156–167, 2014.
13. Subramaniam K, Boisen M, Shah PR, et al.: Mechanical circulatory support for cardiogenic shock, *Best Pract Res Clin Anaesthesiol* 26(2):131–146, 2012.
14. Griffith BP, Anderson MB, Samuels LE, et al.: The RECOVER I: a multicenter prospective study of Impella 5.0/LD for post cardiotomy circulatory support, *J Thorac Cardiovasc Surg* 145 (2):548–554, 2013.
15. Lemaire A, Anderson MB, Yee LY, et al.: The Impella device for acute mechanical circulatory support in patients in cardiogenic shock, *Ann Thorac Surg* 97(1):133–138, 2014.
16. Dangas GD, Kini AS, Sharma SK, et al.: Impact of hemodynamic support with impella 2.5 versus intra-aortic balloon pump on prognostically important clinical outcomes in patients undergoing high-risk percutaneous coronary intervention (from the PROTECT II Randomized Trial), *Am J Cardiol* 113(2):222–228, 2014.
17. Cheng JM, den CA Uil, Hoeks SE, et al.: Percutaneous left ventricular devices vs. intra-aortic balloon pump counterpulsation for treatment of cardiogenic shock: a meta-analysis of controlled trials, *Eur Heart J* 30(17):2102–2108, 2009.
18. Dixon SR, Henriques JP, Mauri L, et al.: A prospective feasibility trial investigating the use of the Impella 2.5 system in patients undergoing high-risk percutaneous coronary intervention (The PROTECT I trial): Initial U.S. experience, *JACC Cardiovasc Interv* 2(2):91–96, 2009.
19. Sarkar K, Kini AS: Percutaneous left ventricular support devices, *Cardiol Clin* 28(1):169–184, 2010.
20. Bagai J, Webb D, Kasabeh E, et al.: Efficacy and safety of percutaneous life support during high-risk percutaneous coronary intervention, refractory cardiogenic shock and in-laboratory cardiac arrest, *J Invasive Cardiol* 23(4):141–147, 2011.
21. Pitsis AA, Visouli AN, Burkhoff D, et al.: Feasibility study of a temporary percutaneous left ventricular assist device in cardiac surgery, *Ann Thorac Surg* 84(6):1993–1999, 2007.
22. Kar B, Gregoric ID, Basra SS, et al.: The percutaneous ventricular assist device in severe refractory cardiogenic shock, *J Am Coll Cardiol* 57(6):688–696, 2011.
23. John R, Long JW, Massey HT, et al.: Outcomes of a multicenter trial of the Levitronix Centrimag ventricular assist system for short-term circulatory support, *J Thorac Cardiovasc Surg* 141 (4):932–939, 2011.
24. Loforte A, Montalto A, Ranocchi F, et al.: Levitronix CentriMag third –generation magnetically levitated continuous flow pump as a bridge to solution, *ASAIO J* 57(4):247–253, 2011.

25. Salaunkey K, Parameshwar J, Valchanov K, et al.: Mechanical support for heart failure, *JICS* 14 (3):220–225, 2013.

26. Takayama H, Takeda K, Doshi D, et al.: Short-term continuous flow ventricular assist devices, *Curr Opin Cardiol* 29(3):266–274, 2014.

27. Worku B, Pak S, van Patten D, et al.: The CentriMag ventricular assist device in acute heart failure refractory to medical management, *J Heart Lung Transplant* 31(6):611–617, 2012.

28. De Robertis F, Birks EJ, Rogers P, et al.: Clinical performance with the Levitronix CentriMag short-term ventricular assist device, *J Heart Lung Transplant* 25(2):181–186, 2006.

29. Takayama H, Naka Y, Jorde U, et al.: Less invasive left ventricular assist device placement for difficult resternotomy, *J Thorac Cardiovasc Surg* 140(4):932–933, 2010.

30. Lidén H, Wiklund L, Haraldsson Å, et al.: Temporary circulatory support with extra corporeal membrane oxygenation in adults with refractory cardiogenic shock, *Scand Cardiovasc J* 43 (4):226–232, 2009.

31. Loforte A, Montalto A, Ranocchi F, et al.: Peripheral extracorporeal membrane oxygenation system as salvage treatment of patients with refractory cardiogenic shock: preliminary outcome evaluation, *Artif Organs* 36(3):E53–E61, 2012.

32. Peek GJ, Moore HM, Moore N, et al.: Efficacy and economic assessment of conventional ventilator support versus extracorporeal membrane oxygenation for severe adult respiratory failure (CESAR): a multicenter randomized controlled trial, *Lancet* 374(9698):1351–1363, 2009.

33. Kagawa E, Dote K, Kato M, et al.: Should we emergently revascularize occluded coronaries for cardiac arrest? Rapid–response extracorporeal membrane oxygenation and intra-arrest coronary intervention, *Circulation* 126(13):1605–1613, 2012.

34. Rastan AJ, Dege A, Mohr M, et al.: Early and late outcomes of 571 consecutive adult patients treated with extracorporeal membrane oxygenation for refractory postcardiotomy cardiogenic shock, *J Thorac Cardiovasc Surg* 139(2):302–311, 2010.

35. Allen SJ, Sidebotham D: Postoperative care and complications after ventricular device implantation, *Best Pract Res Clin Anaesthesiol* 26(2):231–246, 2012.

36. Fernandez AL, Martinez A: Monitoring recovery and weaning from the Thoratec left ventricular assist device, *Ann Thorac Surg* 73(5):1689, 2002.

37. Körfer R, El-Banayosy AM, Arnsoglu L, et al.: Single center experience with the Thoratec ventricular assist device, *J Cardiovasc Surg* 119(3):596–602, 2000.

38. Heilmann C, Geisen U, Benk C, et al.: Haemolysis in patients with ventricular assist devices: major differences between systems, *Eur J Cardiothorac Surg* 36(3):580–584, 2009.

39. Kirklin JK, Naftel DC, Kormos RL: Fifth INTERMACS annual report: risk factor analysis from more than 6,000 mechanical circulatory support patients, *J Heart Lung Transplant* 32(2):141–156, 2013.

40. Miller LW, Guglin M: Patient selection for ventricular assist devices, *JACC* 61(12):1209–1221, 2013.

41. Kirklin JK, Naftel DC, Pagani FD, et al.: Sixth INTERMACS annual report: a 10,000-patient database, *J Heart Lung Transplant* 33(6):555–564, 2014.

42. Thunberg CA, Gaitan BD, Arabia FA, et al.: Ventricular assist devices today and tomorrow, *J Cardiothorac Vasc Anesth* 24(4):656–680, 2010.

43. Slaughter MS, Pagani FD, Rogers JG, et al.: Clinical management of continuous-flow left ventricular assist devices in advanced heart failure, *J Heart Lung Transplant* 29(45):S1–S39, 2010.

44. Patangi SO, George A, Pauli H, et al.: Management issues during HeartWare left ventricular assist device implantation and the role of transesophageal echocardiography, *Ann Card Anaesth* 16(4):259–267, 2013.

45. Uriel N, Morrison KA, Garan AR, et al.: Development of a novel echocardiography ramp test for speed optimization and diagnosis of pump thrombosis in continuous flow left ventricular assist devices: the Columbia ramp study, *J Am Coll Cardiol* 60(18):1764–1775, 2012.

46. Boyle AJ, Russell SD, Teuteberg JJ, et al.: Low thromboembolism and pump thrombosis with the HeartMate II left ventricular assist device: analysis of outpatient anticoagulation, *J Heart Lung Transplant* 28(9):881–887, 2009.
47. Ravichandran AK, Parker J, Novak E, et al.: Hemolysis in left ventricular assist device: a retrospective analysis of outcomes, *J Heart Lung Transplant* 33(1):44–50, 2014.
48. Cowger JA, Romano MA, Shah P, et al.: Hemolysis: a harbinger of adverse outcome after left ventricular assist device implant, *J Heart Lung Transplant* 33(1):35–43, 2014.
49. Najjar SS, Slaughter MS, Pagani FD, et al.: An analysis of pump thrombus events in patients in the HeartWare ADVANCE bridge to transplant and continued access protocol trial, *J Heart Lung Transplant* 33(1):23–34, 2014.
50. Feldman D, Pamboukian SV, Teuteberg JJ, et al.: The 2013 International Society for Heart and Lung Transplantation guidelines for mechanical circulatory support: executive summary, *J Heart Lung Transplant* 32(2):157–187, 2013.
51. Sale SM, Smedira NG: Total artificial heart, *Best Pract Res Clin Anaesthesiol* 26(2):147–165, 2012.
52. Gray NA, Selzman CH: Current status of the total artificial heart, *Am Heart J* 152(1):4–10, 2006.
53. Copeland JG, Copeland H, Gustafson M, et al.: Experience with more than 100 total artificial heart implants, *J Thorac Cardiovasc Surg* 143(3):727–734, 2012.
54. Milano CA, Simeone AA: Mechanical circulatory support: devices, outcomes and complications, *Heart Fail Rev* 18(1):35–53, 2013.
55. Gaitan BD, Thunberg CA, Stansbury LG, et al.: Development, current status, and anesthetic management of the implanted artificial heart, *J Cardiothorac Vasc Anesth* 25(6):1179–1192, 2011.
56. Mankad AK, Tang DG, Clark WB, et al.: Persistent anemia after implantation of the total artificial heart, *J Card Failure* 18(6):433–438, 2012.

Hemodynamic Management Following Cardiac Surgery

16

S. Jill Ley

Astute postoperative monitoring can make the difference between survival and death in a patient after cardiac surgery in the critical care unit. The purpose of this chapter is to provide a conceptual framework for the role of hemodynamic monitoring in postoperative cardiac care across a spectrum of conditions and procedures. First, assessment and management strategies for a routine coronary artery bypass procedure with normal ventricular function are described. Then, key differences in patients with three common difficulties—systolic dysfunction, diastolic dysfunction, and blends of cardiac abnormalities with complex disease—are discussed. Finally, critical steps in the recognition and response for common clinical catastrophes that may occur in postoperative cardiac patients are discussed, including bleeding, ventricular failure, and tamponade.

Optimal postoperative care begins with a formalized hand-off report that details the underlying cardiac disease and history, ventricular function, comorbid conditions, and procedural issues such as bleeding or difficulty weaning from cardiopulmonary bypass (CPB). On admission to the critical care unit, ensuring easy visualization of the hemodynamic monitor, setting appropriate alarm and monitoring parameters, and ensuring hemodynamic accuracy are essential steps. Precise measurements of patient progress toward established, individualized goals of care will guide clinical decisions and interventions thereafter. Each cardiac surgical case carries individualized risks, determined, in part, by the intraoperative course, which can impact postoperative management significantly.

Impact of Cardiac Surgery on Hemodynamics

Although coronary artery bypass is the most common cardiac surgical procedure performed nationwide, aortic valve replacement (AVR) in older adults with aortic stenosis, complex mitral repairs, and "redo" multi-valve replacements occur with increasing frequency. Important variables such as ejection fraction and medical urgency contribute to the potential risks of cardiac surgery, which can be reliably assessed via validated risk prediction models to guide operative decision making.[1,2] Intraoperative monitoring of arterial blood pressure and either central venous pressure (CVP) or pulmonary artery pressures are considered standard of care for patients undergoing cardiac surgery.[3,4] Pulmonary artery catheter (PAC) use has declined in recent decades,[5] with current European guidelines supporting PAC use only in complex procedures, pulmonary hypertension, and severe low output states, particularly when distinguishing right ventricular (RV) versus left ventricular (LV) failure.[3] Current coronary artery bypass guidelines from the United States indicate that PAC use "may be reasonable" in stable patients, after considering the patient's risk profile and other factors.[4] Use of a PAC enables the assessment of numerous valuable parameters of cardiac function via a single device, including cardiac output and cardiac index, calculation of vascular resistances, and pulmonary artery occlusion pressure (PAOP) as an indirect assessment of left heart filling pressures. Catheters that are capable of monitoring saturation of venous oxygen (SvO_2) offer an additional parameter that reflects the overall balance between oxygen supply and consumption. SvO_2 has demonstrated utility in predicting both short-term and long-term mortality after coronary artery bypass surgery.[6]

Cardiac operations are typically performed on an arrested heart with the use of a hyperkalemic cardioplegia solution while maintaining systemic perfusion via the CPB machine. In recent years, minimally invasive approaches have become commonplace in general surgery, and these strategies have been applied to cardiac procedures in the form of small incision or port access techniques (possibly with robotic assistance) and procedures performed without CPB support. Procedural modifications currently permit "off pump" coronary bypass (but not heart valve) approaches, which now comprise approximately 20% of total coronary artery bypass surgical volume nationwide.[4]

Systemic heparinization to prevent embolic events and modest hypothermia to reduce myocardial oxygen demand are routine during CPB. For more complex cardiac surgeries such as aortic arch repair, complete circulatory arrest and profound hypothermia may be required, which contribute to increased coagulopathies and hemodynamic derangements postoperatively. Despite the absence of coronary blood flow during CPB, myocardial protection is accomplished through repetitive antegrade and/or retrograde infusions of cardioplegia into the coronary arteries throughout the procedure. Failure to maintain appropriate protection leads to myocardial ischemia or infarction, with associated reductions in ventricular performance: decreased contractility and decreased compliance (increased stiffness) that may be profound and irreversible. Intraoperative monitoring with transesophageal echocardiography (TEE) is routinely performed to enable prompt detection and management of wall motion or other abnormalities during surgery.[4] On completion of the surgical procedure, patients are rewarmed and weaned from CPB support and heparin is reversed with protamine, with maintenance of sedation and hemodynamic monitoring during transition from the operating room to the critical care unit environment.

All cardiac surgical patients are subject to the potentially adverse effects of anesthesia on ventricular function, causing alterations in vascular tone from cooling and rewarming, acute blood loss and fluid shifts, as well as aberrations in electrolytes or acid–base status, which require careful management.[7] The impact of surgery is generally well tolerated, with mortality rates for most major isolated procedures now reported to be less than 1% to 2% nationwide.[8]

Patient Comfort

Strategies for Surgical Patients

Patients undergoing surgical procedures should anticipate some degree of pain, and efforts to reduce and control pain are essential to recovery. Adverse physiologic effects of pain, particularly tachycardia and vasoconstriction, may negatively affect clinical progress as well as patient satisfaction. Strategies to reduce pain in surgical patients include around-the-clock scheduling of nonopioid agents, such as nonsteroidal anti-inflammatory agents and acetaminophen. Careful timing of analgesic dosing in preparation for painful activities such as physical therapy and pulmonary hygiene is important for optimum patient participation and recovery. Nonpharmacologic therapies, such as guided imagery and anticipatory guidance may be helpful. Patients often voice concerns about pain during removal of tubes and lines, particularly chest tubes. Research by Puntillo and Ley demonstrated that nurses can significantly reduce the perceived pain of this procedure by providing both procedural and sensory information prior to chest tube removal, as well as by coordinating *appropriately timed* analgesic medications.[9] Although it is intuitive that medications should be administered to coincide with tube removal during peak effect, this does not routinely occur. Nurses can significantly reduce pain with chest tube removal by adhering to these practices.

Characteristic hemodynamic changes over subsequent hours should be anticipated postoperatively, including impaired ventricular contractility, typically reaching a downward nadir by the fourth postoperative hour, which will be more profound and prolonged with preoperative dysfunction or perioperative ischemia.[7] Systemic vascular resistance (SVR) is usually elevated initially and decreases with rewarming but may remain persistently elevated in low output states as a compensatory hemodynamic mechanism.

Less often, patients exhibit generalized vasodilation that may be profound and resistant to intervention, particularly when preoperative vasodilator medications are used.[10] The typical postoperative recovery entails gradual rewarming and vaso-dilation and improved ventricular performance and oxygen consumption, with stabilization of hemodynamic aberrations within a few hours after arrival in the critical care unit. This trajectory is largely impacted by underlying pathology and surgical course but may be anticipated and classified according to baseline hemodynamic findings.

Postoperative Hemodynamics in Patients with Normal Ventricular Function

Preoperative cardiac catheterization and echocardiographic findings provide important baseline information to establish the preoperative diagnosis and guide surgical management and postoperative strategies. Echocardiographic parameters, in particular, provide noninvasive data regarding contractile function (ejection fraction and end-diastolic volume), ventricular hypertrophy (wall thickness), and pulmonary artery pressures (based on the velocity of the regurgitant jet from the tricuspid valve).[11] Although some patients experience prompt improvement with surgery, complete ventricular remodeling and hemodynamic normalization often require weeks to months, particularly following cardiac valvular procedures. Baseline parameters are helpful in predicting postoperative hemodynamics and forming individualized treatment plans. The following hemodynamic goals are appropriate for most patients undergoing cardiac surgery:[3]

- $SvO_2 > 65\%$
- Mean arterial pressure (MAP) >65 millimeters of mercury (mm Hg)
- CI >2.0 L/min/m^2
- CVP 8–12 mm Hg
- PAOP 12–15 mm Hg
- Serum lactate level <3 millimoles per liter (mmol/L)

These findings target a "normal" postoperative trajectory, as seen in patient populations experiencing coronary artery disease or early mitral regurgitation with preserved ventricular function, evidenced by an ejection fraction above 55%. The formula: Cardiac output = Heart rate × Stroke volume is a useful hemodynamic equation to differentiate abnormal cardiac parameters and determine appropriate clinical interventions. Stroke volume is further categorized into preload, afterload and contractility or inotropy (see Chapter 1, Figure 1-7).

Postoperatively, cardiac index and SvO_2 may be modestly decreased, particularly in the presence of increased SVR, but prompt normalization is anticipated with rewarming. Filling pressures are relatively low in the presence of hypovolemia; fluid resuscitation leads to increases in both cardiac volume and pressure, as illustrated by the "normal" ventricular compliance curve shown in Figure 16-1.

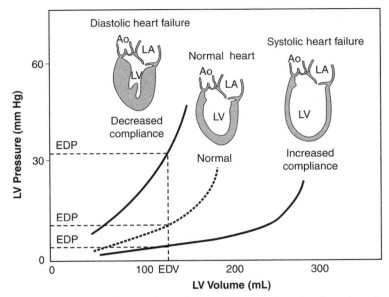

FIGURE 16-1 Ventricular compliance curves for patients with normal cardiac function, decreased compliance (diastolic dysfunction), and increased compliance (systolic dysfunction). The relationship between end-diastolic volume (EDV) and end-diastolic pressure (EDP) in the left ventricle is not linear. In diastolic heart failure with a hypertrophied ventricle, the smaller cardiac chamber volume (EDV) is at a higher pressure, with a steeper ventricular compliance curve, compared with a normal heart. In systolic heart failure, the dilated ventricle requires larger volumes (EDV) and is poorly contractile with lower intra-cardiac pressures (EDP) and a gradually-sloped ventricular compliance curve, compared with a normal heart. *Ao,* Aorta; *EDP,* end-diastolic pressure; *EDV,* end-diastolic volume; *LA,* left atrium; *LV,* left ventricle.

On admission of the patient to the critical care unit, clinicians should anticipate that the patient with a stable hemodynamic profile will look well perfused, produce urine in large amounts, and exhibit hemodynamic data that are either within normal limits or promptly trending in that direction. Should this patient unexpectedly develop a low cardiac index or SvO_2 and elevated filling pressures, clinicians are alerted to immediately explore potential causes such as ischemia or tamponade. Either of these conditions may present with sudden cardiac compromise or even arrest. A more typical scenario is a gradual yet persistent decline in blood pressure, cardiac index, and SvO_2 in combination with compensatory increases in heart rate and SVR. This signals an abnormal trajectory that warrants further assessment. In contrast, patients with either systolic or diastolic dysfunction are expected to display substantially different postoperative presentations and "normal" hemodynamic parameters may not be achievable, as illustrated in Table 16-1. Distinguishing these clinical profiles is essential to developing appropriate postoperative goals and devising optimal strategies to achieve them.

TABLE 16-1　Predicted Hemodynamic Profiles Based on Preoperative Diagnostic Data

	NORMAL	SYSTOLIC DYSFUNCTION	DIASTOLIC DYSFUNCTION	COMPLEX PATHOLOGY
Associated conditions	• Coronary artery disease with preserved LV function • Mitral regurgitation (early)	• Large or multiple MIs • Dilated cardiomyopathy • Aortic insufficiency • Mitral regurgitation (late)	• Aortic stenosis • Hypertension • Restrictive cardiomyopathy	• Aortic stenosis and MI • Multivalve disease
Ejection fraction	>55%	<40%	Varied, often normal	<30%
LV EDV*	Normal	>75 mL/m²	Varied, often normal	Varied, likely increased
LV Wall Thickness*	<1.2 cm	<1.2 cm	>1.2 cm	Varied
LV mass*	44–88 g/m² women 50–102 g/m² men	Increased due to EDV	Increased due to wall thickness	Varied, likely increased
Estimated PAP from TR jet	18–25 millimeters of mercury (mm Hg)	>30 mm Hg	Increased	Varied, likely increased
Anticipated hemodynamics	Within normal limits	↓CO/CI ↓SvO₂ ↑PAP, CVP	CO/CI (normal) SvO₂ (normal) ↑PAP, CVP	↓↓CO/CI ↓↓SvO₂ ↑↑PAP, CVP

*Adjusted for body size.

CI, Cardiac index; *CO*, cardiac output; *cm*, centimeters; *CVP*, central venous pressure; *EDV*, end-diastolic volume; *g/m²*, grams per square meter; *LV*, left ventricle; *MI*, myocardial infarction; *mL/m²*, milliliters per square meter; *PAP*, pulmonary artery pressure; *SvO₂*, mixed venous oxygen saturation; *TR*, tricuspid regurgitation.

Data from Otto CM: *Textbook of clinical echocardiography*, ed 5, Philadelphia, 2013, Saunders.

Clinical Reasoning Pearl

Managing Early Postoperative Instability

When hemodynamic instability occurs following cardiac surgery, the factors that determine cardiac output—heart rate, preload, afterload, and contractility—should be promptly evaluated and a corrective action plan developed on the basis of discrepancies between current and optimal values.

- Optimal heart rate is 80 to 110 beats per minute (beats/min) following cardiac surgery. If the heart rate is lower than this, temporary pacing may be helpful. If high, a compensatory tachycardia may be contributing significantly to cardiac output and should not be counteracted. Instead, additional factors listed below may be considered before attempting to reduce heart rate, unless a life-threatening arrhythmia is present.

- Optimal preload is determined by evaluating volume responsiveness to a fluid challenge. Filling pressures are dynamic, patient-specific surrogates for the true volume status that are quite variable in the early postoperative period. Assessment of the hemodynamic response to administration of a 250- to 500-millilier (mL) aliquot of fluid will confirm hypovolemia if cardiac output increases, or exclude the need for additional volume if hemodynamics fail to improve.

- Optimal afterload of the left ventricle is determined by calculation of SVR and evaluation of vascular tone. Elevated SVR or physical signs of vasoconstriction (cool extremities, diminished peripheral pulses, delayed capillary refill) indicate that afterload is not optimal. Administration of a vasodilator may be helpful to reduce SVR and promote cardiac ejection. Hypovolemia often coincides with vasoconstriction but may be masked by increased SVR that supports blood pressure. In patients lacking an adequate intravascular volume, vasodilator administration may lead to pronounced hypotension. Vasodilators are initiated cautiously, and fluids should be readily available in the event of instability as described in the case study at the end of the chapter.

- Less commonly, reduced SVR and vasodilation occur in the postoperative period and contribute to hypotension. Treatment with a vasoconstrictor such as phenylephrine increases the SVR while exerting minimal effects on heart rate and contractility. When initiating vasoconstrictors, cardiac output and cardiac index are frequently assessed to ensure an appropriate response to therapy. If cardiac output and cardiac index decline after administration of these agents, discontinue and change to a mixed inotrope or vasoconstrictor to optimize contractile function.

- Optimal contractility is not directly measured at the bedside, but if cardiac output and cardiac index and tissue perfusion are inadequate in the presence of an appropriate heart rate, preload, and afterload, impaired contractility is assumed. Pharmacologic therapy using appropriate inotropes, vasopressors, or a combination of both, and possibly mechanical circulatory support devices may be indicated. Refer to Chapter 9 for additional information on use of vasoactive medications and to Chapter 15 for more information on mechanical circulatory support.

- In the initial hours after surgery, hemodynamic volatility and frequent treatment changes are expected. Ongoing assessment of the patient's response to treatment is essential to optimally target therapies at the lowest possible dosage to minimize adverse medication effects and determine needed changes to the plan of care.

Hemodynamics in Systolic Dysfunction: The Volume Overloaded Ventricle

Chronic impairment of systolic function, often accompanying myocardial infarction (MI) or mitral valve regurgitation, leads to an "overstretched" left ventricle and is associated with chamber dilation with reliance on volume loading for optimal contractility (Figure 16-2). Preoperative findings indicative of moderate to severe systolic dysfunction should influence the clinician's estimation of appropriate hemodynamic goals postoperatively. Ejection fraction is a useful gauge of anticipated LV performance; marked reductions in ejection fraction equate to the potential for greater hemodynamic aberrations postoperatively because cardiac output is lower, and filling pressures are higher than normal. Additional findings of systolic dysfunction include increased pulmonary artery pressures and end-diastolic volume, as well as LV mass, which is augmented by increased volume, not wall thickness (see Table 16-1).[11]

The impact of corrective surgery on mitral regurgitation merits special mention, as the procedure eliminates an incompetent mitral valve that was providing a potentially important compensatory release mechanism in the presence of increased LV afterload. Following mitral valve repair or replacement, the blood volume must now correctly exit via the high-pressure forward outflow tract of the left ventricle, placing increased demands on chamber. Postoperatively, this increased afterload typically leads to reduced ventricular performance and a lower ejection fraction. Thus, preoperative ejection fraction measurements will *overestimate* ventricular function in patients with mitral regurgitation.[12] Patients with severe LV contractile dysfunction may be incapable of overcoming even a modest afterload increase without marked pharmacologic and mechanical circulatory support, but this is not always discernible from the preoperative ejection fraction. For this reason, the highest mortality risk is seen in patients undergoing replacement of the mitral valve, particularly if combined with coronary artery bypass or aortic valve replacement.[8]

With chronic volume overload, adequate fluid resuscitation is critically important to optimize systolic function. However, filling pressures become a less sensitive indicator of fluid status in the dilated left ventricle that is accustomed to a large end-diastolic volume. The thin-walled, compliant heart accommodates large increases in chamber

Front View   **View from Above**

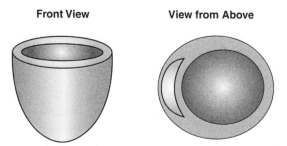

FIGURE 16-2 The volume overloaded left ventricle with systolic dysfunction, illustrated by characteristic thinning of chamber walls, overdistension, and increased end-diastolic volume.

volume, yet hemodynamic monitoring reveals only minimal pressure changes. This is reflected in an abnormal ventricular compliance curve that is relatively low and flat, with a late upstroke in pressure values as shown in Figure 16-1. Absolute numbers are less helpful in determining fluid status than monitoring the hemodynamic response to volume loading: if cardiac performance increases after a fluid bolus, the patient can be considered "volume responsive" regardless of the filling pressures.[7]

Rather than trying to achieve "normal" parameters for patients with LV dysfunction, fluids, medications, and cardiac support devices are titrated to achieve values more realistically aligned to systolic capability and hemodynamic trends. Goals for blood pressure and cardiac index are lower, and those for filling pressures are higher than normal, with exact endpoints targeted initially to intraoperative values that achieved optimal performance. Use of vasodilators and phosphodiesterase inhibitors to reduce afterload may benefit the poorly contracting left ventricle but must be cautiously titrated to avoid causing hypotension. Heart rate is a significant contributor to cardiac index, and the use of temporary pacing to maintain atrioventricular synchrony at a rate of 90 to 110 beats/min may offer hemodynamic benefits for patients with postoperative ventricular dysfunction.

Determination of acceptable hemodynamic targets, particularly when outside of normal ranges, must be clarified with all providers and adjusted frequently based on predetermined hemodynamic endpoints and clinical response. Strategies should achieve continued steady progress toward individualized goals while avoiding rapid rewarming or abrupt adjustments that could lead to acute deterioration of LV function or precipitate arrhythmias. In patients who are incapable of increasing their cardiac output, even modest increases in oxygen demand may precipitate decompensation. These patients derive benefit from frequent reassessment of continuously monitored variables, including cardiac output, cardiac index, and SvO_2. This is to enable careful titration of therapies and facilitate prompt detection of potentially destabilizing conditions such as hypoxia, shivering, seizures, or occult bleeding. A sudden decline in the SvO_2 signals an important, often occult, imbalance between global oxygen supply and demand that warrants immediate assessment and intervention. In a large Swedish trial of coronary artery bypass surgical patients (n = 2755), the mean SvO_2 on arrival to the critical care unit was 66% and values less than 60% were associated with a fivefold increase in early mortality.[6] In patients with aortic stenosis, marked reductions in survival were seen when the initial SvO_2 was less than 55%.[13]

Hemodynamics in Diastolic Dysfunction: The Pressure Overloaded Ventricle

Chronic hypertension, hypertrophic cardiomyopathy, and aortic stenosis are conditions that result in increased LV afterload. With obstruction to LV outflow, hypertrophy of the cardiomyocytes occurs in an attempt to overcome resistive forces to ejection, resulting in increased LV mass (Figure 16-3). The degree of hypertrophy is a significant risk factor for adverse outcomes and has a strong influence on hemodynamic goals.[14] The thickened

View from Front   **View from Above**

Concentric LVH

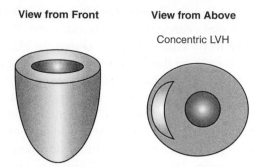

FIGURE 16-3 The pressure overloaded left ventricle with diastolic dysfunction, illustrated by characteristic thickening of chamber walls and reduced cavity size. *LVH,* Left ventricular hypertrophy.

left ventricle can easily generate an adequate systole, but impaired diastolic function and failure to relax contribute to underfilling, which is substantially worsened by atrial fibrillation and loss of atrial kick, or inadequate fluid resuscitation. Echocardiographic findings of diastolic dysfunction include elevated pulmonary artery pressures, greater wall thickness, and LV mass caused by increased muscle mass versus volume overload. Ejection fraction and end-diastolic volume are typically within normal limits in these patients but may be reduced to a modest degree.[11]

Preload assessment is complicated by an atypical relationship between LV pressure and volume in the noncompliant ventricle. In patients with decreased ventricular compliance, the entire curve is shifted to the left, and the slope of this curve is much steeper, reflecting more marked pressure increases with smaller increments of added volume as illustrated in Figure 16-1. Fluid requirements for these patients may be substantially higher than predicted by filling pressure values, and volume may be indicated despite normal or even elevated pulmonary artery pressures when perfusion is inadequate.[7] These patients are subject to impaired cardiac performance from either underfilling or overfilling of the ventricle, which is challenging to manage, with little guidance offered by CVP or pulmonary artery pressure readings. Careful scrutiny of blood pressure, cardiac index, SvO_2, and perfusion is required following each fluid challenge to determine ongoing preload requirements. This situation may change rapidly in the postoperative period, particularly during rewarming as the SVR decreases, and tremendous volatility in blood pressure may occur in some patients despite careful management.

Situations of acute deterioration with signs of shock are challenging in the patient with diastolic dysfunction, as inotropes do not provide a good clinical "match" for this pathophysiology. Repeated boluses of fluid, often in amounts larger than anticipated and possibly including blood products, are the first line of therapy.[7] In cases of continued deterioration, transthoracic echocardiography (TEE) is helpful in determining the presence or absence of cardiac tamponade (discussed below).

Systolic anterior motion (SAM) of the mitral valve leaflet occurs in some hypertrophied hearts when closure of the mitral valve apparatus obstructs LV outflow, especially when the ventricular septum is hypertrophied. This obstruction can lead to significant reductions in the ejected stroke volume and significantly reduce cardiac function (see Figure 16-4).[15]

Following aortic valve replacement, the thickened, hyperdynamic left ventricle can further contribute to obstruction of the left ventricular outflow tract, particularly when septal hypertrophy is present, and this greatly complicates patient management. Mechanical obstruction of aortic blood flow leads to a rapid decline in blood pressure and cardiac index, with dramatic increases in filling pressures as the ventricle fails to empty. Hemodynamics alone cannot distinguish this situation from acute LV failure or tamponade, but TEE is diagnostic and reveals a hyperdynamic left ventricle with a small, underfilled, possibly obliterated cavity.

Management of shock related to systolic anterior motion of the mitral valve is quite different from that of typical systolic failure, with initial efforts being focused on aggressive volume loading and discontinuation of inotropes, if present. The addition of beta-blockers to relax the myocardium and reduce LV outflow tract obstruction may be lifesaving, but appears counterintuitive in the presence of profound hypotension and shock.[15] The early use of TEE to ensure an accurate diagnosis, rule out cardiac tamponade, and direct appropriate interventions is vital to the appropriate management of unresponsive hypotension after surgery.[4,7]

With increasing frequency, patients undergoing cardiac surgery exhibit complex disease processes that are a hybrid of extremes of systolic and diastolic dysfunction, as seen in patients with longstanding aortic stenosis who suffer an acute myocardial infarction or in those with combined aortic stenosis and mitral regurgitation. These patients are not easily categorized but generally demonstrate marked impairments in ventricular function and altered ventricular compliance. Precise and frequent assessment of hemodynamic data is required to determine appropriate targets, to monitor the response to treatment, and to customize optimal therapies. Table 16-1 differentiates characteristic assessment findings seen in patients across a wide variety of cardiac surgical conditions and procedures.

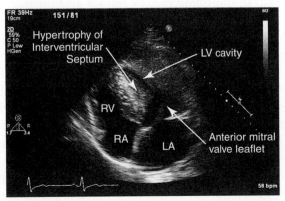

FIGURE 16-4 Echocardiographic image demonstrating systolic anterior motion of the mitral valve and hypertrophy of the interventricular septum, which contribute to dynamic left ventricular outflow tract obstruction.

Important Conditions after Cardiac Surgery: Bleeding, Tamponade, and Ventricular Failure

Absolute or relative hypovolemia resulting from blood or fluid losses, fluid shifts, and effects of rewarming on the peripheral vasculature frequently occur after cardiac surgery. This contributes to a relative mismatch between the circulating blood volume and the size of the vascular compartment. Targeted replacement of intravenous fluids aims to restore cardiac output through augmentation of stroke volume via preload support.[7] Hemodynamic findings of hypovolemia after cardiac surgery are similar to inadequate blood volume in other populations and include: low blood pressure, low cardiac index, and low intracardiac filling pressures, but two important caveats exist as described below.

The first consideration is that postoperative hypovolemia is often associated with bleeding, which may be evident via chest tube output or less obvious when clots obstruct the tubes. Management of chest tube bleeding entails a review of the coagulation profile and complete blood cell count, targeted replacement of blood products, and possibly surgical re-exploration to identify and correct postsurgical bleeding. In patients with signs of a significant fluid deficit or in those unresponsive to therapy, prompt re-exploration to rule out a hemothorax or other source of occult bleeding is indicated. Postoperative bleeding is discussed in more detail later in the chapter.

The second consideration is that identification of optimal volume status using pressure measurements is impacted by numerous variables such as mechanical ventilation, ventricular function, and valvular disease, which further alter interpretation of the hemodynamic profile in postoperative cardiac surgery patients. Sole reliance on pressure readings may inaccurately reflect true volume needs. Goal-directed hemodynamic management to guide volume loading, has been shown to reduce postoperative complications and length of stay.[16]

Despite varying ventricular compliance curves (see Figure 16-1), fluid administration should result in improved cardiac output and cardiac index in patients with true hypovolemia. Lack of improvement or deterioration in cardiac performance should prompt exploration of other causes of ventricular failure. In contrast, the patient with low filling pressures who displays normal perfusion and cardiac index should not receive additional volume simply to achieve an "ideal" CVP or PAOP value.

Cardiac tamponade is a potentially life-threatening complication of cardiac surgery that is often associated with prior bleeding. This condition is characterized by a progressive accumulation of blood in the mediastinal space, causing increased intrapericardial pressure that impairs myocardial filling and outflow.[17] Unlike the "elevation and equalization" of thoracic filling pressures classically described with tamponade, findings after cardiac surgery are unique because bleeding and clotting may occur in a localized manner. In addition, the pericardium has been opened, permitting much larger fluid collections in the mediastinal cavity or chest prior to hemodynamic compromise from "tamponade physiology." Diagnosis of tamponade must always be excluded in the patient with severe heart failure who develops low cardiac index and SvO$_2$ with elevated intrathoracic pressures, particularly when chest tube output is minimal.

Use of transesophageal echocardiography is invaluable for the prompt detection and differentiation of causes of postoperative cardiac dysfunction and should be considered early if compromise is significant or the patient is unresponsive to treatment.[3,4] With cardiac tamponade, all therapies, including cardiopulmonary resuscitation, offer marginal benefit because of mechanical compression of the heart, which impairs filling. In the absence of a pulse, emergently reopening the sternum within 5 minutes will result in optimal neurologic survival.[18] In the presence of tamponade physiology, opening even a portion of the sternum may lower pericardial pressures adequately to permit ventricular filling and can rapidly restore perfusion and improve hemodynamics.

Patient Safety

Resuscitation Management

Clinical instability proceeding to cardiac arrest should be an anticipated event after cardiac surgery, occurring in up to 8% of patients, typically in the critical care environment, where high survival rates are feasible. Astute hemodynamic monitoring enables early detection and optimal management of these life-threatening situations. Although Advanced Cardiac Life Support (ACLS) is an appropriate resuscitation standard for many patients, it can be ineffective, or even harmful, in those who have recently undergone heart surgery. Modifications to standard ACLS management for postoperative cardiac patients have been advocated by the European Resuscitation Council since 2010,[19] and are currently being updated in the United States by the Society of Thoracic Surgeons (STS).

The standard of care in most European countries includes immediate defibrillation or pacing *prior to* external compressions (if available within 1 minute), avoidance of epinephrine during arrest, as it may lead to destabilizing rebound hypertension, and rapid resternotomy by trained providers within 5 minutes if initial resuscitation efforts are unsuccessful. These strategies promote optimal delivery of definitive therapies that are readily available in the critical care environment while avoiding potential damage to the sternotomy incision from compressions that will be minimally effective in tamponade or bleeding.

Although a modest deterioration in postoperative LV function is anticipated in patients with low ejection fraction, pronounced myocardial dysfunction may indicate ischemia caused by graft occlusion or inadequate intraoperative preservation. Alternatively, right ventricular (RV) failure may be present, occurring in approximately 1% of routine cardiac surgeries. For patients who require implantation of a left ventricular assist device (LVAD), up to 43% will experience RV failure, which markedly increases morbidity and mortality.[20] Appropriate management requires differentiation of parameters affecting both right and left ventricular performance, and use of a pulmonary artery catheter or transesophageal echocardiography is essential to guide optimal therapy.[3] Reduced LV performance is accompanied by reductions in blood pressure, cardiac index, and SvO_2 from reduced forward flow, with increased LV end-diastolic volume, LV chamber dilation and reduced compliance. Transesophageal echocardiography graphically reveals the location and extent of wall motion abnormalities and allows evaluation of both left- and right-sided ventricular function.

Treatment strategies for LV failure strive to optimize heart rate and left-sided preload with the use of pacing, volume therapy, or both; reduction in LV afterload with systemic vasodilators; and augmentation of contractility with inotropes.[7] The intraaortic balloon pump (IABP) offers potential benefits of increased coronary perfusion pressure and reduced LV afterload, increasing cardiac output by up to 0.5 liters per minute (L/min), whereas a VAD is capable of providing greater circulatory support, if needed (see Chapter 15 for more detail on mechanical circulatory support).[21] The hemodynamic effects of various vasoactive medications and cardiac mechanical support devices are assessed frequently to determine if desired perfusion goals are achieved.

During right-sided heart failure, CVP increases as a result of inadequate RV emptying, whereas the PAOP is decreased because of inadequate flow from the failing right ventricle. Typically, transesophageal echocardiography images demonstrate a small, contractile left ventricle and a large, akinetic right ventricle. Volume is administered to augment RV preload, and the CVP target range is increased to 10 to 15 mm Hg or higher, to improve cardiac output. During volume loading, failure to increase the cardiac index or the appearance of hypotension with elevated filling pressures warrants cessation of fluids and exploration of other therapies directed at heart rate, afterload, or contractility.[3,15]

Reduction of RV afterload is desirable, targeting pulmonary vascular resistance (PVR) with the use of selective pulmonary vasodilators such as inhaled prostanoids or nitric oxide.[7] Systemic hypotension from RV dysfunction is challenging and requires cautious titration of fluids, inotropes, and vasopressors while carefully monitoring right- versus left-sided filling pressures and the cardiac output or cardiac index response. A variety of mechanical cardiac support devices are currently available for support of right, left, or biventricular cardiac function, should other therapies prove inadequate.[18]

Case Study

Ms. S is a 78-year-old female with a medical history of hypertension, elevated cholesterol, and paroxysmal atrial fibrillation. Preoperative cardiac catheterization showed normal coronary arteries, an ejection fraction of 62%, and left ventricular end-diastolic pressure of 32 mm Hg. She is admitted to the critical care unit following aortic valve replacement (AVR) with a 23-millimeter (mm) bioprosthetic valve. Propofol is infusing at 50 micrograms per kilogram per minute (mcg/kg/min).

Case Study—cont'd

PARAMETERS	INITIAL	AFTER 15 MINUTES	5 MINUTES AFTER START OF NITROPRUSSIDE INFUSION	AFTER NITROPRUSSIDE STOPPED AND 250-mL ALBUMIN BOLUS	AFTER NITROPRUSSIDE RESTARTED AND ANOTHER 250-mL ALBUMIN BOLUS
Temperature	35.2° C				
HR	84	88	102	90	82
Heart rhythm	NSR	NSR	ST	NSR	NSR
BP (mm Hg)	162/90	178/98	82/64	158/88	118/66
MAP	114	125	70	111	75–85
CVP (mm Hg)	8	10	6	9	11
CO (L/min)	3.4			3.3	4.6
CI (L/min/m^2)	1.8			1.6	2.4
SvO$_2$	59%		51%		62%
SVR (dynes·sec/cm^5)	2494			2472	1472
PAOP (mm Hg)	12			13	12

BP, Blood pressure; *CI*, cardiac index; *CO*, cardiac output; *HR*, heart rate; *MAP*, mean arterial pressure; *NSR*, normal sinus rhythm; *PAOP*, pulmonary artery occlusion pressure; *ST*, sinus tachycardia; *SvO₂*, mixed venous oxygen saturation; *SVR*, systemic vascular resistance.

She is cool to the touch and pale, with diminished peripheral pulses. Within 15 minutes, BP rises to 178/98 mm Hg (MAP 125), and nitroprusside is initiated at 0.5 mcg/kg/min.

Within 5 minutes of starting the nitroprusside infusion, her BP falls to 82/64 mm Hg (MAP 70), CVP decreases to 6 mm Hg, and SvO$_2$ decreases to 51%.

The nitroprusside infusion is then stopped, and 250 milliliters (mL) of albumin 5% is administered. The propofol dosage is reduced because of its vasodilation properties.

Following completion of the fluid bolus, the BP has risen to 158/88 mm Hg (MAP 111), CVP 9 mm Hg, PAOP 13 mm Hg, CO/CI are 3.3 and 1.6, respectively, and SVR is 2472. Nitroprusside is restarted at a lower dose of 0.3 mcg/kg/min, and an additional 250 mL of albumin is administered at a slow rate.

Over the next hour, the nitroprusside is gradually titrated upward while additional albumin is administered to achieve the targeted MAP of 75 to 85 mm Hg, as other hemodynamic values stabilize. During the next 5 hours, the patient required upward and downward titration of the vasodilator and received one additional fluid bolus until achievement of a normal body temperature. She remained stable thereafter. ■

Patient Education

Preparation for Discharge

Cardiac surgical patients undergoing elective procedures typically receive detailed information preoperatively about their anticipated hospital course, including expectations for immediate postoperative management in the critical care unit . This includes anticipatory guidance for important activities that promote recovery, including pain management, progressive mobilization, pulmonary hygiene measures, as well as a description of routinely used tubes and lines. Patients should be prepared for awakening with a central line in place and the need for periodic repositioning to obtain hemodynamic measurements. Pulmonary artery catheters are removed after cardiac performance stabilizes, whereas central venous catheters may remain in place outside the critical care environment. Postoperatively, patients should anticipate changes in their medication regimen, which may be continued after discharge. In particular, antihypertensive medications may be reduced or discontinued to permit diuresis. Additionally, beta-blocker therapy may be started to prevent atrial arrhythmias. It is not uncommon for patients to experience postural hypotension during their initial mobilization efforts, and patients should be cautioned to move slowly from the supine to the sitting position and only then to a standing position. Patients are reminded to request assistance until they can safely ambulate independently. Written discharge instructions are provided to promote compliance with the treatment plan and medication regimen at home, as well as after-care appointments to ensure careful follow-up and reinstitution of needed therapies, as appropriate.

Conclusion

Hemodynamic monitoring after cardiac surgery provides essential information about the patient's dynamic recovery progress, but interpretation must include baseline ventricular function and underlying disease processes. Hemodynamic profiles, based primarily on LV function, convey standardized assessment findings that help determine appropriate goals and optimal management strategies across a wide variety of procedures. Although tremendous amounts of numeric data are available regarding postoperative hemodynamic performance, clinicians are cautioned not to focus on isolated numbers, which are "snapshots" in time. Instead, they should look at the "big picture" and overall hemodynamic trends for the patient. Providers describe expected versus actual progress towards intermediate and ultimate goals, enabling interventions that are timely and tailored to individual patient needs to promote recovery. A thorough understanding of hemodynamic assessment and interpretation based on physiology will enable increasingly complex procedures to be performed across a wide variety of conditions while promoting optimal outcomes for a new generation of cardiac surgical patients.

References

1. Society of Thoracic Surgeons: *STS short-term risk calculator.* http://www.sts.org/quality-research-patient-safety/quality/risk-calculator-and-models. Accessed September 1, 2014.
2. euroSCORE Risk Calculator. http://www.euroscore.org/calc.html. Accessed September 1, 2014.
3. Carl M, Alms A, Braun J, et al.: S3 guidelines for intensive care in cardiac surgery patients: hemodynamic monitoring and cardiocirculary system, *Ger Med Sci* 8:1–25, 2010.
4. Hillis LD, Smith PK, Anderson JL, et al.: 2011 ACCF/AHA guideline for coronary artery bypass graft surgery, *J Am Coll Cardiol* 58(24):e123–e210, 2011.
5. Wiener RS, Welch HG: Trends in use of the pulmonary artery catheter in the United States, 1993–2004, *JAMA* 298(4):423–429, 2007.
6. Holm J, Håkanson E, Vánky F, Svedjeholm R: Mixed venous oxygen saturation predicts short- and long-term outcome after coronary artery bypass grafting surgery: a retrospective cohort analysis, *Br J Anaesth* 107(3):344–350, 2011.
7. St. André AC, DelRossi A: Hemodynamic management of patients in the first 24 hours after cardiac surgery, *Crit Care Med* 33(9):2082–2093, 2005.
8. Society of Thoracic Surgeons: Data analyses of The Society of Thoracic Surgeons national adult cardiac surgery database, participant report. April, 2013.
9. Puntillo K, Ley SJ: Appropriately timed analgesics control pain due to chest tube removal, *Am J Crit Care* 13(4):292–302, 2004.
10. Lavigne D: Vasopressin and methylene blue: alternative therapies in vasodilatory shock, *Semin Cardiothorac Vasc Anesth* 14(3):186–189, 2010.
11. Otto CM: *Textbook of clinical echocardiography,* ed 5, Philadelphia, 2013, Saunders, p 159.
12. Huikuri HV: Effect of mitral valve replacement on left ventricular function in mitral regurgitation, *Br Heart J* 49:328–333, 1983.
13. Holm J, Håkanson RE, Vánky F, Svedjeholm R: Mixed venous oxygen saturation is a prognostic marker after surgery for aortic stenosis, *Acta Anaesthesiol Scand* 54:589–595, 2010.
14. Frohlich ED, González A, Diez J: Hypertensive left ventricular hypertrophy risk: beyond adaptive cardiomyocytic hypertrophy, *J Hypertens* 29:17–26, 2010.
15. Ibrahim M, Rao C, Ashrafian H, et al.: Modern management of systolic anterior motion of the mitral valve, *Eur J Cardiothorac Surg* 41(6):1260–1270, 2012.
16. Aya HD, Cecconi M, Hamilton M, Rhodes A: Goal-directed therapy in cardiac surgery: a systematic review and meta-analysis, *Br J Anaesth* 110(4):510–517, 2013.
17. Price S, Prout J, Jaggar SI, et al.: "Tamponade" following cardiac surgery: terminology and echocardiography may both mislead, *Eur J Cardiothorac Surg* 26:1156–1160, 2004.
18. Dunning J, Fabbri A, Koth PH, et al.: Guideline for resuscitation in cardiac arrest after cardiac surgery, *Eur J Cardiothorac Surg* 36(1):3–28, 2009.
19. Nolan JP, Soar J, Zideman DA, et al.: European resuscitation council guidelines for resuscitation 2010 section 1, executive summary, *Resuscitation* 81(10):1219–1276, 2010.
20. Peura JL, Colvin-Adams M, Francis GS, et al.: Recommendations for the use of mechanical circulatory support: device strategies and patient selection: a scientific statement from the American Heart Association, *Circulation* 126:2648–2667, 2012.
21. Kar B, Basra SS, Shah NR, Loyalka P: Percutaneous circulatory support in cardiogenic shock: interventional bridge to recovery, *Circulation* 125:1809–1817, 2012.

Hemodynamic Management of Heart Failure and Cardiogenic Shock

17

Michael Petty

Heart failure is a complex clinical syndrome that begins with an initiating event, such as a myocardial infarction, which results in an inability of the heart to deliver adequate blood flow to meet the metabolic requirements of the tissues.[1] Heart failure can result from a variety of structural or functional disorders of the pericardium, myocardium, endocardium, or great vessels.[2] It affects 5.1 million Americans over the age of 19 years (2.4% of the population), with an additional 825,000 individuals over the age of 44 being diagnosed with heart failure annually.[1] The frequency of heart failure as a diagnosis increases with patient age (Table 17-1).[1] The estimated cost of heart failure to the U.S. economy alone exceeds $34 billion annually (Table 17-2).[3] The most frequently mentioned causes include coronary artery disease, hypertension, diabetes, valvular heart disease, and dilated cardiomyopathy. However, any form of heart disease may result in heart failure symptoms. In addition, factors such as certain cancer treatments, alcohol and drug abuse, human immunodeficiency virus/acquired immunodeficiency syndrome (HIV/AIDS), and obstructive sleep apnea may also result in heart failure (Box 17-1).[4]

The continuum of heart failure has both acute and chronic stages. However, the literature now refers to acute heart failure as acute decompensated heart failure (ADHF), reflecting the progressive nature of the illness.[5] Compensated heart failure describes the condition in a patient who has a heart failure diagnosis but whose symptoms are minimal because of effective pharmacologic and lifestyle management. ADHF represents the failure of those treatment interventions to limit symptoms and often requires hospitalization to optimize therapies and to regain control of the patient's symptoms. At the far extreme of the continuum is cardiogenic shock, in which the heart's ability to support circulation is so impaired that end organ compromise results if rapid and effective interventions are not initiated. Heart failure may impact the left or right ventricle and, not uncommonly, involves both. To understand more about right ventricular (RV) failure, refer to Chapter 18. The rest of this chapter will focus on left heart failure.

In the early stages of left heart failure, a series of compensatory mechanisms are activated to correct blood flow abnormalities. The Starling mechanism yields an increased stroke volume when the left ventricular end-diastolic volume increases because of incomplete emptying of the ventricle. The resulting distention of the ventricle results in stretching of the myocardial fibers and increased ability to contract, thus increasing stroke volume (Figure 17-1).

TABLE 17-1   Prevalence of Heart Failure by Gender and Age

	AGE 20–39		AGE 40–59		AGE 60–79		AGE 80+	
	MALE	FEMALE	MALE	FEMALE	MALE	FEMALE	MALE	FEMALE
Percent of population	0.2	0.4	1.5	0.7	7.8	4.5	8.6	11.5

Data from Go AS, Mozaffarian D, Roger VL, et al.: Heart disease and stroke statistics—2014 update: a report from the American Heart Association, *Circulation* 129:e28–e292, 2013.

TABLE 17-2   Annual Cost of Heart Failure in the United States

CARDIOVASCULAR DISEASE	ESTIMATED DIRECT AND INDIRECT COSTS IN BILLIONS
Coronary heart disease	$108.9
Hypertensive disease	$93.5
Stroke	$53.9
Heart failure	$34.4

Data from Heidenreich PA, Trogdon JG, Khavjou OA, et al.: Forecasting the future of cardiovascular diseases in the United States: a policy statement from the American Heart Association, *Circulation* 123:933–944, 2011.

BOX 17-1   Causes of Heart Failure

- Coronary artery disease
- Hypertension
- Diabetes
- Cardiomyopathy
- Valvular heart disease
- Arrhythmias

- Congenital heart disease
- Outside factors: certain cancer treatments, alcohol and drug use, human immunodeficiency virus/acquired immunodeficiency syndrome (HIV/AIDS)

Data from National Heart, Lung, and Blood Institute: *What causes heart failure?* http://www.nhlbi.nih.gov/health/health-topics/topics/hf/causes.html. Updated 2012. Accessed November 4, 2014.

Neurohormonal responses are activated in heart failure to improve organ and tissue perfusion. The sympathetic nervous system responds to decreased flow with increased concentrations of norepinephrine in the bloodstream. This adrenergic chemical stimulates beta$_1$-receptors, resulting in increases in both heart rate (chronotropy) and myocardial contractility (inotropy). Norepinephrine also stimulates alpha$_1$-receptors in the myocardium increasing contractility. In the arterioles, norepinephrine increases vasoconstriction (afterload), raising blood pressure and shifting blood flow toward the vital organs. Over time, in response to reduced renal blood flow and other stimuli, the renin–angiotensin–aldosterone system (RAAS) converts angiotensinogen,

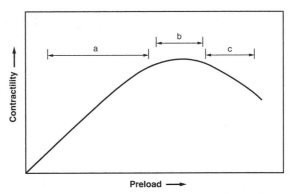

FIGURE 17-1 Starling curve and the impact of preload. a, Increasing preload (volume loading) results in increased contractility. b, Increasing preload does not increase contractility. c, Increasing preload overstretches the myocardial fibers and decreases contractility.

through angiotensin I to angiotensin II, using several pathways. This powerful hormone also contributes to increased arterial vasoconstriction. At the same time, release of aldosterone by the adrenal gland stimulates the renal tubules to retain sodium and, with it, water, to preserve circulating volume (see Chapter 1, Figure 1-17). The third neurohormonal pathway, arginine vasopressin, stimulates a reduction in the excretion of water.[6]

Although initially effective, over time, these compensatory mechanisms may accelerate the rate of decline of cardiac function. The cardiac muscle becomes progressively weaker because of a combination of myocyte necrosis (myocardial infarction), myocyte apoptosis (programmed cell death), cytokines such as tumor necrosis factor alpha (TNF-α), and oxidative stress proteins.[6] This reduced contractility inhibits the heart's ability to increase stroke volume through the Starling mechanism. Similarly, contractile beta-receptors that were initially responsive to norepinephrine lose their sensitivity to the hormone. Vasoconstriction caused by sympathetic stimulation and the RAAS further limit the weakened ventricle from ejecting blood. The backup of blood from inadequate ejection along with continued volume retention stimulated by the RAAS and arginine vasopressin result in fluid volume overload, pulmonary edema, and systemic edema (Figure 17-2).

The myocardium, in response to continued elevation in afterload as a result of vasoconstriction or hypertension, undergoes hypertrophy. When persistently unable to propel enough blood to tissues, the ventricle dilates from the excess volume, and remodeling is complete. Reversal of this remodeling is difficult to achieve, and progression of remodeling accelerates mortality from heart failure. Symptoms often do not appear until after remodeling has begun.

Heart failure is categorized in several ways: (1) type of LV dysfunction: systolic or diastolic; (2) flow pattern: forward flow or backward flow; and (3) severity: heart failure or cardiogenic shock.

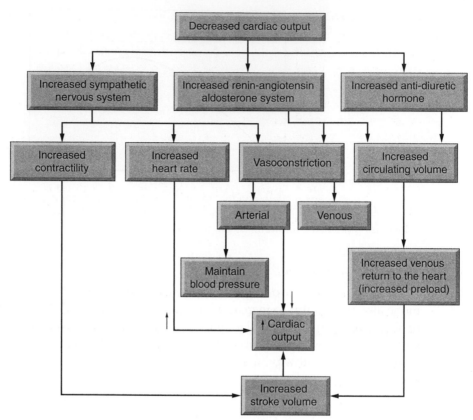

FIGURE 17-2 Neurohormonal compensatory mechanisms in heart failure. (Adapted from Lilly LS (ed).: *Pathophysiology of heart disease*, ed 5, Philadelphia, 2011, Lippincott Williams & Wilkins.)

Subcategories of Heart Failure

Systolic versus Diastolic

To this point, the focus of the discussion has primarily been on systolic heart failure, the inability of the ventricle to eject blood to the tissues because of progressive weakness based on the pathophysiology described. Current literature also classifies this as *heart failure with reduced ejection fraction* (HFrEF). This type of heart failure is the most studied and involves a large percentage of those diagnosed with heart failure. Ejection fraction, calculated as (end-diastolic volume − end-systolic volume) ÷ end-diastolic volume of less than 35% to 40% is classified as heart failure. A normal ejection fraction is 55% to 65%.[7]

However, in recent years, recognition and interest in the role of diastolic dysfunction has grown. In diastolic heart failure, ejection fraction is 45% to 55%, but LV filling is slowed and stroke volume is reduced. Diastolic heart failure accounts for an increasing proportion of all cases of heart failure in the United States.[8] Also referred to as *heart failure with preserved ejection fraction* (HFpEF).[2] Causative mechanisms for this type of heart failure are postulated to include abnormal ventricular relaxation, difficulties with ventricular–vascular coupling, volume overload, chronotropic incompetence, or endothelial dysfunction.[9] The prevalence of HFpEF has been reported to be growing over the last 15 years to now exceed 50% of newly diagnosed patients.[10] Therapeutic options for HFpEF that alter the morbidity and mortality associated with it are limited.

Bursi and colleagues reported rates of diastolic HFpEF of 55% in their sample of 556 participants, associated with increased age and female gender.[11] In this study, isolated diastolic dysfunction was present in 44% of the patients reviewed. Yancy and colleagues in their analysis of the ADHERE (Acute Decompensated Heart Failure National Registry) Database (n = 52,187) identified hypertension as a significant risk factor in those with HFpEF in contrast to patients without preserved ejection fraction. In addition, increased age and female gender were factors more likely to be associated with HFpEF ($p < 0.0001$).[12]

Forward Flow versus Backward Flow

Forward blood flow, measured as cardiac output, is impacted by its basic elements: heart rate and stroke volume ($CO = HR \times SV$), as shown in Figure 1-7 in Chapter 1. Stroke volume may be altered by changes in preload (volume in the ventricle at the end of diastole), contractility (the force exerted against the ventricular contents to propel it out of the ventricle) and afterload (the resistance against which the heart has to pump the blood out of the ventricle and into the arterial circulation). It is important to distinguish this key concept of heart failure—inadequate forward flow to meet the metabolic demands of the tissues—from its most commonly associated symptom: fluid volume overload. As noted above, congestion is the result of inadequate emptying of the left ventricle and the compensatory mechanisms that are intended to correct the acute condition. This will be important to keep in mind during the discussion of interventions to improve cardiac output and reduce congestion.

Cardiogenic Shock

Cardiogenic shock, regardless of cause, represents the most severe form of LV failure. In this severe low cardiac output state, LV volume is elevated, cardiac output and blood pressure are low, and organs demonstrate signs of hypoperfusion: clouded mentation, low urine output, metabolic acidosis and cool extremities.[13] Without rapid and effective intervention, mortality associated with cardiogenic shock has been reported as high as 80% and is associated with about 10% of acute myocardial infarctions.[14]

The key to effective treatment of heart failure lies in recognizing the signs and symptoms of the disease to facilitate diagnosis; characterizing the type and degree of LV failure by utilizing hemodynamic measurement and other assessment tools to guide therapy; and evaluating the interventions undertaken to determine their effectiveness in improving the patient's condition. This chapter will consider each of those elements.

Signs and Symptoms of Acute Decompensated Heart Failure and Cardiogenic Shock

The symptoms most commonly associated with heart failure include shortness of breath, fatigue with resulting exercise intolerance, and fluid retention reflected in edema both in the pulmonary circuit as well as in the periphery. In 1928, the New York Heart Association (NYHA) developed a functional classification system that has been applied to patients with heart failure for more than 80 years. It has undergone modifications over time, and was most recently revised in 1994.[15] Classification is based on functional measures (subjective) as well as objective indicators of cardiac dysfunction (Tables 17-3 and 17-4). However, not all patients experience all of these symptoms. Some may complain of exercise intolerance and dyspnea without evidence of fluid retention; others develop significant edema and yet have no complaints related to exercise or breathing. Some patients are noted to have a severely reduced ejection fraction (HFrEF, systolic heart failure) but are asymptomatic, whereas others with relatively preserved contractility (HFpEF, diastolic heart failure) are symptomatic at rest or with mild exercise. A clear explanation of the physiology of heart failure symptoms remains somewhat elusive.

Physical Examination

As is the case with many health problems, patients with heart failure often present with a constellation of complaints that could represent a variety of disorders. As noted above, although many patients have similar complaints, heart failure may exist

TABLE 17-3   NYHA Functional Classification of Heart Failure

NYHA CLASS	COMFORTABLE AT REST	LIMIT ON PHYSICAL ACTIVITY	MAXIMUM LEVEL OF PHYSICAL ACTIVITY	POTENTIAL CONSEQUENCES OF PHYSICAL ACTIVITY
I	Yes	None	Ordinary	None
II	Yes	Slight	Ordinary	Fatigue, palpitation, dyspnea, or anginal pain
III	Yes	Marked	Less than ordinary	Fatigue, palpitation, dyspnea, or anginal pain
IV	No: symptoms of heart failure or angina syndrome may be present	Fully limited	None	Increased discomfort

NYHA, New York Heart Association.
Source: http://www.heart.org/HEARTORG/Conditions/HeartFailure/AboutHeartFailure/Classes-of-Heart-Failure_UCM_306328_Article.jsp. Accessed September 1, 2014.

TABLE 17-4 Objective Classification of Heart Failure Symptoms

CLASS	OBJECTIVE EVIDENCE	SYMPTOMS	LIMIT ON ORDINARY PHYSICAL ACTIVITY	COMFORTABLE AT REST
I	No	None	No	Yes
II	Minimal cardiovascular disease	Mild	Slight	Yes
III	Moderately severe cardiovascular disease	Moderate	Marked	Comfortable only at rest
IV	Severe cardiovascular disease	Significant	Severe	No

Source: http://www.heart.org/HEARTORG/Conditions/HeartFailure/AboutHeartFailure/Classes-of-Heart-Failure_UCM_306328_Article.jsp. Accessed September 1, 2014.

without all of them being present. In addition, by some estimates, as many as 40% of patients in decompensated heart failure may not demonstrate symptoms detectable purely by physical examination.

However, in those patients exhibiting physical signs and symptoms of heart failure, important insight into their disease and potential initial therapies can be derived. A combination of intentional inquiry about potential symptoms in the patient interview, along with a comprehensive physical examination can yield subtle—and not so subtle—changes in end organ function that reflect an alteration in cardiac output related to heart failure. See Table 17-5 for possible indicators of LV or RV function.

TABLE 17-5 Symptoms of Left and Right Ventricular Failure

LEFT VENTRICULAR FAILURE		RIGHT VENTRICULAR FAILURE	
SUBJECTIVE	PHYSICAL EXAMINATION	SUBJECTIVE	PHYSICAL EXAMINATION
Shortness of breath	Weight gain	Lower extremity heaviness	Weight gain
Cough	Tachycardia	Abdominal distention	Jugular vein distension, pulsation
Weakness, fatigue	Decrease in S1 sound	Gastric distress	Edema
Memory loss	S3, S4, gallop	Nausea, anorexia	Hepatomegaly
Confusion	Crackles in lung fields (rales)		Positive hepatojugular reflux
Palpitations	Pleural effusion		Ascites
Sleeplessness	Diaphoresis		
Anorexia	Pulsus alternans		
Diaphoresis			

Data from Soine LA: Heart failure and cardiogenic shock. In Woods SJ, Froelicher ESS, Motzer SU, Bridges EJ, editors: *Cardiac nursing*, ed 6, Philadelphia, 2010, Wolters Kluwer/Lippincott Williams & Wilkins, p 567.

During the first encounter, patients with ADHF often show evidence of orthopnea and an inability to lie flat, which may be a clue that the patient is experiencing heart failure with volume overload and secondary pulmonary congestion. Other reported symptoms consistent with orthopnea include paroxysmal nocturnal dyspnea, sleeping with multiple pillows or sleeping in a recliner.

Neurologic Signs and Symptoms

During the interview with the patient with ADHF, inadequate cerebral perfusion may be evidenced by somnolence, confusion, and slowness in response to questions as well as complaints of memory impairment. This may be an early subtle sign of deteriorating heart failure in the critical care environment, particularly in the patient being prematurely weaned, or weaned too aggressively from inotropic support. In addition, patients may complain of dizziness or weakness with sudden changes in position (orthostasis). Distinguishing between this and medication side effects is challenging, requiring clinicians to be closely attentive to both current conditions and the trajectory of neurologic functioning over time.

Heart and Vascular Signs and Symptoms

Heart rate and stroke volume are the variables that impact cardiac output. It is common in heart failure for heart rate to be elevated. This response, mitigated by the sympathetic nervous system, is intended to enhance cardiac output by affecting one of its two components (Cardiac Output = Heart Rate × Stroke Volume). This response may be blunted or negligible in patients who are receiving medications such as beta-blockers, which will limit their ability to significantly increase heart rate. Aging may also impair this chronotropic response to reduced blood flow. Patients may report palpitations or an irregular heartbeat. This may be the result of premature contractions of the atria or the ventricles or the development of atrial fibrillation. With those dysrhythmias, the loss of atrial contribution to ventricular filling is another important negative influence on forward flow.

Auscultation and palpation may reveal additional indicators of heart failure. An S3 murmur, reflecting LV distension and severe hemodynamic compromise, may be combined with an S4 murmur, common in diastolic dysfunction, to produce a gallop rhythm.[8] Murmurs associated with either of the atrioventricular valves may provide additional evidence of valvular incompetence associated with volume excess and myocardial dilation disrupting the normal closure of the valve leaflets. Also consistent with cardiac enlargement is the shift of the point of maximal intensity to the left of the midclavicular line and downward toward the fifth intercostal space.[8] Finally, a ventricular heave felt over the precordium provides additional evidence of ventricular enlargement.

Visualization and palpation of the vascular structures provides evidence of inadequate forward flow and volume congestion. Arterial pulses may be diminished. Pulsus alternans, which describes alternating strength of the palpated pulse, is associated with LV systolic dysfunction, and a beat-to-beat variation in ventricular preload.[7] Jugular venous distension, measured with the patient lying at a 45-degree angle and estimated in centimeters of water (cm H_2O), is evidence of the fluid volume excess common in decompensated heart failure.

Kidney Signs and Symptoms

Reduction in perfusion to the kidney stimulates a cascade of neurohormonal responses in the RAAS, which result in a reduction in urine output to control perceived loss of cardiac output. This reflects a decrease in throughput of blood through the nephrons based on both reduced cardiac output and venous congestion that obstructs renal venous outflow. The physiologic goal of this response is to preserve preload in an effort to improve cardiac performance. However, this compensatory mechanism, if left unchecked, may result in an accelerated decompensation of heart failure.

Pulmonary Signs and Symptoms

As forward flow is reduced, renal venous stasis increases, and fluid retention is stimulated by the RAAS, an increase in lung water is inevitable without intervention. LV congestion causes fluid to back up into the lungs. The elevation of hydrostatic pressure in the pulmonary circulation overwhelms the available oncotic pressure, preventing the recruitment of fluid back into the circulation, and instead shifting it into the alveoli. Patients may develop a dry, nonproductive cough and, on auscultation, have fine bi-basilar crackles (rales) that can progress to rhonchi, wheezing, pleural friction rubs, and pulmonary edema, if left untreated. Further fluid pooling may lead to pleural effusion and a notable dullness on chest percussion.

Patient Comfort

The growth of palliative care in hospitals, including in the management of patients with heart failure, has not meant simply an increased focus on end of life. Rather, palliative care specialists have a valuable skill set to help patients manage their symptoms. Pharmacologic interventions such as low-dose opioids do not interfere with the goals of heart failure treatment but will improve the experience of shortness of breath. Low-dose opioids reduce stress and suffering, ultimately decreasing metabolic oxygen demands and improving the match between oxygen requirements with oxygen delivery.

The nurse at the bedside is in a unique position to utilize therapeutic use of self as an intervention to help with shortness of breath, and this is equally as important as pharmacotherapy. When mild symptoms result in panic and anxiety, ensuring a quiet environment, calming reassurance, and use of imagery or muscle relaxation to help break the cycle of catecholamine-driven acceleration of symptoms may be as valuable as medication. Listening and encouraging are important clinical skills. Putting those skills to work in this setting is at the core of nursing practice, is supported in the literature, and is one of the most satisfying ways that a nurse can provide care to a patient and family.

Liver and Gastrointestinal Signs and Symptoms

Right-sided congestion may be associated with liver engorgement and ascites. The edge of the liver is palpable below the right costochondral margin in advanced heart failure, and percussion may reveal hepatomegaly.[7]

Integumentary Signs and Symptoms

The skin, as the body's largest organ, will often reveal an early reduction in perfusion in heart failure as circulation is shunted to supply core organs. This reflects activation of the sympathetic nervous system and the RAAS, both of which stimulate vasoconstriction. Vasoconstriction will strive to raise central blood pressure and improve perfusion of the central organs. The result is cool, pale skin with reduced capillary refill, decreased peripheral pulses, and at times a mottled appearance. Because of significant vasoconstriction, peripheral pulses are often more difficult to detect manually and may require Doppler assessment. Pulse oximetry may be difficult to assess because of inadequate peripheral perfusion. In addition, the augmented afterload increases the workload of the already failing myocardium, again contributing to acceleration of the downward spiral of heart failure if no intervention is attempted.

> **Patient Safety**
>
> The skin is the largest organ in the body and also seems to be the organ to be deprived of circulation in the setting of heart failure. Underperfused capillaries along with prolonged pressure against the skin will unfortunately create the perfect environment for the development of pressure ulcers. Once they develop, persistent hypoperfusion makes pressure ulcer healing more challenging, and the risk of infection increases. If sepsis should develop, the failing heart will be unlikely to meet the increased flow requirements associated with the septic state.
>
> As a result, meticulous attention to the condition of the skin is a core focus of the critical care nurse for the patient in heart failure. Inspection, repositioning, consulting with Wound Ostomy Care nurses, and using all preventive measures possible is the only way to prevent this cascade of patient complications.

Cardiogenic Shock

In cardiogenic shock, the severity of all signs and symptoms is exacerbated. The patient will be unconscious, delirious or irritable and may have a sense of doom. Profound hypotension with narrowed pulse pressure and tachycardia are present, along with pallor, cyanosis, diaphoresis, cool clammy skin, reduced capillary refill, and thready or absent peripheral pulses. Cardiac output may be worsened by dysrhythmias and heart block. Oliguria or anuria may develop quickly. Deteriorating respiratory function is characterized by tachypnea, dyspnea, and irregular breathing patterns. Ventilation–perfusion mismatch leads to hypoxemia. Rapid recognition of these symptoms and initiation of immediate therapies to increase blood flow and restore perfusion to vital organs is essential to increase the likelihood of survival from this critical illness.

Framework for Evaluating Heart Failure

Stevenson and Perloff provided valuable conceptual insights for understanding the four hemodynamic presentations of heart failure.[16,17] Using a 2-by-2 graphic, the presence of the primary features of heart failure—low perfusion and increased venous congestion—were either present or absent[17:]

- Warm and Dry (A)—the patient is experiencing no congestion and has an adequate resting cardiac output
- Warm and Wet (B)—the patient has venous congestion but cardiac output remains adequate
- Cold and Dry (L)—the patient has no evidence of venous congestion but cardiac output is inadequate
- Cold and Wet (C)—the patient has both congestion and inadequate cardiac output.

In 2002, Stevenson and associates expanded the grid to include the principal symptoms that may be seen on physical examination as discussed above[17] (Figure 17-3). The symptoms of congestion were orthopnea, elevated jugular venous pressure, presence of S3 and a loud P2, edema, ascites, rales (crackles), and hepatojugular reflux. Signs of low peripheral perfusion included narrow pulse pressure (the difference between systolic blood pressure and diastolic blood pressure), pulsus alternans (alternating higher and lower systolic pressure),[17] cold forearms and legs, decreased level of consciousness, angiotensin-converting enzyme inhibitor–related symptomatic hypotension,

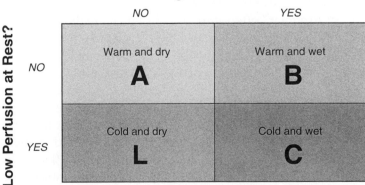

Evidence for Congestion (elevated filling pressure)

Orthopnea
High jugular venous pressure
Increasing S_3
Loud P_2
Edema

Ascites
Rales
Abdominojugular reflux
Valsalva square wave

Congested at Rest?

Evidence for Low Perfusion

Narrow pulse pressure
Pulsus alterations
Cool forearms and legs
Sleepy, obtunded
ACE inhibitor-related
Symptomatic hypotension
Declining serum sodium level
Worsening renal function

Low Perfusion at Rest?

	NO	YES
NO	Warm and dry **A**	Warm and wet **B**
YES	Cold and dry **L**	Cold and wet **C**

FIGURE 17-3 Hemodynamic Profiles for patents presenting in heart failure. (Courtesy Anju Nohria and Lynne Warner Stevenson.)

declining serum sodium level, and worsening kidney function.[18] It is important to note that the vast majority of these signs of heart failure can be determined without a single invasive measurement.

The advantage patients and clinicians have in today's health care environment is the availability of noninvasive technologies that supplement the physical examination in determining the degree of dysfunction associated with a patient's heart failure or cardiogenic shock.

Noninvasive Assessment

Beyond the physical examination, the assessment of blood pressure, cardiac rhythm, and pulse oximetry provide important additional data to better characterize the patient's cardiovascular function. Critically thinking about what each of these tools provides—and does not provide—translates into data to include in the plan of care.

Clinical Reasoning Pearl

A pulmonary artery catheter (PAC) is not required to determine chamber pressures and cardiac output in patients with heart failure. Recent work by Temporelli and colleagues has demonstrated that Doppler echocardiographic analysis of cardiac function can predict right atrial pressure, pulmonary artery pressure, pulmonary artery occlusion pressure (PAOP), pulmonary vascular resistance (PVR), and cardiac output with high reliability ($r = 0.93$–0.97)[19,20] Echocardiography has also been used to estimate left ventricular end-diastolic volume and ejection fraction. This noninvasive method can be used in an outpatient setting, thus avoiding the need for hospital admission to undergo right heart catheterization, while providing clinicians with immediate feedback regarding the effectiveness of changes in therapy.

Cardiac Rate and Rhythm

In addition to the cardiac assessment, which can be performed by auscultatory or palpation methods, understanding the patient's cardiac rhythm beyond rate and "regular or irregular" offers important insights into the possible reasons for reduction in cardiac output as well as possible interventions to improve it.

Flow is most effective when the heart rhythm begins in the sinus node, conducts as a single stimulus through the standard conduction pathways to the atrioventricular node, and then through the bundle branches to the Purkinje fibers. The associated sequential contraction, first of the atria and then of the ventricles, provides an opportunity for optimal filling of the ventricles prior to ejection.

Atrial fibrillation is frequently associated with dilated cardiomyopathy and myocardial infarction. The resultant loss of atrial "kick" reduces ventricular filling and may have a significant negative impact on cardiac output. Bradycardia, persistent supraventricular tachycardia, and ventricular tachycardia will also have a profound negative impact on forward flow. Tachycardia increases myocardial work and myocardial oxygen consumption while reducing coronary artery perfusion time and contributing further to myocardial dysfunction. Thus, monitoring the electrocardiogram (ECG) for signs of dysrhythmias as well as for evidence of myocardial ischemia and bundle branch block facilitates early intervention before permanent myocardial damage has occurred.[21]

Noninvasive Blood Pressure Monitoring. In the early stages of ADHF, systolic blood pressure may be elevated or normal. When heart failure is more advanced because of LV dysfunction, systolic blood pressure is often low. Diastolic blood pressure is frequently elevated owing to the persistent vasoconstriction associated with compensatory mechanisms for heart failure. Pulse pressure is low because of the combination of reduced systolic blood pressure and elevated diastolic pressure. This low pulse pressure is associated with reduced stroke volume.[8] The degree of lowering of systolic blood pressure impacts end organs. Some patients are functional with systolic blood pressure between 80 and 90 millimeters of mercury (mm Hg), whereas others feel light-headed when their pressure is less than 100 mm Hg. Other evidence of the negative sequelae of hypotension may be detected from alterations in laboratory values or reduction in urine output.

Pulse Oximetry

Noninvasive assessment of pulse oximeter oxygen saturation (SpO_2) helps complete the picture of heart failure. Reduced oxygenation may reflect an increase in lung water and associated reduction in gas exchange at the capillary–alveolar interface.

To be accurate, the pulse oximeter must be able to detect a pulse with enough variation to recognize arterial flow and thus appropriately assess the oxyhemoglobin level of the blood passing by. Narrowed pulse pressure, peripheral vasoconstriction, or anemia may reduce the accuracy of the SpO_2 measurement and result in inaccurate data being considered in the treatment plan. Careful monitoring of the waveform displayed by the pulse oximeter is crucial to accurate data collection.

Echocardiography

Transthoracic two-dimensional echocardiography, including two-dimensional Doppler flow studies, has been characterized as the most useful diagnostic tool for evaluating ADHF. This single noninvasive test provides measurements of ventricular chamber size, myocardial wall thickness, valvular function, systolic and diastolic function, and pericardial effusion. Because of its noninvasive nature, rapid patient assessment using a transthoracic echocardiography quickly provides information to guide interventions to improve patient condition.

Echocardiography helps the clinician distinguish between systolic and diastolic heart failure, provides visual evidence of changes in ventricular wall motion and evidence of changes in atrial dimensions. Hemodynamically, patients with diastolic heart failure have elevated filling pressures and reduced cardiac output similar to those with systolic heart failure, but with little reduction in ejection fraction. Thus, the differential diagnosis of diastolic heart failure is made by noting abnormal ventricular filling pressures in the presence of preserved systolic function. In many patients with heart failure, features of systolic and diastolic dysfunction coexist.[2]

Chest Radiography

The 2012 recommendations of the Canadian Cardiovascular Society include obtaining a chest radiograph within the first 2 hours after admission for ADHF. The value of this noninvasive assessment is to assist the clinician in evaluating the lung fields as well as the cardiac silhouette as part of a complete evaluation of the patient with dyspnea.[22]

Invasive Hemodynamic Assessment

Intra-arterial Monitoring

Placement of an arterial catheter in ADHF and cardiogenic shock is usually to facilitate closer monitoring of blood pressure. As mentioned above, pulsus alternans may be an important indication as the ventricle's variable filling, resulting in alternating higher and lower peak systolic pressure tracings on the arterial line display. In addition, narrowed pulse pressure will be reflected in reduced amplitude of the arterial waveform.

Most patients with ADHF requiring hospital admission are hypertensive (SBP > 140 mm Hg). An analysis of the ADHERE (Acute Decompensated Heart Failure National Registry) Database ($n = 52,187$) demonstrated that 44% of patients admitted to the hospital with reduced systolic function had hypertension; an even higher proportion (61%) of those admitted with ADHF with preserved systolic function were hypertensive. DBP was preserved in both groups.[12]

A cardinal finding in cardiogenic shock is hypotension and patients admitted to the critical care area with ADHF often will have a systolic blood pressure less than 90 mm Hg, whereas diastolic blood pressure may remain preserved (70–85 mm Hg), resulting in a narrowed pulse pressure (systolic blood pressure - diastolic blood pressure). In addition, the presence of an arterial catheter and continuous arterial pressure monitoring may provide important feedback about the efficacy of a new therapy. Changes in absolute blood pressure, mean arterial pressure (MAP), and pulse pressure may all be valuable in titrating therapy for the individual patient. Finally, access to arterial blood gas monitoring offers additional clinical information related to the patient's acid–base balance, oxygenation, and ventilatory efficiency.

Intracardiac Pressure Monitoring

Hemodynamically, heart failure is characterized by a low flow state. Patients with compensated heart failure may have adapted reasonably well to this low flow state by increasing oxygen extraction from blood. However, in ADHF, the patient's compensatory mechanisms have become overwhelmed as the cardiac output is insufficient to meet basic oxygen extraction and metabolic needs. Those patients are the ones most likely to be admitted to the critical care unit for stabilization and management of their heart failure symptoms, to reverse the progression of ventricular dysfunction and prolong survival.

Although no single parameter is essential for the diagnosis of ADHF, those most commonly cited include cardiac index below 2.2 liters per minute per square meter ($L/min/m^2$); systolic blood pressure less than 100 mm Hg; pulmonary arterial occlusion pressure (PAOP) greater than 18 mm Hg; and right atrial pressure (RAP) or central venous pressure (CVP) greater than 15 mm Hg.

Congestion is not the cause of heart failure but rather the result of it. Utilizing the information gathered in the hemodynamic assessment, the clinician often can identify the affected ventricle(s) by recognizing which chamber (right ventricle, left ventricle, or both) is congested. This information will permit the clinician to choose the pharmacologic and mechanical therapies that will have the greatest likelihood of improving forward flow and reducing congestion.

Cardiogenic shock is the most extreme form of ADHF, in which tissues are suddenly deprived of blood because of an abrupt failure of the myocardium. Mortality rates of 50% to 100% are not uncommon in this form of shock related to end organ failure. Cardiogenic shock, like ADHF, is a syndrome whose hemodynamic parameters include hypotension defined as MAP <60 mm Hg or systolic blood pressure <90 mm Hg for more than 30 minutes, narrowed pulse pressure, cardiac index of less than 2.0 L/min/m^2 and PAOP >18 mm Hg. The severity of inadequate tissue perfusion is reflected in altered mental status, cool extremities, and low urine output. Disordered laboratory measures include elevated creatinine and serum lactate, metabolic acidosis, and abnormalities in liver tests and pulmonary function.

Clinical conditions that worsen cardiogenic shock may occur as a consequence of acute myocardial infarction. These include dysrhythmias, both tachycardia and bradycardia, and loss of atrial kick with atrial fibrillation. Other potential contributors include major surgery or trauma, and structural abnormalities such as ventricular septal rupture, acute disruption of a cardiac valve, or pulmonary embolism. Likewise, substances that depress myocardial function such as acidemia, drugs, and electrolyte abnormalities may worsen cardiogenic shock.

Cardiac Output Measurement

The standard thermodilution method for cardiac output measurement described in previous chapters and the derived values calculated using cardiac output and other measured hemodynamic values are important in assessing cardiac function in ADHF and cardiogenic shock. The transpulmonary gradient (TPG) and even ventricular stroke work index provide insight into the potential compensatory mechanisms that are causing functional deterioration (Table 17-6).

In heart failure and other low flow states, the Fick method of determining the cardiac index, although less common, is considered more accurate than the thermodilution method. The Fick formula presented here assumes that the rate of oxygen consumption is fixed, a function of the rate of blood flow in liters per minute and the rate at which oxygen is picked up by the hemoglobin molecule.[23] As a result, using a standard rate of oxygen uploading by the red blood cells, and inserting measurements of the patient's arterial oxygen saturation (SaO$_2$), mixed venous oxygen saturation (SvO$_2$), and hemoglobin, a cardiac output measure can be derived. The advantage of the Fick method is that it is free of the issues that affect the shape of the curve derived in thermodilution measurements, thus avoiding common overestimates of cardiac output.[23]

TABLE 17-6	Hemodynamics of Heart Failure and Cardiogenic Shock	
VALUE (UNITS)	**HEART FAILURE**	**CARDIOGENIC SHOCK**
Blood Pressure (mm Hg)	↑→↓	↓
CVP/RAP (mm Hg)	↑→	↑
PAP (mm Hg)	↑	↑
PAOP	↑	↑
SV	↓	↓
HR	↑	↑
SVR	↑	↑
PVR	↑→	↑
RVSWI	↓	↓
LVSWI	↓	↓

CVP, Central venous pressure; *HR*, heart rate; *LVSWI*, left ventricular stroke work index; *mm Hg*, millimeters of mercury; *PAOP*, pulmonary artery occlusion pressure; *PAP*, pulmonary artery pressure; *PVR*, pulmonary vascular resistance; *RAP*, right atrial pressure; *RVSWI*, right ventricular stroke work index; *SV*, stroke volume; *SVR*, systemic vascular resistance.

Laboratory Assessment

Laboratory Signs of Heart Failure

Natriuretic Peptides. Laboratory measurements can be invaluable both in determining the severity of heart failure and cardiogenic shock and in assessing the impact that the low blood flow state has had on other organs. Levels of atrial natriuretic peptide and brain natriuretic peptide are elevated in heart failure. Although ANP is released in response to increases in atrial pressure, brain natriuretic peptide reflects the degree of ventricular wall stress resulting from reduced LV systolic or diastolic function, RV dysfunction, or valvular dysfunction. A brain natriuretic peptide level of less than 100 picograms per milliliter (pg/mL) is a reliable indication that dyspnea symptoms have a source other than heart failure; levels greater than 400 pg/mL rule heart failure into the differential diagnosis for patients with dyspnea. Higher levels can be used as a marker for disease severity and also response to therapy. However, it is important to interpret results in conjunction with potential confounding factors such as age, kidney function, and conditions resulting in myocardial strain such as pulmonary artery hypertension, acute pulmonary embolus, or acute coronary syndrome.[24] The newer measure of brain natriuretic peptide—the N terminal prohormone brain natriuretic peptide (NT pro-brain natriuretic peptide)—has demonstrated significant age-related changes in lower limits of positive findings (Table 17-7). Overall the sensitivity of this measure is

TABLE 17-7 NT Pro-BNP: Cut Points by Age

"Rule in"

AGE STRATA	OPTIMAL CUT-POINT	SENSITIVITY	SPECIFICITY	PPV	NPV	ACCURACY
All <50 years (n=183)	450 pg/mL	97%	93%	76%	99%	95%
All 50-75 years (n=554)	900 pg/mL	90%	82%	82%	88%	85%
All >75 years (n=519)	1800 pg/mL	85%	73%	92%	55%	83%
Overall average		92%	84%	88%	66%	93%

"Rule out"

	OPTIMAL CUT-POINT	SENSITIVITY	SPECIFICITY	PPV	NPV	ACCURACY
	300 pg/mL	99%	62%	55%	99%	83%

NPV, Negative predictive value; *NT pro-BNP*, N terminal pro–brain natriuretic peptide; *pg/mL*, picogram per milliliter; *PPV*, positive predictive value.
Data from Maisel A, Mueller C, Adams K, et al.: State of the art: using natriuretic peptide levels in clinical practice, *Eur J Heart Failure* 10:824–839, 2008.

92% and the specificity 84%, which are excellent characteristics for a laboratory marker.

Sodium. Of all the electrolytes, sodium is an important reflection of the degree of heart failure and is a sensitive indicator of overall compensation. With increases in fluid retention, the sodium level, measured in millimoles per liter (mmol/L), may fall from the normal range of 135 to 145 mmol/L to as low as 120 mmol/L or less. It is important to recognize this electrolyte abnormality not as a reflection of inadequate total body sodium but, rather, as an indication of excessive total body water. Although loop diuretics will stimulate a release of sodium and water in urine, the degree of water loss will far outweigh the loss of sodium. The result is an increase in serum sodium as fluid is removed. Hyponatremia is hazardous; recent studies have reported increases of 52% (heart failure rehospitalization) to 82% (all-cause mortality) in patients with hyponatremia.[25] In a similar analysis performed on Japanese patients with heart failure, the reported all-cause mortality rate for patients with hyponatremia was 15% compared with 5.3% for patients with normal serum sodium levels. [26]

Oxygenation. The impact of congestion in heart failure often is first apparent in a change in blood gas results and increased supplemental oxygen requirements to maintain blood gases in the normal range. As tissues are deprived of the oxygen needed for aerobic metabolism, cellular function will deteriorate further and end organ function will be compromised. See Chapter 6 for more information on oxygenation and arterial blood gas monitoring.

Creatinine. The combination of decreased cardiac output combined with congestion associated with heart failure impairs blood flow through the kidneys. The reduced perfusion will cause creatinine to rise. The action of the RAAS to retain fluid in the face of decreased perfusion to the kidney, if uncontrolled, will make matters worse. Although a moderate increase in the level of serum creatinine (>2 milligrams per deciliter [mg/dL]) may have to be accepted to maintain relief from congestive symptoms, continued increases in serum creatinine require close surveillance. Persistent inadequate perfusion may cause more permanent, irreversible kidney injury. A similar effect on liver perfusion occurs from inadequate blood delivery to the hepatic artery as well as increased venous congestion affecting blood flow in the portal system; this causes a rise in transaminases and bilirubin, attesting to the reduction in blood flow through the liver.

Clinical Reasoning Pearl

Laboratory Values in Acute Decompensated Heart Failure (ADHF):

- *Brain natriuretic peptide:* Elevation in brain natriuretic peptide is the result of ventricular strain. Brain natriuretic peptide greater than 100 has been consistently shown to be highly sensitive and specific to differentiating heart failure from pulmonary disease as a cause of dyspnea. If the patient's brain natriuretic peptide is 89, the cause of shortness of breath is unlikely to be heart failure; if the brain natriuretic peptide is 8900, heart failure is the culprit.

- *Serum sodium:* Serum sodium is a valuable indicator of the degree of fluid volume excess as well as the effectiveness of the fluid removal therapies being applied. If the sodium level is climbing, volume status is improving. Keep in mind that while sodium loss occurs when diuretics are used, water loss is greater than the loss of sodium, so serum sodium will climb.

- *Creatinine:* An elevated serum creatinine may be a consequence of heart failure, the result of excess fluid removal, or an indicator of intrinsic kidney disease. An elevated jugular venous pressure or increased central venous pressure (CVP) reflects congestion in the venous system. In combination with reduced cardiac output, such persistent anomalies may reflect inadequate perfusion to the kidney and may result in permanent kidney injury. Review the patient's history and physical examination data to have a better understanding of the patient's current condition and therapies. Consider the influence of the pharmacologic treatment regimen, perhaps the dosage of angiotensin-converting enzyme inhibitor medications may be reduced or contraindicated with kidney dysfunction.

Laboratory Signs of Cardiogenic Shock

In cardiogenic shock, the sudden loss of blood flow will result in injury to all organs. Lung function is often the first laboratory value to show evidence of severe shock with a precipitous fall in SaO_2 and partial pressure of arterial oxygen (PaO_2). Laboratory evidence of kidney, liver, and other end organ dysfunction follows over the next 1 to 3 days, even with restoration of blood flow. One of the most important laboratory indicators of the restoration of blood flow in shock is the presence of lactate. Lactic acidosis reflects the degree to which tissues have been undersupplied with oxygen because of reduced cardiac output. The resultant shift to anaerobic metabolism increases the blood levels of lactic acidosis. The rise in serum lactate indicates persistence of anaerobic metabolism, reflecting inadequate blood flow to meet the tissues' metabolic needs, see Figure 6-12 in Chapter 6 for additional information. Rising serum lactate indicates failure to restore perfusion to the contributing organs. It is this persistent multi-organ failure that accounts for the high mortality rates associated with cardiogenic shock.

Treatment of Acute Decompensated Heart Failure and Cardiogenic Shock

Find and Treat the Cause of Heart Failure

As in any medical condition, the first goal is to treat and resolve the cause of the disruption of homeostasis. If a structural problem is the cause of the heart failure or cardiogenic shock, then correcting that issue as soon as possible, and when safe for the patient, is of paramount importance.[2] Reperfusion strategies such as thrombolytics, angioplasty, stents, or coronary artery bypass surgery re-establish blood flow to regions of the myocardium deprived by progressive or acute occlusion of one or more coronary arteries. This will most often result in the restoration of myocardial contractility and cardiac output.

Repair or replacement of a stenotic or regurgitant heart valve will facilitate unobstructed, unidirectional forward flow through the heart and to the systemic circulation. Acute ischemic rupture of the interventricular septum needs be repaired quickly to prevent mixing of deoxygenated blood from the right ventricle, with oxygenated blood from the left ventricle. The goal is to optimize the oxygen content of the blood being ejected by the left ventricle into the systemic circulation.

Pulmonary embolism interrupts blood flow in the pulmonary circulation and decreases flow into the left side of the heart causing significant hypotension (refer to the case study in Chapter 3; and refer to Figure 8-7 for the impact of a pulmonary embolism on end tidal CO_2). Treatment may necessitate thrombolytic therapy, or less frequently performing a surgical thrombectomy to remove a large clot. In conjunction with eliminating the offending thrombus, this will permit perfusion of all functional regions of the lung and thus enhance oxygenation of the blood traversing the pulmonary circuit.

Pulmonary arterial hypertension will decrease the amount of blood crossing from the right ventricle to the left ventricle. Regardless of the ability of the lungs to oxygenate blood, the inability to provide LV preload from the right ventricle will reduce cardiac output and increase systemic congestion. Oral and intravenous agents, along with careful diuresis, will significantly improve flow in these patients. See Chapter 18 for additional information on right heart failure and pulmonary hypertension.

One of the most common underappreciated causes of heart failure is hypertension. Aggressive pharmacologic reduction of blood pressure will reduce ventricular afterload, increase stroke volume and cardiac output, and improve perfusion to tissues. Diuretics, angiotensin-converting enzyme inhibitors, angiotensin receptor blockers (ARBs), beta-blockers, and alpha-receptor blockers such as hydralazine, in association with nitrate therapy are used alone and in combination to reduce afterload and increase forward flow.[2] If oral agents are inadequate, parenteral forms of these medications along with nitroprusside and nitroglycerin can improve cardiac function.

Other disease states associated with acute heart failure include anemia and thyroid dysfunction. Adequate blood flow must be combined with adequate oxygen-carrying capacity of blood for tissues to survive. Thus, the treatment for anemia plays an important role in the delivery of oxygen to the cells. As with all therapies, blood transfusions must be balanced with the risk of transfusion-related acute lung injury (TRALI). In addition, if the hemoglobin molecule is not exposed to adequate oxygen concentrations in the lungs, the amount of oxygen available for delivery will be reduced. Metabolic disorders that contribute to heart failure, for example, thyroid dysfunction, may also require detection and treatment to address ADHF seen in the critical care environment.

Following resolution of the acute problem, preventive measures to reduce the likelihood of recurrence are key to effective therapy. Statins to treat hyperlipidemia in patients with coronary artery disease, anticoagulants or antiplatelet agents to prevent recurrent thromboses, antihypertensives to prevent associated recurrence of heart failure are all important interventions. Additional heart-failure–specific interventions as mentioned above, include: loop, thiazide, and spironolactone classes of diuretics; angiotensin-converting enzyme inhibitors, angiotensin receptor blockers; beta-blockers, and vasodilators. All of these medications are intended to prevent or slow the deterioration of cardiac function.[2]

Pharmacologic management is valuable in reducing heart failure re-admissions and improving quality of life. Guidelines published by the American Heart Association and the Centers for Medicare and Medicaid Services (CMS) are examples of continuing efforts to bring increasing focus on the preventive aspects of managing heart failure and cardiogenic shock.[27]

To re-establish blood flow to the systemic circulation, the elements that contribute to cardiac output must be normalized as much as possible. As noted previously, those elements are heart rate and stroke volume. Thus, stabilizing heart rate—and rhythm—will have a significant impact on forward flow in patients with ADHF.

Optimization of Heart Rate and Rhythm

Optimization of heart rate begins with keeping it in an ideal range to permit adequate filling. Tachycardia, although initially compensatory, subsequently contributes to inadequate forward flow simply because the heart does not have enough diastolic time to fill effectively. Bradycardia results in reduced cardiac output because even an enhanced stroke volume may not be adequate to make up for the reduction in the number of ventricular contractions. Maintaining the heart rate in the normal range of 60–100 beats per minute (beats/min) will support filling time and total volume ejected. Beta-blockers are the most common class of medications used to control tachycardia. Their negative chronotropic effects will limit the ability of the heart to achieve a higher rate. Bradycardia contributing to heart failure is most often treated with a permanent pacemaker.

The development of atrial fibrillation in a patient whose cardiac output is already inadequate will result in a significant worsening of flow because of the loss of the atrial contribution to ventricular filling. Atrial fibrillation is common in the patient with cardiac enlargement caused by ventricular remodeling associated with heart failure. It has been reported to occur in up to 50% in patients with severe heart failure symptoms.[28] Monitoring for premature atrial contractions and the onset of atrial fibrillation provides the best opportunity to prevent its development or to restore sinus rhythm.

Restoring sinus rhythm is an important component to managing the hemodynamics of ADHF and cardiogenic shock. The mainstays for intervening in atrial fibrillation are electrical cardioversion, pharmacotherapy, or both. Amiodarone remains one of the most effective agents at controlling both atrial and ventricular dysrhythmias. Other antiarrhythmics such as digoxin and beta-blockers may also be valuable in controlling heart rate even when attempts to convert atrial fibrillation are ineffective. When sinus rhythm cannot be maintained and the ventricular response cannot be controlled pharmacologically, ablation of the atrioventricular node with pacemaker implantation may be indicated.

Once rhythm has been optimized, the next issue to address is management of stroke volume. The three elements that impact stroke volume are preload (volume in the ventricle at the end of diastole), contractility (the force of contraction against the blood in the ventricle during systole), and afterload (the resistance created by arteriolar constriction against which the ventricle must push to eject its volume). The hemodynamic assessment described earlier includes the measurement of preload (PAOP), the calculation of afterload (SVR), and the derivation of contractility assessed via left ventricular stroke work index (LVSWI). These elements are not independent of each other but, rather, constitute a dynamic state that clinicians can influence through an understanding of the hemodynamics of heart failure and cardiogenic shock.

Optimization of Preload

Starling's Law states that as preload increases, myocardial stretch and contractility also increase (Figure 17-1a). However, the law also demonstrates that a point of diminishing returns does occur, and at this juncture, more preload does not yield an increase in cardiac output (Figure 17-1b) and further volume loading will cause a decrease in contractility (Figure 17-1c). Whether a patient is experiencing inadequate or excessive preload, both can negatively impact cardiac output and cause progressive deterioration in heart function and patient condition. It is important to begin management of patients with ADHF or cardiogenic shock by evaluating their fluid status (preload) as illustrated in Figure 17-1.

Hemodynamic assessment is an essential tool in determining the patient's fluid status and planning appropriate interventions in ADHF and cardiogenic shock. Apart from measuring all the central pressures (CVP or right atrial pressure, pulmonary artery pressures and PAOP), evaluating the size and shape of individual waveforms assists with the assessment of the patient's disease process. Changes in the size and slope of the waveforms may indicate other pathologies, including valvular disease, pericardial constriction, or tamponade. For instance, elevation in PAOP may be related to fluid volume excess. However, on examination of the waveform, recognition of a prominent v-wave would more specifically lead to the diagnosis of mitral regurgitation.

Elevated central pressures on both sides of the heart (CVP or right atrial pressure >15 mm Hg, PAOP >18 mm Hg) are indications that the patient has excessive intravascular volume in the right and left ventricles, respectively. Typically, in ADHF, patients with these pressures will benefit from diuresis. Refer again to the 2-by-2 table listing characteristics of heart failure[19] (Figure 17-3). Patients in group B (warm and wet) or group C (cold and wet) both should be treated with volume removal. Loop diuretics and aldosterone inhibitors are the most frequently utilized classes of diuretics for patients with heart failure (see Table 17-6). However, because patients with chronic heart failure already may have been exposed to these medications for an extended period, some will have developed diuretic resistance. In that case, changing to a new medication in the same class, to a new class of medications, or to a combination of diuretics may increase diuretic effectiveness. If these tactics fail to reduce excess fluid volume, then, fluid removal by alternative means such as ultrafiltration is becoming increasingly prevalent.[29] Ultrafiltration refers to the removal of plasma water and recruitment of third spaced fluid into the intravascular space. By maintaining the fluid removal rate at or below the plasma refill rate (rate at which fluid will reenter the bloodstream from the third space), up to 500 milliliters per hour (mL/hr) up to 12 L/day can be removed safely with minimal impact on blood pressure or electrolyte balance. Recent reviews support the use of these approaches to removing excess circulating fluid.[30]

Identifying an imbalance between hemodynamic pressures on the right side and left side of the heart leads to different interventions than with balanced elevation of pressures. When CVP is elevated but PAOP is low, blood is not getting from the right ventricle through the pulmonary circuit to the left atrium. Causes for this imbalance include pulmonary hypertension and pulmonary embolism. In these cases, it is still important to reduce congestion, but fluid removal must be accomplished more slowly, using rates of 50 to 100 mL/hr, which translates to 1.2 to 2.4 L/day fluid removal to prevent excessive underloading of the right ventricle with resultant loss of filling of the left ventricle. The lack of LV preload will lead to systemic hypotension and poor systemic perfusion.

When PAOP is elevated but CVP is normal or low, the prominent feature is LV congestion. As noted earlier in this chapter, if disease of the aortic or mitral valve is the cause of this imbalance, correcting the structural abnormality must be considered. Diuresis is still necessary as well to prevent or rescue the patient from the edge of the "Starling cliff" described as an excess of fluid causing excessive stretch and subsequent reduced contractility. Diuretics are the cornerstone of therapy for LV failure.

Vasodilator therapy is also an important intervention to address congestion in ADHF. Nitroglycerin dilates both the venous and arterial systems. The venous dilation and increased venous capacitance reduces volume returned to the right ventricle and thus provides a degree of unloading.[31] Arterial dilation reduces afterload, permitting enhanced forward flow and decongestion of the left ventricle. It is important to carefully uptitrate nitroglycerin to prevent excessive dilation on either side, as this could result in underfilling and resultant hypotension. More recently, sodium nitroprusside has been used increasingly aggressively to enhance forward flow by significantly reducing afterload while also impacting preload. When successful, this intervention demonstrates that the patient will benefit from oral afterload reducing agents, including angiotensin-converting enzyme (ACE) inhibitors or angiotensin receptor blocker (ARB) and beta-blocker medications[2] (Table 17-8). Finally, intravenous natriuretic agents are supported by multiple studies as valuable in reducing afterload and congestion.[32-34]

In cardiogenic shock, in contrast, vasodilators and diuretics should be avoided. Instead fluid resuscitation and inotropic agents are the hallmark features of medical management. Although inotropic agents will ultimately increase myocardial oxygen demand, their use assists in stabilizing blood pressure and hemodynamics. Serial measurements of cardiac output will aid in the optimization of both fluid and inotropic therapy.[35]

Reduction of Afterload

As previously mentioned in this chapter, the sympathetic nervous system's response to blood flow deficit is to raise heart rate to increase cardiac output. The other major effect of increased sympathetic tone is an increase in afterload, directing flow toward the core organs. The RAAS also increases afterload as a response to persistent renal hypoperfusion. Whether the cause is ADHF or cardiogenic shock, increasing forward blood flow by reducing the resistance to ejection of blood volume from the left ventricle is standard therapy. Although it may appear counterintuitive to give afterload-reducing agents to a relatively hypotensive patient, when carefully titrated, the net effect will be increased blood flow while maintaining or improving the patient's blood pressure.[32] Intravenous

TABLE 17-8 Diuretics by Class	
Loop diuretics	Furosemide
	Bumetanide
	Torsemide
	Ethacrynic acid
Aldosterone inhibitors	Spironolactone
	Eplerenone
	Amiloride
	Triamterene
Thiazide diuretics	Chlorothiazide
	Hydrochlorothiazide
	Metolazone
	Chlorthalidone
	Hydroflumethiazide
	Indapamide
	Methyclothiazide
	Polythiazide
Carbonic anhydrase inhibitors	Acetazolamide
	Dichlorphenamide
	Methazolamide

nitrates, including nitroglycerin and nitroprusside, started in low doses and uptitrated to improve forward flow without compromising blood pressure, have been shown to be highly successful. These medications will reduce the afterload of the right ventricle, left ventricle, or both with a resultant increase in cardiac output. It will also "make room" for more intravascular volume to be administered if needed.[36]

Since afterload is a calculated value, measurement of cardiac output combined with associated hemodynamic parameters, is the only way to directly assess the impact of therapies on afterload. Clinical progress will also be measured by improved peripheral perfusion, with faster capillary refill, warmer arms and legs, improved skin color, and increased urine production.

Increasing Contractility

The last component of cardiac output to be addressed is contractility. In both ADHF and cardiogenic shock, contractility is reduced. Regardless of the reason for this impairment, intravenous inotropic medications can improve contractility with a resultant increase in forward flow. Attention is generally focused on stimulating beta-adrenergic receptors in the heart. Although recent literature favors phosphodiesterase inhibitors such as milrinone and inamrinone over dobutamine for ADHF, all inotropes have been shown to be associated with a significant increase in risk of death in relation to long-term survival of patients suffering from ADHF.[37] Thus, these agents should be reserved for use in patients with hypotension, hypoperfusion, or cardiogenic shock.

Epinephrine, norepinephrine, and vasopressin have also proven valuable in the setting of acute heart failure and cardiogenic shock. Titrating the medications both up and down to optimize the patient's cardiac function while minimizing strain on myocardial oxygen supply and demand is a central part of critical care practice. When multiple agents are in use concurrently, determining which to wean first depends on the preferences of the providers and the plan of care that has been established in collaboration with the bedside caregivers.

Treatment of Cardiogenic Shock

When the patient is in cardiogenic shock, immediate intervention to improve forward flow is the highest priority. Utilizing a combination of inotropic agents and vasodilators, titrated to maintain adequate blood pressure, enhancement of contractility, and reduction of systemic vascular resistance will provide the earliest return of perfusion to the end organs at highest risk. The effectiveness of these therapies can be readily assessed by monitoring vital signs, neurologic function, urine production, and assessing peripheral perfusion by skin temperature and capillary refill. The use of a pulmonary artery catheter (PAC) will provide additional information about central pressures and thermodilution cardiac output. Fine-tuning the therapies once the rescue has been completed may take several days and will involve treating the cause, titrating down the intravenous medications, and uptitrating oral therapy. Whether accomplished in the critical care unit or in a progressive care unit, these stepwise interventions are important to optimize patient outcomes.

Mechanical Circulatory Assistance

In some patients with severe heart failure who present with ADHF, pharmacotherapy will no longer be adequate to decongest and to increase cardiac output. To this end, mechanical circulatory support should be considered, either as a short-term intervention to support the patient awaiting cardiac recovery or as a more permanent intervention to take over for the failing ventricle.

Intra-aortic Balloon Pump

The most widely used mechanical intervention for the treatment of LV dysfunction is intra-aortic balloon pump (IABP) counterpulsation, see Figures 15-2 and 15-3 in Chapter 15. More than 160,000 patients are treated with this therapy worldwide each year. Used in clinical practice since the 1960s, it quickly improves cardiac performance through two effects. First, with inflation, aortic diastolic blood pressure increases, enhancing coronary blood flow by as much as 100% in some reports.[38] Second, with deflation, reductions in left ventricular end-systolic pressure have been demonstrated along with decreases in LV stroke work and left ventricular end-diastolic pressure. At the same time, deflation enhances stroke volume.[38] Hemodynamic improvements are discernible almost immediately after initiation of counterpulsation therapy. Complications of IABP are generally related to vascular compromise of the limb distal to the insertion site.

Although the results of the Shock-II Trial demonstrated no significant survival advantage with the use of the IABP,[39] its continued use is explained by its ease of placement, familiarity, and effectiveness for immediately increasing cardiac output in patients with cardiogenic shock. However, IABP augmentation of cardiac output is significantly less than that achieved by short-term ventricular assist devices such as the Impella and Tandem Heart technologies.[40] These devices are being used increasingly to treat patients with cardiogenic shock as well as to protect patients undergoing high-risk coronary revascularization.

Short-Term Ventricular Assist Devices

When time is of the essence, selecting a ventricular assist device that will provide adequate circulatory and hemodynamic support along with ease of placement is valuable to the clinician. Short-term ventricular assist devices are those technologies that are applied for less than 30 days and require the patient to remain in the critical care environment.

The Impella (Abiomed, Inc., Danvers, MA) is a rotary, axial flow ventricular assist device that is inserted into the femoral artery and advanced across the aortic valve into the left ventricle. The continuous flow impeller contained within the device is powered by an external source and can propel 2.5 to 5 liters per minute (L/min) of blood from the left ventricle into the systemic circulation, see Figure 15-4. The flow capacity is determined by the size of the catheter. Its impact on the acutely failing heart is achieved through ventricular unloading and coronary perfusion as well as through provision of increased blood flow to the end organs.[40] This has been demonstrated to have a positive impact on 30-day outcomes of myocardial infarction and cardiogenic shock.[41] Because of its size (9–13 French [Fr]), complications of the Impella are similar to those of the IABP and are related to vascular obstruction distal to the device insertion.[40]

The Tandem Heart (Cardiac Assist, Inc., Pittsburgh, PA) is a percutaneous centrifugal flow ventricular assist device, see Figure 15-5. It involves placement of two vascular catheters. The first (a 21-Fr catheter) is inserted via the femoral vein into the right atrium. There, a transseptal puncture is performed, and the device is advanced into the left atrium, from which it draws oxygenated blood. That blood is returned to the systemic circulation via a 15-Fr to 17-Fr femoral artery catheter. It can generate flows up to 4.5 L/min. Although the blood infused into the femoral artery is under pressure, which may increase myocardial afterload, the unloading of the ventricle by the device significantly improves cardiac function and provides hemodynamic stabilization.[40]

However, its impact on 30-day outcomes after acute myocardial infarction and cardiogenic shock were similar to those of the IABP.[42]

Centrimag (Thoratec, Inc., Pleasanton, CA) is a centrifugal flow pump that is placed surgically with cannulation of the right atrium and pulmonary artery when used as a right ventricular assist device (RVAD), or into the left atrium and aorta when used as a left ventricular assist device (LVAD), see Figure 15-6. Because of the size of the surgical cannulas placed, this device offers temporary support of up to 10 L/min and optimal unloading of the left ventricle and the right ventricle. In cardiogenic shock, this restoration of forward flow has a rapid and positive impact on both end organ perfusion and function. In contrast to the percutaneous devices, some reports describe use of this technology for more than 100 days before weaning the patient off support, and transitioning to a more permanent ventricular assist device, or performing heart transplant.[43]

If the patient is experiencing cardiorespiratory failure, an oxygenator may be added to larger-volume short-term devices to provide extracorporeal membrane oxygenation (ECMO), see Figure 15-7 in Chapter 15. Both central and peripheral cannulation strategies are used for this therapy. In appropriately selected patients, weaning from ECMO has been reported at rates of up to 60%.[43]

When patients with ADHF do not respond to pharmacologic interventions, or when cardiogenic shock is not resolved with the use of temporary cardiac assist devices, survival is dependent on either replacing the failing heart through heart transplantation or placing a permanent ventricular assist device. Either intervention may increase both quality and quantity of life.

Long-Term Ventricular Assist Devices and Heart Transplantation

Long-term ventricular assist devices use continuous flow technologies. With flow capacity of up to 10 L/min, these pumps can restore hemodynamics to normal levels, decongest the left ventricle, improve end organ function, and allow the patient to be out of bed, active, and discharged home. With electrically powered devices that use wall power, batteries, or power through the outlet in a car, patients experience freedom of movement, mobility, and increased exercise tolerance after recovering from surgery and from the long-term effects of heart failure.[44]

Blood pressure evaluation in a patient with continuous blood flow, in contrast to the pulsatile flow that we are accustomed to, challenges clinicians to think of other ways to evaluate the adequacy of cardiac output. As with ADHF and cardiogenic shock, evaluation of end organ function is a reflection of the adequacy of perfusion. Level of consciousness, urine production, peripheral pulses and temperature are all key when assessing the patient with continuous flow support. Despite the fact that left heart function has been augmented by a mechanical device, the patient still must be treated for heart failure to ensure that the right ventricle remains able to supply blood to the left side of the heart, permitting the LVAD to pump the blood needed by tissues. See Chapter 15 for more information on use of mechanical circulatory assist therapies.

Patient Education

When discussing the patient's current condition and treatments, assess the patient's and family's goals of therapy. Ask what they understand are the treatment options available to improve symptoms and optimize quality of life. Ask what they hope to accomplish and how they perceive quality of life.

For patients who have had recurrent hospitalizations for heart failure, try to assess what interfered with their achievement of the goals set. Ask what they consider to be "success" in their treatment and how likely they think the goals will be achieved.

Break the goals up into achievable steps such as: Today I will stand at the side of the bed for 60 seconds, sit in the chair for 2 hours, or walk to the door twice in the day." Then find out what is the best the patient thinks they could do, and set a goal slightly short of that:

Patient: "I think I could stand at the bedside for 30 seconds."

Nurse: "Okay, let's start with 15 seconds, then progress forward."

Setting an achievable goal will help the patient feel encouraged and be more likely to be engaged in therapy and progress.

Case Study #1

A 64-year-old female with a history of systolic heart failure (ejection fraction 15%) secondary to ischemic cardiomyopathy was admitted to the critical care unit from an outside hospital with acute decompensated heart failure (ADHF). Chronically hypertensive (blood pressure 160/88 mm Hg), she has been complaining of increasing shortness of breath and at the time of presentation to the clinic was able to walk only 1½ blocks before symptoms developed.

	CRITICAL CARE UNIT ADMISSION	AFTER NITROPRUSSIDE THERAPY
Temperature	97.7°F (36.5°C)	98.1°F (36.7°C)
Heart rate (beats/min)	93	85
Respiratory rate (breaths/min)	22	18
Blood pressure	108/77	118/87
SpO$_2$	96%	97%
Cardiac index (L/min/m^2)	1.4	2.9

Case Study #1—cont'd

SVR (dynes·sec/cm^5)	2160	1287
Right atrial pressure (mm Hg)	11	4
Pulmonary artery pressure S/D (mean) mm Hg	52/27 (mean 35)	50/20 (mean 30)
PAOP (mm Hg)	28	18
PVR (dynes·sec/cm^5)	360	88

On physical examination, her blood pressure was 108/77, heart rate 93 beats/min, respiratory rate 22 breaths/min, SpO$_2$ 96%, temperature 97.7°F (36.5°C), and weight 94 kg (207 lb); an increase of 4 kg [8.8 lb] from her previous clinic visit 1 week earlier). On auscultation, her lungs revealed bi-basilar crackles without wheezes or stridor. On ECG, her heart rhythm was paced but irregular with many premature ventricular contractions (PVCs). Jugular venous distension was not present. Her legs and feet were warm, with slightly delayed capillary refill of approximately 4 seconds (sec). She had 3+ edema of her legs and hips. Her heart failure was classified as NYHA Class IIIb (see Table 17-3). Her clinical profile was warm and wet (B) (see Figure 17-3).

On admission, a pulmonary artery catheter (PAC) was placed. Her RAP was 11 mm Hg, pulmonary artery pressure 52/27 mm Hg (mean 35 mm Hg), PAOP 28 mm Hg, CI 1.4 L/min/m^2, SVR 2160 dynes·sec/cm^5, PVR 360 dynes·sec/cm^5.

Laboratory studies in clinic were as follows: sodium (Na$^+$) 126 mmol/L, potassium (K$^+$) 4.1 mmol/L, chloride (Cl$^-$) 94 mmol/L, bicarbonate (HCO$_3^-$) 26 mmol/L, BUN 65 mg/dL, creatinine 2.58 mg/dL, glucose 132 mg/dL, calcium (Ca^{2+}) 9.0 mg/dL. Hematology study results included: hemoglobin 15 grams per deciliter (g/dL), hematocrit 46.5%, white blood cells (WBCs) 8.3 × 10^9/L, platelets 175 × 10^9/L.

Response to interventions: Diuresis—because her weight was increased from her previous evaluation and her PAOP was elevated, administration of intravenous diuretics was initiated because of her unresponsiveness to oral therapy. The treatment plan was to attempt to remove 5 liters of fluid over the next 3 days.

Response to interventions: Afterload reduction—initiation of nitroprusside therapy starting at 0.25 mcg/kg/min and increasing to 1.25 mcg/kg/min resulted in the following: Although she was initially intolerant of low doses of oral afterload reducing agents because of orthostatic hypotension, ultimately she was able to be weaned from nitroprusside and was asymptomatic with a combination of oral nitrates (Imdur) and hydralazine. Although she presented with many PVCs, she remained in sinus rhythm at the time of discharge on amiodarone 200 mg, orally (po), daily. The plan at discharge was to follow up in clinic for further titration of oral heart failure therapy. ■

Case Study #2

A 55-year-old male with a history of dilated cardiomyopathy was admitted to the critical care unit from another hospital in cardiogenic shock; by echocardiogram, the EF was low (<20%) with a LV end-diastolic dimension of approximately 9.5 cm. His heart failure had been first diagnosed 4 years prior to admission and had been successfully managed with oral therapies. However, over the past 2 months, his symptoms became significantly worse. At his last clinic visit, he described being unable to walk from the living room to the kitchen (30 feet) or to perform simple housework without becoming short of breath. He had increasing orthopnea and decreased energy levels. He reported to his local clinic because of worsening symptoms and was found to be in atrial fibrillation. Although successfully converted back to sinus rhythm, his cardiac output remained profoundly depressed. Inotropes were started (dopamine 5 mcg/kg/min and dobutamine 2 mcg/kg/min) and an intra-aortic balloon pump (IABP) was inserted via the right femoral artery with an augmentation ration of 1:1, later reduced to 1:2.

On physical examination, his blood pressure was 98/53 (mean 68) mm Hg (augmented diastolic pressure on IABP 101 mm Hg), heart rate 96 beats/min, respiratory rate 16 breaths/min, SpO_2 94% on oxygen 3 L/min per nasal cannula. On auscultation, his heart tones were irregularly irregular, with noted S1, S2, a S3 gallop with a 3/6 systolic murmur best heard at the cardiac apex. His lungs were diminished bilaterally halfway up the posterior lung fields. He has 4+ peripheral edema, and peripheral pulses were 1+ and symmetric. Extremities were cool and slightly mottled. Weight was 107.2 kg (235.8 lb). He was awake but slow to respond to questions. He was oriented to person, place, and time.

PARAMETERS	CRITICAL CARE UNIT ADMISSION	AFTERLOAD REDUCTION	PEAK DOSE OF SODIUM NITROPRUSSIDE
Temperature	98.2°F (36.8°C)		
Heart rate (beats/min)	96	74	
Respiratory rate (breaths/min)	16		
Blood pressure (systolic/diastolic) (mm Hg)	98/53	76/53	95/48
Mean arterial pressure (MAP) (mm Hg)	68	60	64

Case Study #2—cont'd

SpO$_2$	94% on oxygen 3 L/min per nasal cannula	95% on oxygen at 5 L/min per nasal cannula
Cardiac index (L/min/m^2) Fick Method	1.3	1.8
SvO$_2$	48%	57%
SVR (dynes·sec/cm^5)	2950	1125
Right atrial pressure (mm Hg)	20	9
Pulmonary artery pressure (mm Hg)	50/26	42/22 (mean 29)
PAOP (mm Hg)	34	18
PVR (dynes·sec/cm^5)	123	218

Laboratory studies in clinic were as follows: Na$^+$ 121 mmol/L, K$^+$ 4.9 mmol/L, Cl$^-$ 95 mmol/L, HCO$_3^-$ 26 mmol/L, blood urea nitrogen 21 mg/dL, creatinine 1.73 mg/dL, and glucose 106 mg/dL. Hematology study results were: hemoglobin 11.0 g/dL, hematocrit 33.3%, WBCs 8.3 × 10^9/L, platelets 127 × 10^9/L. International normalized ratio (INR) was 1.58 on Coumadin.

On admission, his right atrial pressure was 20 mm Hg, pulmonary artery pressure (50/26 mm Hg (mean 36), PAOP 34 mm Hg, cardiac Index by Fick method 1.3 L/min/m^2, SVR 2950 dynes·sec/cm^5, PVR 123 dynes·sec/cm^5.

His clinical profile matches cold and wet (C) (see Figure 17-3). His diagnosis is cardiogenic shock.

Response to interventions: Afterload reduction was initiated after discontinuing the dopamine, increasing the dobutamine to 3.0 mcg/kg/min, and adding a sodium nitroprusside infusion that was uptitrated from 0.25 mcg/kg/min to 1.8 mcg/kg/min. His blood pressure initially fell to 76/53 mm Hg (mean 60), and his heart rate remained steady at 74 beats/min; his blood pressure subsequently rebounded to 95/48 mm Hg (mean 64). His SvO$_2$ was 48%, and SaO$_2$ was 95% on oxygen at 5 L/min per nasal cannula. At the peak dose of sodium nitroprusside, his hemodynamics were recalculated by utilizing the Fick calculation:

$$CI\,(L/min/m^2) = \frac{1250}{(SaO_2 - SvO_2) \times 1.34 \times Hemoglobin}$$

Continued

Case Study #2—cont'd

$$1.8\left(L/\min/m^2\right) = \frac{1250}{(95-48) \times 1.34 \times 11.0}$$

Because his hemodynamic response was modest, with a right atrial pressure of 9 mm Hg, pulmonary artery pressure of 42/22 mm Hg (mean 29), PAOP of 18 mm Hg, cardiac index by Fick method 1.8 L/min/m^2, SVR 1125 dynes·sec/cm^5, and PVR 218 dynes·sec/cm^5. The hemodynamic assessment demonstrated that he could respond to improved forward blood flow. However, within the next 48 hours, his condition again deteriorated, and the IABP augmentation was increased to 1:1. Because he demonstrated significant improvements in hemodynamics only with the combination of IABP, intravenous inotropic agents and intravenous vasodilators, it was determined that the best course of therapy for him was to implant a left ventricular assist device (LVAD). He was taken to the operating room, where a Centrimag LVAD was placed. Supported on that device with cardiac indices of 2.1 L/min/m^2, he was able to be diuresed by 15 liters, transferred to the chair twice daily, and showed marked end organ improvements. After 18 days a donor heart became available in his blood group (AB+) and he was successfully transplanted. ■

Conclusion

The population of patients experiencing heart failure is growing steadily in the United States. (Table 17-9). Chronic heart failure is amenable to oral therapy management in many patients. However, in the case of ADHF, hemodynamic monitoring plays an

TABLE 17-9   U.S. Hospital Discharges for Heart Failure

| YEAR | APPROXIMATE NUMBER OF HOSPITAL DISCHARGES | |
	MALE	FEMALE
1980	100,800	200,400
1985	200,600	300,200
1990	300,200	400,000
1995	300,800	500,000
2000	400,200	500,800
2005	400,900	500,800
2010	500,000	500,200

Data from Go AS, Mozaffarian D, Roger VL, et al.: Heart disease and stroke statistics—2014 update: a report from the American Heart Association, *Circulation* 129:228–e292, 2013.

important role in the assessment and ongoing management of this disease. Moreover, in the case of cardiogenic shock, rapid hemodynamic assessment, interventions targeting proximal causes, and attempts to improve forward blood flow and reduce congestion are key to optimizing patient outcomes.

References

1. Go AS, Mozaffarian D, Roger VL, et al.: Heart disease and stroke statistics—2014 update: a report from the American Heart Association, *Circulation* 129:e28–e292, 2013.
2. Yancy CW, Jessup M, Bozkurt B, et al.: 2013 ACCF/AHA guideline for the management of heart failure: a report of the American College of Cardiology Foundation/American Heart Association Task Force on Practice Guidelines, *J Am Coll Cardiol* 62(16):e147–e239, 2013.
3. Heidenreich PA, Albert NM, Allen LA, et al.: American Heart Association Advocacy Coordinating Committee, Council on Arteriosclerosis, Thrombosis and Vascular Biology, Council on Cardiovascular Radiology and Intervention, Council on Clinical Cardiology, Council on Epidemiology and Prevention, Stroke Council: Forecasting the impact of heart failure in the United States: a policy statement from the American Heart Association, *Circ Heart Fail* 6(3):606–619, 2013.
4. National Heart Lung and Blood Institute: *What causes heart failure?* http://www.nhlbi.nih.gov/health/health-topics/topics/hf/causes.html. Accessed September 3, 2014.
5. Piano M: Pathophysiology of heart failure (Chapter 62). In Moser DK, Riegel B, editors: *Cardiac nursing: a companion to Braunwald's heart disease*, St. Louis, MO, 2008, Saunders, p 897.
6. Mann DL: Pathophysiology of heart failure (Chapter 22). In Libby P, Bonow RO, Mann DL, Zipes DP, editors: *Braunwald's heart disease: a textbook of cardiovascular medicine*, ed 8, Philadelphia, 2008, Saunders.
7. Soine LJ: Heart failure and cardiogenic shock. In Woods SL, Froelicher ESS, Motzer SU, Bridges EJ, editors: *Cardiac nursing*, ed 6, Philadelphia, 2010, Wolters Kluwer/Lippincott Williams & Wilkins, p 555.
8. Hess OM, Carroll JD: Clinical assessment of heart failure. In Libby P, Bonow RO, Mann DL, Zipes DP, editors: *Braunwald's heart disease: a textbook of cardiovascular medicine*, ed 8, Philadelphia, 2008, Saunders, p 561.
9. Bhuiyan T, Maurer MS: Heart failure with preserved ejection fraction: persistent diagnosis, therapeutic enigma, *Curr Cardiovasc Risk Rep* 5(5):440, 2011.
10. Owan TE, Hodge DO, Herges RM, et al.: Trends in prevalence and outcome of heart failure with preserved ejection fraction, *N Engl J Med* 355(3):251–259, 2006.
11. Bursi F, Weston SA, Redfield MM, et al.: Systolic and diastolic heart failure in the community, *JAMA* 296(18):2209–2216, 2006.
12. Yancy CW, Lopatin M, Stevenson LW, et al.: ADHERE Scientific Advisory Committee and, Investigators: Clinical presentation, management, and in-hospital outcomes of patients admitted with acute decompensated heart failure with preserved systolic function: a report from the acute decompensated heart failure national registry (ADHERE) database, *J Am Coll Cardiol* 47(1):76–84, 2006.
13. Antman EM: ST-elevation myocardial infarction: management. In Libby P, Bonow RO, Mann DL, Zipes DP, editors: *Braunwald's heart disease: a textbook of cardiovascular medicine*, ed 8, Philadelphia, 2008, Saunders, p 1233.
14. Okuda M: A multidisciplinary overview of cardiogenic shock, *Shock* 25(6):557–570, 2006.
15. The Criteria Committee of the New York Heart Association: *Nomenclature and criteria for diagnosis of diseases of the heart and great vessels*, ed 9, Boston, MA, 1994, Little Brown and Co.
16. Stevenson LW, Perloff JK: The limited reliability of physical signs for estimating hemodynamics in chronic heart failure, *JAMA* 261(6):884–888, 1989.

17. Nohria A, Lewis E, Stevenson LW: Medical management of advanced heart failure, *JAMA* 287 (5):628–640, 2002.

18. Filby S, Chang PP: Heart failure. In Stouffer GA, editor: *Cardiovascular hemodynamics for the clinician*, Malden, MA, 2008, Blackwell Futura, p 169.

19. Temporelli PL, Scapellato F, Eleuteri E, et al.: Doppler echocardiography in advanced heart failure: a non-invasive alternative to Swan-Ganz catheter, *Circ Heart Failure* 3(3):387–394, 2010.

20. Sutton MSJ: A comprehensive non-invasive hemodynamic assessment of systolic heart failure, *Circ Heart Failure* 3:337–339, 2010.

21. Paul S, Vollano L: Care of patients with acute heart failure. In Moser DK, Riegel B, editors: *Cardiac nursing: a companion to Braunwald's heart disease*, St. Louis, MO, 2008, Saunders, p 916.

22. McKelvie RS, Moe GW, Ezekowitz JA, et al.: The 2012 Canadian Cardiovascular Society heart failure management guidelines update: focus on acute and chronic heart failure, *Can J Cardiol* 29 (2):168–181, 2013.

23. Davidson CJ, Bonow RO: Cardiac catheterization. In Libby P, Bonow RO, Mann DL, Zipes DP, editors: *Braunwald's heart disease: a textbook of cardiovascular medicine*, ed 8, Philadelphia, 2008, Saunders, p 439.

24. Maisel A, Mueller C, Adams K Jr., et al.: State of the art: using natriuretic peptide levels in clinical practice, *Eur J Heart Fail* 10(9):824–839, 2008.

25. Gheorghiade M, Rossi JS, Cotts W, et al.: Characterization and prognostic value of persistent hyponatremia in patients with severe heart failure in the ESCAPE trial, *Arch Intern Med* 167 (18):1998–2005, 2007.

26. Sato N, Gheorghiade M, Kajimoto K, et al.: Hyponatremia and in-hospital mortality in patients admitted for heart failure (from the ATTEND registry), *Am J Cardiol* 111(7):1019–1025, 2013.

27. Heidenreich PA, Hernandez AF, Yancy CW, et al.: Get with the guidelines program participation, process of care, and outcome for Medicare patients hospitalized with heart failure, *Circ Cardiovasc Quality Outcomes* 5(1):37–43, 2012.

28. Lardizabal JA, Deedwania PC: Atrial fibrillation in heart failure, *Med Clin North Am* 96 (5):987–1000, 2012.

29. Felker GM, Mentz RJ: Diuretics and ultrafiltration in acute decompensated heart failure, *J Am Coll Cardiol* 59(24):2145–2153, 2012.

30. Freda BJ, Slawsky M, Mallidi J, Braden GL: Decongestive treatment of acute decompensated heart failure: cardiorenal implications of ultrafiltration and diuretics, *Am J Kidney Dis* 58 (6):1005–1017, 2011.

31. Valchanov KP, Arrowsmith JE: The role of venodilators in the perioperative management of heart failure, *Eur J Anaesthesiol* 29(3):121–128, 2012.

32. Joseph SM, Cedars AM, Ewald GA, et al.: Acute decompensated heart failure: contemporary medical management, *Texas Heart Inst J* 36(6):510–520, 2009.

33. Triposkiadis F, Parissis JT, Starling RC, et al.: Current drugs and medical treatment algorithms in the management of acute decompensated heart failure, *Expert Opin Investig Drugs* 18 (6):695–707, 2009.

34. Vilas-Boas F: Modern approach to the treatment of decompensated heart failure, *Exp Rev Cardiovasc Ther* 7(2):159–167, 2009.

35. Gowda RM, Fox JT, Khan IA: Cardiogenic shock: basics and clinical considerations, *Int J Cardiol* 123(3):221–228, 2008.

36. Elkayam U, Janmohamed M, Habib M, Hatamizadeh P: Vasodilators in the management of acute heart failure, *Crit Care Med* 36(1 Suppl):S95–S105, 2008.

37. Heywood JT, Khan TA: The use of vasoactive therapy for acute decompensated heart failure: Hemodynamic and renal considerations, *Rev Cardiovasc Med* 8(Suppl 5):S22–S29

38. Hanlon-Pena PM, Quaal SJ: Intra-aortic balloon pump timing: review of evidence supporting current practice, *Am J Crit Care* 20(4):323–333, 2011.

39. Thiele H, Zeymer U, Neumann FJ, et al.: Intraaortic balloon support for myocardial infarction with cardiogenic shock, *N Engl J Med* 367(14):1287–1296, 2012.
40. Kern MJ: The changing paradigm of hemodynamic support device selection for high-risk percutaneous coronary interventions, *J Invasive Cardiol* 23(10):439–446, 2011.
41. Remmelink M, Sjauw KD, Enriquez JP, et al.: Effects of mechanical left ventricular unloading by Impella on left ventricular dynamics in high-risk and primary percutaneous coronary intervention patients, *Catheter Cardiovasc Interven* 75(2):187, 2010.
42. Burkhoff D, Cohen H, Brunckhorst C, O'Neill WW: TandemHeart Investigators: A randomized multicenter clinical study to evaluate the safety and efficacy of the TandemHeart percutaneous ventricular assist device versus conventional therapy with intraaortic balloon pumping for treatment of cardiogenic shock, *Am Heart J* 152(3):469.e1–469.e8, 2006.
43. Ziemba EA, John R: Mechanical circulatory support for bridge to decision: which device and when to decide, *J Card Surg* 25(4):425–433, 2010.
44. Slaughter MS, Pagani FD, Rogers JG, et al.: Clinical management of continuous-flow left ventricular assist devices in advanced heart failure, *J Heart Lung Transplant* 29(4 Suppl):S1–S39, 2010.
45. Rogers JG, Aaronson KD, Boyle AJ, et al.: Continuous flow left ventricular assist device improves functional capacity and quality of life of advanced heart failure patients, *J Am Coll Cardiol* 55(17):1826–1834, 2010.

Hemodynamics of Acute Right Heart Failure and Pulmonary Hypertension

18

Annette Haynes

The right heart and pulmonary vasculature were once only recognized for supplying volume and oxygenated blood to the left ventricle. Over the last several decades, a deeper understanding of the role of the right ventricle and the pulmonary vascular system has evolved, particularly with recognition of the many causes of right ventricular failure and pulmonary hypertension. This chapter has two parts. The first section is focused on acute right heart failure. The latter section covers pulmonary hypertension.

Clinical Reasoning Pearl

Nonspecific presenting symptoms and signs in both right ventricular failure and pulmonary hypertension make diagnosis difficult. This increases the time to diagnosis and may lead to worse outcomes.

Historical Perspective

In the past, the right heart was seen as a passive conduit bringing deoxygenated blood to the lungs.[1,2] It was perceived as a collection chamber where venous volume returned to the heart and lungs and was only recently recognized for the complex hemodynamics that maintain the continuous movement of blood throughout the cardiovascular system.[3] Failure of the right heart was only seen as the endpoint of injury to the left ventricular and pulmonary arterial systems. Unfortunately, early canine-model investigations supported this misunderstanding,[4] although researchers and surgeons working with human right ventricular hypoplasia in the 1950s to the 1970s expanded baseline knowledge about right ventricular (RV) function.[5,6] Since then, clinicians and researchers working with RV failure, RV myocardial infarction, congenital heart disease, and pulmonary hypertension have highlighted the physiologic importance of the right heart.[2]

Key Physiologic Concepts

The right ventricle is a low-pressure, high-capacitance heart chamber. It can accommodate large volume changes and requires very little pressure to move blood volume forward into the low-pressure pulmonary vasculature. The right ventricle adapts to sudden volume changes with little impact on forward flow. Remarkably, the right heart pumps an identical volume to the left heart at about one sixth of the pressure and with a smaller chamber size.

Volume pressure changes are based on the Starling mechanism, in which myocardial fiber length increases as fibers stretch to accommodate increased volume. Increasing muscle fiber length increases contractility of the myocardial fiber to an endpoint where myofibril function fails.[7] When maximum stretch is reached, myofibrils lose the ability to contract, and the ventricle reacts to the excess volume with dilation.

Right Ventricular Geometry

Structurally the right ventricle is approximately two-thirds the size of the left ventricle with thinner more compliant chamber walls. The right ventricle delivers the same stroke volume as the left ventricle with 25% less work because of low resistance in the pulmonary vasculature and the ability of the pulmonary artery to expand.[1,2]

RV function is dominated by its unique geometry. Anatomically, the RV cavity is shaped like a crescent with a separate infundibulum and prominent trabeculation (structural supports) in the muscular apex.[1] The right ventricle is composed of three different sections: (1) the inlet that comprises the tricuspid valve, chordae tendineae and papillary muscles; (2) the apical section; and (3) the infundibulum (conus) outflow section (Figure 18-1). These sections work in synchrony to eject blood into the pulmonary system.[2,6] RV myocardial fibers are arranged differently in each section, creating a peristaltic-type movement with each contraction. In the RV free wall, the myocytes are

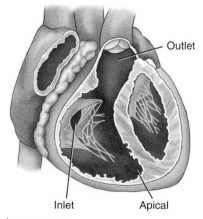

FIGURE 18-1 Right ventricular anatomy.

aligned in a transverse orientation, sometimes called a *transverse constriction*, which causes a bellows-type movement. In the mid-ventricle, the myocyte fibers are aligned in an oblique orientation, which, in combination with the midline septum, creates the twisting ventricular motion necessary to eject against the pulmonary vascular resistance (PVR).[1]

The RV architecture includes the intraventricular septum. The septum divides the two ventricles of the heart and is essential in the motion of ventricular contraction. Both the RV free wall and the intraventricular septum are equally important for normal function of the right ventricle.[2]

Right Ventricular Blood Supply

The RV free wall receives its blood supply from the right coronary artery (RCA). Uniquely, the proximal RCA is perfused in both systole and diastole. Two different arteries supply the septum: (1) the left anterior descending (LAD) artery, which provides blood flow to the anterior two thirds; and (2) the posterior descending artery (PDA), which supplies the inferior–posterior third.[2]

Pericardium

Anatomically, the pericardium plays an important role in the function of the right ventricle. The pericardial sac surrounds the complete heart and restricts excessive ballooning of the compliant right ventricle.

Ventricular Interdependence

The term *ventricular interdependence* describes the situation wherein the size, shape, and compliance of one ventricle may affect the size, shape, and pressure–volume relationship of the other ventricle through mechanical interaction.[6] Ventricular contractile synchrony ensures that a change in one ventricle will be reflected by a change in the other.[8] The constraining effect of the pericardium limits the size of each ventricle and augments the impact of interdependence.

Right Ventricular Volume Overload

The right ventricle, as a high capacitance chamber, can tolerate acute volume overload better than it can tolerate acute pressure overload. Conditions leading to RV volume overload include tricuspid regurgitation and atrial septal defect with a left-to-right shunt. In right heart failure, as the right ventricle progressively dilates, the ventricular cavity changes from the normal crescent shape to an oblong or more rounded shape. This geometric change impacts both the left ventricle and the pericardial sac via ventricular interdependence, as demonstrated in Figure 18-2.

The intraventricular septum bows into the left ventricle as increased RV pressure or volume forces the RV chamber to dilate. This change in RV chamber shape, and increase in RV pressure, affects the ability of the left ventricle to fill and eject. The

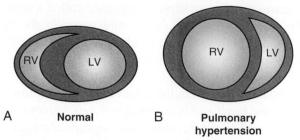

FIGURE 18-2 A, Normal right and left ventricle size and shape. **B,** Impact of pulmonary hypertension on the right and left ventricle size and shape.

progressive RV dilation also increases pressure against the constraining effects of the pericardial sac. With these geometric imbalances, the left ventricle is challenged to accommodate a normal preload volume and generate a normal stroke volume.[6,8] The result is a decreased left ventricular (LV) stroke volume and decreased cardiac output.

Right Ventricular Dilation

RV dilation results in distortion of the tricuspid annulus, causing tricuspid regurgitation. Tricuspid regurgitation increases RV preload and decreases cardiac output. Thinning of the walls as occurs in myocardial infarction, leads to higher local wall tension and increased risk of further RV free wall dysfunction.[9]

Right Ventricular Pressure Overload

Pressure overload on the ventricular myocytes, as seen with pulmonary valve stenosis, pulmonary embolism, pulmonary hypertension, and left heart failure, leads to cellular replacement by connective tissue. Pressure overload decreases RV contractility and decreases forward movement of blood into the pulmonary vascular bed. With progressive hypertrophy, RV function continues to deteriorate. Ejection becomes less complete, and wall tension remains elevated throughout the cardiac cycle. Coronary arterial perfusion is impaired and contributes to RV ischemia.[10] The patient demonstrates increasing symptomatology and decreasing functional reserve.

Acute Pulmonary Embolism

Massive pulmonary embolism may lead to acute right heart failure and is considered the most frequent cause of acute RV pressure overload.[11] Major emboli are usually bilateral, widespread, and involve large territories of the pulmonary vasculature.[12] With pulmonary embolism, the sudden increase in afterload pressure for the right ventricle leads to initial myocardial hypertrophy and contractile dysfunction. This obstructive pressure is further increased with the release of pulmonary vasoconstrictors and hypoxemia.[12] The RV chamber dilates to maintain stroke volume with rising filling pressures. This leads to diastolic dysfunction, decreased cardiac output, and tricuspid regurgitation.[2] Other signs of acute pulmonary embolism include hypotension, as described in the case study at the end of Chapter 3, and a decrease in the partial pressure of end tidal carbon dioxide ($PetCO_2$) as described in Chapter 8 (see Figure 8-7).

Right Ventricular Hypertrophy

Hypertrophy of the right ventricle occurs in response to increased resistance to ejection. The law of Laplace is used to describe the relationship of the tension (T) in the walls of a container with its radius (R) and the pressure (P) of its contents.[9] Tension is proportional to the product: Pressure × Radius as described in Chapter 1 (Table 1-2). The thickening of ventricular walls tends to reduce the tension. Injury or conditions that generate increased pulmonary vascular resistance force the right ventricle to generate higher pressures to eject blood into the pulmonary vasculature. Hypertrophy ultimately limits RV diastolic filling ability and restricts cardiac output.[8] Initially, this lowers wall tension. However, as RV failure progresses, ventricular diameter increases, causing increased stress on the RV wall.

Neurohormonal reactions to the decreased flow include activation of the sympathetic system that increases both heart rate and contractility. Continued decrease in cardiac output activates the renin-angiotensin-aldosterone system (RAAS) resulting in sodium and fluid retention.[13] RAAS activation leads to a vicious cycle of volume overload and increased work for the failing right ventricle (see Figure 1-17 in Chapter 1).

Right Ventricular Infarction

Infarction of the right ventricular impacts its contractility. Right ventricular myocardial infarction (RVMI) is identified with increasing frequency with reports of RV involvement in 40% to 50% of acute myocardial infarctions.[14] Classic signs of RVMI include hypotension, with elevated jugular venous pressure, and clear lung fields.[13] Studies identify increased risk of mortality, cardiogenic shock, malignant ventricular arrhythmias, and atrioventricular block in the patient with an acute RVMI. Occlusion of the RCA proximal to the marginal branches leads to hypokinesis in the lateral and inferior right ventricle, whereas ischemia of the left anterior descending artery (LAD) usually results in anterior RV wall hypokinesis.[1] The right ventricle has been known to exhibit spontaneous recovery with aggressive support. This recovery post ischemic injury is theorized to be secondary to the thinner muscular wall and dual arterial perfusion.[6]

Right Ventricular Failure

RV function is dependent on the classic factors that govern cardiac output: preload or the amount of volume in the right ventricle at the end of diastole; afterload or the

TABLE 18-1	Causes of Right Heart Failure
PHYSIOLOGIC IMPACT ON RIGHT VENTRICLE	**CLINICAL CONDITION**
Increased preload	Atrial septal defect Acute tricuspid regurgitation Volume overload
Decreased contractility	Myocardial infarction Myocarditis Cardiomyopathy Congenital heart disease (some conditions impact preload and afterload)
Increased afterload	Pulmonary hypertension Pulmonary embolism Interstitial lung disease Acute respiratory distress syndrome Left heart failure Acute mitral valve regurgitation Ventricular septal defect or rupture

resistance the right ventricle is ejecting against, contractility, and heart rate.[15] Failure of the right ventricle occurs as a result of structural or functional disorders that alter the ventricle's ability to fill or eject blood.[6,10] The causes of RV failure are categorized under three areas that affect right ventricular function: preload, afterload, and contractility, and listed in Table 18-1.

Most or all of these conditions result in increased volume or pressure in the right ventricle. Initially, the right ventricle tolerates increased pressure or volume with increased myocardial stretch and increased contractility. When these adaptive mechanisms are overwhelmed, the ventricle compensates in one of two ways: (1) by hypertrophy in response to increased pressure, and (2) by dilation in response to increased volume. Either of these conditions decreases ventricular function, as described earlier.

Acute decompensation, in which normal mechanisms are overwhelmed, occurs with an increase in cardiac demand such as sepsis or with an increase in afterload, as seen with arrhythmias, pulmonary embolism, or pulmonary hypertension.[15]

Right Ventricular Dysfunction in Left Heart Failure

Many studies on heart failure focus on impairment of the left ventricle as the main pump of the body.[16] Chapter 17 discusses heart failure that alters left ventricular function in detail. In left heart failure, right heart work increases from afterload transmitted in a retrograde fashion through the pulmonary venous system with an increased transpulmonary gradient. Ischemia generated injury may affect both ventricles, depending on the culprit lesion, as the right heart is perfused by both RCA and LAD vessels. Left heart failure results in decreased cardiac output with concomitant decreased perfusion of the RCA. The RCA fills during systole and diastole and is sensitive to any fall in cardiac output. This impairment of RCA perfusion is compounded by the restricted pericardial compartment.[2] The other component of left heart failure that impacts the right heart is related to the dilation of the LV chamber. This causes compression of the right ventricle in the limited pericardial space and results in decreased RV filling.

End-Stage Right Ventricular Failure and Pulmonary Hypertension

Pulmonary hypertension generates increased afterload in the right ventricle as explained in the next part of this chapter. The increased resistance causes RV hypertrophy, which results in decreased RV filling. This results in decreased RV stroke volume that results in decreased LV filling with concomitant hypotension and reduced cardiac output.

Diagnosis

Right heart failure was historically difficult to evaluate given the right ventricle's geometry, interrelationship with the left ventricle, and sensitivity to alterations in pulmonary pressure.[1] Right heart failure is diagnosed on the basis of signs and symptoms, laboratory tests, imaging techniques, and right heart catheterization, as described below.

Signs and Symptoms

Signs of right heart failure include fluid retention, peripheral edema, ascites, anasarca, exercise intolerance, fatigue, dyspnea, and atrial and ventricular arrhythmias.[11] As RV failure worsens, the liver becomes engorged with a positive hepatojugular reflex. If severe, the patient may have discomfort or pain in right upper quadrant or epigastrium with a pulsatile enlarged liver.[17] Auscultation may reveal an RV S3 gallop, and the murmur of tricuspid regurgitation. A parasternal RV lift may be observed. An RV "heave" may be felt when a clinician places the palm of the hand on the patient's chest, over the area of the right ventricle. When present, this signifies RV hypertrophy.

Patient Comfort

Patient comfort measures in advanced right heart failure include administration of morphine to treat dyspnea, as morphine decreases the anxiety of air hunger and provides some pulmonary vasodilation.

Advanced right heart failure results in hypotension resulting from elevated filling pressures and low cardiac output. As the systolic reserve or the ability to maintain adequate forward flow with ejection decreases, patient symptoms progression can be tracked using the New York Heart Association (NYHA) functional classification system, as described in Chapter 17 (see Table 17-3).

Laboratory Tests for Right Heart Failure

Laboratory tests used in the diagnosis of heart failure are similar for both left-sided and right-sided heart failure. B-type natriuretic peptide, abbreviated as BNP, is a useful diagnostic test as levels increase as heart failure-related volume overload progresses. Natriuretic peptides correlate with right atrial and RV volume increase, and excessive stretching of the cardiac muscle. Serial measurements may help with diagnosis and treatment evaluation as discussed in Chapter 17 (see Table 17-7). Other laboratory abnormalities in right heart failure include hematology, chemistry, and anticoagulation measures.

With increased antidiuretic hormone (ADH) release, fluid retention and hyponatremia occur.[17] Sodium levels less than 130 milliequivalents per liter (mEq/L) indicate significant fluid retention, which causes some patients to present with a decreased level of consciousness. Potassium is also an important electrolyte to monitor in right heart failure.

Creatinine levels, which are used to monitor for kidney insult, may be misinterpreted in this population. Although most would consider increased creatinine levels a sign of progressive kidney impairment, in right heart failure, it may be related to venous congestion rather than decreased perfusion from impaired cardiac output.[10] Decrease in central venous pressure (CVP) may improve renal artery perfusion and clear the rising creatinine. Other dilutional effects include decreased hemoglobin and hematocrit levels.

With significant hepatic engorgement, impaired liver function may be detected from elevated liver biomarkers; impaired coagulation function is detected from elevated prothrombin time, international normalized ratio (INR), and activated partial thromboplastin time (aPTT).

Intracardiac Pressure Measurements

An estimation of CVP can be obtained from inspection of the internal jugular veins as described in Chapter 2 (Figure 2-3). This technique may be challenging and difficult to achieve in obese patients or with the presence of fluid or pressure lines in these vessels.[10] Direct measurement of CVP or right atrial pressure (RAP) with invasive pressure lines assist with baseline and ongoing measurement of treatment effectiveness (see Chapter 4 for more details about CVP monitoring).

As mentioned later in this chapter, diagnostic right heart catheterization in the cardiac catheterization laboratory is considered the gold standard for the diagnosis of pulmonary hypertension. In the critical care unit, continuous monitoring with a pulmonary artery catheter (PAC) measures changes in pulmonary pressures in response to treatments. PAC measurements include pulmonary artery occlusion pressures (PAOP) or 'wedge' pressure, as an indirect measure of the LV end-diastolic pressure. However, whenever possible, noninvasive assessment of RV function is recommended.

Right Ventricular Diagnostic Tests

Chest Radiography

In the right heart failure picture, chest radiography may reflect an enlarged heart with increased major vessels. Because the right heart is positioned mostly behind the sternum, the enlargement may only be seen as LV displacement.[18]

Echocardiography and Doppler Imaging

In clinical practice, echocardiography is the most frequent evaluation method of the right ventricle. Transthoracic echocardiography is challenging because the retrosternal position of the right ventricle limits direct views.[6] The increasing use of more advanced echocardiography modalities has helped improve recognition and evaluation of right ventricular function and failure.

Vena Cava Collapsibility

Because inferior vena cava collapsibility is a surrogate measure for filling volumes, findings related to inferior vena cava collapsibility may assist with assessment and treatment. The mechanics of breathing significantly influence superior vena cava flow, hepatic vein flow, and RV inflow velocities. Inspiration increases venous return, whereas exhalation decreases venous flow by up to 20%. With normal breathing, an inferior vena cava decrease in size greater than 50% suggests the RAP is less than 10 millimeters of mercury (mm Hg).[1] A small inferior vena cava with spontaneous collapse indicates intravenous volume depletion, whereas no collapse suggests that the RAP is greater than 15 mm Hg.[1] See Chapter 11 for a more detailed discussion on the use of bedside ultrasound.

2D Doppler Imaging

Two-dimensional transthoracic echocardiography (TTE) is a noninvasive measure that is easy to perform at the bedside. Advances in portable devices, including the newer hand-held models, permit rapid assessment of ventricular fill and function.

Echocardiography and Doppler imaging has evolved with combination methods and use of computer models that can recreate the geometric complexities of the right ventricle. These various modalities can all be performed from a single echocardiography assessment and are described below.

Tissue Doppler Imaging

Tissue Doppler imaging is a quantitative assessment of RV systolic and diastolic function, which measures velocities of flow across the atrioventricular (mitral and tricuspid) valves. This measure helps detect low velocity and high amplitudes, determine systolic and diastolic time intervals, and estimate cardiac output.[1] Velocity is the speed of flow into each chamber over time and is used to estimate the cardiac output. A low systolic annular velocity through the pulmonic valve may predict right ventricular dysfunction.

Speckle Tracking Imaging

Speckle tracking imaging is an update of two-dimensional echocardiography, which uses a pattern-matching technology to combine ultrasound and cine data from cardiac catheterization. D'Andrea et al. found that this approach could quantify regional myocardial function and predict response to cardiac resynchronization using biventricular pacing.[19]

Three-Dimensional Echocardiography

Three-dimensional (3D) echocardiography with analysis eliminates reliance on geometric modeling.[1] This method uses both short-axis and long-axis views to calculate RV volumes and ejection fraction.[1]

Transesophageal Echocardiography and Doppler

Transesophageal echocardiography (TEE), with the probe inserted in the esophagus, measures the size, function, contractility, and dilation of the right ventricle, as well as the flow through the valves.

Transesophageal Doppler probes calculate cardiac output by measuring stoke volume in the descending aorta. Esophageal probes are typically referred to as minimally invasive. See Chapter 10 for a more detailed discussion on the use of transesophageal Doppler.

Hemodynamic Values Derived from Echocardiography and Doppler

Unique hemodynamic measures are derived from the echocardiographic and Doppler modalities described above; these help with comprehensive RV evaluation, as described below:

- Right ventricular ejection fraction (RVEF) calculates the amount of volume ejected from the right ventricle with each heartbeat. This measure has the disadvantage of being volume related and is difficult to evaluate in the right ventricle. Normal values are 46 ± 7 percent of the RV volume.[1]
- Right ventricular fractional area change (RVFAC) looks at changes in the areas of the ventricle in relationship to the cardiac cycle.[4] With the complex geometry of the right ventricle, impairment in one section, for example, acute ischemic injury, will significantly affect function. Normal values for this measurement are greater than $51\% \pm 11\%$ change in the ventricle during each cardiac cycle.[1]
- Myocardial performance index (MPI) is a geometry-dependent index of RV global function, with the advantages of being unaffected by heart rate, loading conditions, and tricuspid regurgitation.[1] MPI is a ratio of the sum of isovolumic contraction time

(IVCT) and isovolumic relaxation time (IVRT) divided by ejection time (ET). Increasing values correlate with decreasing ventricular function.[1] Refer to the equation in Table 18-2. Normal values for this measure are 0.28 to 0.04.[6]

- Tricuspid annular plane systolic ejection (TAPSE) is a measure of the level of systolic excursion of the lateral tricuspid annulus toward the apex. This estimates RV function and is a strong predictor of heart failure. Normal TAPSE values are 15 to 20 millimeters (mm).[1,2]

TABLE 18-2 Hemodynamic Equations used in the Diagnosis of Pulmonary Hypertension

HEMODYNAMIC EQUATIONS	NORMAL VALUES	HOW OBTAINED	SIGNIFICANCE
MPI (TEI) $MPI = (IVCT + IVRT) / ET$	0.32 ± 0.03[2]	2D echocardiography	Greater than 0.4 in RV dysfunction[2]
TPG $TPG = mPAP - mPAOP$	<10 mm Hg[56]	PA catheter or RHC	Increases because of retrograde transmission of LV pressure into PV system[56]
Bernoulli equation $PAP = 4 \times (TR\ velocity)^2$		PA catheter or RHC	Signs of increased pressure in the pulmonary system and diagnostic of pulmonary hypertension
PVR Wood units	70 (20–130) dynes·sec/cm[5] <3	PA catheter or RHC	Measure of RV afterload
RVEF	$46 \pm 7\%$[2]	2D echocardiography	Prognostic value in cardiopulmonary disorders[7]
RVFAC	$51 \pm 11\%$[2]	2D echocardiography	Correlates with RVEF prognostic value in MI[7]
TAPSE	15–20 mm[2]	2D echocardiography measures maximal systolic velocity at the tricuspid annulus	Strong predictor of heart failure prognosis[2]

CHD, Congenital heart disease; *ET*, ejection time; *IVCT*, isovolumetric contraction time; *IVRT*, isovolumetric relaxation time; *MI*, myocardial infarction; *MPI*, myocardial performance index or tricuspid systolic excursion index; *PVR*, pulmonary vascular resistance; *RHC*, right heart catheterization; *RVEF*, right ventricular ejection fraction; *RVFAC*, right ventricular fractional area change; *TAPSE*, tricuspid annular plane excursion; *TPG*, transpulmonary gradient.

Cardiac Magnetic Resonance Imaging

Cardiac magnetic resonance imaging (cMRI) is being used more often to measure dimensions and function of the right ventricle. cMRI evaluates blood flow, stroke volume, cardiac output, and dimensions of the right ventricle noninvasively.

Exercise Testing

Cardiopulmonary exercise testing is useful in assessing RV function as maximum oxygen consumption (VO_2 max) correlates with prognosis and quality of life. Exercise tolerance, which can be measured using the 6-minute walk distance (6MWD), is a simple measure to test exercise ability. The 6MWD test is easy to repeat over time to evaluate progression of right heart failure. With implementation of treatment, repeated measures indicate ventricular function progression or deterioration.

A functional class system for the right heart has been developed. Haddad et al. (2008) created a four-level continuum of right heart failure, with stages A and B denoting risk for chronic failure, and stages C and D demonstrating chronic right heart failure. Structural changes and increasing needs for management progress along this continuum.[11]

> ### Patient Safety
>
> The right heart is preload dependent and afterload sensitive, which necessitates careful management to ensure there is sufficient venous return to promote functional contractility.

Treatment of Right Heart Failure

Goals of treatment for right heart failure are focused on optimizing preload, decreasing afterload, improving contractility, and stabilizing heart rates.

Optimizing Right Ventricular Preload

Decreasing volume and resistance to pumping are the key concepts in right heart failure management. Increased preload may be the initiating problem and is often the first focus of treatment. The aim of treating right heart failure is to optimize preload rather than initiate aggressive diuresis.[7] Aggressive diuresis may result in hypovolemia and generate a vicious cycle of neurohormonal stimulation that results in further fluid and sodium retention. Removing excess volume load will decrease RV preload and pericardial constraint, optimize LV preload, and improve cardiac output. Progressive diuresis with doses of diuretics matched to a goal rate of diuresis is used for patients with marked volume overload. The goal is to generate diuresis while avoiding hypotension that may lead to RV ischemia. If this approach is not successful and the patient progresses to acute RV failure, more advanced fluid removal efforts include ultrafiltration and dialysis.[7] For the patient with RV ischemia and hypotension, acute volume loading is started with a slow initial challenge of 500 milliliters (mL). If this careful fluid bolus does not improve blood pressure, further loading may escalate hemodynamic compromise.[7] Continued judicious use of diuretics is designed to minimize fluid retention and limit preload. Other efforts include moderate sodium restriction (2 grams per day [g/day]) with daily weight monitoring to track progress of fluid removal over time.

Patient Safety

With nitroglycerin, careful titration is necessary to prevent profound hypotension with sudden preload reduction.

Reducing Right Ventricular Afterload

Reducing afterload is the second goal in the treatment of right heart failure. Again, careful management of hemodynamics is essential to prevent worsening failure as a consequence of treatment. The two primary causes of increased afterload for the right ventricle are pulmonary hypertension and left heart failure, Understanding the inter-relationship and interdependence of these systems is essential to understanding the hemodynamics of RV failure.[20]

Pulmonary vascular vasodilation is essential treatment to manage the pulmonary hypertension process. The three classes of medications used to treat pulmonary hypertension are (1) endothelin receptor antagonists, (2) phosphodiesterase inhibitors, and (3) prostanoids. These agents work to decrease the proliferation of endothelial cells and promote vasodilation of the pulmonary arteries.[7] Oral and intravenous vasodilator medications are discussed in more detail later in this chapter.

Inhaled vasodilators: Inhaled nitric oxide may alleviate RV ischemia associated with cardiogenic shock. Inhaled nitric oxide has potent selective pulmonary vasodilatory effects that promote reduction in RV afterload. It is used following cardiac surgery in patients with acute right heart failure to treat exacerbations of pulmonary hypertension. The cost and serious side effects, including the risk of rebound pulmonary hypertension and methemoglobinemia, are limiting factors for routine use of inhaled nitric oxide.[7] More recently, nebulized epoprostenol is being trialed to treat acute right heart failure exacerbations with results similar to using inhaled nitric oxide.[21,22] Limitations of inhaled epoprostenol include side effects of hypotension, bradycardia, headache, or flushing.[20] Dopamine or epinephrine may be considered in patients with severe hypotension and used with caution, as the increase of arrhythmic side effects of these inotropic medications may result in worsening RV failure.

Improving Right Ventricular Contractility

The third focus for treating right heart failure is improving contractility. In the acute hemodynamically compromised right ventricle, the use of a combination of inotropes, vasopressors, and vasodilators is beneficial. Dobutamine and milrinone are the agents of preference with right heart failure.[1,10,15] Both dobutamine and milrinone have vasodilatory effects that promote decreasing afterload while improving contractility. Dobutamine improves myocontractility while decreasing both systemic vascular resistance (SVR) and pulmonary vascular resistance (PVR).[7] Dobutamine is less likely to cause arrhythmias than dopamine. If the patient is already experiencing tachyarrhythmias, the inodilator milrinone, a phosphodiesterase III inhibitor, is preferred to improve RV contractility.[20] Milrinone vasodilates pulmonary and systemic vessels and increases inotropy by increasing cyclic adenosine monophosphate and decreasing afterload.[15] The combination effects of inotropy and vasodilation promote increased cardiac output and stroke volume while maintaining preload.

Clinical Reasoning Pearl

Pulmonary vasodilators are useful to reduce RV afterload in several patient scenarios including pulmonary hypertension and RV failure after cardiac surgery.

Heart Rhythm Management

The fourth aspect of treatment for right heart failure focuses on heart rhythm management. High-degree atrioventricular block or atrial fibrillation will have profound hemodynamic effects on right heart function. Loss of AV synchrony may significantly decrease cardiac output in patients with right heart failure because the RV preload is essential for function.[20] Treatments include sequential atrioventricular pacing and cardioversion of unstable tachyarrhythmias.[11] Biventricular pacing, also known as *cardiac resynchronization therapy*, may improve symptoms and survival.[10]

Implantable cardioverter defibrillators are considered for patients with acute RVMI who are at risk of sudden cardiac death. This includes patients who survived a cardiac arrest, have a history of sustained ventricular tachycardia, or who have demonstrated inducible ventricular tachycardia in the electrophysiology laboratory. Campbell et al. (2013) reviewed data from the MADIT-CRT trial and reported that treatment with cardiac resynchronization therapy improved RV function and generated a reduction in tricuspid regurgitation velocity.[23]

For patients with inducible monomorphic ventricular tachycardia, catheter ablation that interrupts the ventricular tachycardia circuit may be an effective treatment.

Preventing Complications

Other pharmacologic treatments are focused on prevention of complications associated with right heart failure including use of anticoagulation to prevent clot formation.

Supplemental oxygen therapy is used to reverse hypoxemia and its side effect of vaso-constriction. In acute respiratory failure with right heart failure, ventilator support is challenging, as discussed in Chapter 14. It is important to avoid high levels of positive end-expiratory pressure (PEEP), maintain plateau pressures less than 30 mm Hg, and avoid acidosis and alveolar hypoxia. These actions will minimize the positive pressure effects of mechanical ventilation on intrathoracic pressures, which increase the workload of the right heart.

Surgical Procedures

Surgical procedures in right heart failure include correction of underlying causes such as tricuspid regurgitation, ventricular septal defect, or ventricular aneurysm repair.[1] For end-stage right heart failure, a palliative measure of atrial septostomy may decompress the right ventricle by creating a right-to-left shunt.[20] The atrial septostomy procedure (Figure 18-3) is performed in the interventional cardiac catheterization suite to decrease RV preload and decrease RV pressures.[20] Decreasing preload improves symptoms of right heart failure. The major side effect is that deoxygenated blood passes into the left atrium, which increases systemic hypoxia.

Right ventricular assist devices (RVAD) are used to treat right heart failure refractory to medical treatment. Mechanical circulatory assist devices may be used as a bridge to transplantation or as destination therapy. A number of devices can be inserted percutaneously for short-term use or implanted surgically.[10] The hemodynamic effects of RVAD and other mechanical circulatory assist devices are discussed in detail in Chapter 15.

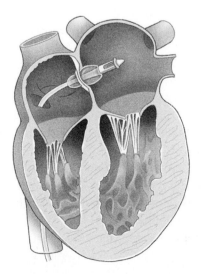

FIGURE 18-3 Atrial septostomy.

Outpatient Treatments

In the outpatient setting, medications to treat right heart failure are similar to those used to manage left heart failure. Beta-blockers and angiotensin-converting enzyme inhibitors or angiotensin receptor blockers are used to lower blood pressure and limit ventricular remodeling. Arrhythmia control will continue with the use of oral antiarrhythmic medications. Maintaining anticoagulation will be driven by the diagnosis and decisions of the patient and clinical management team. With recovery after the initial insult and as heart failure progresses, graded physical activity may improve functional capacity and quality of life.

It is important for patients with right heart failure to avoid isometric exercises, as these may be associated with syncope. Patient symptoms are what drive changes in patient management. Education for patients and caregivers include symptoms to report, ongoing weight management, moderate sodium restriction, medications, and regular office visits essential to follow-up. Verifying patients' understanding of treatments and knowledge of whom to access for questions decreases hospital readmissions and improves satisfaction.

Case Study #1

S.K., a 75-year-old female, was admitted emergently with severe back pain and shortness of breath. She reported awakening with this pain and that her condition did not improve with repositioning and the aspirin her daughter told her to take. She had an impending sense of doom by the time her daughter came to check on her, so she agreed to take an ambulance to the emergency room. Prehospital electrocardiogram (ECG) demonstrated inferior ST elevation myocardial infarction (STEMI), and she was transported to the nearest center for treatment of STEMI. In the emergency room, S.K. was found to have hypertension and tachycardia. After administration of one dose of sublingual nitroglycerin, she complained of dizziness. Her blood pressure dropped from 132/86 to 90/50 mm Hg and subsequently increased to 110/70 mm Hg with a 500-mL normal saline intravenous (IV) bolus. She continued to have back pain and increasing shortness of breath. Her pain subsided with IV morphine. The repeat 12-lead ECG showed increased ST elevation in the inferior leads and frequent ventricular arrhythmias. The STEMI team was activated, and she received a drug-eluting stent to the proximal right coronary artery after a cardiac catheterization showed a 98% occlusion of this vessel.

S.K. spent the night in a monitored unit recovering from this initial insult and procedure. During the night, she woke up with increasing shortness of breath and complained of dizziness. The ECG monitor showed a conversion from sinus rhythm of 72 with premature atrial contractions, to atrial fibrillation with rapid ventricular response, with heart rate at 126. Clinical assessment revealed distended jugular veins, decreased bi-basilar aeration, and blood pressure of 90/56 mm Hg. S.K. denied chest pain and said she was feeling very anxious. Amiodarone 150 mg IV bolus was administered, and an IV dobutamine infusion was started. Defibrillator pads were applied and the defibrillator was stationed at the bedside in anticipation of the need for cardioversion.

Case Study #1—cont'd

Symptoms persisted for 45 minutes. Electrolytes (potassium and magnesium) were within normal limits, and the 12-lead ECG did not demonstrate new signs of ischemia. Using a hand-held ultrasound device, the intensivist observed adequate RV filling with impaired RV contraction. With the addition of a second 150-mg IV amiodarone bolus and continuous IV amiodarone infusion at 1.0 mg/min, S.K. converted to sinus rhythm with heart rates in the 90s. The dobutamine infusion was titrated up to 5 micrograms per kilogram per minute (mcg/kg/min), and improved her blood pressure to 110/58 mm Hg. S.K. reported less shortness of breath.

Over the next 2 days, S.K. was weaned off the IV medications, started on oral amiodarone, and continued on her oral clopidogrel and aspirin. She began progressive walking in the critical care unit but tired easily. She also found that she had limited appetite. As her blood pressure stabilized, an angiotensin-converting enzyme inhibitor was added to her medication regime.

S.K. and her daughter reviewed the discharge information on heart failure with her nurses. This included heart failure videos, handouts, and discussions on changes she needed to make in her diet and activity at home plus the new medications. She was discharged home after 3 days with instructions for cardiology evaluation in 1 week and emergency contact information. ■

Connections Between Right Heart Failure and Pulmonary Hypertension

The right heart accommodates increases pressure by RV hypertrophy, which decreases RV filling. As the heart works harder to pump against the increased resistance, RV stroke volume and LV filling decrease, with resultant pulmonary hypotension and reduced cardiac output. Pulmonary hypertension increases resistance to right heart ejection. Management of right heart failure and of pulmonary hypertension requires specialized knowledge as discussed in the rest of this chapter.

Hemodynamics of Pulmonary Hypertension

Pulmonary hypertension is a complex, chronic, incurable, and progressively debilitating syndrome involving the pulmonary vascular system.[24] This syndrome results from restricted flow through the pulmonary circulation causing increased PVR and ultimately right heart failure.[25] Pulmonary hypertension may develop from several different etiologies, all with similar clinical presentations and endovascular pathology. This disorder includes changes at the endothelial membrane, smooth muscle, and adventitia; vascular remodeling with smooth muscle proliferation, hyperplasia, and in-situ thrombus.[26] Pulmonary hypertension exists in different forms with similar clinical presentations and endovascular changes. Irrespective of the cause, pulmonary hypertension is a progressive disorder resulting in right ventricular dysfunction, leading to right heart failure and death.

The five classifications of pulmonary hypertension identified by the World Health Organization (WHO) criteria[27] are listed in Table 18-3. These criteria, first described in 1973, have evolved over time as research evidence became available. The most recent revisions were completed in the 2008 Dana Point conference.[25] Patient diagnosis, treatment, and prognosis are guided by these criteria. A brief description of the five classifications of pulmonary hypertension, with a specific focus on group I pulmonary arterial hypertension (PAH) and group II pulmonary hypertension with left heart disease, is given below.

Historical Milestones

Pulmonary hypertension was first identified in the late nineteenth century in patients presenting with severe dyspnea and cyanosis.[28] Autopsy reports of the classic obstructive small pulmonary arteries and right ventricular hypertrophy were published by Kolb in 1865 and Romberg in 1891.[28] Developments in the early 1900s included the nickname "black heart disease," because of the associated cyanotic appearance. At that time, syphilis was eliminated as the cause. Introduction and development of the right heart catheterization procedure from 1929 to 1956 explained the hemodynamic basis of pulmonary hypertension. The first documented case was a high altitude–related incident in a physician working at the Mont Blanc observatory in the European Alps.[29,30]

Clinical reports of pulmonary hypertension in the literature surfaced in the early 1950s, including articles by Dr. Paul Wood in his discussion of congenital heart disease[31] and Eisenmenger syndrome.[32] By 1957, the primary underlying causes of all five classes were identified. In 1968, Switzerland experienced an epidemic of pulmonary hypertension related to the increased use of appetite suppressants. This epidemic spread as the use of popular appetite suppressants increased, including aminorex fumarates in Germany and Austria, fenfluramine in Europe, and the combination of fenfluramine and phentermine (Fen-Phen) in the United States.[28]

Pulmonary hypertension was initially classified at a World Health Organization (WHO) international meeting in 1973. The intense international focus supported by these periodic meetings led to identification and successful treatment development. Introduction of Doppler echocardiography in the late 1970s expanded the diagnostic predictability of pulmonary artery pressures and RV structural information. The National Institutes of Health (NIH) introduced the National Registry for pulmonary hypertension in 1981.

A new era of treatments began in 1984 with the introduction of prostacyclin. Epoprostenol, identified for potent antiplatelet aggregation and pulmonary vascular dilation, demonstrated a successful decrease in endothelial cells. These findings led to introduction of prostacyclin as an additional therapy.

TABLE 18-3 Clinical Classification of Pulmonary Hypertension

Group 1	Pulmonary arterial hypertension (PAH) Idiopathic PAH Heritable *BMPR2* gene Activin receptor-like kinase 1 (*ALK1*) gene Endoglin (with or without hereditary hemorrhagic telangiectasia) Unknown Drugs and toxins induced Associated with pulmonary arterial hypertension (APAH) Connective tissue diseases Human immunodeficiency virus infection Portal hypertension Congenital heart disease Schistosomiasis Chronic hemolytic anemia Persistent pulmonary hypertension of the newborn
Group 1′	Pulmonary veno-occlusive disease (PVOD), pulmonary capillary hemangiomatosis (PCH), or both
Group 2	Pulmonary hypertension caused by left heart disease Systolic dysfunction Diastolic dysfunction Valvular disease
Group 3	Pulmonary hypertension caused by lung diseases, hypoxia, or both Chronic obstructive pulmonary disease Interstitial lung disease Other pulmonary diseases with mixed restrictive and obstructive pattern Sleep-disordered breathing Alveolar hypoventilation disorders Chronic exposure to high altitude Developmental abnormalities
Group 4	Chronic thromboembolic pulmonary hypertension
Group 5	Pulmonary hypertension with unclear and multifactorial mechanisms Hematologic disorders: myeloproliferative disorders, splenectomy Systemic disorders: sarcoidosis, pulmonary Langerhans cell histiocytosis, lymphangioleiomyomatosis, neurofibromatosis, vasculitis Metabolic disorders: glycogen storage disease, Gaucher disease, thyroid disorders Other: tumoral obstruction, fibrosing mediastinitis, chronic renal failure on dialysis

Data from Simmoneau G, Robbins IM, Beghetti M, et al.: Updated clinical classification of pulmonary hypertension, *J Am Coll Cardiol* 54(Suppl 1):543–554, 2009.

Physiologic Concepts in Pulmonary Hypertension

Group 1 Pulmonary Arterial Hypertension

Group 1 PAH presents with pathologic changes resulting from both genetic and environmental factors that affect the structure and function of the pulmonary artery.[33] The heritable type of group 1 PAH is predominately related to mutations in the *BMPR2* gene in combination with other less frequently identified gene mutations. *BMPR2* works to help regulate the number of cells in specific tissues. Mutations are passed to offspring in an autosomal dominant pattern meaning that both males and females are equally affected if one parent carries the mutated gene. [34] However, not all affected children will manifest symptoms; therefore a watch-and-wait approach is recommended with ongoing monitoring.

Medial hypertrophy, intimal proliferation and fibrosis, with adventitial thickening, as well as plexiform and thrombotic lesions, are found in the pulmonary arteries of affected patients (Figure 18-4).[35,36] Abnormal endothelial function drives some of these

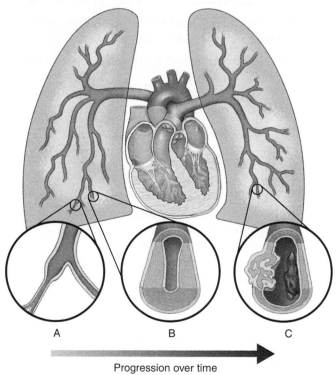

FIGURE 18-4 Pulmonary hypertension is a progressive disease. **A,** Vasoconstriction. **B,** Hypertrophy and hyperplasia of all three layers of the arterial wall (adventitia, media, intima). The thickening of the arterial media is found in all pulmonary arteries. **C,** Development of plexiform lesions and in-situ thrombosis. These changes result in the progressive narrowing of the peripheral vessels leading to the pruned tree appearance seen on chest radiography, and to right ventricular enlargement and dysfunction. PAH is a progressive disease with medial hypertrophy, intimal proliferation, fibrosis, adventitial thickening, plexiform and thrombotic lesions.

changes. The endothelium generally functions to balance constriction and dilation actions.[24,37] Factors involved in this vascular dysfunction include the following:

1. Excess of endothelin-1, which promotes vasoconstriction and smooth muscle proliferation
2. Overproduction of thromboxane a potent vasoconstrictor
3. Decrease in production of endogenous prostacyclin a vasodilator and antiproliferative
4. Decreased production of nitric oxide also a vasodilator and antiproliferative[35]

The mediators produced by the endothelium to regulate this balance are listed in Table 18-4.

Dysfunction of the pulmonary endothelium promotes a triad of vasoconstriction, thrombosis, and tissue proliferation. In patients with PAH, these changes promote medial hypertrophy, intimal proliferation, fibrotic changes, adventitial thickening with plexiform (perivascular inflammatory infiltrate complexes) and thrombotic lesions. These changes result in excessive vasoconstriction and proliferative and obstructive remodeling with abnormal endothelium. However, pulmonary veins are typically not affected.[26]

Group 1' (one prime) was added to this section with the 2008 revisions to capture the similar pathologic changes of pulmonary veno-occlusive disease and pulmonary capillary hemangiomatosis. The similarities in clinical presentation, risk factors, and familial association suggest these are components of the same disease spectrum.[24,25]

The hemodynamics of PAH are related to the narrowed lumen of the pulmonary vessels. Normally, the pulmonary arteries accommodate the increased flow needs related to exercise, illness, and stress. With PAH intraluminal narrowing, the decreased diameter results in flow restriction through the pulmonary arteries. The right ventricle must deliver the normal volume with increased pressure to advance it through the lung vasculature, where gas exchange normally occurs. This increased resistance to flow causes an increased workload for the right ventricle. Over time, this extra workload results in RV hypertrophy. As PAH evolves, this hypertrophy leads to right ventricular dilation and ultimately right heart failure.

TABLE 18-4 Endothelial Balance Mediators

VASODILATES	VASOCONSTRICTS
Prostacyclins	Thromboxane A_2
Nitric oxide	Endothelin-1
Adenosine	Hypoxia
Endothelium-derived hyperpolarizing agents	Serotonin Interleukin

Data from Badesch DB, Abman SH, Simonneau G, et al.: Medical therapy for pulmonary arterial hypertension: updated ACCP evidence-based clinical practice guidelines, *Chest* 131:1917–1928, 2007.

Group 2 Pulmonary Hypertension

Group 2 pulmonary hypertension **is** caused by left heart disease and has multiple mechanisms responsible for elevating PVR, including LV systolic dysfunction, diastolic dysfunction, and valvular disease. The elevation mechanism is passive backward transmission of pressure (postcapillary). This is measured as transpulmonary pressure gradient (TPG), which is determined by the difference between mean pulmonary arterial pressure and mean PAOP (wedge pressure).[24] Refer to Table 18-2 for this equation. The TPG is affected by pressure changes in both the pulmonary arterial and pulmonary venous systems, including reactive and fixed components. Reactive pulmonary hypertension is reversible under pharmacologic testing, whereas nonreactive or fixed obstructive components are not. Mechanisms may include reflexes from stretch receptors in left atrium and pulmonary artery.[13] Increased stretch initially promotes an increased vasoconstriction reflex.

Endothelial dysfunction of the pulmonary arteries favors vasoconstriction and proliferation of endothelial cells. The differences in PAH and pulmonary hypertension type 2 are illustrated in Figure 18-5.

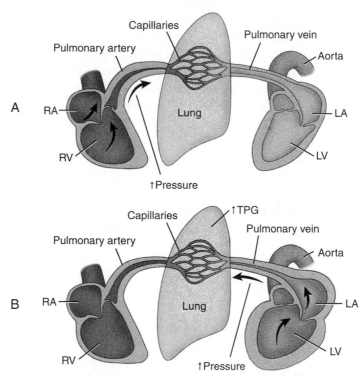

FIGURE 18-5 Differences between PAH and PH type 2. **A,** Pulmonary arterial hypertension Group 1. Group 1 PAH vasoconstriction and hyperplasia of the pulmonary artery results in increased resistance to flow and increases workload of the right ventricle leading to failure. **B,** Pulmonary hypertension secondary to Left heart disease Group 2. With left heart disease passive backward transmission of pressure results in increased LA pressure, increased pulmonary vein pressure, pulmonary vein fibrosis, and increased transpulmonary gradient.

Group 3 Pulmonary Hypertension

Group 3 pulmonary hypertension is caused by chronic lung disease and chronic hypoxemia. In this classification, pulmonary hypertension is related to alveolar hypoxemia and hypoventilation. Respiratory diseases most frequently associated with pulmonary hypertension include chronic obstructive pulmonary disease (COPD), interstitial lung disease, and sleep-disordered breathing. Less commonly, chronic hypoventilation conditions and high altitude exposure are associated with pulmonary hypertension.

Group 4 Chronic Thromboembolic Pulmonary Hypertension

Group 4 chronic thromboembolic pulmonary hypertension is the result of gradual formation of organized thromboembolism after deep venous thromboembolism or pulmonary embolism. Elevation of mean pulmonary arterial pressure is caused by thromboemboli in the pulmonary arterial system.

Group 5 Pulmonary Hypertension

Group 5 pulmonary hypertension with unclear, multifactorial mechanisms includes a variety of conditions affecting the pulmonary vasculature. Hematologic, systemic, metabolic, and other disorders are included in this group. Sarcoidosis, histiocytosis X, lymphangiomatosis, and compression of pulmonary vessel by adenopathy, tumor, or fibrosing mediastinitis are mechanisms included in this group.

Grouping the wide variety of causes for pulmonary hypertension with similar conditions helps focus the diagnosis and treatment regimens of this complex disease.

Diagnosis of Pulmonary Hypertension

Pulmonary hypertension is often a diagnosis of exclusions. Many of the symptoms are nonspecific, which explains why time to definitive diagnosis is often almost 3 years.[38] Typical symptoms are dyspnea on exertion, fatigue, nonproductive cough, syncope, angina pectoris, peripheral edema, and hemoptysis.[36] Physical assessment clues are listed in Table 18-5. Persistent symptoms without an easy explanation necessitate a number of diagnostic procedures ranging from physical examination through multiple diagnostic tests including serology, radiology, and pulmonary function testing.

Laboratory Tests

Laboratory testing includes use of biomarkers of cardiopulmonary disease such as troponin and B-type natriuretic protein, thyroid function tests, antinuclear antibody, coagulation factors, and serologies.

TABLE 18-5   Physical Assessment Clues in Pulmonary Hypertension

CARDIAC	PULMONARY	GASTRO-INTESTINAL	VASCULAR	SKIN
Left parasternal lift	SOB	Loss of appetite	Cyanosis	Telangiectasis
Accentuated pulmonary component of second heart sound (P2)	Lung sounds usually normal	Hepatomegaly	Jugular vein distention (JVD)	Sclerodactyly
Pansystolic murmur of TR	Inspiratory crackles of interstitial disease	Ascites	Peripheral edema	Digital ulceration
Diastolic murmur of Pulmonic insufficiency	Digital clubbing may indicate PVOD or CHD	Stigmata of liver disease	Cool extremities	Palmer erythema
RV third heart sound (S3)	Pulmonary edema suggests LV dysfunction			Spider nevi

CHD, Congenital heart disease; *JVD*, Jugular vein distention; *LV*, left ventricle; *PVOD*, pulmonary veno-occlusive disease; *RV*, right ventricle; SOB, shortness of breath; *TR*, tricuspid regurgitation.
Data from Zamanian RT, Haddad F, Doyle RL, Weinacker AB: Management strategies for patients with pulmonary hypertension in the intensive care unit, *Crit Care Med* 35:2037–2050, 2007; and Galie N, Hoeper MM, Humbert M, et al.: Guidelines for the diagnosis and treatment of pulmonary hypertension: the task force for the diagnosis and treatment of pulmonary hypertension of the European Society of Cardiology (ESC) and European Respiratory Society (ERS), endorsed by the International Society of Heart and Lung Transplantation (ISHLT), *Eur Heart J* 30:2493–2537, 2009.

Laboratory clues to pulmonary hypertension diagnosis and the WHO group identification include the following:

- Polycythemia, suggesting chronic hypoxemia
- Thyroid dysfunction, which is often associated with PAH
- Liver function abnormalities, which may indicate portal hypertension and reflect right heart failure
- Serologic markers of connective tissue disease (lupus, scleroderma)
- Human immunodeficiency virus (HIV)
- Elevated cardiac biomarkers (troponins), which may indicate RV distension, ischemia, or pulmonary embolism[25,37]

Further questioning leads to a cascade of cardiopulmonary testing measures.

Methods used to diagnose and evaluate pulmonary hypertension include pulse oximetry, 12-Lead ECG, radiology, echocardiography, and right heart catheterization, which is considered the gold standard. Oximetry is often the first measure of discord between oxygen demand and delivery. Symptoms of dyspnea and chest pain escalate concerns of inadequate oxygenation, leading to more diagnostic procedures. 12-Lead ECG clues to pulmonary hypertension diagnosis include classic signs of right axis deviation, RV hypertrophy, right atrial dilation, and arrhythmias.[25,37] Tachyarrhythmias may be associated with atrial and ventricular dilation and hypertrophy. Table 18-6 lists the diagnostic tests that help clinicians identify the appropriate WHO class for treatment.

Radiography

Radiologic testing begins with chest radiography. Classic changes seen with PAH include right atrial and right ventricular enlargement, RV hypertrophy, and central pulmonary artery dilation with pruning.[24,37] *Pruning* refers to the narrowing of small end arteries and sparse branching producing a pruned-tree appearance (Figure 18-6).[18] In group 2 pulmonary hypertension with left heart disease, increased pulmonary

TABLE 18-6 Diagnostic Tests for Pulmonary Hypertension

TEST	FINDINGS	SIGNIFICANCE
Troponin	Ischemic heart disease	May indicate left heart disease
B-type natriuretic peptide	Biomarker to evaluate heart failure	May indicate right heart disease, pulmonary embolism
Thyroid function	Abnormal in thyroid disease	Thyroid abnormalities are frequently associated with pulmonary hypertension
Antinuclear antibody	Elevated in connective tissue diseases	Identify other causes of pulmonary hypertension
Coagulation factor	Abnormal elevation in clot formation	May be elevated in Chronic thromboembolism
Serologies	Human immunodeficiency virus, lupus, scleroderma markers	Indicate other causes for pulmonary hypertension
Electrocardiography	Right axis deviation, arrhythmias	Right heart distension, right ventricular hypertrophy and strain
Radiology	• Right atrial and ventricle enlargement; • Central pulmonary artery dilation with pruning • Interstitial disease • Embolism	• Pulmonary arterial hypertension (PAH) • PAH • WHO group III (add perfusion scan to rule out) • WHO group IV
Computed tomographic angiography (CTA)	Pulmonary perfusion	• Reversible decreased perfusion with IV adenosine (PAH) • Perfusion blocks in CTEPH

Continued

TABLE 18-6   Diagnostic Tests for Pulmonary Hypertension—cont'd

TEST	FINDINGS	SIGNIFICANCE
Cardiac magnetic resonance imaging (cMRI)	Assessment of size, morphology, and function of right ventricle and pulmonary artery	• Evaluation of flow effect of pulmonary vascular resistance (PVR); • Three-dimensional image re-creation for structural definitions
Echocardiography	Identification of size and function of heart chambers and valves	Calculation of indexes to measure cardiac performance
Oximetry	Identification of supply and demand mismatch	• Identification of tolerance to activity • Progression of pulmonary hypertension–related hypoxemia
Bioimpedance	Differences in impedance during diastole and systole are closely related to decrease in PVR	Hypoxic vasoconstriction will increase impedance
Right heart catheterization	Specific measurement of intracardiac pressures, oxygenation, and hemodynamics	Verification of diagnosis with intracardiac chamber pressures clarification of right and left heart influences PAOP and PVR.

CTEPH, Chronic thromboembolic pulmonary hypertension; *IV,* intravenous; *PAH,* pulmonary arterial hypertension; *PAOP,* pulmonary artery occlusion pressure; *PVR,* pulmonary vascular resistance; *WHO,* World Health Organization.

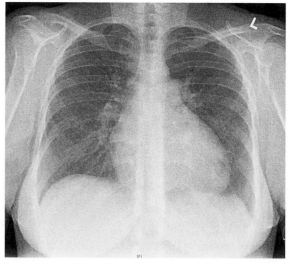

FIGURE 18-6 Chest radiography showing enlarged right ventricle, central pulmonary artery dilation with narrowing of small arteries and decreased branching to give a "pruned tree" appearance.

venous pressure is reflected by prominence and thickening of the upper lobe blood vessels and decreased prominence of the lower lobe vessels plus haziness of the hilar vessels.[18] Other radiographic signs of interstitial lung disease and embolism help exclude group 3 and 4 causes of pulmonary hypertension. If pulmonary embolism is still on the differential diagnosis list, radionuclide perfusion scanning will help rule out this cause. Surprisingly, in group 4, only 50% of patients with chronic thromboembolic pulmonary hypertension have any prior history of pulmonary embolism.[25]

Computed Tomography Angiography

Computed tomography angiography (CTA) helps quantify blood flow through the pulmonary vascular bed. The diagnostic value is increased with faster multi-detector electron beam scanners.[39] Findings include markedly decreased perfusion that may reverse with administration of IV adenosine. In group 4 chronic thromboembolic pulmonary hypertension, decreased perfusion may also be seen as perfusion blocks of the lung. Disadvantages of CTA include radiation exposure and the need for supine positioning of the patient for prolonged periods. These factors limit its usefulness as a monitoring tool.

Cardiac Magnetic Resonance Imaging

cMRI is used to assess the size, morphology, and function of the right ventricle.[36] cMRI evaluates blood flow, stroke volume, cardiac output, and dimensions of the distended pulmonary artery and right ventricle noninvasively.[24] Poor function is indicated by the following:

- Stroke volume less than or equal to 25 mL/m^2
- Right ventricular end-diastolic pressure 84 mL/m^2 or greater
- RV dilation
- Left ventricular end-diastolic pressure 40 mL/m^2 or less
- Pulmonary artery stiffness measured by cross-sectional area change, with less than 16% change indicating increased mortality[25]

Contrast-enhanced MRI using gadolinium helps visualize chamber abnormalities and identify shunts or other congenital malformations. A gated technique, in which ECG-triggered measurements are made in the same phase of the cardiac cycle displays perfusion per heartbeat. Increased PVR leads to slower passage of contrast fluids through peripheral lung vasculature, resulting in the regional distribution no longer being determined by gravity.[40,41] An advantage of MRI is its ability to recreate a 3D image of the anatomy.[40] Rotating the 3D model provides views of the vascular structures from different directions and separates individual vascular structures from overlapping vessels.[18]

Echocardiography has both invasive (transesophageal) and noninvasive (transthoracic) techniques as previously described. In PAH, both methods can identify right atrial and RV enlargement, decrease in RV function, displacement of the septum,

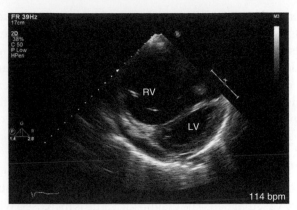

FIGURE 18-7 Echocardiogram in pulmonary hypertension with right heart dilation and flattened septum.

tricuspid regurgitation, pericardial effusion, and general appearance of the heart chambers (Figure 18-7).[42]

For group 2 pulmonary hypertension with left heart disease, Doppler examination is used to evaluate the mitral valve flow profile, mitral annulus tissue, and left atrium and LV dilation. Calculated indices include tricuspid excursion index (TEI), which is a measure of myocardial performance. TEI is an index of combined systolic and diastolic function obtained by dividing the sum of isovolumetric contraction and relaxation intervals by ejection time.[39] See Table 18-2 for this equation.

Transthoracic echocardiography, in which a noninvasive probe is moved across the chest, gives a view of structural changes and flow measurements in the heart and across cardiac valves. With transesophageal echocardiography the probe is positioned in the esophagus behind the heart and allows a clear picture of the left heart and pulmonary vein structures. Pulmonary arterial pressure is estimated on peak velocity of the tricuspid valve regurgitant jet by using the Bernoulli equation. See Table 18-2 for this equation. The equation describes the relationship of tricuspid valve velocity and peak pressure gradient of the tricuspid valve.[24] RV systolic pressure can then be estimated by adding this pressure gradient to the right atrial pressure. RV systolic pressure can be equated to the systolic pulmonary arterial pressure in the absence of pulmonic stenosis.[43,44] The measurement of pulmonary artery diameter is an early sign of the increased pressure in the pulmonary system and diagnostic of pulmonary hypertension. Indicators of PAH progression identified by echocardiography include right atrial enlargement septal bowing and pericardial effusion.[42]

Electrical bioimpedance tomography is another noninvasive measure used in some centers to quantify blood flow through the pulmonary vascular bed. Measuring the change in electrical impedance during the cardiac cycle reflects pulmonary blood volume changes. This procedure uses 8 to 16 electrodes in a ring around the chest at the third intercostal level. A constant current of 5 milliamperes (mA) or less is used to measures differences in electrical impedance. By measuring the differences between the electrodes, an image of impedance is constructed.[41] A systolic increase in blood volume will decrease impedance and decrease end-diastolic volume. Impedance changes are closely related to changes in PVR. Hypoxic vasoconstriction creates significantly increased impedance that will decrease with 100% oxygen administration without stroke volume or heart rate changes.[41]

Right Heart Catheterization

The combination of patient history, physical assessment and noninvasive diagnostic testing ideally lead to an accurate pulmonary hypertension diagnosis. However, for other patients, confirmation by right heart catheterization may be needed.[25] Although right heart catheterization is more invasive, it provides specific measurement of intra-cardiac pressures, hemodynamics, and oxygenation in the cardiopulmonary system. Normally, the pulmonary circulation is a high flow and low-pressure circuit.[45] The flow-directed pulmonary artery catheter (PAC) measures pressures in each heart chamber as it progresses from the vena cava through the right atrium across the tricuspid valve into the right ventricle across the pulmonary valve and into the pulmonary artery. See Chapter 5 for more information on pulmonary artery catheter insertion.

Right heart catheterization of patients with severe pulmonary hypertension necessitates unique technical requirements because of the high pressures and changes in these chambers.[46] Use of a flow-directed PAC, with a balloon tip that floats into the pulmonary arteriole, allows measurement of PAOP in several sections of the lung.[25,46] Right heart catheterization verifies if the patient meets criteria for diagnosis of PAH, which is defined as follows:

- Baseline mean PAP of greater than 25 mm Hg at rest
- PAOP, left atrial pressure, or LV end-diastolic pressure of 15 mm Hg or less
- PVR greater than 3 Wood units[25]

Wood units are the original or "hybrid" measure of PVR. The calculation of Wood units uses mm Hg/L/min/m^2 for calculation. Multiplying this result by 80 converts the number into pressure measures in dynes·sec/cm^5. Refer to Table 18-2 for this equation. PVR is based on Ohms law calculating a ratio of decrease in pressure between two points and flow through a segment. Previous definitions of PH included mPAP 30 mm Hg or greater with exercise; however, research has not validated that definition, so the simpler definition of "increase at rest" is used currently.[22] A PAOP value below 15 mm Hg will rule out LV and pulmonary venous disease for group identification.[42]

With right heart catheterization, clarification of pressures, structural changes, and oximetry measurements throughout the heart, as well as results of the acute vasodilator test help identify the cause of pulmonary hypertension and identification of the most effective treatments.[25] Precise analysis of mixed venous oxygen saturations during passage through the heart chambers helps with intracardiac shunt diagnosis. Fick determination of cardiac output using these measures of oxygen consumption is more accurate in patients with tricuspid regurgitation.[37]

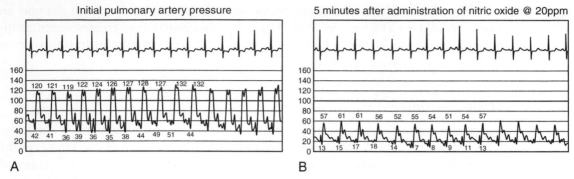

FIGURE 18-8 Vasoreactivity test. **A,** Initial elevated pulmonary artery pressures, indicative of pulmonary hypertension. **B,** Fall in pulmonary artery pressures five minutes after administration of inhaled nitric oxide at 20 parts per million (ppm). This result, where the mean pulmonary artery pressure is less than 40 mm Hg, indicates the patient is a responder to the vasoreactivity test.

Acute Vasoreactivity Test

The acute vasodilator (vasoreactivity) test is performed during right heart catheterization by administering a potent vasodilator such as inhaled nitric oxide or IV adenosine and measuring the resultant difference in pulmonary artery pressure, as shown in Figure 18-8. Acute vasoreactivity is defined as a fall in mPAP of at least 10 mm Hg to an absolute mean value less than 40 mm Hg and an unchanged or increased cardiac output.[33,38] Vasoreactivity is an important factor to identify in patients who will benefit from administration of long-acting oral calcium channel blockers.

Right heart catheterization is an invasive procedure and precautions to ensure patient safety are essential. The rate of serious complications in patients with pulmonary hypertension about 1% in settings with experienced practitioners.[47] The most frequent complications are related to venous access (hematoma or pneumothorax), followed by tachyarrhythmias and hypotension as a consequence of a vasoreactivity test or a vasovagal reaction.[47]

Treatment of Pulmonary Hypertension

Treatments include anticoagulation, diuresis, digoxin, oral vasodilators, and oxygen. Once the diagnosis is verified, treatment focuses on controlling symptoms with medications, monitoring disease progression, adapting to the long-term progressive disease, and planning for the possibility of lung transplantation in some scenarios. A treatment algorithm for pulmonary hypertension is shown in Figure 18-9. The goals of treatment include the following:

- Improvement in symptoms
- Improvement in functional class
- Lowering of pulmonary arterial pressure
- Normalization of cardiac output
- Delaying disease progression
- Improving survival

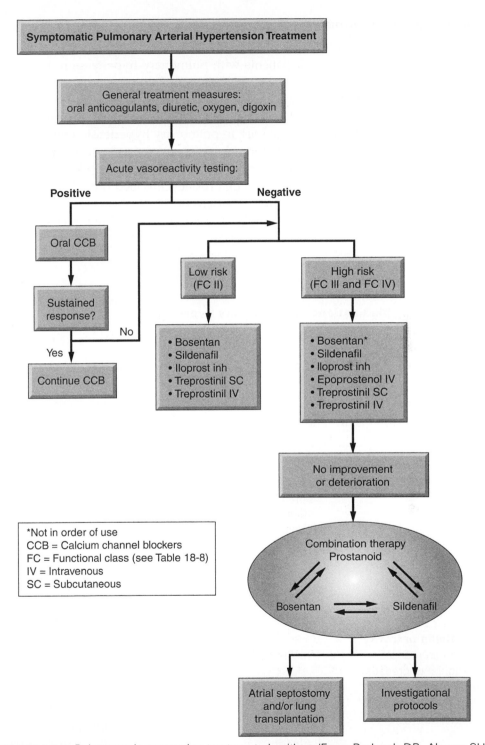

FIGURE 18-9 Pulmonary hypertension treatment algorithm. (From Badesch DB, Abman SH, Simonneau G, et al.: Medical therapy for pulmonary arterial hypertension: updated ACCP evidence-based clinical practice guidelines, *Chest* 131:1917–1928, 2007.)

Medications in Pulmonary Hypertension

Identification of vasoreactivity with initial right heart catheterization directs medication treatment choices for patients with pulmonary hypertension. Patients with a positive vasoreactivity test will benefit from the use of long-acting calcium channel blockers. Routine use without testing is discouraged as calcium channel blockers can cause potentially fatal cardiogenic shock in nonresponders.[48] The smooth muscle relaxation effects from calcium channel blockers work in pulmonary hypertension by decreasing PVR.

Medication treatments for pulmonary hypertension exist in three categories based on the areas of impaired endothelial function: (1) phosphodiesterase type 5 (PDE-5), (2) endothelin antagonist, and (3) prostacyclins. See Table 18-7 for a list of medications used in treating pulmonary hypertension.

All the medication classifications for pulmonary hypertension treatment work to promote vasodilation and decrease cellular proliferation. Phosphodiesterase type-5 inhibitors work by blocking cellular enzymes that regulate vascular tone, which results in vasodilation and antiproliferative effects.

TABLE 18-7   Medications for Pulmonary Hypertension

DISEASE PATHWAY	MEDICATION: GENERIC (TRADE) NAME	ROUTE	SIDE EFFECTS
Prostacyclin pathway Dilates pulmonary and systemic vessels; inhibits platelet	Iloprost (Ventavis)	Inhaled	Flushing, hypotension, cough, headache; jaw pain, trismus
	Treprostinil (Tyvaso)	Inhaled	Headache, cough, flushing, epistaxis, throat irritation
	Epoprostenol sodium (Flolan; Veletri)	Intravenous (IV) infusion	Rebound pulmonary hypertension if abrupt decrease or stop the epoprostenol infusion; headache, nausea and vomiting, jaw pain, flushing, hypotension
	Treprostinil sodium (Remodulin)	IV or subcutaneous infusion	Headache, nausea and vomiting, infusion site pain, headache, rash, jaw pain, flulike symptoms
Endothelin pathway Endothelin receptor antagonist decreases pulmonary vascular resistance (PVR)	Bosentan (Tracleer)	Oral	Respiratory tract infections, hepatic failure, headache, edema, anemia, chest pain, syncope, teratotoxicity, decreased sperm count
	Ambrisentan (Letairis)	Oral	Edema, flushing, nasal congestion, palpitations, decreased sperm count, potential hepatotoxicity, teratotoxicity

TABLE 18-7 **Medications for Pulmonary Hypertension—cont'd**			
DISEASE PATHWAY	**MEDICATION: GENERIC (TRADE) NAME**	**ROUTE**	**SIDE EFFECTS**
Nitric oxide pathway Phosphodiesterase-5 inhibitor, vasodilator	Tadalafil (Adcirca)	Oral	Hypotension, headache, flushing, myalgia, respiratory tract infections, hearing or vision loss
	Sildenafil (Revatio)	Oral	Dyspnea, hypotension, headache, flushing, epistaxis, hearing loss
Calcium channel blockers block calcium influx into cell, relax smooth muscle, decrease PVR	Nifedipine (Procardia XL)	Oral	Angina, hypotension, edema, headache, fatigue
	Diltiazem (Cardizem CD)	Oral	Bradycardia, hypotension, syncope, headache, rash, heart block
	Amlodipine (Norvasc)	Oral	Angina, hypotension, edema, headache, fatigue, palpitations

Data from Paul J: *AHA Pulmonary arterial hypertension study guide*, Overland Park, KS, 2010, Ascend Integrated Media.

Endothelin receptor antagonists block the potent effects of vasoconstriction and mitogenesis of endothelin-1. This action leads to a release of vasodilator and antiproliferative substances that decrease the narrowing of pulmonary arteries and obstructive lesions of pulmonary hypertension.

Prostacyclin is a potent vasodilator with platelet aggregation inhibition and antiproliferative actions. These medications improve pulmonary hypertension by decreasing resistance and the narrowing of affected vessels. The initial preparations of epoprostenol had a very short half-life (3–5 minutes) and were stable at room temperature for only 8 hours. Newer preparations, including treprostinil (Remodulin) and epoprostenol (Veletri), have improved both of these limitations.[24]

Combination therapies of pulmonary hypertension medications improve hemodynamics and delay disease progression. Many patients report improvement in their symptoms and activity with combination therapy regimens.[49]

Group 2 pulmonary hypertension caused by left heart disease starts as pulmonary venous hypertension with increase in pulmonary artery resistance over time[25] (see Figure 18-5). Usual causes of left heart failure include systolic dysfunction, diastolic dysfunction, or mitral valve dysfunction, each leading to acute left ventricular end-diastolic pressure elevation measured as an elevated PAOP pressure. Left heart failure is measured by changes in transpulmonary gradient, with results of greater than 12 mm Hg reflecting changes in pulmonary circulation. Persistent transpulmonary gradient elevations greater than 15 mm Hg pose an increased risk for RV failure and early postcardiac surgical mortality.[24] Treatments focus on underlying left heart disease and includes diuretics, nitrates, hydralazine, angiotensin-converting enzyme inhibitors, beta blockers, nesiritide, inotropic support, left ventricular assist device (LVAD) support, and heart transplantation.[24,25]

Pulmonary hypertension following cardiac and thoracic surgery is thought to be the result of endothelial and parenchymal insult from cardiopulmonary bypass or reperfusion injury. Treatments include use of inhaled nitric oxide, sildenafil, and prostacyclin. If the failure includes hypotension, dobutamine and milrinone have been used.

Monitoring Symptom Progression in Pulmonary Hypertension

Progression is measured by symptoms and activity intolerance as defined by the WHO functional class for pulmonary hypertension shown in Table 18-8. This classification system is modeled after the NYHA functional class system[50] (see Table 17-3 in Chapter 17). The patient's ability to perform activities of daily living drives this model. The pulmonary hypertension–specific classification is designed to focus evaluation of progression and treatments. In general, patients with more severe pulmonary hypertension tend to have a higher functional class, indicating greater disease severity.[50,51] Some limitations exist for using functional class, as it can be difficult to quantify and assessment can vary among patients and care givers. It has shown correlation with outcomes, yet may not always correlate with other measures of disease severity. Health care professionals need to consider other variables, including signs and symptoms of right heart failure, hemodynamics, 6MWD, and side effects of treatments when evaluating disease progression.[33] Measuring the distance walked in 6 minutes is a simple measure of exercise capacity that is inexpensive, reproducible, and used as standardized measure for pulmonary hypertension patients progression.[24] Standardizing differences in age, height, and weight may improve the usefulness of this test for calculating predicted 6MWD.[35]

Patient Safety

It is important to verify the normal oximetry range for the patient with pulmonary hypertension, as some patients may be hypoxic by normal standards. Additional oxygen may worsen their clinical condition by decreasing the trigger to breathe.

Surgical Treatments for Pulmonary Hypertension

Worsening right heart failure leads to more advanced treatment decisions. Graded atrial balloon dilation septostomy is used as an emergency treatment or as a bridge to transplantation. This procedure creates a right-to-left shunt, which decreases right

TABLE 18-8	**WHO Functional Class for Pulmonary Hypertension**
CLASS	**SYMPTOMS**
Class I	Patients with pulmonary hypertension but without resulting limitation of physical activity—ordinary physical activity does not cause undue dyspnea or fatigue, chest pain, or near syncope.
Class II	Patients with pulmonary hypertension resulting in slight limitation of physical activity—comfortable at rest; ordinary physical activity causes undue dyspnea or fatigue, chest pain, or near syncope.
Class III	Patients with pulmonary hypertension resulting in marked limitation of physical activity—comfortable at rest; less than ordinary activity causes undue dyspnea or fatigue, chest pain, or near syncope.
Class IV	Patients with pulmonary hypertension with inability to carry out any physical activity without symptoms—manifest signs of right heart failure; dyspnea, fatigue, or both may be present even at rest; discomfort is increased by any physical activity.

Modified from Barst RJ, McGoon M, Torbicki A, et al.: Diagnosis and differential assessment of pulmonary arterial hypertension, *J Am Coll Cardiol* 43:40S–47S, 2004.

heart filling pressure and improves right heart function and left heart filling.[24] See Figure 18-3. The procedure uses intracardiac catheters to open the atrial septum in the area of the foramen ovale with progressively larger dilation catheters or a balloon dilation catheter to create a shunt.[42] Atrial septostomy carries a considerable risk, with a procedural mortality averaging 15% (5%–50%).[25]

Right ventricular assist device (RVAD) may be useful in acute postoperative heart failure or as a bridge to transplantation. Lung transplantation remains the gold standard for the treatment of pulmonary hypertension once medical therapy has failed and in most centers is discussed early in treatment planning.[52] Decline in functional status and hemodynamics to the point where survival without transplantation is unlikely leads to the transplantation decision. The options include single lung transplantation, bilateral lung transplantation, or heart–lung transplantation. With either single or bilateral lung transplantation, the right heart recovers quickly with a rapid decrease in PVR.[52] Although single lung transplantation is technically easier with less ischemic time and bypass time, which results in early graft survival, bilateral lung transplantation is preferred. Bilateral lung transplantation increases functional reserve with less ventilation–perfusion mismatch and, according to the International Society of Heart and Lung Transplantation, has a significantly better survival rate.[52] The number of organs available for transplantation is significantly lower than the number of patients who need transplantation. This scarcity of available lungs for transplantation results in few patients having this option for treatment.

TABLE 18-9 Infection Prevention Tips for Central Venous Catheter Care with Prostanoids

General	Cuffed or tunneled catheter with minimal lumens or ports. Sterile barriers with insertion or aseptic technique for care. Do NOT submerge catheter in water; NO SWIMMING. Remove catheter if central line–associated bloodstream infection (CLABSI) documented. Negative blood culture before new central catheter inserted; verify clearance of bacteremia with blood cultures 4 days after start of antibiotic treatment.
Hand hygiene	Soap and water or waterless gel or foams before and after palpation of insertion sites; replacing, accessing, repairing, or changing dressing. Use of gloves does NOT obviate need for hand hygiene.
Catheter hub	Closed hub with needleless intravenous (IV) device recommended. Split valve type preferred over mechanical. Change hub device weekly and with blood draw. Minimize contamination by wiping with 70% alcohol. Access port ONLY with sterile device. Clean threads of central venous catheter (CVC) only when visibly soiled Be sure connection is dry before changing.
Catheter site	Aseptic technique for site care. Replace gauze dressing every 2 days; at least every 7 days if transparent. New tunneled CVC dressing no more than 1 time a week until healed. Gauze dressing preferred if patient is perspiring, or if site is leaking or oozing. Disinfect clean skin with antiseptic before insert and during dressing changes. 2% chlorhexidine–based preparation is preferred. Do not use topical antibiotics on insertion sites.
Prostanoid preparation	Unopened vials stored at room temperature; do not use beyond expiration date. Opened vials—Epoprostenol: single dose only; use manufacturer diluent Treprostinil: multi-use vials stable for 30 days; sterile normal saline or sterile water for diluent, limit number of vial punctures, store opened vial in refrigerator.
Prostanoid administration	Replace administration sets at least every 72 hours. Filters are recommended to remove particulate matter and air. Do NOT use catheter for administration of blood or total parenteral nutrition. Epoprostenol may be administered up to 48 hours after reconstitution if kept cold for total of 48 hours (24 hours in refrigerator and 24 hours with ice packs around cassette). Treprostinil may be administered up to 48 hours after reconstitution at room temperature.
Line flushes	Normal saline or heparin flushes single-dose vials are preferred. Prefilled syringes may be used on if "ready for sterile field."
Antibiotic lock solutions	Do NOT use routinely. Use only in special circumstances (multiple CLABSI with optimal treatments).
Prophylactic antibiotics	Do NOT administer intranasal or systemic prophylaxis routinely before insertion or during use of intravenous catheters.

Data from Doran AK, Ivy DD, Barst RJ, et al.: Guidelines for the prevention of central venous catheter-related blood stream infections with prostanoids therapy for pulmonary arterial hypertension, *Int J Clin Pract Suppl* 160:5–9, 2008.

Patient and Caregiver Considerations

Patients with pulmonary hypertension and their caregivers have many learning needs related to understanding the disease process, long-term effects of a progressive syndrome, and treatment options. For the newly diagnosed patient, education about the diagnostic procedures and preparation related to each procedure is important. These patients have often endured years of symptoms without a definitive diagnosis, and gaining their trust is vital for successful treatment planning. Centers of excellence for pulmonary hypertension have physician experts and nursing staff specially trained for complex patient care; multi-disciplinary support is essential.[25]

Patient care focuses on managing the typical symptoms of pulmonary hypertension including shortness of breath and fatigue. Once the initial diagnosis is made, re-admissions for patients with pulmonary hypertension are generally related to increased symptoms, disease progression, further testing, and infections. These patients and their family or other caregivers are active participants responsible for complex care outside of the hospital. This involvement requires ongoing emotional support and education of the care requirements during the patient's hospitalization.

As with any progressive end-stage disease, it is essential to develop a multi-disciplinary plan of care, with input from the team of physicians, nurses, pulmonary hypertension specialists, respiratory therapists, pharmacists, social workers, discharge planners, and palliative care specialists. Caregivers need support, as they provide emotional, medical and often financial support to the patient with pulmonary hypertension. These responsibilities, may increase the risk of depression in family caregivers.[53,54]

Case Study #2

D.J. is a 46-year-old female diagnosed with WHO group 1 pulmonary hypertension secondary to past use of the appetite suppressant medication fenfluramine (Anorexigen)[55] and a stimulant (methamphetamine). She was initially seen by her primary care physician for vague pulmonary symptoms and decreased exercise tolerance and had been treated for asthma in the outpatient setting. After several years of respiratory complaints, she was admitted with acute right heart failure symptoms and diagnosed with pulmonary hypertension. Her initial studies showed enlarged right atrial and right ventricular chambers with dilated pulmonary arteries on chest radiography.

Right heart catheterization revealed her RV systolic pressure was 68 mm Hg; right atrial pressure 12 mm Hg; with 1+ tricuspid regurgitation. She had a positive response to vasoreactivity testing and was started on nifedipine, sildenafil, warfarin, furosemide, and potassium. On discharge, she was classified as WHO functional class II. Within a few months, her 6MWD decreased from 500 meters (m) to 325 m, and her WHO functional class

Continued

Case Study #2—cont'd

progressed to III with symptoms on minimal exertion. Her pulmonary hypertension specialist added iloprost inhalation treatment, six times a day, which improved functional capacity, decreased her symptoms, and increased her ability to complete activities of daily living.

D.J. presented at her routine clinic visit with significantly increased symptoms, including shortness of breath with any activity. She had been frustrated by her inability to complete her grocery shopping without needing to sit down frequently. She was admitted to the intermediate critical care unit for further assessments and initiation of an IV prostacyclin infusion. Echocardiographic findings demonstrated markedly reduced RV systolic function, mild to moderate tricuspid regurgitation with an estimated RV systolic pressure of 108 mm Hg; right atrial pressure was 20 mm Hg. LV size and function were normal.

On admission, D.J. was visibly short of breath and anxious. Her husband was at her side and quickly explained that his wife was extremely tired, as she had not slept for days. He showed the nurse the iloprost inhalation materials and stated that he would continue to help his wife with these treatments. Nurses on this unit knew the couple and quickly made them comfortable. D.J.'s husband filled out the admission record of her current pulmonary hypertension medications. A new peripherally inserted central catheter (PICC) was placed for initiation of intravenous epoprostenol (Flolan).

The nurse practitioner, pharmacist, and bedside nurse spent time explaining the plan for initiating this infusion, including graduated increases with the goal of decreasing her symptoms and improving activity tolerance. Teaching included information about the possible side effects of headache, nausea, and vomiting, as well as jaw pain, flushing, and chest pain, that must be reported if they occur.

After several days, D.J. was ready to return home. Her mother, who was their backup support, came with inhalation treatment supplies from home, eager to ensure that these were used before the expiration date. The pharmacist was able to sit down with D.J.'s mother to make sure that she understood the need for aseptic techniques for the IV medication preparation and need for icing the solution to prolong its effectiveness. After final review of symptom management, instructions for IV infusion, line management, follow-up appointment, activity tolerance, low-salt diet, and other medications, D.J. was discharged home with her husband and mother. ■

Conclusion

Right heart failure is recognized as a significant cardiac condition independent of the left heart. Symptomatology and specific ECG changes are the primary defining differences between right and left heart failure, as the laboratory results are similar for both conditions. Early recognition is hampered by the vague nature of the initial symptoms.

Early recognition with treatments focused on optimizing preload, decreasing afterload, improving contractility, and addressing arrhythmias improve outcomes in this condition. Right heart failure may be caused by a variety of conditions, including pulmonary hypertension. Left heart failure is the leading cause of right heart failure.

Pulmonary hypertension is a complex, multi-disciplinary disorder with restricted blood flow through the pulmonary circulation. This results in increased PVR and ultimately heart failure. Multiple cellular pathways and tissues have been identified as potential target for research into treatments for pulmonary hypertension, including genetics, smooth muscle and endothelial cellular function. Identification, treatment, patient and caregiver education, and ongoing evaluation of prognosis are essential in this disease state. Noninvasive hemodynamic measures are useful in early diagnosis. Right heart catheterization remains the gold standard for definitive diagnosis, group identification, and treatment evaluation. With this progressive and potentially fatal disease, early recognition and treatment are essential to improving patient prognosis. The evolution of hemodynamic measures, and treatment may improve patient outcomes.

Patient Education

Pulmonary Hypertension

- Medications and side effects
  - Anticoagulation (warfarin with goal INR of 1.5–2.5)
  - Diuretics to manage RV volume overload
  - Oxygen to maintain saturation greater than 90%
  - Digoxin for right heart failure, low cardiac output, and atrial arrhythmias
  - Calcium channel blockers, if positive vasoreactivity test (see Figure 18-8)
- Symptoms to report to care providers
- Prevention of infection
- Exercise training
  - Avoidance of heavy physical activities or isometrics that may cause exertional syncope
- Hypoxic pulmonary vasoconstriction at high altitudes
- Sodium restriction
- Avoidance of pregnancy
  - Birth control preferences: surgical sterilization or barrier methods[23]

  For patients on continuous infusions, education specifics include the following:

1. Sterile preparation of solution
2. Storage
3. Pump function
4. Backup pump and supplies

Continued

Patient Education—cont'd

5. Need for light and temperature protection

6. Line maintenance

7. Site infection prevention techniques

8. Contact information for medication supplier or company representative

References

1. Vitarelli A, Terzano C: Do we have two hearts? New insights in right ventricular function supported by myocardial imaging echocardiography, *Heart Failure Rev* 15(1):39–61, 2010.

2. Voelkel NF, Quaife RA, Leinwand LA, et al.: Right ventricular function and failure: report of a National Heart, Lung, and Blood Institute working group on cellular and molecular mechanisms of right heart failure, *Circulation* 114(17):1883–1891, 2006.

3. Funk DJ, Jacobsohn E, Kumar A: Role of the venous return in critical illness and shock: part II-shock and mechanical ventilation, *Crit Care Med* 41(2):573–579, 2013.

4. Kagan A: Dynamic responses of the right ventricle following extensive damage by cauterization, *Circulation* 5(6):816–823, 1952.

5. Dell'Italia LJ: The right ventricle: anatomy, physiology, and clinical importance, *Curr Probl Cardiol* 16(10):653–720, 1991.

6. Haddad F, Hunt SA, Rosenthal DN, Murphy DJ: Right ventricular function in cardiovascular disease, part 1: Anatomy, physiology, aging, and functional assessment of the right ventricle, *Circulation* 117(11):1436–1448, 2008.

7. Price LC, Wort SJ, Finney SJ, et al.: Pulmonary vascular and right ventricular dysfunction in adult critical care: current and emerging options for management: a systematic literature review, *Crit Care* 14(5):R169, 2010.

8. Chin KM, Coghlan G: Characterizing the right ventricle: advancing our knowledge, *Am J Cardiol* 110(6 Suppl):3S–8S, 2012.

9. Basford JR: The law of Laplace and its relevance to contemporary medicine and rehabilitation, *Arch Phys Med Rehabil* 83(8):1165–1170, 2002.

10. Greyson CR: Right heart failure in the intensive care unit, *Curr Opin Crit Care* 18(5):424–431, 2012.

11. Haddad F, Doyle R, Murphy DJ, et al.: Right ventricular function in cardiovascular disease, part II: pathophysiology, clinical importance, and management of right ventricular failure, *Circulation* 117(13):1717–1731, 2008.

12. Castillo C, Tapson V: Right ventricular responses to massive and submassive pulmonary embolism, *Cardiol Clin* 30:233–241, 2012.

13. Braunwald E: Heart failure: an update, *Clin Pharmacl Thera* 94(4):430–432, 2013.

14. Linqvist P, Calcutteea A, Henein M: Echocardiography in the assessment of right heart function, *Eur J Echocardiogr* 9(2):224–234, 2008.

15. Hoeper MM, Granton J: Intensive care unit management of patients with severe pulmonary hypertension and right heart failure, *Am J Respir Crit Care Med* 184(10):1114–1124, 2011.

16. Funk DJ, Jacobsohn E, Kumar A: The role of venous return in critical illness and shock- part I: physiology, *Crit Care Med* 41(1):255–262, 2013.

17. Wilson SR, Ghio S, Scelsi L, et al.: Pulmonary hypertension and right ventricular dysfunction in left heart disease (group 2 pulmonary hypertension), *Prog Cardiovasc Dis* 55(2):104–118, 2012.

18. Novelline RA: The heart. In *Squires's fundamentals of radiology*, ed 6, Cambridge, MA, 2004, Harvard University Press, pp 192–193.

19. D'Andrea A, Salerno G, Scarfile R, et al.: Right ventricular myocardial function in patients with either idiopathic or ischemic dilated cardiomyopathy without clinical sign of right heart failure: effects of cardiac resynchronization therapy, *Pacing Clin Electrophysiol* 32(8):1017–1029, 2009.

20. Green EM, Givertz MM: Management of acute right ventricular failure in the intensive care unit, *Curr Heart Fail Rep* 9(3):228–235, 2012.

21. Jerath A: The successful management of severe protamine-induced pulmonary hypertension using inhaled prostacyclin, *Anesth Analg* 110:376–379, 2010.

22. Haraldsson A: The additive pulmonary vasodilatory effects of inhaled prostacyclin and inhaled milrinone in postcardiac surgical patients with pulmonary hypertension, *Anesth Analg* 93:1439–1445, 2001.

23. Campbell P, Takeuchi M, Bourgoun M, et al.: Right ventricular function, pulmonary pressure estimation, and clinical outcomes in cardiac resynchronization therapy, *Circ Heart Fail* 6 (3):435–442, 2013.

24. Galie N, Hoeper MM, Humbert M, et al.: Guidelines for the diagnosis and treatment of pulmonary hypertension: the Task Force for the Diagnosis and Treatment of Pulmonary Hypertension of the European Society of Cardiology (ESC) and the European Respiratory Society (ERS), endorsed by the International Society of Heart and Lung Transplantation (ISHLT), *Eur Heart J* 30(20):2493–2537, 2009.

25. McLaughlin VV, Archer SL, Badesch DB, et al.: ACCF/AHA 2009 expert consensus document on pulmonary hypertension: a report of the American College of Cardiology Foundation Task Force on Expert Consensus Documents and the American Heart Association: developed in collaboration with the American College of Chest Physicians, American Thoracic Society, and the Pulmonary Hypertension Association, *Circulation* 119(16):2250–2294, 2009.

26. Gupta V: Inhalation therapy for pulmonary hypertension, *Crit Rev Ther Drug Carrier Syst* 27 (4):313–370, 2010.

27. Simonneau G, Robbins IM, Beghetti M, et al.: Updated clinical classification of pulmonary hypertension, *J Am Coll Cardiol* 54(1 Suppl):S43–S54, 2009.

28. van Wolferen SA, Grunberg K, Vonk Noordegraaf A: Diagnosis and management of pulmonary hypertension over the past 100 years, *Respir Med* 101(3):389–398, 2007.

29. Gensini GF, Conti AA: A historical perspective on high altitude pulmonary edema, *Monaldi Arch Chest Dis* 60(1):45–47, 2003.

30. Richalet JP: The scientific observatories on Mont Blanc, *High Alt Med Biol* 2(1):57–68, 2001.

31. Wood P: Congenital heart disease; a review of its clinical aspects in the light of experience gained by means of modern techniques, II, *Br Med J* 2(4881):693–698, 1950.

32. Wood P: The Eisenmenger syndrome or pulmonary hypertension with reversed central shunt, *Br Med J* 2(5099):755–762, 1958.

33. Badesch DB, Abman SH, Simonneau G, et al.: Medical therapy for pulmonary arterial hypertension: updated ACCP evidence-based clinical practice guidelines, *Chest* 131(6):1917–1928, 2007.

34. *Genetics Home Reference website*, National Library of Medicine, National Institute of Health. http://ghr.nlm.nih.gov/condition/pulmonary-arterial-hypertension. Accessed September 6, 2014.

35. Rich S: Clinical insights into the pathogenesis of primary pulmonary hypertension, *Chest* 114(3 Suppl):237S–241S, 1998.

36. Widlitz AC, McDevitt S, Ward GR, et al.: Practical aspects of continuous intravenous treprostinil therapy, *Crit Care Nurse* 27(2):41–50, 2007.

37. Zamanian RT, Haddad F, Doyle RL, et al.: Management strategies for patients with pulmonary hypertension in the intensive care unit, *Crit Care Med* 35(9):2037–2050, 2007.

38. Badesch DB, Raskob GE, Elliott CG, et al.: Pulmonary arterial hypertension: baseline characteristics from the REVEAL Registry, *Chest* 137(2):376–387, 2010.

39. Peacock A, Keogh A, Humbert M: Endpoints in pulmonary arterial hypertension: the role of clinical worsening, *Curr Opin Pulm Med* 16(Suppl 1):S1–S9, 2010.

40. Benza R, Biederman R, Murali S, et al.: Role of cardiac magnetic resonance imaging in the management of patients with pulmonary arterial hypertension, *J Am Coll Cardiol* 52 (21):1683–1692, 2008.

41. Vonk-Noordegraaf A, van Wolferen SA, Marcus JT, et al.: Noninvasive assessment and monitoring of the pulmonary circulation, *Eur Respir J* 25(4):758–766, 2005.

42. Berkowitz DS, Coyne NG: Understanding primary pulmonary hypertension, *Crit Care Nurs Q* 26(1):28–34, 2003.

43. Janda S, Shahidi N, Gin K, et al.: Diagnostic accuracy of echocardiography for pulmonary hypertension: a systematic review and meta-analysis, *Heart* 97(8):612–622, 2011.

44. Zhang RF, Zhou L, Ma GF, et al.: Diagnostic value of transthoracic Doppler echocardiography in pulmonary hypertension: a meta-analysis, *Am J Hypertens* 23(12):1261–1264, 2010.

45. Naeije R: Pulmonary vascular function. In Peacock A, Naeije R, Rubin LJ, editors: *Pulmonary circulation, diseases and their treatment*, ed 3, London, 2011, Hodder Arnold, pp 5–13.

46. Bull TM, Bertron MG, Badesch DB: Cardiac catheterization of patients with pulmonary hypertension. In Peacock A, Naeije R, Rubin LJ, editors: *Pulmonary circulation, diseases and their treatment*, ed 3, London, 2011, Hodder Arnold, pp 159–168.

47. Hoeper MM, Lee SH, Voswinckel R, et al.: Complications of right heart catheterization procedures in patients with pulmonary hypertension in experienced centers, *J Am Coll Cardiol* 48:2546–2552, 2006.

48. Paul J: *Pulmonary arterial hypertension study guide*, Overland Park, 2010, American Heart Association Ascend Integrated Media.

49. Iheagwara NL: Pharmacologic treatment of pulmonary hypertension, *US Pharm* 35(8): HS11–HS22, 2010.

50. Barst RJ, McGoon M, Torbicki A, et al.: Diagnosis and differential assessment of pulmonary arterial hypertension, *J Am Coll Cardiol* 43(12 Suppl):40S–47S, 2004.

51. Doran A, Harris S, Goetz B: Advances in prostanoid infusion therapy for pulmonary arterial hypertension, *J Infus Nurs* 31(6):336–345, 2008.

52. Long J, Russo MJ, Muller C, et al.: Surgical treatment of pulmonary hypertension: Lung transplantation, *Pulm Circ* 1(3):327–333, 2011.

53. Hwang B, Howie-Esquivel J, Fleischmann KE, et al.: Family caregiving in pulmonary arterial hypertension, *Heart Lung* 41(1):26–34, 2012.

54. Doran AK, Ivy DD, Barst RJ, et al.: Guidelines for the prevention of central venous catheter-related blood stream infections with prostanoid therapy for pulmonary arterial hypertension, *Int J Clin Prac Suppl* 160:5–9, 2008.

55. Brown-Beasley MW: After fen-phen/Redux: cardiac and pulmonary sequelae implications for patient assessment, *J Emerg Nurs* 24(1):62–65, 1998.

56. Dadfarmay S, Berkowitz R, Kim B, et al.: Differentiating pulmonary arterial and pulmonary venous hypertension and implications for therapy, *Congest Heart Fail* 16:287–291, 2010.

Hemodynamic Management in Hypovolemia and Trauma

Paul Thurman, Kathryn Truter Von Rueden, and Roy Ball

19

Nearly constant evaluation of the severely injured trauma patient is vital during the resuscitation and critical care phases. Patients respond to the stress of traumatic injury with many physiologic changes. The trauma patient may deteriorate and fail to achieve physiologic stability as a result of systemic inflammatory response syndrome (SIRS) from the initial injuries. Additionally, instability may result from the massive fluid resuscitation or from injuries that may have been missed on admission. The potential for life-threatening complications demands early detection for prevention or treatment to increase the chances of survival.

Utilization of hemodynamic data is an important aspect of caring for trauma patients during the resuscitation and critical care phases. Hemodynamic assessment focuses on assessing adequacy of oxygen delivery to meet oxygen requirements and determining the endpoints of resuscitation. Ongoing monitoring of hemodynamic assessment data can serve as validating criteria for accurate diagnoses and the patient's tolerance of, and response to, interventions.

Initial admission and resuscitation parameters may include parameters such as heart rate; systolic, diastolic, and mean arterial pressure (MAP); central venous pressure (CVP); arterial waveform based cardiac output; dynamic volumetric parameters such as stroke volume variation (SVV) or pulse pressure variation (PPV); and tissue perfusion indices such as tissue oxygen saturation (StO_2) or sublingual capnometry. Through the perioperative and critical care phase, additional hemodynamic data may be acquired through a pulmonary artery catheter to evaluate the adequacy of oxygen delivery, oxygen utilization, and end organ tissue perfusion.

Epidemiology

Historically, trauma was considered a disease of young adults and teens. However, as the population of older adults in the United States continues to grow, the average

age of trauma patients has steadily increased with increasing numbers of older adult trauma patients.[1] For example, in a large academic medical center, of 6591 admissions in 2013, 20.2% were 65 years or older, compared with 14.3% in 2008.[2] Over 25% of patients in the 2013 National Trauma Data Bank were 65 years or older, compared with 19% in the 2008 Annual Report.[3] Because of the increased age of trauma patients, particular attention needs to be paid to the normal physiologic changes associated with aging, as well as the multiple comorbid conditions and related medication regimes that may be present.[4] Older patients, particularly those with pre-existing cardiovascular disease, may have significantly less cardiac reserve and tolerance for fluid overload or increased myocardial demands related to tachycardia, increased intravascular volume (preload), and elevated metabolic rate.[5]

The unique needs of this population necessitate alterations to the typical approaches to resuscitation and critical care practices. In the general population, a high percentage of older patients have comorbid conditions that affect cardiovascular function. From 2007 to 2010, over 70% of persons 60 to 79 years old and over 83% of those 80 years and older were reported to have hypertension, coronary heart disease, stroke, or heart failure.[6]

Table 19-1 shows the difference in the prevalence of cardiovascular diseases as the population ages.[6] Thus, the likelihood of older trauma patients having cardiovascular disease is very high and cardiac pharmacologic management can have a profound impact on the hemodynamic status and response to therapy following injury.[4,7] Pharmacologic considerations specifically relate to treatment of comorbid cardiovascular conditions, with medications such as aspirin and anticoagulants, beta-blockers, angiotensin-converting enzyme inhibitor or angiotensin receptor blocker (ARB) medications. These medications affect the patient's cardiovascular system, their ability to mount a physiologic stress response, and their hemodynamic status.[7]

These multiple issues in the aging trauma population have important implications for the reconsideration of resuscitation goals or endpoints, and specific, targeted management throughout their hospitalization.[4] The following case study is used as a basis of discussion throughout this chapter.

TABLE 19-1   Prevalence of Common Cardiovascular Diseases by Age, U.S.

	AGE 18–44 YEARS	AGE 45–64 YEARS	AGE ≥ 65 YEARS
Heart failure		2.7%	7.8%
Stroke		1.9%	9.7%
Congenital heart disease (CHD)	1.2%	8.7%	19.1%
Hypertension	12.7%	42.7%	71.8%

Data from National Institutes of Health: National Heart, Lung, and Blood Institute: *NHLBI fact book, fiscal year 2012* (February 2013). Bethesda, MD, 2012, NHLBI.

Case Study

J.W. is a 70-year-old male, who has been involved in a motor vehicle crash. He was a front-seat passenger of a car that sustained a side impact. Emergency medical services (EMS) arrived to find J.W. awake, complaining of right-side chest and abdominal pain and right lower extremity (RLE) deformity. He denied any loss of consciousness and is worried about his wife, who was a back-seat passenger. He had been extricated from the vehicle, with maintenance of spinal immobilization. EMS had noted a MedicAlert bracelet with a past medical history of coronary artery disease and the medications listed below.

J.W.'s Medications Prior to Admission
Aspirin
Metoprolol
Atorvastatin
Enalapril
Glucophage
Clopidogrel

His vital signs at the scene indicated hemorrhagic shock. Two large bore intravenous lines were started, and his right lower extremity was immobilized. He was transported to a Level I trauma center for evaluation and treatment.

J.W. arrives in the trauma resuscitation area in the emergency department (ED). He is awake but confused. His vital signs on admission indicate he is decompensating. He is intubated to protect his airway. His breath sounds are decreased on the right side. Chest radiography shows multiple rib fractures and a pneumothorax. A chest tube is placed, and breath sounds and his oxygen saturation improve. He remains hypotensive. A massive transfusion protocol is initiated. Focused abdominal sonography for trauma (FAST) reveals no fluid in J. W.'s abdomen and an extremity radiograph reveals a femur fracture. His vital signs are responding to the transfusion of blood products. His laboratory values confirm hemorrhagic shock is present. A large central line is placed for resuscitation, along with an arterial pressure line for continuous blood pressure monitoring.

J.W. is transported to radiology for computed tomography (CT) of his brain, spine, chest, abdomen, and pelvis. Injuries found include small remaining right pneumothorax, grade II liver laceration, pelvic fracture with hemorrhage, and right femur fracture. He is transported to the interventional radiology suite for angiography of the liver and pelvis. He undergoes embolization of bleeding pelvic blood vessels; however, his pelvic fractures

Continued

Case Study—cont'd

and femur fracture require immobilization. Because of his unstable condition, external fixation is performed to minimize anesthesia and operating time.

Following fracture immobilization, he is transported to the critical care unit for continued resuscitation and care. His injury had occurred 12 hours ago. He is assessed from head to toe to ensure no injuries were missed. His initial and 1-hour hemodynamic parameters and laboratory values indicate continued shock, as well as acidosis, coagulopathy, and hypothermia. An oximetric central venous catheter is placed, and the arterial pressure transducer is exchanged for an arterial-based continuous cardiac output transducer to assess oxygen delivery and supply-demand balance. These are connected to the monitoring equipment, which will provide additional information to guide his continued resuscitation.

His hemodynamic data indicate decreased cardiac output and hypovolemia. Additional blood products are administered to correct the hypovolemia. All fluids and blood products are warmed through a high-flow fluid warmer. He is also being warmed with a forced-air blanket. His cardiac output improves, although, he remains hypotensive. A vasopressor is added for blood pressure support.

As J.W. emerges from anesthesia, he follows all commands and indicates he is in pain. An opiate infusion, along with sedation, is initiated for comfort. This causes a decrease in blood pressure. His vasopressor is titrated to support arterial blood pressure, and an inotrope is titrated to support cardiac output, as the hypovolemia has resolved. His hemodynamic profile is improving, as are oxygen supply and demand. Laboratory values indicate his shock is resolving.

At 24 hours after J.W.'s motor vehicle crash, his heart rate begins to rise with a decrease in blood pressure. His hematocrit is stable; however, his hemodynamic parameters indicate hypovolemia. His abdomen is now tense. Intra-abdominal pressure, obtained from the urinary catheter, is elevated. The trauma surgeon performs a laparotomy for abdominal compartment syndrome. J.W.'s hemodynamic profile improves following this procedure.

After 4 days in the critical care unit, J.W.'s hemodynamic status has stabilized. He has been weaned off the vasopressor and the inotrope. His pain is controlled, and he is awake and calm. His chest drain, which reveals no air leak, is placed to water seal. The critical care team has cleared him for operative repair of his pelvic and femur fractures and closure of the laparotomy. After surgery, he returns to the critical care unit on a vasopressor. His hemodynamic values indicate some hypovolemia with hypotension. Blood products and fluids are administered because of marginal anemia. His vital signs improve with the transfusion, and he is weaned off the vasopressor. J.W. begins to awake. He indicates he has some pain. His opiate infusion is resumed.

The following morning, he is fully awake, mechanically ventilated, and has stable hemodynamic parameters. He passes a spontaneous breathing trial. J.W. is extubated and received supplemental oxygen via a facemask. He is able to state his name and is asking about his wife. He is told that his wife will be in to see him in the afternoon. J.W. is transferred to a rehabilitation facility 12 days after the motor vehicle crash. ∎

J.W.'S VITAL SIGNS AND HEMODYNAMIC PARAMETERS

TIME	RESUSCITATION			CRITICAL CARE										
	SCENE	ED ADMISSION	AFTER TRANSFUSION	INITIAL	ONE HOUR	TRANSFUSION	VASOPRESSOR	SEDATION AND ANALGESIA	INOTROPE	24 HOURS	POST LAPAROTOMY	4 DAYS	POST-OPERATIVE	5 DAYS
HR	92	98	86	96	94	82	78	71	82	96	78	80	89	78
Systolic/diastolic blood pressure (BP) mm Hg	94/70	86/68	102/74	89/53	88/54	90/52	110/66	90/62	108/60	84/56	112/64	110/66	88/58	124/72
Mean arterial pressure (MAP)	78	74	83	65	65	64	80	71	76	65	80	81	68	89
Pulse oximeter oxygen saturation (SpO$_2$)	92%	88%	99%	96%	96%	98%	98%	98%	98%	92%	98%	99%	96%	99%
Temperature (°C)	36°	36°	35°	34°	35°	36°	36.5°	37°		37.5°		37°	37°	
Central venous pressure (CVP) mm Hg				8	8	11	12	10	10	15	8	10	6	8
Cardiac output (L/min)/cardiac index (L/min/m^2)					4.2/2.1	5.4/2.8	5.1/2.6	4.4/2.2	5.8/2.9	3.8/1.9	5.9/3	5.8/2.9	4.3/2.2	5.7/2.9
Stroke volume variation (SVV) %					16%	8%	6%	7%	8%	18%	9%	8%	14%	6%
Central venous oxygen saturation (ScvO$_2$)					52%	60%	68%	64%	72%	51%	68%	74%	62%	76%
Arterial oxygen delivery (DaO$_2$)					432	716			731	440		692	465	726
Hemoglobin mg/dL		9.2		8.4	10.1				9.6	9.4		9.0	8.4	9.6
Hematocrit %		29		24	29				28	28		27	24	30
Lactate mmol/L		6.2		7.8	5.2				3.1	6.1		0.8	2.2	0.6

Continued

J.W.'S VITAL SIGNS AND HEMODYNAMIC PARAMETERS—CONT'D

TIME	RESUSCITATION							CRITICAL CARE						
	SCENE	ED ADMISSION	AFTER TRANSFUSION	INITIAL	ONE HOUR	TRANS-FUSION	VASO-PRESSOR	SEDATION AND ANALGESIA	INOTROPE	24 HOURS	POST LAPAROTOMY	4 DAYS	POST-OPERATIVE	5 DAYS
Prothrombin time (PT) seconds		22			16			14				14		
Partial thromboplastin time (PTT) seconds		34			28			24				25		
International normalized ratio (INR)		1.9			1.2			1.1				1.1		
pH		7.11			7.18			7.32		7.28	7.34	7.39	7.32	7.41
Partial pressure of arterial oxygen (PaO$_2$) mm Hg		68			72			84		64	86	92	78	89
Partial pressure of arterial carbon dioxide (PaCO$_2$) mm Hg		28			30			34		48	36	38	38	41
Bicarbonate (HCO$_3^-$) mEq/L		16			14			20		19	20	24	18	26
Base deficit		−12			−13.7			−5.6		−6.8	−4.5	−0.41	−8.2	1.8
Intra-abdominal pressure (IAP) mm Hg										26	11	8		
Body surface area				1.93										

Etiology of Traumatic Injuries

Injury without interruption of skin integrity is considered *blunt trauma*. Blunt trauma may be life threatening because the extent of the injury may be covert, making diagnosis difficult. Blunt forces transfer energy that causes tissue deformation. The nature of the injury is related to both the transfer of energy and the anatomic structures involved.[8]

Penetrating trauma refers to injury sustained by the transmission of energy to body tissues from a moving, projectile object that interrupts skin integrity, whereas blunt trauma produces tissue deformation by the transfer of energy. Penetrating trauma produces actual tissue penetration and may also cause surrounding tissue deformation based on the energy transferred by the penetrating object.[8]

Key Physiologic Concepts

Hemorrhagic Shock

Hemorrhagic shock is caused by a sudden loss of intravascular volume, as experienced in blood loss related to injury. Venous return to the heart is decreased, and this results in reduced cardiac output. Stimulation of the sympathetic nervous system and neurohormonal responses increases circulating blood volume to compensate for the blood loss (Figure 19-1). Until the hemorrhage is controlled and circulating volume is restored, the existing blood volume is shunted to the vital organs (heart, lungs, and brain), causing hypoperfusion to other organs such as the liver, stomach, and kidneys. Eventually, compensatory mechanisms become ineffective, causing cellular hypoperfusion and inability to meet cellular oxygen requirements for metabolism. The cells use anaerobic metabolism in an effort to meet their cellular adenosine triphosphate (ATP) requirements, resulting in lactic acidosis.

> **Clinical Reasoning Pearl**
>
> Trauma patients may present with or develop other shock etiologies such as cardiogenic shock. However, hemorrhagic shock is the most common shock state seen in this patient population.

Sympathetic stimulation to increase heart rate, contractility, and systemic vascular resistance (SVR) escalates the workload of the heart. Ejection of a higher volume of blood against an increased afterload further stresses the myocardium, causing an increase in myocardial metabolism and myocardial oxygen consumption (MvO_2). The continued lack of circulating volume reduces oxygen delivery to the heart, creating a vicious cycle. Circulatory collapse fails to provide end organ perfusion, with reduction in oxygen delivery, and forces a conversion to anaerobic (without oxygen) metabolism to meet cellular energy needs. Anaerobic metabolism cannot provide sufficient

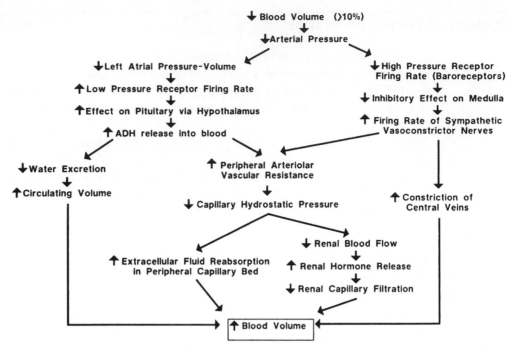

FIGURE 19-1 Compensatory mechanisms after loss of greater than 10% blood volume. (From McQuillan KA, Flynn MB, Whalen E, editors: *Trauma nursing: from resuscitation through rehabilitation*, ed 4, Philadelphia, 2008, WB Saunders.)

adenosine triphosphate (ATP) to meet energy demands; for further discussion on the impact of anaerobic metabolism see Chapter 6 and Figure 6-12. If the situation continues, myocardial fatigue, circulatory collapse, inadequate cell perfusion and ischemic damage may result in end organ failure (Figure 19-2).

Systemic Inflammatory Response Syndrome

Once a shock state develops, the subsequent course may have more to do with the physiologic response to shock, including activation of the sympathetic nervous system, the inflammatory response, and the immune system, rather than with the initial cause of the shock. Thus, shock can be considered a derangement of compensatory mechanisms that results in further circulatory and respiratory dysfunction with subsequent multiple organ damage.

Activation of the inflammatory response causes the release of cytokines from macrophages such as tumor necrosis factor-alpha (TNF-α) and interleukin-1 (IL-1). Normally, tight junctions exist between the endothelial cells that line blood vessels. Proinflammatory cytokines disrupt these tight junctions, causing the endothelial cells to separate, increasing capillary permeability and plasma leak into the interstitial spaces. The coagulation system is activated because of the endothelial cell separation and exposure of the sub-basement endothelial membrane. Platelets aggregate and adhere to endothelial cells and sub-basement membrane, forming platelet plugs.

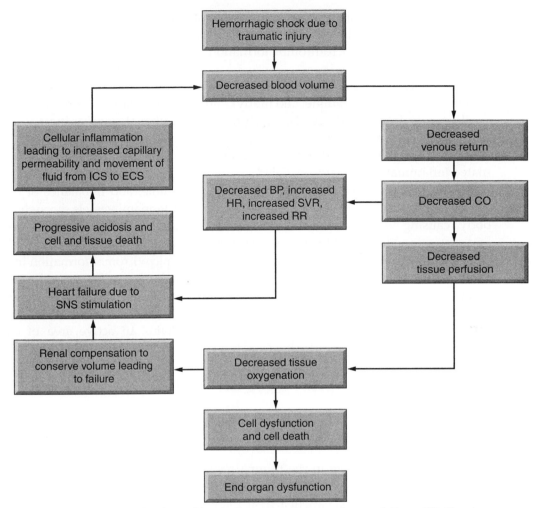

FIGURE 19-2 Hemorrhagic shock resulting in decompensation and organ failure. *BP*, Blood pressure; *CO*, cardiac output; *ECS*, extracellular space; *HR*, heart rate; *ICS*, intracellular space; *RR*, respiratory rate; *SNS*, sympathetic nervous system; *SVR*, systemic vascular resistance. (Adapted from Von Rueden KT, DesChamps E, Johnson K: SIRS, sepsis and shock. In Morton PG, Fontaine DK, Hudak CM, Gallo BM, editors: *Critical care nursing: a holistic approach,* ed 10, Philadelphia, 2013, Lippincott Williams & Wilkins.)

Fibrin, the end product of the coagulation cascade, forms strands around the clot to give it stability and strength.

Proinflammatory cytokines also attract phagocytic white blood cells (WBCs) to the area and activate the complement cascade. The combination of WBC activity and complement proteins may result in elimination of the invading microorganism.[9]

Endothelial cells that line blood vessels are central to the development of a local inflammatory response. Endothelial cells provide an anticoagulant surface and control permeability of vessels.[10] In a local inflammatory response, endothelial cells near the site of inflammation become activated as a result of mediators released by injured tissue cells. The activated endothelial cells express cell surface proteins that attract platelets and neutrophils. A procoagulant endothelial surface is formed in the area. Thus, in SIRS, increased coagulation, neutrophil aggregation, and impaired fibrinolytic mechanisms lead to microthrombi formation and reduced or obstructed capillary blood flow.[11]

WBCs, platelets, and activated endothelial cells release vasodilating substances such as nitric oxide (NO), histamine, and bradykinin. These substances promote additional capillary leak from blood vessels, which result in additional extravasation of plasma and coagulation factors.

In SIRS, the inflammatory response is systemic. The result is an overwhelming, unregulated inflammation with uncontrolled coagulation, disruption of capillaries, intravascular volume loss, maldistribution of circulating volume, and imbalance of oxygen supply and demand.[9] Endothelial cells are activated in many vessels throughout the body, causing widespread extravasation of fluid into the interstitial compartment and systemic activation of the immune system and coagulation cascade (Figure 19-3).

Substantial extravascular fluid accumulation and microthrombi formation in capillaries and in the interstitium decreases circulating blood volume, This cascade of events results in reduced perfusion of vital organs increasing the likelihood of multiple organ dysfunction syndrome (MODS) and death.

The complex interaction of SIRS mediators remains an active area of clinical research. Multiple mediators are believed to play a role in the maldistribution of blood flow, oxygen delivery and the consumption imbalance associated with SIRS and sepsis. Table 19-2 lists the key cellular mediators of SIRS and summarizes their activity.

Trauma Resuscitation Phase

Hemodynamic assessment in the trauma resuscitation area begins with a few basic indicators. Heart rate, noninvasive (cuff) blood pressure, and oxygen saturation measurements are taken upon patient arrival. Other hemodynamic parameters that can be measured in the trauma resuscitation area include central venous pressure (CVP), cardiac output and tissue oxygen saturation (StO_2). Clinical laboratory tests are frequently obtained in the trauma resuscitation area. Common tests include a basic chemistry panel, complete blood cell count (CBC), coagulation profile, arterial blood gas (ABG) and lactate.

Hemodynamic Assessment Parameters

Heart rate is one of the simplest vital signs to measure in the trauma resuscitation area. Of the three hemodynamic parameters measured upon patient arrival in the trauma resuscitation area, heart rate is the most sensitive to blood loss and actual or potential hemodynamic instability. Because the sympathetic nervous system and neurohormonal responses are activated to increase circulating blood volume and compensate for the blood loss, as previously described (see Figure 19-1), even small volume losses can result in an increase in heart rate.[8] Hemorrhage is not the only factor that can

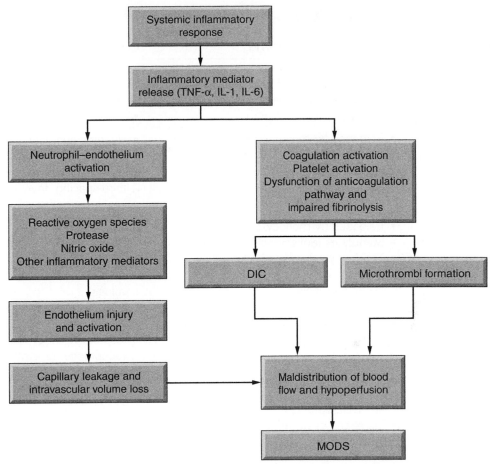

FIGURE 19-3 Inflammation, coagulation, and impaired fibrinolysis in systemic inflammatory response syndrome (SIRS) and multiple organ dysfunction syndrome. *DIC,* Disseminated intravascular coagulation; *IL,* interleukin; *MODS,* multiple organ dysfunction syndrome; *TNF-α,* tumor necrosis factor-alpha. (Adapted from Von Rueden KT, DesChamps E, Johnson K: SIRS, sepsis and shock. In Morton PG, Fontaine DK, Hudak CM, Gallo BM, editors: *Critical care nursing: a holistic approach,* ed 10, Philadelphia, 2013, Lippincott Williams & Wilkins.)

cause heart rate elevation in trauma patients. Pain is an expected complaint of any trauma patient and will cause an elevation in heart rate. Persistent tachycardia in the presence of adequate pain control should be interpreted as significant for volume loss until proven otherwise.

Blood pressure is not a reliable measure of actual end organ perfusion because of the multiple compensatory mechanisms activated by hypovolemia. In the resuscitation area noninvasive blood pressure via automated cuff blood pressure devices does help establish an important surrogate marker of perfusion until specific markers such as serum lactate, are obtained. Unlike heart rate, blood pressure abnormalities may not appear until significant blood loss has occurred.[8] A patient who presents to the trauma

TABLE 19-2 **Mediators of Inflammation**

MEDIATOR	DESCRIPTION OF ACTIVITY	CLINICAL RESPONSE
Endotoxin	• Activates complement system and coagulation cascades • Activates macrophages, which release TNF-α and IL-1	• Increased microvascular permeability, vasodilation, third-spacing, microthrombi formation • Inflammatory response
Tumor necrosis factor alpha (TNF-α)	• Released by monocyte–macrophages • Multiple effects locally and systemically • Stimulates other mediator activity	• Hypotension, tachycardia, myocardial depression, tachypnea, hyperglycemia, metabolic acidosis, third-spacing, fever, microvascular vasoconstriction
Interleukin-1 (IL-1)	• Released by monocyte–macrophages • Stimulates leukocytosis • Triggers production of acute phase proteins and release of amino acids from skeletal muscle • Activates procoagulant activity • Decreases vascular responsiveness to catecholamines	• Increased white blood cells • High urinary nitrogen excretion and muscle wasting • Elevated coagulation laboratory values • Decreased systemic vascular resistance (SVR), which is not as responsive to low dosages of vasopressor or synthetic catecholamine agents
Interleukin-6 (IL-6)	• Released by monocytes, helper T cells, and macrophages • Increases inflammatory response • B-cell stimulation and differentiation • Synergistic with IL-1	• Fever • Antibody secretion
Complement cascade	• Inflammatory process • Opsonization and lysis of foreign particles and cells • Stimulates neutrophils (and oxygen radicals) and IL-1 • Degranulation of mast cells and basophils	• Edema formation, vasodilation, vascular permeability, third-spacing • All effects of IL-1
Platelet aggregating factor (PAF)	• Released by mast cells, basophils, macrophages, neutrophils, platelets, and damaged endothelium • Increases platelet aggregation • Increases neutrophil adhesion • Increases vascular permeability and bronchoconstriction • Negative inotropic effects on the heart	• Microthrombi formation interfering with perfusion • Third-spacing • Bronchoconstriction, rhonchi, and wheezes, increased pulmonary airway pressures • Decreased heart contractility and force, which is not as responsive to low dosages of vasopressor and inotropic agents

TABLE 19-2	**Mediators of Inflammation—cont'd**	
MEDIATOR	**DESCRIPTION OF ACTIVITY**	**CLINICAL RESPONSE**
Arachidonic acid metabolites (AA)	• Stimulation of AA causes the release of metabolites prostaglandins (PG), thromboxanes (TX), and leukotrienes (LT) • PGF and TXA2 cause pulmonary hypertension, vasoconstriction, and platelet activation and aggregation • PGE, PGD, and prostacyclin cause vasodilation and decreased platelet aggregation • Leukotrienes increase neutrophil chemotaxis, vascular constriction, and vascular permeability • Increase gastric permeability to gram-negative bacteria • Inhibits leukocyte adhesion and platelets	• Oxygenation and ventilation difficulties, increased airway resistance, wheezing • Third-spacing and edema formation • Vasodilation, increased capillary permeability, and hypotension
Oxygen radicals	• Generate metabolites (O_2^-, H_2O_2, OH^-) during the respiratory burst of the neutrophils • Damage cell structure and interfere with cell activities • Damage endothelial cells, which stimulate the coagulation system • Increase permeability	• Inflammatory response, edema formation, fever • Microthrombi formation • Third-spacing

Adapted from Morton PG, Fontaine DK, et al., editors: *Critical care nursing: a holistic approach*, ed 10, Philadelphia, 2013, Lippincott Williams & Wilkins.

resuscitation area with hypotension should be assumed to be in profound shock. Transient blood pressure changes in the trauma patient should be viewed as a marker of intravascular volume status, as opposed to end organ perfusion. The normotensive trauma patient who develops transient hypotension with the administration of analgesia or sedation is likely to be hypovolemic. Analgesics and sedatives blunt the sympathetic nervous system response to trauma and hypotension. If the patient has sustained significant blood loss, hypotension will result.

Clinical Reasoning Pearl

Automatic blood pressure readings may overestimate blood pressure in hypotensive patients. Manual measurement is more accurate, but the procedure may be challenging during the resuscitation.

Davis J, Davis I, Bennink L, et al.: Are automated blood pressure measurements accurate in trauma patients? *J Trauma* 55(5):860–863, 2003.

Direct arterial blood pressure measurement via an arterial catheter and pressure monitoring system is an option in the trauma resuscitation area, although not a practical early monitoring strategy. Arterial cannulation may be challenging in some patients who are in hypovolemic shock, as vasoconstriction, low blood pressure, and low intravascular volume all conspire to raise the difficulty of the procedure. While inserting the catheter, direct arterial blood pressure monitoring may be challenging. The advantage of arterial pressure monitoring is that it provides continuous and more accurate data regarding blood pressure than noninvasive automated blood pressure devices.[12]

Indirect automated cuff pressures overestimate blood pressure in hypotensive states. Arterial pressure monitoring may also provide information at lower blood pressure than noninvasive devices are able to measure. As will be discussed later, there are direct arterial pressure systems that can be utilized to monitor cardiac output.

Practitioners need to be cognizant of the trauma patient's pre-existing medical conditions. For example, a patient with uncontrolled or untreated hypertension may experience the effects of hypotension at a significantly higher blood pressure than expected. Additionally, medications used to manage pre-existing conditions may significantly alter baseline hemodynamic parameters. A typical example is the patient taking a beta-blocker medication. A patient appropriately dosed on beta-blockers will not be able to elevate his or her heart rate as a compensatory response to blood loss.

Arterial Oxygenation Assessment

Arterial oxygen saturation is an important determinant of oxygen delivery. Assessment of arterial oxygen saturation by pulse oximetry (SpO_2) provides additional information related to the patient's hemodynamic status in the trauma resuscitation area. Oxygen saturation measurement reflects the amount of oxygen bound to hemoglobin that is available to the tissues and allows an estimation of the partial pressure of oxygen (PaO_2) dissolved in the plasma. Blood loss does not shift the oxyhemoglobin dissociation curve, so on initial presentation, a saturation of 90% still correlates with a PaO_2 of 60 mm Hg.[13] Because oxygen saturation is not impacted by blood loss, a reading of 100% simply means that even in the face of severe hemorrhage, the available hemoglobin is fully saturated with oxygen. This should not be misinterpreted as adequate perfusion. In a profound shock state, the body can deliver fully saturated hemoglobin to the tissues, but it may be insufficient to meet metabolic requirements or the cells may not extract the oxygen. New technology that helps measure the oxygen levels of peripheral tissue has been developed and will be discussed later in this chapter.

SpO_2 may also be misleading in other conditions. Oxygen saturation via SpO_2 may be difficult to assess in the patient with significant vasoconstriction, as most monitors are designed to measure the saturation in peripheral digits such as fingers. As arteries constrict, blood flow to the digits is reduced, and the sensor may not be able to detect an adequate signal. Hypothermia causes similar difficulties with accurate measurement.

Modern pulse oximeters include both waveform and signal quality indicators; oxygen saturation is most accurate in the presence of an appropriate waveform and high signal quality index. Another condition that impacts SpO_2, measurement in trauma patients, particularly if involved in a fire, is carbon monoxide inhalation and the formation of dyshemoglobins. In carbon monoxide poisoning cases, hemoglobin preferentially binds to carbon monoxide rather than to oxygen. As all of the hemoglobin's binding sites are filled, the oxygen saturation sensor will report a saturation level near 100%, even though the hemoglobin is bound with a compound that cannot contribute to tissue oxygen metabolism. Refer to Figure 6-7 and Table 6-2 in Chapter 6 for more information about measurement of oxygen saturation and carbon monoxide. ABG measurement via co-oximetry in the laboratory will provide accurate information about oxygen availability in these patients.[13]

Tissue Oxygen Assessment

Tissue oxygen saturation (StO_2) is a relatively new parameter for use in trauma patients. Similar to SpO_2, this technology uses near-infrared spectroscopy to measure the oxygen saturation via a noninvasive, single-use sensor placed on the thenar eminence (thumb muscle). Unlike SpO_2, which evaluates the percent hemoglobin saturated with oxygen in the arterial circulation, StO_2 evaluates the hemoglobin saturation of blood cells in the capillary beds of underlying tissues where cellular gas exchange occurs.

This parameter provides an assessment of perfusion as it evaluates oxygen uptake at the tissue level rather than oxygen delivery. A normal value for StO_2 is in the range of 86% to 90%; the lower the value, the more severe is the hypoperfusion of the tissue bed being monitored. Values in the range of 40% to 55% suggest severe shock in trauma patients.[14] Tissue oxygen saturation is well correlated with other markers of perfusion such as lactate and base deficit.[15] Recent studies have shown a correlation between StO_2 and mortality in patients requiring a massive transfusion.[16] Because it is noninvasive, StO_2 may be useful in the prehospital setting by paramedics or military medics. A recent study that examined the feasibility of prehospital use of StO_2, reported that baseline StO_2 measurements did not differ between survivors and nonsurvivors. However, when a vascular occlusion test was incorporated, a comparison of the pre- and postocclusion StO_2 was predictive of in-hospital mortality.[17]

Central Venous Pressure Assessment

Less commonly measured hemodynamic parameters during the resuscitation include CVP and cardiac output. CVP can provide some information about intravascular volume status and preload; however, it is not a reliable source of data to predict the patients need for additional volume as described in the Critical Care Phase section of this chapter. In addition, the upper torso is not a preferred site for central venous access during resuscitation. The relative complexity of vascular venous access makes the subclavian approach less than ideal and many patients present with the potential for cervical injury, thus eliminating the internal jugular as a site for cannulation.

TABLE 19-3   Estimated Blood Loss[1] Based on Patient's Initial Presentation

	CLASS			
	I	II	III	IV
Blood loss (mL)	up to 750	750–1500	1500–2000	>2000
Blood loss (% blood volume)	up to 15%	15%–30%	30%–40%	>40%
Pulse rate (BPM)	<100	100–120	120–140	>140
Systolic blood pressure	Normal	Normal	Decreased	Decreased
Pulse pressure (mm Hg)	Normal or increased	Decreased	Decreased	Decreased
Respiratory rate	14–20	20–30	30–40	>35
Urine output (mL/hr)	>30	20–30	5–15	Negligible
Central nervous system/ mental status	Slightly anxious	Mildly anxious	Anxious, confused	Confused, lethargic
Initial fluid replacement	Crystalloid	Crystalloid	Crystalloid and blood	Crystalloid and blood

BPM, Beats per minute; *hr*, hour; *mL*, milliliters.
[1]For a 70 kg man
From American College of Surgeons. Advanced trauma life support (ATLS®): the ninth edition, Chicago, IL, 2012, American College of Surgeons.

Case Study Discussion of Hemodynamic Assessment

The case study highlighted several potential pitfalls in the hemodynamic assessment of a seriously injured trauma patient. Emergency medical system (EMS) personnel reported vital sign of: heart rate, 92; BP 94/70; MAP 78; SpO_2, 92%. J.W.'s initial heart rate and blood pressure do not appear overly concerning; however, knowing that he is on beta-blocker and angiotensin-converting enzyme inhibitor medications for hypertension management changes the interpretation. J.W. will not be able to mount a normal tachycardic response to blood loss; thus, heart rate cannot be used as a reliable indicator of hypovolemia. Although a BP of 94/70 mm Hg may be normal in many trauma patients, for J.W., it is not normal and should be considered as hypotensive. Reviewing the EMS vital signs in light of J.W.'s medical history paints a picture of a patient who may be in class II or III shock (Table 19-3). On his arrival to the trauma center, J.W.'s shock is worsening: heart rate, 98; BP 86/68; MAP 74; SpO_2, 88%. J.W. still has not mounted a tachycardic response but is now hypotensive, secondary to significant blood loss, inadequate intravascular volume, and cardiac preload. The decreased oxygen saturation is likely caused by J.W.'s worsening pneumothorax. On

Case Study Discussion of Hemodynamic Assessment—cont'd

the basis of these vital signs, J.W. is diagnosed as being in hypovolemic shock, with insufficient intravascular volume to support cardiac output. He has decreased hemoglobin and inadequate arterial oxygen to support oxygen delivery to his tissues and vital organs.

Volume resuscitation with blood and blood components is indicated and discussed in the management section. The initial negative focused abdominal sonography for trauma (FAST) should not preclude the use of blood products for J.W.'s resuscitation. As identified by computed tomography (CT), J.W.'s liver injury and pelvic fracture are both sources of significant blood loss. J.W.'s confusion on admission could indicate a mild traumatic brain injury (TBI), so head CT is indicated. Yet, because the brain is acutely sensitive to reduced perfusion, any alterations in level of consciousness may also be an indicator of shock.

After transfusion in the resuscitation phase, J.W.'s vital signs improve, demonstrating the desired response to volume and blood administration therapy. Although the bleeding continues, the increase in blood pressure and decrease in heart rate support the appropriateness of the interventions and are positive signs. ∎

Cardiac Output Assessment

Cardiac output monitoring in trauma patients is more often implemented in the critical care unit. Use of arterial pressure waveform-based, less-invasive cardiac output monitoring (described in the Critical Care Phase) has not yet been widely adopted in the trauma resuscitation area. However, in trauma patients with pre-existing cardiovascular disease, monitoring cardiac output and stroke volume variation via an arterial catheter may be useful to avoid complications of overly aggressive volume administration. See Chapter 12 for more information on arterial waveform–based cardiac output monitoring.

Laboratory Assessments

Evaluation of shock in the trauma patient requires assessment of multiple laboratory tests in conjunction with hemodynamic monitoring. A typical battery of laboratory tests in the trauma resuscitation area includes basic chemistries, a CBC, and a coagulation panel consisting of partial thromboplastin time (PTT), prothrombin time (PT), and international normalized ratio (INR). These blood tests provide valuable information about a patient's baseline status but should not be utilized as the sole guideline for management in a severely injured trauma patient. The decision to transfuse is based on clinical presentation, heart rate, and blood pressure, as well as hemoglobin and hematocrit. Similarly, the decision to use fresh frozen plasma and platelets in the severely injured trauma patient is not determined by the results of the INR or the platelet count. An exception may be the patient with a severe traumatic brain injury. Brain tissue damage could activate the coagulation cascade, which may lead to clotting factor consumption and coagulopathies. Brain injured patients may require directed interventions with recombinant factor VII, fresh frozen plasma, and platelets to prevent or reduce further intracranial bleeding.[11]

Initial laboratory studies provide a measure of the adequacy of cellular oxygenation through evaluation of serum lactate or base deficit. These laboratory tests provide an early indication of end organ perfusion. Hypoperfusion of tissues leads to cellular hypoxia that results in anaerobic metabolism (which produces 2 ATP molecules versus 36 in aerobic metabolism), and pyruvate. Pyruvate is converted into lactic acid. Large quantities of hydrogen ions are generated in this process causing serum pH to decrease. As oxygen availability decreases to below metabolic requirements with hemorrhage, lactic production increases, and serum lactate measurements rise above the normal 2.2 millimeters per liter (mm/L). Elevated serum lactate levels in a severely hypovolemic patient may indicate the severity of shock, which is especially useful in patients who may show little hemodynamic evidence of their shock state, for example, those in compensated shock or on beta-blocker therapy.

Serum lactate levels in patients in shock have been demonstrated to correlate with outcome and have been utilized to guide resuscitation. A recent study found that in a wide variety of traumatized patients, both initial lactate and lactate clearance provide important prognostic information over and above traditional clinical predictors of mortality.[18] As reported, one of every eight patients who are not hypotensive but have a lactate of 4.0 milligrams per deciliter (mg/dL) or greater die, as do patients who have poor lactate clearance. A significant decrease in mortality is seen among patients whose lactate returns to normal levels within 24 hours of injury compared with those whose serum lactate level requires longer than 24 hours to normalize.[19]

Other physiologic conditions associated with traumatic injuries in addition to shock may cause an elevation in lactic acid levels. For example, alcohol toxicity or traumatic brain injury could cause seizures and result in an increased lactate level.[20,21] Thus, evaluation of the serum lactate level of a seriously injured patient who presents with post-injury seizures may be challenging.

Base deficit is another useful marker of end organ perfusion in the severely injured patient. Base deficit represents the actual deficit of base in the bloodstream in a patient with compensated or uncompensated acidosis. The production of lactic acid by tissues in anaerobic metabolism causes metabolic acidosis, and thus a base deficit, to develop. Even patients with compensated metabolic acidosis may have a measurable base deficit. Because base deficit is a component of ABG analysis, practitioners will also gain valuable information from the other components of blood gas analysis, including pH and PaO_2.[13] See Chapter 6 for additional information about arterial oxygen and acid–base monitoring.

Case Study Discussion of Serum Lactate and Base Deficit

J.W.'s laboratory values in the case study provide valuable insight into his condition. His lactate of 6.2 millimoles per liter (mmol/L) and base deficit of −12 are indicators of profound shock and are predictive of a high likelihood of death in light of his age.[22]

Case Study Discussion of Serum Lactate and Base Deficit—cont'd

As noted earlier, J.W.'s vital signs, in isolation, are not indicative of profound shock and hemodynamic instability. His laboratory values clearly show the depth of his shock and are not altered by his premorbid medication regime. Complicating J.W.'s assessment and management is his prior use of aspirin and clopidogrel, both of which impair platelet function, predispose him to additional intravascular volume loss and hypovolemia. Although J.W. will need platelet transfusions as part of his massive transfusion, his practitioners appreciate that his hemorrhage will be more difficult to control because of his medication regime. ■

Resuscitation Strategies to Optimize Hemodynamic Status

Hemodynamic management of the trauma patient is directed toward ensuring the adequacy of preload, cardiac output, SaO_2, and hemoglobin (the components of oxygen delivery as diagramed in Figure 7-2) to re-establish end organ perfusion. The two most common shock states in trauma— hypovolemic and distributive (neurogenic) shock— are both treated initially with volume resuscitation. This widely accepted principle has been the basis of trauma resuscitation management for decades and remains well supported by evidence.[11] More recent research studies have shown value in volume resuscitation. Damage control resuscitation, first described in 2007, encapsulates two key principles in the management of hemorrhagic shock in trauma: (1) permissive hypotension and (2) resuscitation with blood products.[23]

Permissive Hypotension

Permissive hypotension involves resuscitation of the severely bleeding trauma patient to a minimum blood pressure sufficient to ensure perfusion of critical organs and yet low enough to limit bleeding. Many severely injured trauma patients present to the trauma resuscitation area with active noncompressible hemorrhage such as intraabdominal bleeding, which can only be controlled by interventional radiology or surgical interventions. In this population, volume resuscitation to the traditionally normal blood pressure of 120/80 mm Hg could increase the rate of hemorrhage. Elevated blood pressure does not promote homeostasis because the higher pressures and increased blood flow may disrupt clot formation in damaged vessels. Permissive hypotension, usually resuscitation to a lower MAP, for example, a systolic blood pressure of 80 to 100 mm Hg (MAP approximately 60 mm Hg), will ensure adequate perfusion to critical organs while limiting the rate of hemorrhage.[8,24,25]

Permissive hypotension is a temporizing measure; it does not reverse a patient's shock state and so must be accompanied by definitive control of hemorrhage. Resuscitation to appropriate therapeutic endpoints occurs after definitive control of hemorrhage has been obtained. Exceptions to its use also exist. Patients with traumatic brain injury are acutely sensitive to hypotension, and any episodes of hypotension may worsen outcome. In the setting of acute hemorrhage with traumatic brain injury, the use of permissive hypotension cannot be recommended as a routine practice.

Clinical Reasoning Pearl

Facilities that receive severely injured patients should have a supply of "universal donor" packed red blood cells and thawed group AB or low-titer anti-B group A plasma available for immediate use.

Resuscitation with Blood Products

A second key component of damage control resuscitation is the use of blood and blood products rather than crystalloid. During the recent U.S. military engagements, blood component availability was limited, and injured soldiers were often resuscitated with whole blood rather than blood components. This experience highlighted the benefits of early blood use in resuscitation and the benefits of using whole blood or approximated whole blood.[26] Subsequent research has shown that utilizing blood components in a ratio that approximated whole blood, one unit of packed red blood cells with one unit of plasma and one unit of platelets, reduces mortality compared with resuscitation with large volumes of packed red blood cells with limited or no plasma and platelets.[23]

Patient Safety

Un–Cross-Matched versus Type-Specific versus Cross-Matched Blood Products

- During an emergency, un–cross-matched blood can be transfused while the blood bank performs the necessary tests for cross-matching. Type O blood is always used for un–cross-matched transfusions.

  - Type O negative blood should be reserved for women of childbearing age.

  - Type O positive blood should be used for all others.

- Type-specific blood products are matched to blood type and Rh status, a process that requires approximately 10 minutes. In an emergency, type-specific blood may be given to preserve the supply of un–cross-matched blood.

- Blood products are considered fully cross-matched when blood type (A, B, O), Rh status, and antigen screening have been established. Fully cross-matched products are the least likely to cause a transfusion reaction.

  - This process may require up to 1 hour or more to complete and may be complicated if the patient has received numerous transfusions in the past.

- Current recommendations from the American College of Surgeons state that resuscitation with blood products should utilize un–cross-matched units to begin, switch to type-specific blood, when available, then to cross-matched products.[1]

---

[1]American College of Surgeons Trauma Quality Improvement Program (TQIP): Massive transfusion in trauma guidelines, Chicago, 2013, American College of Surgeons.

Patient Safety

Emergency Line Placement

- Rapid placement of vascular access in the hemodynamically unstable patient may be extremely challenging.

  - Patients may already have vasoconstriction, which makes peripheral access with large-bore needles impossible.

  - The need for speed and the multitude of procedures required, especially in trauma or medical emergencies encountered in the ED, may make it difficult to follow the best practices for sterile line placement.

  - In these cases, central access may be achieved in less than ideal conditions.

- The use of intraosseous access should be considered as a bridge to central access.

  - The ability to initiate intraosseous access is limited by body habitus, not volume status or vasoconstriction.

  - Use of manual impact-driven or drill powered intraosseous devices has been recommended across a variety of clinical situations.[1]

- Central vascular access, including femoral arterial lines, placed emergently and without full sterile precautions, should be exchanged for an access placed under sterile conditions as soon as possible (within 48 hours).[2]

- Central vascular access placed emergently or without full sterile precautions should be marked as such. For example:

  - Use of a different dressing for emergently placed lines

  - Intravenous (IV) tubing marked or highlighted

---

[1]The Consortium on Intraosseous Vascular Access in Healthcare Practice: Recommendations for the use of intraosseous vascular access for emergent and nonemergent situations in various health care settings: a consensus paper, *Crit Care Nurse* 30(6), e1–e7, 2010.
[2]O'Grady N, Alexander M, Burns L, et al. and the Healthcare Infection Control Practices Advisory Committee: Guidelines for the prevention of intravascular catheter-related infections, *Am J Infect Control* 39: S1–S34, 2011.

Hemorrhage Control

As mentioned earlier, the severely injured trauma patient will require definitive control of hemorrhage before the shock state can be completely reversed. Traditionally, definitive control of hemorrhage was achieved in the surgical suite with time-consuming procedures to halt the hemorrhage and repair all identified injuries. In the past, on a surprisingly frequent basis, these patients would subsequently die in the critical care unit postoperatively.[27] During a damage control surgery, the surgeon focuses on halting any active hemorrhage and performs only the minimum procedures required to stabilize the patient. The patient is then transported to the critical care unit where resuscitation continues before the patient ultimately undergoes definitive repair of their injuries. This practice has become standard among trauma surgeons.[8]

Percutaneous interventional radiology procedures, once used only as a diagnostic tool, have become an important adjunct in the definitive control of hemorrhage. The use of interventional procedures for the definitive management of traumatic injuries was postulated in the 1970s[28] and is now a standard of care.[8]

Case Study Discussion of Hemorrhage Control

In the case study, J.W.'s management in the trauma resuscitation area follows current standard practices. He is resuscitated with blood via a massive transfusion protocol, has a chest tube placed for his pneumothorax, and undergoes appropriate diagnostic imaging. Prior to the widespread use of percutaneous catheter-based interventional radiology, J.W. would have required a laparotomy to evaluate his liver injury for ongoing bleeding and to pack his pelvis for hemorrhage control. Utilization of interventional radiology procedures spares J.W. from a complex open procedure. Thus, the only immediately necessary surgical procedure is the orthopedic stabilization of J.W.'s fractures. ■

Use of vasoconstrictor and positive inotropic agents is not commonly required in the resuscitation phase and is appropriate only after adequate intravascular volume replacement. In hemorrhagic shock, these vasoactive medications may worsen perfusion to end organs if intravascular volume is not restored prior to use.

Patient Comfort

Temperature Regulation
- Maintenance of normothermia is both essential and challenging in trauma patients, especially during the initial evaluation and resuscitation.[1]
  - A comprehensive trauma assessment requires removing all clothing to assess for occult injuries, thus exposing the patient to the environment.
  - Clothing may have been removed by prehospital care providers.
  - Administration of room-temperature intravenous fluids and refrigerated blood products may rapidly decrease the core temperature.
- Routine use of measures to maintain normothermia and prevent hypothermia.
  - Store intravenous fluids and blankets in a warming cabinet.
  - Use warm blankets for all admissions.
    - Remove any wet clothing or blankets.
  - Be prepared to use forced-air warming blankets, conductive-fabric warmers, or water-circulating warmers.

> **Patient Comfort—cont'd**
>
> - Consider the use of an underbody forced-air warming blanket to prevent chill from exposure.
>
> - Infuse all blood products and large volumes of crystalloid via a fluid warmer.
>
> - If the patient is intubated, use a warmed and humidified ventilator circuit.
>
> ---
>
> [1]Mizushima Y, Wang P, Cioffi W, et al.: Should normothermia be restored and maintained during resuscitation after trauma and bleeding? *J Trauma* 48(1):58–65, 2000.

Severely injured trauma patients are at significant risk for hypothermia, and the impact of hypothermia on resuscitation and hemodynamic status is an important consideration. The trauma patient may have been exposed to cool environmental temperature prior to admission, their clothing will have been removed as part of the primary assessment, and blood products or other fluids may have been infused at room temperature or lower until fluid-warming devices are attached to the infusions. Additionally, hemorrhage and shock can lower the core body temperature as circulating blood volume decreases and peripheral vasoconstriction occurs. As the core temperature is lowered, the coagulation cascade becomes less effective, causing hemorrhage to worsen and potentially leading to more profound hypovolemic shock and hemodynamic instability.

Case Study Discussion of Hypothermia

Early measurement of temperature showed J.W. to be hypothermic, and use of multiple warming methods are vital in his case. ◾

A final aspect in the resuscitation phase that will impact a patient's hemodynamic status is the administration of analgesics, sedatives, and anesthetic agents for pain relief and to perform the needed procedures and diagnostic tests. These medications may blunt the response of the sympathetic nervous system; therefore, trauma patients in hypovolemic shock may experience transient or prolonged hemodynamic sequela following sedative and opiate administration. Providers administering these medications must be cognizant of their effects and be prepared to respond to the resulting hemodynamic instability.

The hemodynamic-related parameters most frequently utilized to determine the end of resuscitation in the trauma resuscitation area are the aforementioned laboratory-based measures, lactate, and base deficit. These parameters, in addition to normalization of blood pressure and heart rate, are necessary to identify the re-establishment of adequate oxygen delivery to meet oxygen requirements. Frequently, severely injured patients require a definitive surgical or other intervention to control hemorrhage, and resuscitation may continue into the critical care phase. Thus, management of the severely injured patient often revolves around preventing further deterioration while the diagnostic workup is completed and injuries are identified.

Critical Care Phase

Hemodynamic Assessment Parameters

Clinical findings are directly related to the severity and acuity of volume loss (see Table 19-3). Some patients, especially older patients or those who have chronic diseases, have more subtle compensatory responses (Table 19-4), which may be overlooked. Serial assessments of physical and laboratory findings may uncover trends that guide treatment and mitigate SIRS, vascular collapse, and organ failure.

Heart rate increases because of the activation of the sympathetic nervous system. Severely injured patients with severe blood loss may continue to have an elevated heart rate despite adequate resuscitation for a number of reasons, including the inflammatory response to shock, pain and anxiety, fever, and many medications, especially sympathomimetic infusions. Trending the heart rate will provide a better picture than any one number in isolation.

Case Study Discussion of Heart Rate

In J.W.'s case, his heart rate is not greater than 100 beats per minute (beats/min). This most likely is related to his age and long-term use of a beta-blocker medication.[7] ■

TABLE 19-4   Considerations in Older Adult Trauma Patients That Impact Hemodynamic Status

Cardiovascular changes	Increased dysrhythmias, increased atrial size and irritability, left ventricular myocardial thickening leading to decreased compliance and lower ejection fraction; thickened heart valves that interfere with forward flow; decreased response to sympathetic nervous system; decreased sensitivity of baroreceptors; generalized stiffening of arterial vessels, including aorta
Pulmonary changes	Decreased tidal volume and respiratory muscle strength, decreased alveolar surface area, increased dead space at end expiration, decreased elastic recoil of lungs, increased resting respiratory rate, increased risk for infection as a result of decreased number of cilia, blunted response to hypoxemia, decreased gag and cough reflex leading to increased risk for infection, aspiration
Hematologic changes	Decreased ability of bone marrow to produce cells (red blood cells, white blood cells, platelets), increased anemia, decreased immune function (decreased production of T and B lymphocytes) leading to increased infections, lower baseline temperature, gradual changes in temperature in older adults versus spikes, increased risk for adverse drug reactions

Adapted from Morton PG, Fontaine DK, et al., editors: *Critical care nursing: a holistic approach*, ed 10, Philadelphia, 2013, Lippincott Williams & Wilkins.

Tachycardia shortens ventricular filling time, which negatively affects cardiac output. As heart rate increases, the diastolic period shortens, and preload is decreased. When heart rate is greater than 120 beats/min, diastole may become shorter than systole. This results in a reduction in ventricular filling volume and reduced cardiac output.

Continuous monitoring of arterial blood pressure provides useful information about the patient throughout resuscitation in the critical care unit. The MAP is used to evaluate organ perfusion. Vasoactive medications are titrated to achieve low-normal MAP, around 70 mm Hg. Most organ perfusion measurements can be estimated by subtracting the organ pressure from MAP such as intracranial pressure (ICP), intra-abdominal pressure (IAP), and pulmonary artery occlusion pressure (PAOP). Pulse pressure, defined as the difference between the systolic and diastolic blood pressure, is proportional to the patient's stroke volume and inversely related to compliance of the aorta. This measurement aids the clinician to determine cardiac function and fluid status. The narrower the pulse pressure, the lower is the stroke volume.

CVP traditionally has been used to gauge the patient's intravascular volume status and preload. The CVP is believed to be an indicator of right-ventricular end-diastolic volume index, which in turn, is believed to be an indicator of preload responsiveness. Trending CVP values may assist with assessing preload; however, this pressure may be affected by many factors. As vasoconstriction occurs, the venous reserve supports preload, so CVP may not decrease as expected in hypovolemia. Conversely, increases in intrathoracic pressure caused by mechanical ventilation, tension pneumothorax, cardiac tamponade, or, as in J.W.'s case, increased intra-abdominal pressure, may result in an increase in CVP that is reflective of intrathoracic pressure, not of intravascular volume. In hypervolemia, the CVP may not be elevated until the right ventricle fails.[29]

A recent meta-analysis concluded that no data exist to support the widespread use of CVP to guide fluid therapy and that utilizing CVP during fluid resuscitation lacks a scientific basis and thus should be abandoned.[30] This meta-analysis examined 43 studies that reported the correlation between the CVP and change in cardiac performance following a fluid challenge, passive leg raise maneuver, postural change, or positive end-expiratory pressure (PEEP) challenge.

Because of the challenges that the curvilinear shape of the pressure–volume curve presents, interest in measuring other surrogates of preload in trauma and other

Case Study Discussion of Fluid Administration and Ventricular Compliance

Because of the curvilinear shape of the ventricular pressure–volume curve, a poor relationship exists between ventricular filling pressure and ventricular volume (preload), as illustrated in Figure 16-1 in Chapter 16. This relationship is further disturbed by diastolic dysfunction and altered ventricular compliance that could occur because of J.W.'s coronary artery disease and critical illness. ∎

populations has increased. Ultrasonography has been suggested as a useful noninvasive tool for the detection of hypovolemia and assessment of the response to volume administration. Two possible sonographic markers as a surrogate for hypovolemia are the diameters of the inferior vena cava and the right ventricle. The inferior vena cava is a highly collapsible major vein, and its diameter closely correlates with right-sided preload and cardiac function (see Figure 11-12 in Chapter 11). The inferior vena cava diameter is not affected by the normal compensatory vasoconstrictor response to volume loss. Zengin et al. found that the inferior vena cava and RV diameters may be beneficial for the early detection of hypovolemia and in trending the impact of fluid replacement. The inferior vena cava and RV diameters are more sensitive compared with conventional parameters of blood pressure and heart rate in diagnosing hypovolemia.[29]

Cardiac Output Monitoring

Cardiac output provides clinicians with additional information to ensure adequate resuscitation. Cardiac output, along with hemoglobin and SaO_2, is a major determinant of oxygen delivery. Cardiac output is increased or decreased as oxygen demands increase or decrease. An increased or decreased cardiac output provides global information only and needs to be evaluated in light of the components affecting heart rate and stroke volume, which are determined by preload, contractility, and afterload. Clinicians may administer fluid boluses while monitoring cardiac output to determine adequate preload. If cardiac output increases, this indicates that the trauma patient is inadequately volume resuscitated. A "normal" cardiac output may be inadequate to meet oxygen demands in some trauma patients. Those with adequate intravascular fluid volume may require the addition of an inotrope to increase cardiac output if indicators of hypoperfusion such as lactate or low venous oxygen saturation persist.

In the past, cardiac output required the use of a pulmonary artery catheter (PAC), making it difficult to obtain at times. A marker (thermodilution, dye, or lithium) was injected, and the concentration of the marker was measured as it passed by a sensor on the catheter. A thermodilution cardiac output waveform was generated, and the monitor calculated the output from it.

Uses of arterial pressures, arterial waveforms, or both are newer methods for determining cardiac output and stroke volume. The basic premise relates to the proportional relationship of pulse pressure to stroke volume and the inverse relationship of pulse pressure to aortic compliance. These methods determine the stroke volume through interpretation of the arterial pressure or waveform, which is multiplied by heart rate to obtain the cardiac output. General components required for these methods are an existing arterial line, a special sensor, and specific monitor that uses a unique algorithm for the stroke volume and cardiac output determinations. Arterial-based cardiac output systems are described in more detail in Chapter 12.

These systems can be quickly set up without the need for additional invasive lines. They also provide "dynamic" hemodynamic parameters such as stroke volume variation (SVV), pulse pressure variation (PVV), taking advantage of the natural phenomenon that occurs during the normal respiratory cycle when the arterial pressure falls during inspiration and rises during expiration because of intrathoracic pressure changes. The reverse occurs in the patient who is mechanically ventilated. SVV and PVV have been shown to be better predictors of fluid responsiveness compared with static measures such as CVP and right atrial pressure in the critically ill.[31]

Patient Safety

Hemodynamic Considerations during Patient Transport

- Trauma patients will frequently need to leave the supportive environment of the critical care unit for diagnostic tests and procedures, including CT, interventional radiology procedures, and surgery, even when they are hemodynamically unstable or are maintained on high levels of hemodynamic and ventilatory support.

- Accurate monitoring of key hemodynamic parameters is vital during patient transport and time out of the critical care environment.

  - Care should be taken when selecting parameters to monitor during transport, even though not every parameter will need to be monitored.

- Important parameters to consider monitoring during transport are as follows:

  - Electrocardiography (ECG) for heart rate and rhythm

  - SpO_2

  - Arterial blood pressure and waveform

  - Pulmonary artery pressure and waveform for immediate identification of accidental PA occlusion. The PAC may migrate forward, and a spontaneous wedge pressure waveform may be seen, or it may slip backward into the right ventricle and a classic RV waveform may be observed.

- It may be necessary to add additional monitoring prior to the initiation.

  - For example, the patient with a traumatic brain injury may need an intracranial pressure monitor or ventriculostomy prior to the initiation of an interventional radiology procedure, as clinical neurologic assessments will not be possible in this situation.

Case Study Discussion of Cardiac Output

J.W.'s cardiac output initially increases with the administration of fluid, and subsequently preload improves. As he becomes euvolemic, the cardiac output no longer increases with additional volume administration. Because he continues to show signs of hypoperfusion, an inotrope is initiated to improve oxygen delivery. ■

Venous Oxygen Saturation Monitoring

Mixed venous oxygen saturation (SvO_2) traditionally has been used to evaluate oxygen consumption. The mixed venous oxygen content could be subtracted from the arterial oxygen content to estimate oxygen consumption, which approximates 25% of available oxygen. Normal SaO_2 is 100% and SvO_2 approximates 75%. When oxygen supply is reduced or the demand is increased, SvO_2 will fall, reflecting the increased oxygen extraction to meet metabolic requirements. Obtaining true mixed SvO_2 requires the use of a pulmonary artery catheter. Oxygen saturation from a central venous catheter (CVC) may be used as a surrogate. Oxygen saturation levels from the CVC are influenced by the catheter tip location; the closer the location to the right atrium, the more closely the central SvO_2 ($ScvO_2$) correlates with the mixed SvO_2 levels.[32] See Chapter 7 for more information on venous oxygen monitoring (SvO_2 and $ScvO_2$).

Case Study Discussion of Venous Oxygen Saturation Monitoring

The use of cardiac output, hemoglobin, SaO_2, and SvO_2 measurements provides the clinician with the determinants of oxygen delivery and consumption. On the basis of J.W.'s low cardiac output, oxygen delivery is considered inadequate for the demand, resulting in a compensatory increase in oxygen extraction, as suggested by the low $ScvO_2$. Increasing J.W.'s hemoglobin through blood transfusion, improves the oxygen-carrying capacity of his blood. This, coupled with improved cardiac output from both increased preload that decreased his SVV and use of a positive inotrope, results in reduced compensatory oxygen extraction yielding a higher $ScvO_2$. ▪

Capnography Monitoring

Capnography, an adjunct assessment strategy, is the measurement of exhaled carbon dioxide, measured by sampling the partial pressure of end-tidal carbon dioxide ($PetCO_2$). To simply detect the presence of carbon dioxide, a single-use colorimetric detector may be attached to the tracheal tube to ensure correct endotracheal placement following intubation. Additionally, the $PetCO_2$ value should be continuously monitored, as discussed in Chapter 8 (see Figure 8-3 and Figure 8-6.).

ABG analysis enables $PetCO_2$ to be calibrated against $PaCO_2$; the capnometer can then be used for indirect, continuous monitoring of $PaCO_2$ and, thus, ventilation. Decreases in cardiac output caused by hypovolemia or cardiac dysfunction reduce pulmonary perfusion and increase the alveolar dead space, thus reducing $PetCO_2$ independently of any change in ventilation. This parameter may assist in the assessment of volume status and cardiac output.

> **Clinical Reasoning Pearl**
>
> Capnography, the graphical representation of the partial pressure of end-tidal carbon dioxide ($PetCO_2$), is useful in the evaluation of respiratory function, especially for monitoring restrictive airway diseases or evaluating for changes in airway diameter in response to bronchodilator therapies.

Laboratory Assessment Parameters

Laboratory data help the clinician to identify and interpret deviations from normal hemodynamic values and to use the information to develop an effective plan of care to optimize oxygen delivery and utilization.

Hemoglobin, a protein found in red blood cells, is necessary for oxygen transport. Generally, low hemoglobin levels are well tolerated by patients as long as their cardiac output is able to increase to compensate. The strongest evidence guiding transfusion policy in critically ill adult patients comes from the Transfusion Requirements In Critical Care (TRICC) study, which recommended that critically ill patients receive red blood cell transfusions when their hemoglobin concentrations fall below 7 grams per deciliter (g/dL) and that hemoglobin concentrations should be maintained between 7 and 9 g/dL.[33] The study showed that the mortality rate during hospitalization was significantly lower in patients in the restricted transfusion group (transfused for hemoglobin below 7 g/dL and maintained at 7 to 9 g/dL) compared with patients who received transfusions when their hemoglobin concentration fell below 10 g/dL and was maintained at 10 to 12.0 g/dL.[33] However, this was not the case in patients who had clinically significant cardiac disease, and may have been the rationale for the additional red blood cell transfusion administered to J.W. when his hemoglobin was 8.4 g/dL on admission to the critical care unit.

Normal hemostasis is dependent on the complex interactions among plasma coagulation and fibrinolytic proteins, platelets, and the blood vasculature. A variety of blood tests, most commonly prothrombin time (PT) with INR and activated partial thromboplastin time (aPTT) or PTT, are performed to assess the status and function of the varied processes implicated in coagulation. PT measures the time required for a fibrin clot to form when the extrinsic pathway for coagulation is initiated. PT values are useful in the evaluation of trauma patients with deficiencies in the extrinsic or common pathway of the coagulation cascade. aPTT and PTT assess the intrinsic pathway of the coagulation cascade, which is composed of factors XII, XI, IX, VIII, X, V, prothrombin, and fibrinogen. These tests are useful to identify patients with deficiencies in the intrinsic pathway or the common pathway of the coagulation cascade. Coagulopathies in the critical care phase are multifactorial in trauma patients, and precipitating events such as hypothermia, acidosis, liver dysfunction, SIRS, and hemodilution must be recognized and treated as early as possible to prevent further blood loss in the severely injured patient.

Both serum lactate and base deficit are measurable through laboratory studies. Careful assessment must continue in the critical care unit to detect continued hypoperfusion. In the setting of severe liver injury with reduced liver function, lactate interpretation may be more challenging because it is converted by the liver.

Base deficit is defined as the amount of base required to raise one liter of whole blood to the predicted pH based on the $PaCO_2$. It has also been used as a surrogate marker of metabolic acidosis. As J.W.'s oxygen delivery improves and cellular oxygen requirements are met, his lactate and base deficit return to normal.

Critical Care Phase Management

Fluid Management

Crystalloid fluid administration is a mainstay to replace intravascular volume. Typically, an isotonic solution (e.g., 0.9% saline, lactate Ringer) is administered until adequate preload is reached. As 0.9% saline has equal parts of sodium and chloride, patients may develop a hyperchloremic acidosis. Other solutions (e.g., Plasma-Lyte A Injection 7.4, Normosol-R pH 7.4) that more closely resemble the electrolyte composition of human plasma are commercially available and may reduce electrolyte abnormalities associated with crystalloid volume expansion.

Clinicians continue to debate the use of colloidal solutions for volume expansion in critical care. The largest study of colloid use in critically ill patients was performed by the Saline Versus Albumin Fluid Evaluation (SAFE) investigators. SAFE was a prospective, multicenter, randomized, and double-blind trial that compared the effects of 4% albumin versus 0.9% sodium chloride (saline) on mortality in a heterogeneous critical care unit population ($n = 6997$). The investigators found no significant differences in mortality between the two groups. A subgroup analysis found that trauma patients with a traumatic brain injury had a significantly higher chance of death when albumin was used versus saline, but there was no difference in the outcomes of trauma patients without brain injury. The investigators did find that patients in the saline group received slightly more fluid than the albumin group. They concluded that albumin and saline should be considered clinically equivalent treatments for intravascular volume resuscitation.[34]

Considering that most fluid administered leaks out of the vascular space, interstitial edema should be anticipated. If considerable edema is present, hypertonic solutions or colloids may be considered for fluid administration. Hypertonic solutions and colloids raise the intravascular osmotic and oncotic pressure, which moves fluid from the interstitial space to the vascular space, reducing the amount of volume administered.

Pharmacologic Management

Once adequate intravascular volume has been achieved, trauma patients in the critical care unit may still exhibit hypoperfusion caused by the inflammatory process. It may be necessary to support perfusion through pharmacologic methods.

Vasopressors raise global perfusion pressures through vasoconstriction. This is accomplished through stimulating alpha- and vasopressin receptors. Norepinephrine occurs naturally in humans and stimulates both alpha- and beta-receptors, with a greater affinity for the alpha-receptor, resulting in vasoconstriction, increased SVR, and some increase in cardiac output from beta-stimulation. Phenylephrine is a pure alpha-agonist and purely vasoconstrictive. Vasopressin accomplishes vasoconstriction through stimulating vasopressin receptors in the endothelium. Because of the cardiac effects of norepinephrine, tachydysrhythmias may occur.

Positive inotropes are used to raise cardiac output through enhanced myocardial contractility. This is accomplished through stimulation of $beta_1$- and $beta_2$-receptors or inhibiting phosphodiesterase, resulting in increased action of cyclic adenosine monophosphate in cardiac and vascular muscle cells. This action results in increased contractility of cardiac muscle and vasodilation. Dobutamine stimulates beta-receptors. Tachycardia should be anticipated with its use. Milrinone inhibits the action of phosphodiesterase. It may cause considerable vasodilation, which could cause a drop in blood pressure. As inotropes increase myocardial oxygen consumption, monitoring for myocardial ischemia is important in patients with coronary artery disease.

Debate regarding the use of vasopressors and inotropes to improve blood flow in the microcirculation continues. The ideal MAP and cardiac output are different for each patient, depending on baseline physiologic status and extent of traumatic injury. To date, no data are available in support of the idea that increasing MAP is beneficial from the perspective of microcirculatory perfusion, oxygenation, or both, and such an idea is not in line with the physiologic theory of the microcirculation as a low-pressure vascular compartment.[35] Further research is necessary to evaluate the microcirculation and establish new therapies.

Pain and anxiety are considerable challenges to the care team in the management of the trauma patient. Pain is traditionally treated with opiates and anxiety with sedatives. These medications alter the patient's perception of pain and anxiety. As mentioned, these medications result in reduced sympathetic response and may result in a decreased cardiac output and blood pressure.

Once J.W.'s volume status is adequate, vasopressors and inotropes are used to maintain perfusion pressures and cardiac output, which are impacted related to the vasodilation associated with systemic inflammation and use of opiates and sedatives.

Mechanical Ventilation Management

Mechanical ventilation is often utilized to support critically injured patients, either because the primary injury involved the lung or because of other injuries. Critically injured patients are at high risk for the development of acute respiratory distress syndrome (ARDS) caused by the inflammatory processes associated with trauma. The increased intrathoracic pressure associated with mechanical ventilation may make interpretation of hemodynamic data difficult. Refer to Chapter 14 for a complete description of the effects of mechanical ventilation on hemodynamics.

Early Mobilization

Immobility and bedrest play an important role in the development of muscular weakness and other complications. Early mobilization of patients is aimed at preventing these complications. Immobility alters the performance of the circulatory system, thus mobilizing patients after a period of immobility predisposes patients to postural hypotension.

Changing the patient's position alters the level of the phlebostatic axis impacting hemodynamic pressure readings unless the transducer is re-leveled. Refer to the chapters on the fundamentals of hemodynamic monitoring for appropriate actions described in Chapters 3, 4, and 5.

Complications of Trauma in the Critical Care Phase

Rewarming

Hypothermia is frequently observed following critical injury. Considering the complications associated with hypothermia, rewarming the patient is a priority. Rewarming patients is accomplished through warming the fluid and blood products administered and forced-warm-air blankets. As patients are rewarmed, vasodilation will occur, increasing vascular capacity and causing a relative hypovolemia. As the patient rewarms, blood pressure may fall, necessitating administration of fluid. As J.W. is rewarmed, vasodilation and administration of additional fluid or titration of vasopressors will be anticipated by the trauma team.

Intra-abdominal Hypertension and Abdominal Compartment Syndrome

Intra-abdominal hypertension (IAH) and abdominal compartment syndrome (ACS) are significant concerns in the postresuscitative phase. The intra-abdominal pressure can be measured via the patient's urinary catheter. Transducer systems are now commercially available (e.g., AbViser and Bard Intra-abdominal Pressure Monitoring Device) that facilitate monitoring of intra-abdominal pressure (IAP) while maintaining a closed urinary catheter drainage system.

Definitions and guidelines for IAH and ACS have been established by the World Society of the Abdominal Compartment Syndrome.[36] Abdominal perfusion pressure (APP) may be obtained by subtracting intra-abdominal pressure from mean arterial pressure (MAP – IAP = APP). A normal APP should be greater than 60 mm Hg. Intra-abdominal hypertension describes any intra-abdominal pressure greater than 12 mm Hg, and ACS occurs when intra-abdominal pressure is greater than 20 mm Hg (see Table 19-5). Severity of IAH is determined by the degree of intra-abdominal pressure (IAP) measured inside the abdomen

Grade I: IAP 12–15 mm Hg;
Grade II: IAP 16–20 mm Hg;
Grade III: IAP 21–25 mm Hg;
Grade IV: IAP >25 mm Hg.

Intra-abdominal pressure may occur primarily with abdominal catastrophes such as devastating liver injuries. Operative abdominal packing and retroperitoneal hematomas are examples of conditions that physically fill the abdominal space. Or more frequently, secondary intra-abdominal hypertension or ACS is caused by shock, massive fluid resuscitation, and systemic inflammation, which result in the combination of visceral and parietal edema, ascites, and paralytic ileus. Increased intra-abdominal pressure is associated with cardiovascular dysfunction, including increased SVR, decreased preload and venous return, and reduced ventricular compliance and cardiac output. Pulmonary complications include increased dead space ventilation, shunt and decreased compliance, and reduced lung volumes. The dysfunction of cardiovascular and pulmonary systems caused by intra-abdominal hypertension further impacts the patient's organ dysfunction.

Treatment strategies for intra-abdominal hypertension and ACS are directed at the causes of increase intra-abdominal pressure: conditions decreasing abdominal wall compliance, increasing intraluminal contents, related to abdominal collections (fluid, air and blood) and related to capillary leak and fluid resuscitation. Trauma is a major risk factor for intra-abdominal hypertension or ACS, particularly when requiring massive resuscitation and emergent abdominal surgery. In some cases, abdominal laparotomy is needed to relieve intra-abdominal hypertension and ACS. Table 19-5 describes treatment strategies related to the intra-abdominal pressure.

Sepsis

Patient Safety

- During trauma resuscitation, it may not be possible to use sterile technique when inserting a resuscitative catheter.

  - Central venous catheters (CVCs) placed under less-than-sterile conditions should be replaced as soon as possible within 48 hours.[1]

- CVCs may become sources of nosocomial infection in trauma patients.[2]

  - Because of injury pathophysiology, or comorbid diseases, trauma patients may require CVCs for an extended period

- Use of a best practice bundle for preventing central line–associated bloodstream infections (CLABSI) is important to reduce the number and rate of infections:[3]

  - Use a checklist for every CVC insertion.

  - Empower nurses to stop procedures if an error in technique occurs.

  - Assess daily if the CVC can be removed.

  - Develop policies related to the use and maintenance of CVCs.

  - Audit CVC maintenance on an ongoing basis.

  - Investigate every CLABSI, and use the results to improve infection prevention processes.[4]

[1]The Consortium on Intraosseous Vascular Access in Healthcare Practice: Recommendations for the use of intraosseous vascular access for emergent and nonemergent situations in various health care settings: a consensus paper, *Crit Care Nurse* 30(6):e1–e7, 2010.
[2]Ong A, Dysert K, Herbert C, et al.: Trends in central line-associated bloodstream infections in a trauma-surgical intensive care unit, *Arch Surg* 146(3):302–307, 2011.
[3]Emerick M, Standiford H, McQuillan M, et al.: Reduction of CLABSI in the trauma population, *Am J Infect Control* 39(5):e50, 2011.
[4]Agency for Healthcare Research and Quality: *Tools for reducing central line-associated blood stream infections.* http://www.ahrq.gov/professionals/education/curriculum-tools/clabsitools/index.html, 2012. Accessed September 15, 2014.

TABLE 19-5   Treatment Strategies for Increased Intra-abdominal Pressure

	IAP GRADE I	IAP GRADE II	IAP GRADE III	IAP GRADE IV
Intra-abdominal pressure measurement (mm Hg)	12–15	16–20	21–25	IAP >25 and/or APP <50 and new organ dysfunction or failure is present; or intra-abdominal hypertension or abdominal compartment syndrome is refractory to medical management
Evacuate intraluminal contents	NG tube or rectal tube Gastroprokinetic and colonoprokinetic agents Minimize enteral feeding	Enemas	Consider colonoscopic decompression Stop enteral feeding	Strongly consider surgical decompression
Evaluate intra-abdominal space-occupying lesion	Lesions on ultrasonography	Lesions on CT Percutaneous catheter drainage of lesions	Surgical evaluation of lesions	
Improve abdominal wall compliance	Sedation and anesthesia Remove constrictive elements	Avoid prone position Elevate head of bed >20 degrees Consider reverse Trendelenberg position	Neuromuscular blockade	
Optimize fluid administration	Avoid excess Aim: zero to negative fluid balance by day 3	Hypertonic saline resuscitation Judicious diuresis	Hemodialysis or ultrafiltration	
Optimize tissue perfusion	Goal-directed fluid resuscitation Maintaining APP >60 mm Hg correlates with improved survival from IAH/ACS	Hemodynamic monitoring	Vasoactive medications	

ACS, Abdominal compartment syndrome; APP, abdominal perfusion pressure; CT, computed tomography; IAH, intra-abdominal hypertension; IAP, intra-abdominal pressure; NG, nasogastric.
Adapted from Rizoli SM, Scarpelini A, Sandro AK: Abdominal compartment syndrome in trauma resuscitation, *Curr Opin Anaesthesiol* 23(2):251–257, 2010.

Trauma patients are at high risk for the development of sepsis. The critically injured have multiple portals of entry for organisms, including invasive lines and tubes, wounds from injury, and surgical incisions. Trauma patients are also immunosuppressed because of SIRS and from receiving blood products. The hemodynamic effects associated with sepsis are discussed in Chapter 20.

Conclusion

The trauma patient presents considerable challenges in both the resuscitative and critical care phases. Utilization of hemodynamic data, especially during the resuscitation and critical care phases, is essential for treating the patient with multiple injuries. Focusing on the adequacy of oxygen delivery to meet oxygen requirements and determining the endpoints of resuscitation provide the critically injured patient with the best chance for survival and reduced complication rate from injuries.

References

1. Bonne S, Schuerer DJ: Trauma in the older adult: epidemiology and evolving geriatric trauma principles, *Clin Geriatr Med* 29(1):137–150, 2013.
2. Kramer B: *Shock trauma registry*, Baltimore, MD, 2013, R Adams Cowley Shock Trauma Center. University of Maryland Medical Center.
3. American College of Surgeons: *National trauma data bank annual report 2008*, 2013. http://www.facs.org/trauma/ntdb/pdf/ntdb-annual-report-2013.pdf. Accessed September 14, 2014.
4. Dimitriou R, Calori G, Giannoudis P: Polytrauma in the elderly: specific considerations and current concepts of management, *Eur J Trauma Emerg Surg* 37(6):539–548, 2011.
5. Pisani MA: Considerations in caring for the critically ill older patient, *J Intensive Care Med* 24 (2):83–95, 2009.
6. National Institutes of Health National Heart, Lung, and Blood Institute: *NHLBI fact book, fiscal year 2012*. http://www.nhlbi.nih.gov/about/factbook/toc.htm. Updated 2013. Accessed August 17, 2013.
7. Fleg JL, Aronow WS, Frishman WH: Cardiovascular drug therapy in the elderly: benefits and challenges, *Nat Rev Cardiol* 8(1):13–28, 2011.
8. American College of Surgeons: Advanced trauma life support (ATLS(R)): the ninth edition, *J Trauma Acute Care Surg* 74(5):1363, 2013.
9. McQuillan KA, Flynn-Makic MB, Whalen E, editors: *Trauma nursing: from resuscitation through rehabilitation*, ed 4, St. Louis, MO, 2009, Saunders.
10. Nanas S, Gerovasili V, Renieris P, et al.: Non-invasive assessment of the microcirculation in critically ill patients, *Anaesth Intensive Care* 37(5):733–739, 2009.
11. Gando S: Microvascular thrombosis and multiple organ dysfunction syndrome, *Crit Care Med* 38(Suppl 2):S35–S42, 2010.
12. Lehman LW, Saeed M, Talmor D, et al.: Methods of blood pressure measurement in the ICU, *Crit Care Med* 41(1):34–40, 2013.
13. Marino PL, Sutin KM: *The ICU book*, Philadelphia, 2007, Lippincott Williams & Wilkins.
14. Crookes BA, Cohn SM, Bloch S, et al.: Can near-infrared spectroscopy identify the severity of shock in trauma patients? *J Trauma* 58(4):806–813, 2005.
15. Santora RJ, Moore FA: Monitoring trauma and intensive care unit resuscitation with tissue hemoglobin oxygen saturation, *Crit Care* 13(Suppl 5):S10, 2009.

16. Moore FA, Nelson T, McKinley BA, et al.: Massive transfusion in trauma patients: tissue hemoglobin oxygen saturation predicts poor outcome, *J Trauma* 64(4):1010, 2008.

17. Guyette FX, Gomez H, Suffoletto B, et al.: Prehospital dynamic tissue oxygen saturation response predicts in-hospital lifesaving interventions in trauma patients, *J Trauma Acute Care Surg* 72(4):930–935, 2012.

18. Odom SR, Howell MD, Silva GS, et al.: Lactate clearance as a predictor of mortality in trauma patients, *J Trauma Acute Care Surg* 74(4):999–1004, 2013.

19. Abramson D, Scalea TM, Hitchcock R, et al.: Lactate clearance and survival following injury, *J Trauma* 35(4):584–588, 1993.

20. Hulme JS, Sherwood N: Severe lactic acidosis following alcohol related generalised seizures, *Anaesthesia* 59(12):1228–1230, 2004.

21. Baba R, Zwaal JW: Severe metabolic acidosis after a single tonic-clonic seizure, *Anaesthesia* 60(6):623–624, 2005.

22. Callaway DW, Shapiro NI, Donnino MW, et al.: Serum lactate and base deficit as predictors of mortality in normotensive elderly blunt trauma patients, *J Trauma* 66(4):1040–1044, 2009.

23. Holcomb JB, Jenkins D, Rhee P, et al.: Damage control resuscitation: directly addressing the early coagulopathy of trauma, *J Trauma* 62(2):307, 2007.

24. Jansen JO, Thomas R, Loudon MA, Brooks A: Damage control resuscitation for patients with major trauma, *Br Med J* 338:b1778, 2009.

25. Rossaini R, Bouillon B, Cerny V, et al.: Management of bleeding following major trauma: an updated European guideline, *Crit Care* 14(2):R52, 2010.

26. Chandler MH, Roberts M, Sawyer M, Myers G: The US military experience with fresh whole blood during the conflicts in Iraq and Afghanistan, *Semin Cardiothorac Vasc Anesth* 16(3):153, 2012.

27. Mattox KL: Introduction, background, and future projections of damage control surgery, *Surg Clin North Am* 77(4):753, 1997.

28. Chuang VP, Reuter SR: Selective arterial embolization for the control of traumatic splenic bleeding, *Invest Radiol* 10(1):18, 1975.

29. Zengin S, Al B, Genc S, et al.: Role of inferior vena cava and right ventricular diameter in assessment of volume status: a comparative study: ultrasound and hypovolemia, *Am J Emerg Med* 31(5):763–767, 2013.

30. Marik PE, Cavallazzi R: Does the central venous pressure predict fluid responsiveness? An updated meta-analysis and a plea for some common sense, *Crit Care Med* 41(7):1774–1781, 2013.

31. Kalantari K, Chang JN, Ronco C, Rosner MH: Assessment of intravascular volume status and volume responsiveness in critically ill patients, *Kidney Int* 83(6):1017–1028, 2013.

32. Kopterides P, Bonovas S, Mavrou I, et al.: Venous oxygen saturation and lactate gradient from superior vena cava to pulmonary artery in patients with septic shock, *Shock* 31(6):561–567, 2009.

33. Hébert PC, Wells G, Blajchman MA, et al.: A multicenter, randomized, controlled clinical trial of transfusion requirements in critical care. transfusion requirements in critical care investigators, Canadian critical care trials group, *N Engl J Med* 340(6):409–417, 1999.

34. Finfer S, Bellomo R, Boyce N, et al.: A comparison of albumin and saline for fluid resuscitation in the intensive care unit, *N Engl J Med* 350(22):2247–2256, 2004.

35. Boema MA, Ince C: The role of vasoactive agents in the resuscitation of microvascular perfusion and tissue oxygenation in critically ill patients, *Intensive Care Med* 36(12):2004–2018, 2010.

36. Kirkpatrick AW, Roberts DJ, De Waele J, et al.: Intra-abdominal hypertension and the abdominal compartment syndrome: updated consensus definitions and clinical practice guidelines from the World Society of the Abdominal Compartment Syndrome, *Intensive Care Med* 39(7):1190–1206, 2013.

Hemodynamics of Sepsis

20

Barbara McLean

Infectious diseases have been a leading cause of death throughout the history of the human race, but only recently have we begun to therapeutically intervene to lower mortality rates.

Historical Milestones

Ancient Greek and Roman philosophers viewed sepsis as a form of biological decay.[1] It was not until the seventeenth and eighteenth centuries that the germ theory of disease ushered in the eras of infection control and modern microbiology. The discovery of antibiotics during the first half of the twentieth century finally provided a specific weapon to fight infection.

The 1992 joint statement from the American College of Chest Physicians (ACCP) and the Society of Critical Care Medicine (SCCM) introduced the term *systemic inflammatory response syndrome* (SIRS) to describe the nonspecific inflammatory process that develops in response to significant physiologic insults such as infection, trauma, burns, and other systemic disease processes (Figure 20-1).[2]

In 2001, Rivers and colleagues reported that among patients with severe sepsis or septic shock in a single urban emergency department, mortality was significantly lower among those who were treated according to a 6-hour protocol of early goal-directed therapy (EGDT) than among those who were given standard therapy (30.5% compared with 46.5% mortality).[3] The EGDT protocol is shown in Figure 20-2.

The clinical targets in this trial included achieving a central venous pressure (CVP) of greater than 8 millimeters of mercury (mm Hg) in spontaneously breathing patients or greater than 12 mm Hg in patients who were mechanically ventilated;[3] maintaining mean arterial pressure (MAP) above 65 mm Hg,[3] and attaining a central venous oxygen saturation (ScvO₂) greater than 70%, or a mixed-venous oxygen saturation (SvO₂) greater than 65%.[3] Early goal-directed sepsis management has led to one of the greatest reductions in sepsis-related morbidity and mortality over the past 50 years.

On the basis of this and other studies, the Society of Critical Care Medicine (SCCM) and European Society of Intensive Care Medicine (ESICM) created the "Surviving Sepsis Campaign" (SSC) in October 2004 with a vision of decreasing sepsis mortality by

Relationship of Infection, SIRS, Sepsis, Severe Sepsis, and Septic Shock

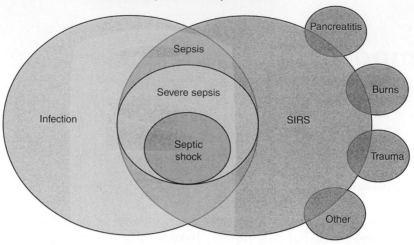

FIGURE 20-1 Relationship of infection, systemic inflammatory response syndrome (SIRS), sepsis, severe sepsis, and septic shock. (Adapted from Bone RC, et al.: Definitions for sepsis and organ failure and guidelines for the use of innovative therapies in sepsis, *Chest* 101(6): 1644–1655, 1992.)

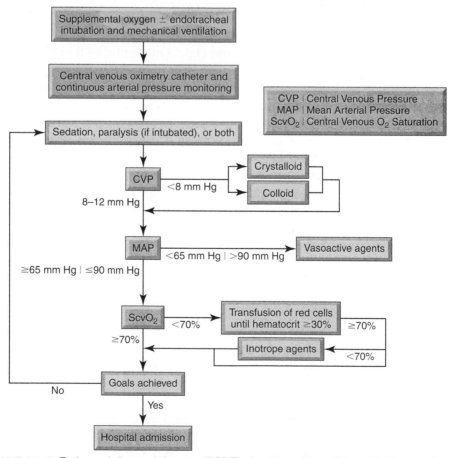

FIGURE 20-2 Early goal-directed therapy (EGDT) algorithm. (From Rivers E, Nguyen B, Havsted S, et al.: Early goal directed therapy in the treatment of severe sepsis and septic shock. *N Engl J Med* 345(19):1368–1371, 2001.)

TABLE 20-1 Signs of Systemic Inflammatory Response Syndrome (SIRS) and Sepsis

SIRS	SEPSIS
Clinical	**General**
• Body temperature greater than 38°C or less than 35°C • Heart rate greater than 90 beats per minute • Respiratory rate higher than 20 breaths per minute	• Fever (>38.3°C) • Hypothermia (core temperature <36°C) • Heart rate > 90 per minute or more than two so above the normal value for age • Tachypnea • Altered mental status • Significant edema or positive fluid balance (>20 mL/kg over 24 hours) • Hyperglycemia (plasma glucose >140 mg/dL or 7.7 mmol/L) in the absence of diabetes
Laboratory	**Inflammatory**
• $PaCO_2$ below 32 mm Hg • White blood cell count of greater than 12,000/mm^3 or less than 4000/mm^3 • >10% immature neutrophils (bands)	• Leukocytosis (white blood cell count >12,000 per liter) • Leukopenia (white blood cell count <4000 per liter) • Normal white blood cell count with greater than 10% immature forms • Plasma cross-reactive protein ≥2 above the normal value • Plasma procalcitonin ≥2 the normal value

25% over the following 5 years.[4,5] One of the most important contributions of the campaign was clarification of the definitions for sepsis and for systemic inflammatory response syndrome (SIRS) as listed in Table 20-1.

The most recent guidelines update was published in 2013. Early identification, antibiotics, and source control, as well as initial volume resuscitation remain as the foundation of sepsis management.[6,7] The current recommendations for the resuscitation timeframe are listed as the Surviving Sepsis Campaign bundles (Box 20-1).

For most patients with sepsis syndrome, the failure of three or more organ systems results in a mortality rate above 90%. The mortality rate for patients with acute kidney injury in the setting of sepsis ranges from 50% to 80%. Recent research and innovation has focused on the molecular mechanisms and hemodynamics of sepsis and septic shock.[8]

Identifying the very generic presentation of systemic inflammatory response syndrome offers little guidance for clinicians, as many disease processes present in a similar fashion. As sepsis progresses, however, the syndrome may spiral into a generalized

---

BOX 20-1 **Surviving Sepsis Campaign Bundles**

To Be Completed within 3 Hours
1. Measure lactate level.
2. Obtain blood cultures prior to administration of antibiotics.
3. Administer broad spectrum antibiotics.
4. Administer 30 milliliters per kilogram (mL/kg) crystalloid for hypotension or lactate ≥ 4 millimoles per liter (mmol/L).

To Be Completed within 6 Hours
1. Apply vasopressors (for hypotension that does not respond to initial fluid resuscitation to maintain a mean arterial pressure [MAP] ≥ 65 mm Hg).
2. In the event of persistent arterial hypotension despite volume resuscitation (septic shock) or initial lactate ≥ 4 mmol/L (36 milligrams per deciliter [mg/dL]):
   - Measure central venous pressure (CVP).[*]
   - Measure central venous oxygen saturation ($ScvO_2$).[*]
3. Remeasure lactate if initial lactate was elevated.[*]

[*]Targets for quantitative resuscitation included in the guidelines are CVP ≥ 8 mm Hg, $ScvO_2 \geq 70\%$, and normalization of lactate. From Dellinger RP, Levy MM, Rhodes A, et al.: Surviving sepsis campaign: International guidelines for management of severe sepsis and septic shock: 2012, *Crit Care Med* 41(2): 580–637, 2013.

---

circulatory, immune, coagulopathic, and neuroendocrine response, that ultimately promotes vascular dysfunction, failure of oxygen delivery, and inability to meet tissue oxygen consumption needs. This forms the continuum of SIRS to septic shock.

Clinical Reasoning Pearl

The signs and symptoms of sepsis are sensitive but not specific and range from tachycardia and tachypnea to life-threatening lactic acidosis and hypotension, as well as low or high venous oxygen ($ScvO_2$) values.

Epidemiology of Sepsis to Septic Shock

The significance of septic shock associated mortality continues to be a worldwide health issue. In the United States (U.S.) alone, 2% of all hospital admissions have a diagnosis of severe sepsis, which represents 10% of all patients admitted to critical care units.[9] The incidence of severe sepsis (sepsis-induced organ dysfunction) in the European Union has been estimated at 90.4 cases per 100,000 populations, compared to 58 per 100,000 for breast cancer.[10] In a comprehensive U.S. National Hospital Discharge Survey published in 2011, the incidence of sepsis-related hospitalizations increased from 221 to 337 cases per 100,000 per year between 2000 and 2008.[10a]

Older age is a significant risk factor. The risk of a sepsis-related hospitalization for people over 85 years of age is 30 times that of people under 65 years of age.[10a]

Septic shock is defined as a state of acute circulatory failure characterized by persistent hypotension that is unexplained by other causes despite adequate fluid resuscitation, and its incidence is increasing. Mortality from septic shock in critical care is estimated to range between 45% and 63% in observational studies.[11–14] The average sepsis survivor requires 7 to 14 days of critical care unit support with much of this time spent on a ventilator. An additional 10- to 14-day hospital stay is typical, creating an average hospital length of stay for survivors of up to 3 to 5 weeks.[15] Hospital charges in excess of tens of thousands of dollars for individual patients are typical, resulting in annual expenditures of nearly $17 billion in the U.S.[16] In 2009, sepsis was the sixth most frequent and the single most expensive U.S. hospital admission diagnosis. In 2011, the Agency for Healthcare Research and Quality (AHRQ) listed sepsis as the most expensive condition treated in U.S. hospitals, costing more than $20 billion in that year.[7] One estimate is that treatment of sepsis costs $44,600 for the initial admission alone, with costs increasing dramatically with prolonged hospital stays and any complications arising from the sepsis sequelae.[17]

Sepsis Pathophysiology

In its most fundamental presentation, sepsis is a clinical syndrome characterized by SIRS, or a presumed or documented infection and tissue injury. It represents a continuum of severity that results in a cascade of biochemical and pathophysiologic events. If left unabated, microbial toxins together with a dysfunctional host immune response quickly lead to tissue damage, shock, organ failure, and death.

The major pathways involved in sepsis include the innate immune response, inflammatory cascades (cytokine and arachidonic), procoagulant and antifibrinolytic pathways, alterations in cellular metabolism and signaling, as well as an ultimate acquired immune dysfunction. The pathways and their effects are shown in Figure 20-3.[18–21]

Sepsis is characterized by the cardinal signs of inflammation (vasodilation, leukocyte accumulation, increased microvascular permeability) occurring in tissues that are remote from the site of stimulation along with the suspicion or confirmation of infection. In certain patients, the normal innate immune response, stimulated by invading pathogens may augment the cascade of sepsis pathophysiology. Cytokines regulate multiple inflammatory responses, including localizing and controlling infection. Deregulated cytokine release may lead to endothelial dysfunction, vasodilation, and increased capillary permeability. The resulting cellular leakage syndrome disrupts regulatory mechanisms and leads to profound intravascular hypovolemia, cellular dysfunction, and, ultimately, cell death. Hemodynamic alterations in sepsis are directly related to endothelial derangements, tissue hypoxia, mitochondrial dysfunction, decreased oxygen delivery, and alterations in blood flow.[22]

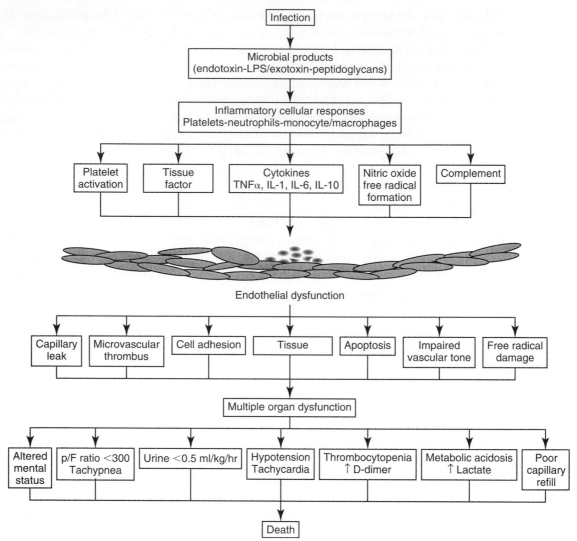

FIGURE 20-3 Pathophysiologic cascade of events in sepsis. (From Cunneen J, Cartwright M: The puzzle of sepsis: Fitting the pieces of the inflammatory response with treatment, *AACN Clin Issues* 15(1): 18–44, 2004.)

The ultimate result may be systemic vasodilation, heart failure, and microcoagulopathy, all contributing to a significant alteration of microvascular blood flow, decreased oxygen delivery, and profound dysoxia at the mitochondrial level.[23]

In addition, circulating or expressed mediators promote a loss of arterial vasomotor tone and myocardial depression. Cardiac output cannot increase because of the myocardial depression; nor can the stroke volume maintain a constant driving blood flow in the face of the dilated vasculature, which is presented as refractory hypotension. This cascade of events is partly responsible for the imbalance between systemic oxygen delivery and oxygen demand, leading to global tissue hypoxia.

Severe sepsis and septic shock are characterized at different points on a continuum and integrate signs and symptoms of hypovolemic shock, cardiogenic shock, and distributive shock. Patients with severe sepsis and septic shock often exhibit all three states simultaneously, making effective diagnosis and therapeutic interventions difficult to standardize and achieve. In clinical practice, the terms sepsis, severe sepsis, and septic shock are generally used interchangeably to describe a myriad of events along this continuum of presentations.

Sepsis Definitions

The diagnosis of sepsis requires clinical evidence of infection and the presence of SIRS, which is characterized by specific physiologic alterations, including changes in temperature, white blood cell count, heart rate, and respiratory rate.[24,25]

The terms *SIRS*, *sepsis*, and *severe sepsis*, and *septic shock* are not interchangeable, although often presented as such. The definitions are discussed in more detail below. These definitions drive the interventions, as recommended in the Surviving Sepsis Campaign guidelines.[6,22]

Systemic Inflammatory Response Syndrome

SIRS may result from numerous conditions but is only defined as sepsis when the etiology includes infection (Figure 20-1). SIRS presents as a deregulated inflammatory response, regardless of origin, when two or more clinical signs are present. The salient signs of SIRS and sepsis are listed in Table 20-1. This SIRS response has been criticized for a lack of specificity for sepsis because the signs represent a clinical response to acute inflammation.[26] The pathogenesis of SIRS may be associated with the release of bacterial toxins and cellular mediators that cause systemic instability.[27]

Clinical Reasoning Pearl

Increased minute ventilation and tachypnea are present in 80% of critical care patients presenting with sepsis. Fever presents in 60% of patients.[28]

Sepsis

Sepsis is defined as infection accompanied by two or more of the following signs of systemic inflammation: hypothermia or hyperthermia, tachycardia, tachypnea, and elevated or depressed leukocyte count. The laboratory diagnosis may be supported by positive cultures, tissue stain, or polymerase chain reaction tests as listed in Table 20-2.

TABLE 20-2 **Surviving Sepsis Campaign 2012 Guidelines for Identification**

SEPSIS	SEVERE SEPSIS	SEPTIC SHOCK
Suspected or documented infection plus some of the following:	Criteria from previous column plus any of the following thought to be caused by the infection:	All of the criteria from previous columns plus:

General and Hemodynamic Sepsis Variables

• Heart rate >90 beats per minute • Temperature >101°F (38.3°C) or <96.8°F (36°C) • Altered mental status • Significant edema or positive fluid balance (>20 mL/kg over 24 hours) • Hyperglycemia (plasma glucose >140 mg/dL in the absence of diabetes)	• Sepsis-induced hypotension • Acute lung injury with $PaO_2/FiO_2 < 250$ in the absence of pneumonia as infection source • Acute lung injury with $PaO_2/FiO_2 < 200$ in the presence of pneumonia as infection source • Serum creatinine >2.0 mg/dL • Bilirubin >2 mg/dL • Platelet count <100,000/mm³	• Systolic blood pressure <90 mm Hg or • MAP <70 mm Hg or • Systolic blood pressure decrease >40 mm Hg or less than two standard deviations below normal for age in the absence of other causes of hypotension

Inflammatory variables

- White blood cell count >12,000/mm³ or <4000/mm³
- Normal white blood cell count with >10% immature forms (bands)
- Plasma cross-reactive protein more than two standard deviations above the normal value
- Plasma procalcitonin more than two standard deviations above the normal value

Procalcitonin

The utilization of the peptide procalcitonin, which is released in response to proinflammatory stimuli, is a biomarker for infection and may have a higher diagnostic accuracy compared with other traditional biomarkers of inflammation.[29,30] The findings of several meta-analysis present conflicting evidence as to the benefits of procalcitonin levels and early recognition of sepsis.[31–34]

In general, evidence supports procalcitonin as more helpful for making individualized decisions regarding antibiotic stewardship, including discontinuation and withholding of antibiotics. The initiation of antibiotics in the presence of hypotension remains the single-most important therapeutic intervention for improving outcomes of patients with sepsis.[35]

Severe Sepsis

Severe sepsis requires the presence of at least one new organ dysfunction. Or an acute injury may be superimposed on chronic organ dysfunction.

Septic Shock

Septic shock is defined as hypotension with organ system dysfunction that is not correctable by intravenous fluid resuscitation and requires the addition of vasopressors. Shock is a clinical diagnosis defined by inadequate end-organ perfusion in the setting of hemodynamic instability (Figure 20-4).

Hemodynamics of Sepsis: Variability in Oxygen Delivery, Vascular Tone, and Arterial Volume

The cardiovascular and endothelial systems play a key role in the pathophysiology of severe sepsis and septic shock, and both are central and critical. Distinguishing between the direct effects of sepsis on the myocardium, endothelial alterations, and cardiac responses to changes in preload, afterload, and neurohumoral activity is challenging.

Hemodynamic monitoring endpoints for therapeutic interventions focus on five primary areas:

1. Inadequate volume (low preload)
2. Loss of vascular tone (low afterload)
3. Myocardial depression (decreased contractility)
4. Alterations in microvascular blood flow
5. Oxygen-demand supply balance assessed by the comparison of SaO_2 and $ScvO_2$ or SvO_2

Preload: Volume Status in Severe Sepsis and Septic Shock

Determining the optimal preload level in sepsis is challenging. A patient who is not considered fluid responsive may be potentially harmed by aggressive fluid resuscitation. In fact, in non–fluid responsive patients, the volume may exacerbate acute respiratory distress syndrome (ARDS), acute kidney injury, and intra-abdominal hypertension. Traditional methods for monitoring, namely the CVP, and pulmonary

Diagnosis is made when findings are caused by infection

Sepsis: infection with some of the following findings including SIRS criteria
OR infection with 2 SIRS criteria

Exam findings
• Temperature: >38.3°C
• Altered mental status
• Significant edema
• Positive fluid balance: >20 mL/kg over 24 hr

Lab findings
• Glucose (NO diabetes): >120 mg/dL or
                          >7.7 mmol/L
• C-reactive protein: >2 SD above normal
• Procalcitonin: >2 SD above normal

End-organ dysfunction
(criteria not mentioned elsewhere or
different from other criteria):
• Creatinine: increase 0.5 mg/dL
• Ileus: absent bowel sounds
• Total bilirubin: >4 mg/dL or
                   >70 mmol/L
• PaO$_2$/FiO$_2$: <300
• aPTT: >60sec

Tissue perfusion findings
• Decreased capillary refill
• Mottling
• Lactate: >1 mmol/L

SIRS criteria
• Temperature: >38°C or <36°C
• Heart rate: >90 beats/min
• Respirations: >20 breaths/min, or
                PaCO$_2$ <32 mm Hg
• WBC: >12,000/μL, or
                <4,000/μL, or
                >10% immature forms

Severe sepsis: sepsis with end-organ damage
• PaO$_2$/FiO$_2$: <250 with NO pneumonia
• PaO$_2$/FiO$_2$: <200 WITH pneumonia
• Creatinine: >2.0 mg/dL (176.8 μmol/L)
• Bilirubin: >2 mg/dL (34.2 μmol/L)
• Lactate: >normal
• Coagulopathy: INR >1.5
• Platelet count: <100,000/μL

Sepsis-induced hypoperfusion
• Hypotension*
• Lactate: ≥4 mmol/L
• Oliguria**

Septic shock
Hypotension in
spite of adequate
fluid resuscitation

*Hypotension: Systolic blood pressure (SBP) <90 mm Hg
            Mean arterial pressure (MAP) <70 mm Hg
            SBP decrease >40 mm Hg, ≤2 SD below normal for age
**Oliguria: <0.5 mL/kg/hr for more than 2 hours despite adequate fluid resuscitation

FIGURE 20-4 Identification of sepsis, severe sepsis, and septic shock. (From Reifel Saltzberg, JM: Fever and signs of shock: The essential fever, *Emerg Med Clin N Am* 31(4): 907–926, 2013.)

artery occlusion pressure (PAOP), were used to gauge volume resuscitation, however, the utility of these methods is now considered dubious even when high or low. CVP and PAOP are considered static hemodynamic measurements, as they are obtained under a single ventricular loading condition.

Central Venous Pressure

The CVP is used to obtain a static measurement of preload. The validity of CVP measurement in patients with severe sepsis or septic shock is widely debated. There is no known threshold value of CVP that identifies patients whose cardiac output will increase in response to fluid resuscitation.[36] Recent evidence negates the value of the CVP-driven protocol endpoint in the Surviving Sepsis Campaign guidelines, as new findings suggest that fluid management utilizing CVP-targeted resuscitation contributes significantly to morbidity and mortality.[37–39]

The Surviving Sepsis Campaign both acknowledges the limitations of CVP monitoring and accepts that a low CVP generally indicates low intravascular volume although there has been evidence to the contrary. Current Surviving Sepsis Campaign guidelines recommend fluid resuscitation of patients presenting with sepsis-induced tissue hypoperfusion to a targeted CVP of 8 to 12 mm Hg (or 12 to 15 mm Hg in mechanically ventilated patients) within 6 hours of sepsis identification. The rationale behind this CVP-targeted fluid resuscitation is to ensure adequate cardiac preload and maintain cardiac output and organ perfusion. However, absolute levels or changes in CVP poorly predict cardiovascular response to volume resuscitation or fluid responsiveness.[40]

Pulmonary Artery Catheter

The pulmonary artery catheter (PAC) measures or calculates intrapulmonary pressures, cardiac output, and, on particular types of PACs, mixed venous oxygen saturation (SvO$_2$). A systematic review of the use of PAC catheters, which included 13 studies and 5686 patients, revealed that the use of the PAC did not alter mortality, or critical care unit length of stay of these patients.[19] The PAC-Man (Pulmonary Artery Catheters in Patient Management) trial, performed between 2001 and 2004, provided the strongest evidence to date that PAC use conferred neither benefit nor harm to critical care patients.[41] Consequently, a PAC is not routinely inserted for volume guidance in sepsis management.

Dynamic Measures of Fluid Responsiveness

Today, dynamic or volumetric measures may offer a better guide to fluid responsiveness. This indicator is evaluated across the thoracic inspiratory and expiratory pressure changes that affect the volume loading and compliance of the right ventricle immediately and the left ventricle thereafter, related to the pulmonary transit of blood.

Heart–lung interactions during mechanical ventilation are used to evaluate the variations in stroke volume, systolic pressure, and pulse pressure. Pulse pressure variation estimated from the arterial waveform, stroke volume variations from pulse contour analysis, pulse oximeter plethysmographic waveform, and thoracic bioreactance have been found to be reliable predictors of fluid responsiveness when patients receive a volume challenge test such as a passive leg raise.[42,43]

Multiple methods exist for evaluating a volume challenge. It is possible to view arterial waveform variability with the bedside monitor by setting the sweep speed for the arterial pressure at 6.25 millimeters per second (mm/sec), allowing for a more compressed time view as shown in Figure 20-5. Although quantifying the variability can be somewhat difficult, the presence of variability is helpful when observed.

Other ways to evaluate volume responsiveness or variability are to utilize minimally invasive, arterial-based stroke volume variation (SVV), or arterial-based pulse pressure variation (PPV). These techniques, measured via specialized arterial transducers or bioreactance electrodes, correlate volume changes to positive pressure breathing, which increases intrathoracic pressure during inspiration in a predictable pattern. Minimally invasive, arterial-based systolic pressure variation (SPV) can be measured on

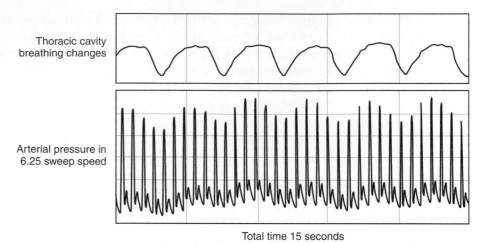

Thoracic cavity
breathing changes

Arterial pressure in
6.25 sweep speed

Total time 15 seconds

FIGURE 20-5 Arterial pressure wave with variability.

any patient regardless of ventilation status.[44,45] The impact of mechanical ventilation on hemodynamic monitoring is discussed in detail in Chapter 14.

Volume responsiveness can be assessed noninvasively with plethysmography variation, to generate a perfusion index (Philipps) or a perfusion variability index (Massimo). In combination with one of these measurement technologies, the passive leg raise can help to determine whether or not the patient is likely to be fluid responsive (Figure 20-6).[46,47] More information about the passive leg raise maneuver is presented in Chapters 3 and 12.

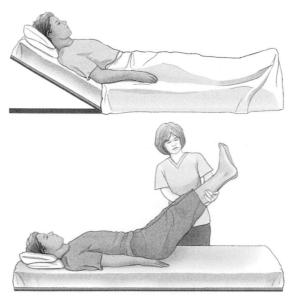

FIGURE 20-6 Passive leg raise maneuver.

> **Clinical Reasoning Pearl**
>
> Patients with septic shock often have fluid deficits of 6 to 10 liters and require aggressive fluid resuscitation.

Afterload and Loss of Vascular Tone

Blood Pressure Monitoring in Severe Sepsis and Septic Shock

High-level evidence does not exist to support the most effective mean arterial pressure (MAP) target for resuscitation of patients with septic shock. When patients experience hypotension, cerebral blood flow may fall below 50 mm Hg. The consequence of inadequate organ perfusion is ischemic injury to the brain, kidney, gut, and myocardium, followed by multiple organ dysfunction and death. The presence of a prolonged hypotensive state is of significant concern.

The goal of cardiovascular resuscitation of septic shock is to improve organ perfusion, often by increasing the MAP above 65 mm Hg. Adequate fluid resuscitation is limited when the administration of fluids is associated with distributive shock and causes third-spacing of fluid and tissue edema. This is of particular concern given the need to avoid increasing extra lung water in acute lung injury. Vasopressors are added if fluid resuscitation does not restore adequate perfusion, but doses are limited by the side effects of vasoconstriction and organ ischemia. Distinguishing between ischemia that is caused by inadequate resuscitation, and ischemia that is caused by excessive vasoconstriction, is a difficult clinical challenge. [48]

One of the major pathophysiologic characteristics of sepsis and a primary indicator of septic shock is loss of control of the vascular tone. The balance between locally produced vasoconstrictors and vasodilators is disrupted in sepsis. The vasodilation is not uniform across tissue beds; nor is it simply an increase in the baseline vessel caliber. The major cause of vasodilation in sepsis appears to be created by stimulation of cell membrane potassium channels in smooth muscle. The result is increased permeability of vascular smooth muscle cells to potassium. Additionally, hyperpolarization of the cell membranes inhibits muscle contraction leading to vasodilation. A second concern is an increased production of nitric oxide, which causes a generalized vasodilation and resistance to alpha-based vasoconstrictors: norepinephrine, epinephrine, and phenylephrine. Nitric oxide is a powerful vasodilator, and its excessive production may contribute to the vasodilation, which is a hallmark of septic shock. In addition to the sensitized potassium channels and inducible nitric oxide, vasopressin levels fall to very low levels often an expression of pituitary dysfunction.[49]

A MAP between 65 and 90 mm Hg describes the lower limit of autoregulation in healthy persons, and the same level appears to be present in critically ill patients with sepsis without a history of hypertension. Accordingly, the Surviving Sepsis Campaign recommends a MAP target of greater than 65 mm Hg.

> **Clinical Reasoning Pearl**
>
> For refractory hypotension, consider the following possibilities: an overwhelming systemic inflammatory state, adrenal insufficiency, and a mixed physiologic condition such as sepsis and acute heart failure, or neurogenic shock.

Myocardial Depression and Decreased Contractility

Although many theories regarding the causative factors of myocardial dysfunction exist, one issue is not controversial: The heart is one of the most frequently affected organs in sepsis, and patients who exhibit myocardial dysfunction are more likely to die. Of the many possibilities, it appears that a combination of decreased myocardial contractility, ventricular-arterial decoupling, and decreased coronary blood flow creates a situation where it is almost impossible for the heart to support optimal oxygen delivery and achieve adequate perfusion pressures.[50] Although a number of mediators and pathways have been shown to be associated with myocardial depression in sepsis, the precise cause remains unclear. Tumor necrosis factor–alpha (TNF-α) and interleukin 1 (IL-1) show significant cardiovascular depressive effects.[50,51] Biomarkers of heart failure such as N-terminal pro–B-type natriuretic peptide hormone are elevated in patients with sepsis who have systolic cardiac dysfunction.[52]

High sympathetic stress is also implicated in sepsis-induced myocardial depression. Patients with sepsis often remain tachycardic, even after excluding expected causes such as hypovolemia, anemia, agitation, and medication effects. Beta-adrenergic blockade may control the heart rate and improve cardiovascular performance, whereas beta-adrenergic stimulation may improve stroke volume and tissue perfusion. However, concerns that beta-blocker or beta-adrenergic stimulation in septic shock may lead to cardiovascular decompensation must be considered.

A reduction in heart rate variability in sepsis is a measure of autonomic dysregulation, which reflects a loss of the balance between sympathetic and parasympathetic tone.[53,54] Because tachycardia frequently signals a response to increasing tissue demand for oxygen, the ability to respond by increasing the heart rate may be lifesaving.

When critical care clinicians estimate the cardiac output and systemic vascular resistance (low, normal, or high) of patients in a medical or respiratory critical care units and these estimates were compared with values obtained by pulmonary artery catheterization, the physicians were correct about 50% of the time.[55] After the objective hemodynamic data was obtained, the information promoted the alteration of planned therapy in 58% of cases and the addition of unanticipated therapy in 30% of individuals studied.[55] Myocardial function can be evaluated via echocardiography to identify sepsis-induced cardiomyopathy. The impact of severe sepsis on the heart and cardiovascular system is shown in Figure 20-7.[53]

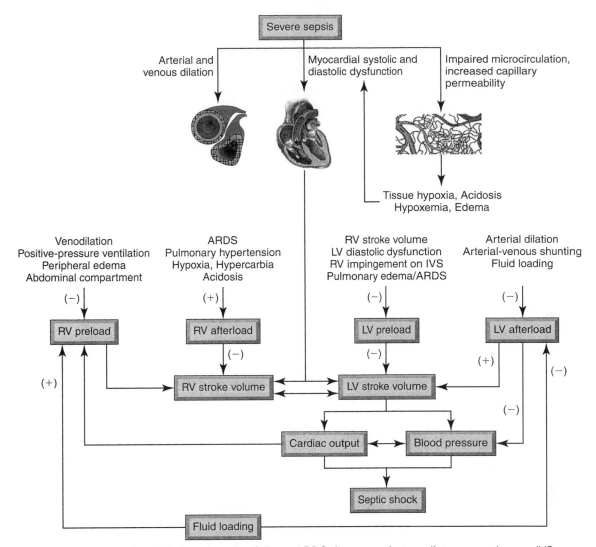

FIGURE 20-7 Sepsis-induced cardiac failure. *ARDS*, Acute respiratory distress syndrome; *IVS*, intraventricular septum; *LV*, left ventricular; *RV*, right ventricular. (From Hochstadt A, Meroz Y, Landesberg G: *Myocardial dysfunction in severe sepsis and septic shock: more questions than answers? J Cardiothorac Vasc Anesth* 25(3):526–535, 2011.)

Alterations in Microvascular Blood Flow Oxyhemoglobin Dissociation and Mixed Venous and Central Venous Oxygen Saturations

As discussed in other chapters, mixed venous and central venous oxygen saturations reflect the balance between oxygen demand and oxygen delivery and may be used to assess the adequacy of tissue oxygenation. Measurement of SvO_2 involves placement of a fiberoptic pulmonary artery catheter and typically is not the first choice to manage sepsis. Measuring $ScvO_2$ requires a fiberoptic central venous catheter, which, is a preferable alternative, as the multi-lumen catheter can also be used for monitoring the CVP and for administration of vasoactive medication and antibiotics.

In principle, the $ScvO_2$ value reflects the amount of oxygen consumption in the upper part of the body, including the brain. The $ScvO_2$ obtained from the superior vena cava may be slightly lower or higher than right atrial and mixed venous SvO_2. The difference is typically less than 5% and with normal physiology is an excellent surrogate. For more information about the relationship of $ScvO_2$ and SvO_2 see Figure 7-11 in Chapter 7. For patients in shock, a consistent reversal of the normal relationship occurs, and $ScvO_2$ of the superior vena cava becomes significantly higher than the SvO_2 of the pulmonary artery. The difference may range from 5% to 18%.[56] This difference reflects the change in SvO_2 as indicative of the mixing of splanchnic and coronary venous blood flow, which in this state is significantly desaturated.

Declines in $ScvO_2$ and SvO_2 predict the onset of inadequate myocardial compensation and may precede cardiogenic shock, capillary blood flow failure, or the development of arrhythmias, even though other vital signs remain relatively normal.[57]

In early compensatory sepsis, the oxyhemoglobin curve shifts to the right often with an $ScvO_2$ value as low as 30% to 40%; later, decompensated sepsis frequently presents with features of cardiogenic shock. However the SvO_2 is normal to high, in the presence of significant lactic acidosis (see Figure 6-5 and Table 20-3). The presence of a pathologically low $ScvO_2$ or SvO_2 is clinically important because a consistent $ScvO_2$ below 60% is linked with cardiac shock and increased mortality.[58–61] Applying strategies to treat the inadequate oxygen delivery are essential. If allowed to persist, the patient's oxygen debt will present with evolving metabolic acidosis related to anaerobic metabolism (lactic acidosis), although this may occur early or late in the process. Although intermittent venous blood gas evaluation is considered by some to be adequate, only continuous measurement of $ScvO_2$ or SvO_2 has been associated with beneficial outcomes.[25,62]

A decrease in SvO_2 or $ScvO_2$ is a global index of an inadequate oxygen delivery to oxygen demand relationship. In this setting, a therapeutic decision to improve determinants of SvO_2 should be considered within the context of all other hemodynamic parameters.

Clinical Reasoning Pearl

$ScvO_2$ should never be used as the primary measure of tissue oxygen adequacy but combined with other cardiocirculatory indicators of organ perfusion such as serum lactate concentration and urine output.

Lactate Monitoring in Severe Sepsis and Septic Shock

The serum lactate level is suggested as a marker of global hypoperfusion and tissue hypoxia in sepsis. Even before patients develop frank hypotension, tissue perfusion is impaired by myocardial depression, relative hypovolemia from a leaky

TABLE 20-3 Hemodynamic Features of Compensated and Decompensated Severe Sepsis and Septic Shock

MEASURES	COMPENSATORY SEVERE SEPSIS OR SHOCK	DECOMPENSATED SEVERE SEPSIS OR SHOCK
Cardiac index	↑↑	↓↓
Stroke volume index	↑↑	↓↓
Stroke volume variation (SVV)	↑↑	↓↓
Mean arterial pressure (MAP)	↑	↓↓
Central venous pressure (CVP)	↓	↑↑
Saturation of central venous oxygen (ScvO$_2$)	↓↓	↑↑
Lactic acid	↑↑	↑↑↑

endothelium, increased metabolic demands, and impaired vasoregulatory mechanisms. Consequently, oxygen demand exceeds supply, and anaerobic (without oxygen) production of lactate ensues. Refer to the discussion on aerobic and anaerobic lactic acid levels later in this chapter.

When all of the compensatory mechanisms are exhausted, the appearance of metabolic acidosis associated with increased plasma lactate concentration signifies failure of both the endogenous compensation and the exogenous support. Not all agree that lactate production is a reliable marker of global hypoxia in sepsis.[60,61]

In adults with severe sepsis, an increased lactate level of greater than 4 millimoles per liter (mmol/L), in the presence of acidosis, and not necessarily an acidotic pH, is a negative prognostic indicator and should trigger aggressive resuscitation according to the Surviving Sepsis Campaign guidelines.[22]

Elevated lactate levels, although typically thought of as a marker of inadequate tissue perfusion with concurrent shift toward increased anaerobic metabolism, may be present in patients in whom systemic hypoperfusion is not present and therefore should be evaluated in conjunction with an arterial blood gas and an ScvO$_2$ or SvO$_2$ measurement profile. Refer to Table 6-9 in Chapter 6 for normal lactic acid values.

An increase in circulating lactate in critically ill patients, in the setting of poor oxygen delivery, is an ominous sign. If cellular perfusion is restored quickly, cellular and mitochondrial function may resume, and cell function may return to a healthy state. If hypoperfusion is allowed to persist, cellular death (apoptosis) will begin, inevitably leading to organ dysfunction.

A recent study of 9,179 patients with sepsis, who had serum lactate levels between 2.0 and 4.0 mmol/L and a predicted hospital mortality of 10.3%, found that early administration of fluids lowered lactate levels and decreased mortality.[63,64] In addition, early lactate clearance, defined as a decrease in serum lactate level by 10% or more after initial fluid resuscitation, was associated with improved outcomes in severe sepsis and septic shock.[65–68]

Other frequent causes of metabolic acidosis include ketosis and inability of the kidney to regulate acid. When there is more than one cause of acidosis in the patient with severe sepsis, this makes accurate diagnosis and intervention more difficult.

Managing the Hemodynamics of Sepsis, Severe Sepsis, and Septic Shock

EGDT for patients with severe sepsis or septic shock, which included treatment goals for MAP, CVP, and $ScvO_2$, was the first study to significantly and reliably reduce mortality in severe sepsis; however, the target endpoint of CVP has recently been questioned.[7] The results of the large multi-center Protocolized Care in Early Septic Shock trial (ProCESS) also has the potential to alter another tenet of the resuscitation phase of sepsis management, namely the $ScvO_2$. For this reason the ProCESS trial will be described in some detail.[69] ProCESS enrolled 1,341 patients from 31 emergency departments in the U.S. and randomized the patients to one of three groups for the first 6 hours of sepsis resuscitation.[69]

Group 1: EGDT protocol[3] as outlined in Figure 20-2 and Box 20-1, which included use of an $ScvO_2$ fiberoptic central venous catheter.
Group 2: Protocol-driven care, which included use of peripheral venous catheters for volume resuscitation. A central line was inserted only if peripheral venous access was inadequate.
Group 3: Usual care, as directed by the physicians in the local emergency department.

Patients in all three groups received similar amounts of intravenous fluids, averaging 2.8 L, 3.3 L, and 2.3 L for Groups 1, 2, 3, respectively. Mortality at 60 days was 21.0%, 18.2%, and 18.9% for Groups 1, 2, 3, respectively.[69] These results have led many to conclude that a fiberoptic central venous catheter may not be required for early resuscitation in severe sepsis and septic shock. Others consider that a direct comparison between ProCESS and the original EGDT trial[3] in 2001 cannot be made because patients in the ProCESS study had already received approximately 2 liters of fluid prior to randomization, and more than 75% had received antibiotics prior to randomization.[70]

In patients who are found to initially have elevated lactate levels, targeting resuscitation to normalize lactate is a tangible endpoint, with equal weight given to the $ScvO_2$. Where both technologies are available, both targets are valuable.[68]

Crystalloid Fluid Resuscitation in Sepsis

Crystalloid fluid resuscitation is the first intervention guided by preload, afterload, and tissue hypoxia in severe sepsis and septic shock. Initial fluid challenge in patients with sepsis-induced tissue hypoperfusion should include a minimum of 30 milliliters per kilogram (mL/kg) of crystalloids. More rapid administration and greater amounts of fluid may be needed in some patients. Fluid challenge techniques should continue as long as hemodynamic improvements are based either on dynamic parameters (change in pulse pressure, stroke volume variation, systolic pressure variation) or static parameters (CVP, arterial pressure, heart rate).

It is also of value to recall that maintenance fluids are provided in low volume and minimally affect acid–base and electrolyte balance. In contrast, resuscitation fluids are aggressively administered and have an impact on organ function and acid–base balance.

The choice of resuscitation fluid has also been studied. A Cochrane Database systematic review of perioperative fluids that were buffered with bicarbonate versus non-buffered fluids found both types of fluids to be safe and effective, although buffered fluids were associated with less metabolic derangement.[71]

Raghunathan et al. evaluated the difference between balanced crystalloid of lactated Ringer's solution and isotonic (0.9%) normal saline for resuscitation in sepsis.[72] Among the 6,730 patients studied, administration of a balanced fluid (lactated Ringer's solution) was associated with a lower in-hospital mortality (19.6% versus 22.8%). Mortality was progressively lower among patients receiving larger proportions of balanced fluids.[72]

Blood pressure is considered a secondary monitoring parameter, although the Surviving Sepsis Campaign guidelines recommend achieving a target MAP of 65 mm Hg or higher in the management of septic shock. With refractory hypotension to both fluids and vasopressors, the clinician should consider the following possible causes: an overwhelming systemic inflammatory state, adrenal insufficiency, a mixed physiologic condition such as sepsis or acute heart failure, receptor site paralysis, and loss of response to exogenous vasopressor administration, which occurs in the face of severe metabolic acidosis (pH <7.25), as well as neurogenic shock.

Vasopressor Therapy in Sepsis

Vasopressor therapy is used only when volume replacement alone has not achieved a target MAP above 65 mm Hg. Norepinephrine is the first-choice of vasopressor. When norepinephrine fails to achieve the MAP target, vasopressin, up to 0.03 units per minute, may be added to norepinephrine.[6,73,74] Epinephrine is also considered a second line vasopressor in septic shock when norepinephrine does not raise the MAP above 65 mm Hg.

The use of intravenous steroids or sodium bicarbonate in patients with persistent vasopressor-dependent septic shock is controversial but may be considered for refractory shock.[75] Laboratory testing of serum cortisol levels is no longer recommended.[76]

The degree of myocardial dysfunction may determine whether a patient survives. In survivors, ventricular compliance is increased with a higher end-diastolic volume that contributes to the maintenance of an adequate stroke volume.

Inotropic Therapy in Sepsis

Current therapy for sepsis-induced cardiac dysfunction is based on aggressive treatment of underlying sepsis with antibiotics and source control as well as hemodynamic support.[77] It is possible that adequate volume resuscitation leads to an elevation in cardiac index, via manipulation of stroke volume, which may obscure the evolving myocardial dysfunction that occurs in severe sepsis regardless of the SvO_2 or $ScvO_2$. Dobutamine may be used to increase oxygen delivery via increased stroke volume in the presence of ongoing signs of hypoperfusion evidenced by lactic acidosis. Following initial resuscitation of patients with sepsis-induced hypoperfusion utilizing fluids and vasopressors, a trial of the inodilator dobutamine, with an infusion up to 20 micrograms per kilogram per minute (mcg/kg/min) may be added to the initial vasopressor in the setting of reduced stroke volume.

Antimicrobial Therapy in Sepsis

Antimicrobials administered within the first hour of recognition of severe sepsis and septic shock should be a key treatment goal.

Case Study
SIRS to Severe Sepsis and Back

A 31-year-old man came to the emergency department (ED) with complaints of flulike symptoms after exposure to his son who had had similar complaints for 4 days. He denied smoking and alcohol and substance abuse. He had taken 600 milligrams (mg) of acetaminophen 2 hours ago. Vital signs were evaluated, and the patient was asked to wait in triage waiting area.

Four hours after initial evaluation, the patient stated that he felt very hot and dizzy. After re-evaluation, he was sent immediately back to the acute medical zone in the ED for intervention and evaluation.

PARAMETERS	TRIAGE IN ED	4 HOURS AFTER TRIAGE IN ED	6 HOURS AFTER TRIAGE IN ED	EMERGENCY ADMISSION TO CRITICAL CARE UNIT	36 HOURS LATER
Saturation of peripheral oxygen (SpO_2)	99%	92%	89%	94%	98%
Heart rate	131	144	132	112	104
Respiratory rate	22	34	36	25 (vent)	18 (vent) (10 ventilator, 8 spontaneous)
Temperature (Centigrade)	37.9	39	39.9	40.0	37.8
Blood Pressure (mm Hg)	100/62	92/55	80/32	128/71	140/82

Case Study
SIRS to Severe Sepsis and Back—cont'd

PARAMETERS	TRIAGE IN ED	4 HOURS AFTER TRIAGE IN ED	6 HOURS AFTER TRIAGE IN ED	EMERGENCY ADMISSION TO CRITICAL CARE UNIT	36 HOURS LATER
Abnormal Laboratory Results					
White blood cells	—	15.2		17.8	11.4
% Neutrophils	—	92%		90%	60%
Bands	—	11.6%		12%	3%
Saturation of arterial oxygen (SaO_2)	—	91%	87%	90%	100%
Partial pressure of arterial oxygen (PaO_2) (mm Hg)	—	90	80	88	120
Partial pressure of arterial carbon dioxide ($PaCO_2$) (mm Hg)	—	22	20	35	35
pH	—	7.36	7.22	7.35	7.38
Base deficit/bicarbonate (HCO_3^-)	—	−9 (18)	−11 (15)	−8 (18.5)	−4 (21)
Fraction of inspired oxygen (FiO_2)	—	Nasal cannula (NC) at 4 L	Emergency intubation	1.0/positive end-expiratory pressure (PEEP) 18	0.4/PEEP 5
$ScvO_2$	—	—	—	41%	68%
Central venous pressure (CVP) (mm Hg)	—	—	—	13	15
Stroke volume (SV) (mL)	—	—	—	36	48
Stroke volume variation (SVV)	—	—	—	18%	
Chloride (Cl^-) (mEq/L)	—	99	—	105	101
Sodium (Na^+) (mEq/L)	—	138	—	140	138
Anion gap	—	26	—	17	15
Prothrombin time (PT) seconds	—	12.9	14.3	15.0	9.1
Platelets/mm^3	—	120	80	91	200
Serum lactate (mmol/L)	—	5.9	8.1	7.2	3.9

Continued

Case Study
SIRS to Severe Sepsis and Back—cont'd

Initial Triage in ED. Patient has flulike symptoms but appears relatively healthy and has normal vital signs. In fact, the patient is presenting with systemic inflammatory response syndrome (SIRS).

4 Hours after Triage with Second ED Assessment. A significant change in vital signs requires urgent treatment in the ED. A large bore peripheral catheter and radial arterial catheter are successfully inserted.

Interventions: He receives two 30 mL/kg intravenous (IV) fluid boluses totaling approximately 3 liters in 1.2 hours via the large bore peripheral access. Blood cultures and laboratory values are obtained, and the patient receives IV broad-spectrum antibiotics. The plan is to continue to monitor vital signs and laboratory results, which reveal acute metabolic acidosis and hyperlactatemia. The patient is hyperventilating in response to the metabolic acidosis, as his $PaCO_2$ has decreased to 22 mm Hg.

6 Hours after Triage with Third ED Assessment. Acute respiratory failure, acute cardiovascular collapse, hematologic dysfunction, and acute respiratory and metabolic acidosis are identified. The patient is now recognized as having severe sepsis to septic shock. Emergency intubation is performed and the patient is initially supported with bag mask ventilation.

Transfer to the Critical Care Unit. He is transferred to the critical care unit, where arterial-based cardiac output monitoring is initiated. A central venous oximetry catheter is inserted. Balanced fluids using lactated Ringer's solution are infused at 50 mL/kg and a norepinephrine infusion is started. Positive pressure mechanical ventilation is initiated for acute respiratory failure.

36 Hours Later. Severe sepsis and shock are resolving and gas exchange has improved. The patient is successfully weaned from the ventilator. Norepinephrine is discontinued. The serum lactate is clearing. ■

Conclusion

The singular and most important issue in sepsis continues to be early identification. The aggressive, protocol-driven management of patients who do not yet have shock has likely lowered the mortality rates of severe sepsis and septic shock since the inception of the Surviving Sepsis Campaign.

Sepsis remains a critical problem with significant morbidity and mortality even in the modern era of critical care management and advanced hemodynamic options. Multiple derangements exist in sepsis, involving several organs and systems. Previously, it was believed that sepsis merely represented an exaggerated, hyperinflammatory response, with death occurring from inflammation-induced organ injury. More recent data indicate that substantial heterogeneity exists in the inflammatory responses of patients with sepsis, with some appearing immunostimulated and others appearing immunosuppressed. Several factors initiate and perpetuate the inflammatory process in sepsis, including cytokines and endothelial dysfunction. Sepsis is a complex syndrome characterized by increased systemic coagulation, inflammation, and fibrinolysis. At this time, the literature does not support the concept of a single mediator, system, pathway, or pathogen that drives the pathophysiology of sepsis.

Management of sepsis and septic shock includes respiratory support, aggressive fluid resuscitation, inotropic support, vasopressor therapy, and early antibiotic therapy. In the future, less invasive methods of optimizing patients' fluid status and hemodynamics, along with monitoring of the microcirculatory dysfunction that is so prevalent in sepsis, may be routinely utilized.

Clinical Reasoning Pearl

Sepsis is a complex disease process.

Early resuscitation substantially reduces mortality substantially.

Administration of empirical antibiotics within an hour reduces mortality.

Resuscitation should address the multiple possible clinical manifestations of sepsis.

References

1. Geroulanos S, Douka ET: Historical perspective of the word "sepsis," *Intensive Care Med* 32:2077, 2006.
2. Bone RC, Balk RA, Cerra FB, et al.: Definitions for sepsis and organ failure and guidelines for the use of innovative therapies in sepsis. The ACCP/SCCM Consensus Conference Committee. American College of Chest Physicians/Society of Critical Care Medicine, *Chest* 101:1644–1655, 1993.
3. Rivers E, Nguyen B, Havsted S, et al.: Early goal directed therapy in the treatment of severe sepsis and septic shock, *N Engl J Med* 345(19):1368–1371, 2001.
4. Slade E, Tamber PS, Vincent JL: The surviving sepsis campaign: raising awareness to reduce mortality, *Crit Care* 7:1–2, 2003.
5. Levy MM, Fink MP, Marshall JC, et al.: 2001 SCCM/ESICM /ACCP/ATS/SIS international sepsis definitions conference, *Crit Care Med* 31:1250–1256, 2003.
6. Dellinger RP, Levy MM, Rhodes A, et al.: Surviving sepsis campaign: international guidelines for management of severe sepsis and septic shock: 2012, *Crit Care Med* 41(2):580–637, 2013.
7. Yealy DM, et al.: A randomized trial of protocol-based care for early septic shock, *N Engl J Med* 370(18):1683–1693, 2014.
8. Funk DJ, Parrillo JE, Kumar A: Sepsis and septic shock: a history, *Crit Care Clin* 25(1):83–101, 2009, viii.
9. Angus D, Van der Poll T: Severe sepsis and septic shock, *N Engl J Med* 369(21):2063, 2013.
10. Davies A, Green C, Hutton J: Severe sepsis: a European estimate of the burden of disease in ICU, *Int Care Med* 27:S284, 2001.
10a. Hall MJ, Williams SN, DeFrances CJ, Golosinskiy A: *Inpatient care for septicemia or sepsis: a challenge for patients and hospitals. NCHS data brief, no 62*, Hyattsville, MD, 2011, National Center for Health Statistics. http://www.cdc.gov/nchs/data/databriefs/db62.pdf. Accessed January 8, 2015.
11. Brun-Buisson C, Meshaka P, Pinton P, Vallet B: EPISEPSIS: a reappraisal of the epidemiology and outcome of severe sepsis in French intensive care units, *Intensive Care Med* 30:580–588, 2004.

12. Pittet D, Rangel-Frausto S, Li N, et al.: Systemic inflammatory response syndrome, sepsis, severe sepsis and septic shock: incidence, morbidities and outcomes in surgical ICU patients, *Intensive Care Med* 21:302–309, 1995.

13. Salvo I, de Cian W, Musicco M, et al.: The Italian SEPSIS study: preliminary results on the incidence and evolution of SIRS, sepsis, severe sepsis and septic shock, *Intensive Care Med* 21 (Suppl 2):S244–S249, 1995.

14. Mayr FB, Yende S, Angus DC: Epidemiology of severe sepsis, *Virulence* 5(1):4–11, 2014.

15. Martin GS, Mannino DM, Eaton S, Moss M: The epidemiology of sepsis in the United States from 1979 through 2000, *N Engl J Med* 348(16):1546–1554, 2003.

16. Angus DC, Linde-Zwirble WT, Lidicker J, et al.: Epidemiology of severe sepsis in the United States: analysis of incidence, outcome, and associated costs of care, *Crit Care Med* 29 (7):1303–1310, 2001.

17. Chalupka AN, Talmor D: The economics of sepsis, *Crit Care Clin* 28(1):57–76, 2012.

18. Cunneen J, Cartwright M: The puzzle of sepsis, *AACN Clin Issues* 15(1):18–44, 2004.

19. Baron RM, Baron MJ, Perrella MA: Pathobiology of sepsis: are we still asking the same questions? *Am J Respir Cell Mol Biol* 34:129–134, 2006.

20. Robertson CM, Coopersmith CM: The systemic inflammatory response syndrome, *Microbes Infect* 8:1382–1389, 2006.

21. Aird WC: The role of the endothelium in severe sepsis and multiple organ dysfunction syndrome, *Blood* 101(10):3765–3777, 2003.

22. Levinson AT, Casserly BP, Levy MM: Reducing mortality in severe sepsis and septic shock, *Semin Resp Crit Care Med* 32:195–205, 2011.

23. Ait-Oufella H, Maury E, Lehoux S, et al.: The endothelium: physiological functions and role in microcirculatory failure during severe sepsis, *Intensive Care Med* 36:1286–1298, 2010.

24. Mohammed I, Nonas S: Mechanisms, detection, and potential management of microcirculatory disturbances in sepsis, *Crit Care Clin* 26:393–408, 2010.

25. Dugas AF, Mackenhauer J, Salciccioli JD, et al.: Prevalence and characteristics of nonlactate and lactate expressors in septic shock, *J Crit Care* 27(4):344–350, 2012.

26. Hotchkiss RS, Karl IE: The pathophysiology and treatment of sepsis, *N Engl J Med* 348 (2):138–150, 2003.

27. Mayer S, Yasir A, Oaqaa KP: Definitions and pathophysiology of sepsis, *Curr Probl Pediatric Adoles Health Care* 43:260–263, 2013.

28. Sprung CL, Sakr Y, Vincent JL, et al.: An evaluation of systemic inflammatory response syndrome signs in the Sepsis Occurrence in Acutely ill Patients (SOAP) study, *Intensive Care Med* 32(3):421–427, 2006.

29. Becker KL, Nylén ES, White JC, et al.: Procalcitonin and the calcitonin gene family of peptides in inflammation, infection, and sepsis: a journey from calcitonin back to its precursors, *J Clin Endocrinol Metab* 89:1512–1525, 2004.

30. Reinhart K, Bauer M, Riedemann NC, Hartog CS: New approaches to sepsis: molecular diagnostics and biomarkers, *Clin Microbiol Rev* 25:609–634, 2012.

31. Agarwal R, Schwartz DN: Procalcitonin to guide duration of antimicrobial therapy in intensive care units: a systematic review, *Clin Infect Dis* 53:379–387, 2011.

32. Schuetz P, Müller B, Christ-Crain M, et al.: Procalcitonin to initiate or discontinue antibiotics in acute respiratory tract infections, *Cochrane Database Syst Rev* 9, 2012, CD007498.

33. Matthaiou DK, Ntani G, Kontogiorgi M, et al.: An ESICM systematic review and meta-analysis of procalcitonin-guided antibiotic therapy algorithms in adult critically ill patients, *Intensive Care Med* 38:940–949, 2012.

34. Wacker C, Prkno A, Brunkhorst FM, Schlattmann P: Procalcitonin as a diagnostic marker for sepsis: a systematic review and meta-analysis, *Lancet Infect Dis* (12):70323–70327, 2013.

35. Kumar A, Roberts D, Wood KE, et al.: Duration of hypotension before initiation of effective antimicrobial therapy is the critical determinant of survival in human septic shock, *Crit Care Med* 34:1589–1596, 2006.

36. Preisman S, Kogan S, Berkenstadt H, et al.: Predicting fluid responsiveness in patients undergoing cardiac surgery: functional hemodynamic parameters including the Respiratory Systolic Variation Test and static preload indicators, *Br J Anaesth* 95:746–755, 2005.

37. Legrand M, Dupuis C, Simon C, et al.: Association between systemic hemodynamics and septic acute kidney injury in critically ill patients: a retrospective observational study, *Crit Care* 17(6): R278, 2013.

38. Boyd JH, Forbes J, Nakada T, et al.: Fluid resuscitation in septic shock: a positive fluid balance and elevated central venous pressure are associated with increased mortality, *Crit Care Med* 39:259–265, 2011.

39. Marik PE, Baram M, Vahid B: Does central venous pressure predict fluid responsiveness? A systematic review of the literature and the tale of seven mares, *Chest* 134:172–178, 2008.

40. Osman D, Ridel C, Ray P, et al.: Cardiac filling pressures are not appropriate to predict hemodynamic response to volume challenge, *Crit Care Med* 35:64–68, 2007.

41. Harvey S, Harrison DA, Singer M, et al.: PAC-Man study collaboration: Assessment of the clinical effectiveness of pulmonary artery catheters in management of patients in intensive care (PACMan): a randomised controlled trial, *Lancet* 366(9484):472–477, 2005.

42. Bridges E: Using functional hemodynamic indicators to guide fluid therapy, *Am J Nurs* 113 (5):45–50, 2013.

43. Gattinoni L, Carlesso E: Supporting hemodynamics: what should we target? What treatments should we use? *Crit Care* 17(Suppl 1):S4, 2013.

44. Marik PE, Cavallazzi R, Vasu T, Hirani A: Dynamic changes in arterial waveform derived variables and fluid responsiveness in mechanically ventilated patients: a systematic review of the literature, *Crit Care Med* 37:2642–2647, 2009.

45. Cannesson M, Aboy M, Hofer CK, Rehman M: Pulse pressure variation: where are we today? *J Clin Monit Comput* 25:45–56, 2011.

46. Jabot J, Teboul JL, Richard C, et al.: Passive leg raising for predicting fluid responsiveness: importance of the postural change, *Intensive Care Med* 35:85–90, 2009.

47. Michard F, Teboul J: Predicting fluid responsiveness in ICU patients, *Chest* 121:2000–2008, 2002.

48. Asfar P, Meziani F, Hamel JF, et al.: High versus low blood-pressure target in patients with septic shock, *N Engl J Med* 370(17):1583–1593, 2014.

49. Landry DW, Levin HR, Gallant EM, et al.: Vasopressin pressor hypersensitivity in vasodilatory septic shock, *Crit Care Med* 25:1279–1282, 1997.

50. Zaky A, Deem S, Bendjelid K, et al.: Characterization of cardiac dysfunction in sepsis: an ongoing challenge, *Shock* 41(1):12–24, 2014.

51. Fernandes Jr CJ, de Assuncao MS: Myocardial dysfunction in sepsis: a large, unsolved puzzle, *Crit Care Res Pract*: 9 pages, 2012, Article ID 896430.

52. Turner KL: Identification of cardiac dysfunction in sepsis with B-type natriuretic peptide, *J Am Coll Surg* 213(1):139–146, 2011.

53. Hochstadt A, Meroz Y, Landesberg G: Myocardial dysfunction in severe sepsis and septic shock: more questions than answers? *J Cardiothorac Vasc Anesth* 25(3):526–535, 2011.

54. Schmidt H, Müller-Werdan U, Hoffmann T, et al.: Autonomic dysfunction predicts mortality in patients with multiple organ dysfunction syndrome of different age groups, *Crit Care Med* 33 (9):1994–2002, 2005.

55. Eisenberg PR, Jaffe AS, Schuster DP: Clinical evaluation compared to pulmonary artery catheterization in the hemodynamic assessment of critically ill patients, *Crit Care Med* 12:549–553, 1984.

56. Martin C, Auffray JP, Badetti C, et al.: Monitoring of central venous oxygen saturation versus mixed venous oxygen saturation in critically ill patients, *Intensive Care Med* 18:101–104, 1992.

57. Wo CC, Shoemaker WC, Appel PL, et al.: Unreliability of blood pressure and heart rate to evaluate cardiac output in emergency resuscitation and critical illness, *Crit Care Med* 21:218–223, 1993.

58. Reinhart K, Rudolph T, Bredle DL, et al.: Comparison of central-venous to mixed-venous oxygen saturation during changes in oxygen supply/demand, *Chest* 95:1216–1221, 1989.

59. Rady MY, Rivers EP, Martin GB, et al.: Continuous central venous oximetry and shock index in the emergency department: use in the evaluation of clinical shock, *Am J Emerg Med* 10:538–541, 1992.

60. James JH, Luchette FA, McCarter FD, et al.: Lactate is an unreliable indicator of tissue hypoxia in injury or sepsis, *Lancet* 354(9177):505–508, 1999.

61. Jansen TC, van Bommel J, Schoonderbeek FJ, et al.: LACTATE study group: Early lactate-guided therapy in intensive care unit patients: a multicenter, open-label, randomized controlled trial, *Am J Respir Crit Care Med* 182:752–761, 2010.

62. Rivers EP, Ander DS, Powell D: Central venous oxygen saturation monitoring in the critically ill patient, *Curr Opin Crit Care* 7:204–211, 2001.

63. Mikkelsen M, Miltiades A, Gaieski D, et al.: Serum lactate is associated with mortality in severe sepsis independent of organ failure and shock, *Crit Care Med* 37(5):1670–1677, 2009.

64. Liu V, Moorehouse J, Soule J, et al.: Fluid volume, lactate values, and mortality in sepsis patients with intermediate lactate values, *Ann Am Thorac Soc* 10(5):466–473, 2013.

65. Arnold RC, Shapiro NI, Jones AE, et al.: multicenter study of early lactate clearance as a determinant of survival in patients with presumed sepsis, *Shock* 32(1):35–39, 2009.

66. Nguyen HB, Rivers EP, Knoblich BP, et al.: Early lactate clearance is associated with improved outcome in severe sepsis and septic shock, *Crit Care Med* 32(8):1637–1642, 2004.

67. Arnold RC, Shapiro NI, Jones AE, et al.: Emergency Medicine Shock Research Network (EMShockNet) Investigators: multi-center study of early lactate clearance as a determinant of survival in patients with presumed sepsis, *Shock* 32:35–39, 2009.

68. Jones AE, Shapiro NI, Trzeciak S, et al.: Lactate clearance vs central venous oxygen saturation as goals of early sepsis therapy: a randomized clinical trial, *JAMA* 303(8):739–746, 2010.

69. The ProCESS Investigators: A Randomized Trial of Protocol-Based Care for Early Septic Shock, *N Engl J Med* 370(18):1683–1693, 2014.

70. Surviving Sepsis Campaign: Surviving sepsis campaign responds to the ProCESS trial. http://www.survivingsepsis.org/SiteCollectionDocuments/SSC-Responds-Process-Trial.pdf. Updated May 19, 2014. Accessed September 15, 2014.

71. Burdett E, Dushianthan A, Bennett-Guerrero E, et al.: Perioperative buffered versus non-buffered fluid administration for surgery in adults, *Cochrane Database Syst Rev 12: CD004089*, 2012.

72. Raghunathan K, Shaw A, Nathanson B, et al.: Association between the choice of IV crystalloid and in-hospital mortality among critically ill adults with sepsis, *Crit Care Med* 42(7):1585–1591, 2014.

73. De Backer D, Biston P, Devriendt J, et al.: SOAP II Investigators: comparison of dopamine and norepinephrine in the treatment of shock, *N Engl J Med* 362:779–789, 2010.

74. Russell JA, Walley KR, Singer J, et al.: VASST Investigators: vasopressin versus norepinephrine infusion in patients with septic shock, *N Engl J Med* 358:877–887, 2008.

75. Annane D, Bellissant E, Bollaert PE, et al.: Corticosteroids in the treatment of severe sepsis and septic shock in adults: a systematic review, *JAMA* 301:2362–2375, 2009.

76. Sprung CL, Annane D, Keh D, et al.: CORTICUS Study Group: hydrocortisone therapy for patients with septic shock, *N Engl J Med* 358:111–124, 2008.

77. Zanotti-Cavazzoni SL, Hollenberg SM: Cardiac dysfunction in severe sepsis and septic shock, *Curr Opin Crit Care* 15(5):392–397, 2009.

Hemodynamic and Intracranial Dynamic Monitoring in Neurocritical Care

21

Patricia A. Blissitt

As with other critically ill patients, patients with catastrophic neurologic illness or injury require hemodynamic monitoring. However, unique to the management of the critically ill patient with neurologic diagnoses such as severe traumatic brain injury (TBI), acute ischemic stroke, aneurysmal subarachnoid hemorrhage (aSAH), and spontaneous intracerebral hemorrhage (ICH) is consideration for intracranial dynamics. Management of both hemodynamic and intracranial dynamics is critical to minimizing secondary neuronal injury and maximizing neurologic outcomes. This chapter will (1) describe intracranial dynamics and the various physiologic methods of measurement; and (2) provide practical application of that knowledge and technology in the care of the critically ill neuroscience patient.

Historical Milestones

Prior to a discussion of physiology and physiologic methods, a brief history of neuromonitoring is warranted. Hemodynamic monitoring, specifically the pulmonary artery catheter, was first conceptualized in the 1960s by R.D. Bradley in collaboration with M.A. Branthwaite. The work of H.J.C. Swan and William Ganz soon followed.[1] Although less well known, neurologic monitoring began with J. Guillaume and P. Janny in the early 1950s. They used an electromagnetic transducer to measure cerebrospinal fluid (CSF) pressure in the ventricles of patients with intracranial pathology.[2] In the 1960s, Nils Lundberg's seminal work with the intraventricular catheter and external strain gauge transducer and identification of intracranial pressure (ICP) waveforms A, B, and C followed. Of particular significance is the A wave (plateau wave), which is described as an elevated ICP of 25 to 75 millimeters of mercury (mm Hg) lasting for 5 to 20 minutes.[3] Lundberg's work was followed by the development of additional ICP monitoring devices, including those placed outside of the ventricles, using fiberoptics, electronic internal strain gauge sensors, or air pouch technologies. After the development of ICP monitoring, other devices, both internal and external, were developed to measure additional intracranial dynamics, including brain oxygenation, indirect and direct measurement of cerebral blood flow, and biomarkers of cerebral ischemia.

Central Nervous System Multimodality Monitoring

In the past 20 years, the term *multimodality monitoring* has been used with increasing frequency with regard to the application of multiple physiologic methods to monitor the brain of the critically ill neuroscience patient. The use of additional monitoring modalities, both neurologic and systemic, and the resultant increase in data have added to the complexity of clinical decision making in this patient population. In a critically ill neuroscience patient, a number of intracranial and extracranial devices, both continuous and intermittent, as well as systemic devices are used to obtain clinical information. This plethora of information may confound patient assessment and management. While clinicians await such innovations as computer-assisted neurophysiologic decision support systems to assist them clinically, current knowledge and experience with intracranial and systemic multimodality monitoring are critical in maximizing neurologic outcomes.[4]

Key Physiologic Concepts

Intracranial Pressure and Cerebral Perfusion Pressure

Intracranial Pressure

The skull is a rigid container. Normally, the intracranial volume is composed of 80% brain tissue, 10% arterial and venous blood, and 10% CSF.[5] As a result of neurologic illness or injury, the volume of each may increase. Cerebral edema or tumor may increase brain tissue volume; hydrocephalus may increase CSF volume; and hemorrhage and hyperemia may increase cerebral blood volume (CBV). Hyperemia is defined as an excess of arterial blood flow to tissues as shown in Figure 21-1.

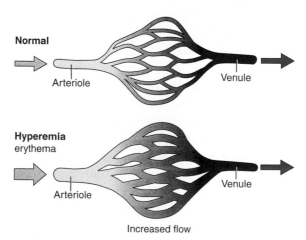

FIGURE 21-1 Hyperemia.

Small volume increases in one or two of the intracranial contents can be tolerated with a reciprocal decrease in the other one or two volumes. This compensation for small increases in volume between the three components—blood (arterial and venous), CSF, and brain tissue—is known as the *Monro-Kellie Doctrine*.[5,6] In pathological states, as the intracranial volume increases, the brain has limited compensatory mechanisms, including (1) shunting of the CSF out of the ventricular system and into the lumbar subarachnoid space and perioptic subarachnoid space, and (2) return of venous blood out of the brain through the internal jugular veins and back to the heart. Once these compensatory mechanisms are exhausted, ICP begins to increase (Figure 21-2). With an increasing ICP, pressure gradients are generated which will result in herniation of brain tissue, if effective emergency interventions are not undertaken.

Although an ICP greater than 20 mm Hg is generally considered elevated requiring treatment, patients herniate at various values for reasons that are not completely understood. Herniation may be subfalcine (cingulate), transtentorial (central and uncal), tonsillar (at the foramen magnum), or extracranial (through a traumatic or surgical defect) (Figure 21-3).

Normal ICP is 5 to 15 mm Hg[5,6] (Table 21-1). Although a systolic and diastolic component to the ICP waveform is evident, ICP is read as a mean value (Figure 21-4). The ICP waveform consists of three components—cardiac, respiratory, and vasogenic—as determined by spectral analysis.[7] ICP is influenced by a number of cerebral regulatory mechanisms, including the partial pressure of arterial carbon dioxide ($PaCO_2$), cerebral blood flow (CBF), cerebral metabolism coupling, and pressure autoregulation. The $PaCO_2$ is a potent vasodilator. As a result, as the $PaCO_2$ increases, CBF increases,

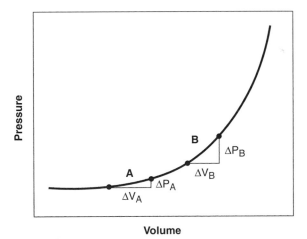

FIGURE 21-2 Volume pressure response curve. Each change in volume (ΔV) is associated with an associated change in pressure (ΔP) within the rigid cranium (skull). At point *A*, the intracranial pressure (ICP) is low and the increase in volume (ΔV$_A$) produces only a small change in pressure (ΔP$_A$). At point *B*, the ICP is higher indicating that the normal compensatory mechanisms are no longer effective, consequently the same small increase in volume (ΔV$_B$) is associated with a steep rise in ICP (ΔP$_B$). (From Padayachy LC, Figaji AA, Bullock MR: Intracranial pressure monitoring for traumatic brain injury in the modern era, *Childs Nerv Syst* 26(4): 442, 2010.)

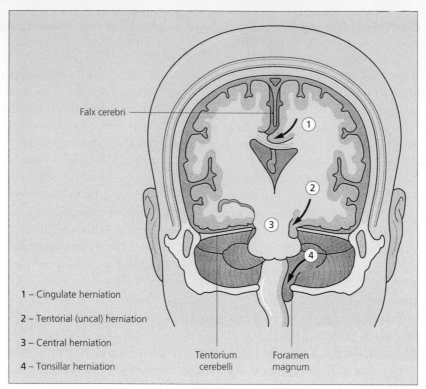

FIGURE 21-3 Types of brain herniation. (From Rengacharry SS, Ellenbogen RG: *Principles of neurosurgery*, ed 2, Philadelphia, 2005, Elsevier.)

Labels within figure:

Falx cerebri

1 – Cingulate herniation

2 – Tentorial (uncal) herniation

3 – Central herniation

4 – Tonsillar herniation

Tentorium cerebelli

Foramen magnum

TABLE 21-1   Normal Values

PARAMETER	NORMAL VALUES	COMMENTS
ICP	5-15 mm Hg	Intraventricular catheter represented the gold standard for obtaining the ICP waveform and mean value.
CPP	60-160 mm Hg	$CPP = MAP - ICP$
CBF (global)	50-100 mL/100 g/min (global brain CBF) 80 mL/100 g/min (gray matter) 20 mL/100 g/min (white matter)	Calculated as: $CBF = CPP \div$ cerebrovascular resistance
$CMRO_2$	3.2 mL/100 g/min (global brain $CMRO_2$) 6 mL/100 g/min (gray matter) 2 mL/100 g /min (white matter)	
$PbtO_2$	25-30 mm Hg	A specialized fiberoptic tipped catheter placed into brain tissue is required to measure brain tissue oxygen levels.
$SjvO_2$	55%-70%	A specialized fiberoptic catheter inserted into the jugular vein
$AjvDO_2$	4-8 mL/dL	Calculated value

AjvDO₂, Arteriojugular venous oxygen difference; *CBF*, cerebral blood flow; *CMRO₂*, cerebral metabolic rate of oxygen; *CPP*, cerebral perfusion pressure; *g/min*, grams per minute; *ICP*, intracranial pressure; *MAP*, mean arterial pressure; *mL*, milliliters; *mL/dL*, milliliters per deciliter; *PbtO₂*, brain tissue oxygenation; *SjvO₂*, jugular venous oxygen saturation.

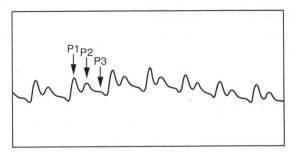

FIGURE 21-4 Normal intracranial pressure waveform with characteristic P1, P2, and P3 components of decreasing amplitude (P1 >P2 > P3). (From Kirkness CJ, Mitchell PH, Burr RI, et al.: Intracranial pressure waveform analysis: clinical and research implications, *J Neurosci Nurs* 32(5): 273, 2000.)

resulting in increased CBF and CBV (Figure 21-5). In contrast, lowering of the $PaCO_2$, such as through hyperventilation, decreases CBV and CBF and may result in ischemia.[8]

Normally, a decrease in cerebral metabolic rate (CMR) results in a decrease in CBF; however, this mechanism may not be intact in neurologically injured or ill patients.[5,9] Systemic blood pressure and ICP also have a dynamic interplay. In the presence of intact cerebral autoregulation (discussed later), increased blood pressure may accompany increased ICP spontaneously or be induced pharmacologically. This will result in a compensatory decrease in the diameter of cerebral blood vessels, lower CBV, and consequently decreased ICP.[3]

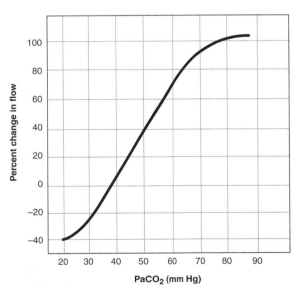

FIGURE 21-5 The relationship between partial pressure of arterial carbon dioxide ($PaCO_2$) and percentage change in cerebral blood flow (CBF). (From Padayachy LC, Figaji AA, Bullock MR: Intracranial pressure monitoring for traumatic brain injury in the modern era, *Childs Nerv Syst* 26(4): 442, 2010.)

Cerebral Perfusion Pressure

Cerebral perfusion pressure (CPP) has been defined as the pressure that drives CBF into the brain's microcirculation.[10] Clinically, it is calculated as mean arterial pressure (MAP) minus ICP. Adequate CPP provides some protection against secondary ischemia. However, to date, adequate CPP for each patient is not known. Evidence-based guidelines such as the Brain Trauma Foundation's *Guidelines for the Management of Severe Traumatic Brain Injury* support a CPP range of 50 to 70 mm Hg for adults.[11] However, the CPP threshold may vary from patient to patient, depending on such factors as autoregulatory status and intracranial compliance.[10] *Intracranial compliance* is defined as a change in ICP in relationship to the change in intracranial volume.[5,6] Elevated CPP in neurological injury or illness does not necessarily result in improved outcomes.[12,13]

Cerebral Blood Flow

The brain normally receives 15% to 20% of the cardiac output in the healthy adult.[14–16] CBF has been defined as CPP divided by cerebrovascular resistance. In the uninjured brain, increases in CPP and cerebrovascular resistance (vasomotor tone) result in controlled increases or decreases in CBF, as needed, to protect the brain against cerebral ischemia and hyperemia (Figure 21-6). The average global normal CBF is 50 to 100 mL/100 g/min.[14–16] Flow varies in white and gray matter, with gray matter (the

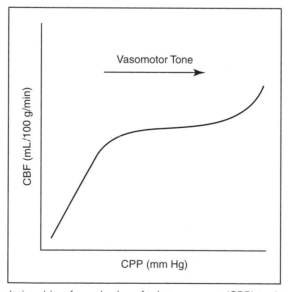

FIGURE 21-6 The relationship of cerebral perfusion pressure (CPP) and cerebrovascular resistance to cerebral blood flow (CBF).

cell bodies of the neurons) being more metabolically active and having greater energy (oxygen and glucose) requirements. The average CBF to white matter is 20 mL/100 g/min, whereas the average CBF to gray matter is 80 mL/100 g/min.[14–16]

CBF is regulated by a number of factors, including metabolism, $PaCO_2$, partial pressure of arterial oxygen (PaO_2), blood viscosity, and cerebral autoregulation. The relationship with the $PaCO_2$ is linear; as the $PaCO_2$ increases from 20 to 80 mm Hg, CBF increases. In contrast, as the $PaCO_2$ decreases, CBF decreases. CBF is unaffected by PaO_2 when the PaO_2 is greater than 50 mm Hg. However, when the PaO_2 is less than 50 mm Hg, as the PaO_2 decreases, CBF increases.[6] CBF is inversely related to blood viscosity. As viscosity increases, CBF diminishes. Viscosity is primarily influenced by hematocrit. Hemodilution enhances CBF by improving the rheology (flow).[16] The role of cerebral metabolism and cerebral autoregulation in CBF is described below.

Cerebral Metabolism

CBF and cerebral metabolism are normally tightly coupled. A change in cerebral metabolism and the cerebral metabolic rate of oxygen ($CMRO_2$) normally results in a corresponding change in CBF. If the metabolic needs are heightened, CBF increases. If the metabolic demands are lessened, CBF decreases both globally and regionally in the brain. The average $CMRO_2$ globally in the brain is about 3.2 mL/100 g/min.[16] Similar to CBF, $CMRO_2$ also varies in white and gray matter, with white matter $CMRO_2$ averaging 2 mL/100 g/min and gray matter averaging 6 mL/100 g/min.[16] The primary source of energy for the brain is glucose. Oxygen is required for aerobic metabolism.

Cerebral Autoregulation

Cerebral autoregulation is the ability of the cerebral blood vessels to constrict and dilate as needed to maintain adequate cerebral perfusion. In the normal adult, cerebral autoregulation is considered operational over a range of MAP between 60 and 160 mm Hg or CPP between 50 mm Hg and 150 mm Hg (accounting for a normal ICP of 10 mm Hg)[15–17] (Figure 21-7). Cerebral autoregulation protects the brain from injury related to ischemia or hyperemia. If autoregulation is impaired regionally or globally or MAP or CPP is outside these limits, the brain is dependent on the systemic blood pressure and may be at risk for secondary injury. Cerebral autoregulation is impacted by metabolic, myogenic, and neurogenic mechanisms.[15] Possible chemical mediators include adenosine, nitric oxide, protein kinase C, melatonin, prostacyclin, and activated potassium channels.[16] The term *myogenic mechanism* refers to the response of vascular smooth muscle to changes in perfusion or transmural pressure. The neurogenic response of the cerebral blood vessels may involve such neurotransmitters as norepinephrine, neuropeptide Y, cholecystokinin, acetylcholine, and peptides. The blood pressure range for intact cerebral autoregulation may be different for patients who are chronically hypertensive. They may require a higher range of MAP or CPP to maintain CBF, and their autoregulatory curve is said to be "shifted to the right."[16,17]

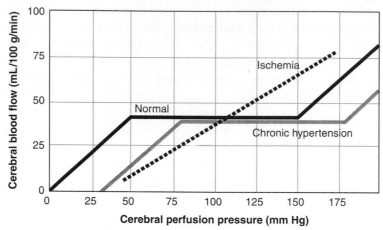

FIGURE 21-7 Cerebral autoregulation ranges from 50 to 150 mm Hg for the healthy brain. In chronic hypertension the autoregulation range is shifted to the right, and may be 75 to 175 mm Hg or higher, with considerable individual variation. Autoregulation is impaired in ischemia and hyperemia, leaving brain tissues unprotected against a pathological increase in cerebral blood flow (CBF) and increase in cerebral perfusion pressure (CPP). (From Rose JC, Mayer SA: Optimizing blood pressure in neurological emergencies, *Neurocrit Care* 1(3): 289, 2004.)

Following catastrophic brain injury or illness, autoregulation may be impaired or abolished regionally or globally.

Cerebral Ischemia

Cerebral ischemia has been defined as a CBF of 18 to 20 mL/100 g/min.[14] Ischemia may lead to cerebral infarction. Neuronal death has been found to occur at a CBF of 8 to 10 mL/100 g/min.[14] Inadequate CBF may be global or regional and relative or absolute. Whenever the CBF does not meet the cerebral metabolic demands, the brain is at risk. At a cellular level, an ischemic cascade has been hypothesized; in this cascade, increased levels of toxic excitatory neurotransmitters are released; calcium moves intracellularly; and free radicals injure the neuronal cell membrane in a process known as *lipid peroxidation*.[10] Although much of the damage may occur with primary brain injury or insult, secondary brain injury such as hypotension, hypoxia, fever, hypoglycemia, hyperglycemia, hypernatremia, hyponatremia, hypercapnia, hypocapnea, hyperemia, increased ICP, and decreased ICP may compound the damage.[5]

Cerebral Hyperemia

Cerebral hyperemia, an absolute or relative excess of blood flow, occurs when CBF exceeds the brain's metabolic demand. Excess CBF results in increased cerebral blood volume and may contribute to increased ICP and decreased CPP. Cerebral hyperemia sometimes follows TBI in children or young adults and may contribute to secondary injury. Cerebral hyperemia is thought to represent an impairment of cerebral autoregulation. As with other derangements of cerebrovascular physiology, hyperemia may be absolute or relative, associated with a regional or global decrease in metabolic demand.[14,15]

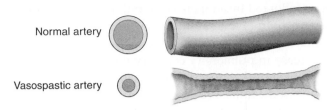

FIGURE 21-8 Cerebral vasospasm: normal artery versus spasm.

Cerebral Vasospasm

Cerebral vasospasm is a sustained narrowing of cerebral arteries (Figure 21-8). It is thought to be the result of vasoconstriction, edema of the vascular endothelium, remodeling of the tunica media (the muscular layer of the vessel), subendothelial fibrosis, or a combination of all these factors.[18] As a result of the narrowing, the total blood volume flowing through the vessel is compromised, resulting in decreased CBF and a fall in oxygen and glucose delivery, which leads to cerebral ischemia and infarction. The inadequate blood supply associated with cerebral vasospasm has been termed *delayed cerebral ischemia* (DCI).[19]

Vasospasm may be radiographically visualized on angiography or quantified indirectly by the measurement of flow velocities by transcranial Doppler (TCD). A patient who has vasospasm may or may not present clinically with neurologic deficits. Also, a patient with clinical deterioration that is thought to be related to vasospasm may not show radiographic evidence. Cerebral vasospasm is most frequently associated with aSAH but is also associated with traumatic SAH. Following aSAH, cerebral vasospasm occurs after day 3 but ends before day 21. It most commonly occurs between days 4 and 14, with a peak incidence on day 7.[18] Vasospasm may involve multiple vessels both proximal and distal to the ruptured aneurysm. Vasospasm with delayed cerebral ischemia (DCI) is associated with cerebral infarction and increased morbidity and mortality.[20–22] Cerebral vasospasm after subarachnoid hemorrhage is a major cause of secondary neuronal injury.

Neurogenic Pulmonary Edema

Following severe brain injury or illness, some critically ill neuroscience patients are at risk for neurogenic pulmonary edema, which may be abbreviated as NPE. Onset is rapid and may further compromise the critically ill neuroscience patient. Hypoxia from the sudden increase in interstitial and alveolar pulmonary fluid contributes to secondary brain injury.[23,24] Neurogenic pulmonary edema is most often associated with aSAH and severe TBI and has also been reported with status epilepticus and cerebellar hemorrhage.[23,24] The pathophysiology is not clear. At least three different etiologies are thought to be responsible for the development of neurogenic pulmonary edema: (1) a dramatic increase in ICP and corresponding decrease in cerebral perfusion globally; (2) cerebral hemorrhage; or (3) focal ischemia in specific areas of the brain, including the vasomotor centers located in the dorsal medulla of the brainstem such as the area postrema, and the solitarius tractus nuclei or the posterior hypothalamus. These areas provide input and output to the pulmonary system.[23,25] As a result of increased ICP or cerebral ischemia, one of two mechanisms may occur: (1) the cerebral injury results in a sympathetic response followed by an increase in pulmonary hydrostatic pressure, which leads to an increase in pulmonary capillary permeability, or (2) the cerebral injury results in an inflammatory response such as the release of cytokines and chemokines, which leads to an increase in pulmonary capillary permeability[23] (Figure 21-9).

The clinical presentation of neurogenic pulmonary edema varies. It typically occurs at the time of the initial brain injury; however, it may also present with neurologic deterioration. In its purest form, it presents as pulmonary edema in the absence of left ventricular failure. Increased heart and respiratory rates, pulmonary crackles in the bases, respiratory failure, and the absence of a cardiac gallop are more frequently reported. Unilateral neurogenic pulmonary edema has been reported as well.[23]

The diagnostic workup for neurogenic pulmonary edema includes chest radiography, echocardiography, electrocardiography (ECG), and central venous pressure (CVP). The chest radiography reveals bilateral pulmonary infiltrates. Echocardiography, ECG, and

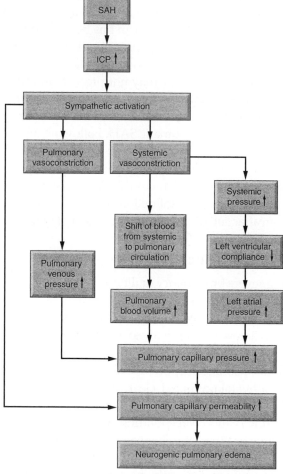

FIGURE 21-9 The proposed mechanism of neurogenic pulmonary edema. *ICP*, Intracranial pressure; *SAH*, subarachnoid hemorrhage. (From Muroi C, Keller M, Pangalu A, et al.: Neurogenic pulmonary edema in patients with subarachnoid hemorrhage, *J Neuorsurg Anesthesiol* 20(3): 191, 2008.)

CVP are typically normal. If a pulmonary artery catheter is in place, it may reveal a transient increase in pulmonary artery occlusion pressure (PAOP). Neurogenic pulmonary edema must be differentiated from aspiration pneumonia, ventilator-associated pneumonia (VAP), ventilator-induced lung injury, and acute respiratory distress syndrome (ARDS).[23]

The management of neurogenic pulmonary edema includes treatment of the catastrophic brain injury with normalization of the ICP and CPP, mechanical ventilation, and diuretic therapy with maintenance of adequate CPP. If needed for blood pressure support, norepinephrine (Levophed) and epinephrine have not been found to worsen neurogenic pulmonary edema as these medications increase pulmonary capillary pressure but not pulmonary vascular permeability. Although neurogenic pulmonary edema is of non-cardiac origin, dobutamine (Dobutrex) has been reported to provide beneficial effects such as improvement in the cardiac index (CI), left ventricular stroke work index (LVSWI), pulmonary artery pressure (PAP), and P/F ratio, without a decrease in cerebral oxygenation.[23] The P/F ratio is calculated as PaO_2 divided by the FiO_2 (fraction of inspired oxygen). However, caution is advised, as dobutamine may lower blood pressure, and attention to maintenance of adequate CPP is imperative.[26] Beta-blockers are not recommended.[23]

Neurogenic Stunned Myocardium

Severe brain injury or illness has also been associated with neurogenic stunned myocardium, also referred to as *neurogenic stress cardiomyopathy*. Neurogenic stunned myocardium has most often been associated with aSAH but has also been reported in association with increased ICP, stroke, seizures, and meningitis.[27] As with neurogenic pulmonary edema, the pathophysiology is not clear. The general areas of the brain responsible for the clinical presentation may be similar to neurogenic pulmonary edema, including the brainstem and diencephalon, incorporating the thalamus and hypothalamus, and also the insular cortex between the temporal and frontal lobes. The specific area in the medulla oblongata that is thought to be responsible for neurogenic stunned myocardium includes the nucleus tractus solitarius (Figure 21-10). One postulated mode of transmission includes a sympathetic mediated response at the insula and hypothalamus with connections through the medulla oblongata of the brainstem and lateral horn of the spinal cord where the sympathetic nervous system sends input to the heart via the thoracic nerve roots and the cervical ganglia[27] (Figure 21-10).

At least three mechanisms have been proposed in neurogenic stunned myocardium. They are (1) ischemia induced coronary artery spasm; (2) cardiac microvascular dysfunction; and (3) the sympathetic-mediated hypothesis. Neither the first nor the second mechanism has been supported by substantial evidence. The release of catecholamine into the bloodstream as a result of the catastrophic brain injury is associated with increased cardiac enzymes creatine kinase–MB (CK-MB) and troponin T (cTnT). In addition the local release of norepinephrine directly into the heart from sympathetic nervous system nerve terminals may contribute to resultant necrosis of the myocardial contraction bands as well (Figure 21-10).[27]

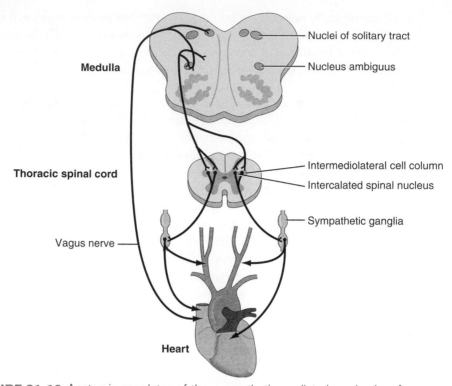

FIGURE 21-10 Anatomic correlates of the sympathetic-mediated mechanism for neurogenic stunned myocardium: nucleus tractus solitarius (nuclei of the solitary tract) of the medulla of the brainstem and its projections through the spinal cord to the heart.

Clinical manifestations of neurogenic stunned myocardium including regional wall motion abnormalities (RWMA), abnormalities on echocardiography, pulmonary edema on chest radiography, cardiac biomarker elevation, and ECG changes but with normal coronary arteries.[28] Cardiac arrhythmias may cause hemodynamic instability, resulting in sudden death. In addition to arrhythmias, ECG abnormalities may include QT prolongation, ST segment changes, new Q waves, U waves, and ECG criteria diagnostic for left ventricular (LV) hypertrophy. With regard to cardiac biomarkers, CK-MB may increase more slowly and peak lower than is seen in myocardial infarction.[28] Troponin I (cTnI) may be a more sensitive indicator for LV dysfunction. In neurogenic stunned myocardium, LV dysfunction is sometimes reversible. The degree of permanent cardiac injury, especially myocardial necrosis, is related to the severity of the neurologic injury. Elevated brain natriuretic peptide may also rise as an indicator of the dysfunction of the myocardium. On echocardiography, regional wall abnormalities may manifest differently with neurogenic stunned myocardium compared with myocardial changes related to coronary artery disease.[27] Neurogenic stunned myocardium may progress to low ejection fraction with acute heart failure sometimes manifesting as *Tako-tsubo cardiomyopathy*, with left apical ballooning[27] (Figure 21-11).

As with neurogenic pulmonary edema, management of neurogenic stunned myocardium includes appropriate management of the underlying neurologic injury. If

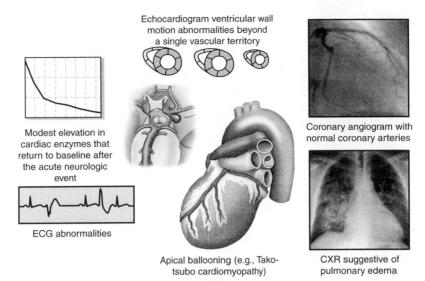

Echocardiogram ventricular wall motion abnormalities beyond a single vascular territory

Modest elevation in cardiac enzymes that return to baseline after the acute neurologic event

ECG abnormalities

Apical ballooning (e.g., Tako-tsubo cardiomyopathy)

Coronary angiogram with normal coronary arteries

CXR suggestive of pulmonary edema

FIGURE 21-11 Clinical manifestations of stunned neurogenic myocardium following an acute neurological event include pulmonary edema, cardiac wall motion abnormalities, elevation in cardiac biomarkers, ECG abnormalities and normal coronary arteries. Acute heart failure with left atrial ballooning may develop. (From Lee VH et al.: Mechanisms in neurogenic stress cardiomyopathy after aneurysmal subarachnoid hemorrhage, *Neurocrit Care* 5(3): 243-249, 2006.)

the neurogenic stunned myocardium progresses to wall abnormalities and ventricular failure, this may prove difficult, as management of the neurologic illness or injury and that of the neurogenic stunned myocardium may be in direct conflict. Use of a pulmonary artery catheter to guide management of fluids and vasoactive agents may be necessary, and in rare instances, intra-aortic balloon counterpulsation may be required to support the patient's systemic and cerebral hemodynamics.[27]

Central Nervous System Measurement Methods

Overview

A number of measurement methods are available for monitoring the brain in catastrophic brain injury or insult. Although nothing can be done to reverse primary neuronal injury, the goal is prevention or minimization of secondary neuronal injury. Secondary insults include hypoxia, hypercapnia, hypotension, hypertension, hyperglycemia, hypoglycemia, hypernatremia, hyponatremia, fever, increased ICP, decreased CPP, and cerebral vasospasm. No amount of intracranial dynamic monitoring negates the need for the bedside assessment; however, monitoring the brain can provide additional data to assist in clinical decision-making. This section discusses various methods of ICP and CPP monitoring, including the external ventricular catheter drain (EVD), transducer-tipped catheters, both fiberoptic and electronic strain gauge, and air pouch technology. Methods of brain oxygen monitoring to be included are brain tissue oxygenation ($PbtO_2$), the fiberoptic retrograde jugular bulb catheter (jugular venous oxygen saturation [$SjvO_2$]), and near-infrared spectroscopy (NIRS).

Application of transcranial Doppler (TCD), as an indirect measurement of CBF will be discussed. Although less commonly used to quantify CBF, thermal diffusion flowmetry (TDF) and laser Doppler flowmetry (LDF) will also be reviewed.

Cerebral microdialysis is another tool that will be briefly discussed. Additional adjuncts are temperature measurement, partial pressure of end-tidal carbon dioxide ($PetCO_2$) monitoring, and pupillometry. Each measurement method will be discussed with regard to clinical procedure, technical considerations, indications setup, establishing a baseline assessment, maintenance, troubleshooting, and patient safety, comfort, and education.

Intracranial Pressure Monitoring and Cerebral Perfusion Pressure Monitoring

External Ventricular Drain

The external ventricular catheter, or ventricular drain with an external strain gauge transducer is considered the gold standard for ICP monitoring.[2,29] Compared with other ICP monitoring systems, it is said to be the least expensive, most accurate, and most reliable.[29] A catheter is inserted into the anterior horn of one of the two lateral ventricles of the brain, preferably on the nondominant side.[2,29] The ventricular catheter is attached to an fluid-filled external strain gauge transducer and drainage system. The external ventricular catheter has the added advantage of allowing CSF drainage as a method of controlling ICP in addition to ICP monitoring. The ventriculostomy catheter is radiopaque and is magnetic resonance imaging (MRI) compatible.

Clinical Procedure

The external ventricular catheter may be inserted in the operating room or at the bedside in the critical care unit. Sterile technique must be maintained regardless of the location. The critical care unit environment must be held to the standard of an operating room with use of sterile gowns and gloves, hair covers, face masks, and sterile draping; minimal movement in and out of the room; and a closed door. Approximately 30 minutes to an hour before beginning the procedure, an antibiotic may be ordered for prophylaxis. Prior to draping, the patient's hair may be clipped, and the skin prepared. The use of chlorhexidine is controversial because of possible neurotoxicity associated with chlorhexidine.[30] Povidone iodine is preferred. The physician will make the skin incision and burr hole, open the dura, and insert the catheter toward the opposite nare. Once CSF is obtained, the primed external ventricular drainage system will be connected to the catheter (Figure 21-12). The catheter is tunneled to exit a few centimeters away from the burr hole and the incisions are closed. If cerebral edema with midline shift or collapse of the lateral ventricle is present, insertion of the catheter may be more complicated.

Indications

Indications for ICP monitoring in general include TBI, ICH, SAH, hydrocephalus, hepatic failure with encephalopathy, acute ischemic stroke with large infarction, and

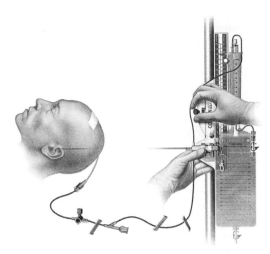

FIGURE 21-12 External ventricular drain. (Courtesy of Codman Neuro. EDS 3 is a trademark of Codman Neuro.)

meningitis.[2–6] The Brain Trauma Foundation's *Guidelines for the Management of Severe Traumatic Brain Injury* recommend ICP monitoring for the following reasons:

(1) post-resuscitation Glasgow Coma Scale (GCS) of 8 or less, with an abnormal computed tomography (CT) (Level II of III recommendation); or (2) a post-resuscitation GCS of 8 or less with a normal CT with at least two of the following: hypotension defined as a systolic blood pressure less than 90 mm Hg, age over 40 years, and decorticate or decerebrate posturing (Level III of III recommendation, the lowest quality of evidence) [31,32] (Table 21-2).

The patient who has a GCS of 9 or greater may also be considered for ICP monitoring, particularly if the patient is unable to participate in the bedside assessment for any reason[33] (Table 21-3). The American Heart Association and American Stroke Association (AHA/ASA) have recommended ventriculostomy and insertion of an external ventricular drain after acute aneurysmal SAH with decreased level of consciousness, which is a Class I out of III (highest quality of evidence) recommendation related to the communicating hydrocephalus associated with aSAH[34–36] (Table 21-4).

The AHA/ASA recommendation also includes ICP monitoring and maintenance of a CPP of 50 to 70 mm Hg for spontaneous ICH (patients with a GCS of ≤ 8 with intraventricular hemorrhage, hydrocephalus, or evidence of transtentorial herniation). This is a Class IIb out of III recommendation[37,38] (Table 21-5). Ventricular drainage is specifically recommended for hydrocephalus associated with spontaneous ICH.[39,40] In contrast, the AHA/ASA recommendation does not include routine ICP monitoring for acute ischemic stroke, even though the patient may have a focal area of cerebral edema. ICP monitoring is not considered helpful in large hemispheric infarcts, since herniation is the greater concern and definitive therapy such as decompressive craniectomy is effective. This is a Class I out of III recommendation based on the highest quality of evidence[41] (Table 21-6).

TABLE 21-2   Brain Trauma Foundation Evidence-Based Guidelines for Severe Traumatic Brain Injury (TBI)

PARAMETER		CLASSIFICATION OF RECOMMENDATION AND LEVEL OF EVIDENCE
Blood pressure	In severe TBI, systemic blood pressure must be monitored, and hypotension, defined as a systolic blood pressure <90 mm Hg, must be avoided.	Class of Evidence: Moderate Quality Randomized Controlled Trial, Good Quality Cohort Study or Good Quality Case Control Study. Recommendation: Level II
Intracranial pressure	In severe TBI, intravenous mannitol (Osmitrol) at a dose range of 0.25–1.0 gram per kilogram (g/kg) is effective in reducing increased intracranial pressure (ICP).	Class of Evidence: Moderate Quality Randomized Controlled Trial, Good Quality Cohort Study, or Good Quality Case Control Study. Recommendation: Level II
Intracranial pressure	In severe TBI, the use of intravenous mannitol should be restricted prior to ICP monitoring to patients with neurologic deterioration or transtentorial herniation.	Class of Evidence: Poor Quality Randomized Controlled Trial. Recommendation: Level III
Intracranial pressure	In severe TBI, a patient should have ICP monitoring with a Glasgow Coma Scale score of ≤ 8 after resuscitation or an abnormal head computed tomography (CT), demonstrating hematomas, contusions, edema, herniation, or compressed basal cisterns.	Class of Evidence: Moderate Quality Randomized Controlled Trial, Good Quality Cohort Study, or Good Quality Case Control Study. Recommendation: Level II
Intracranial pressure	In severe TBI, patient should have ICP monitoring with a normal head CT and two or more of the following: >40 years old, motor posturing, or systolic blood pressure <90 mm Hg.	Class of Evidence: Poor Quality Randomized Controlled Trial. Recommendation: Level III
Intracranial pressure	In severe TBI, ICP >20 mm Hg should be treated.	Class of Evidence: Moderate Quality Randomized Controlled Trial, Good Quality Cohort Study, or Good Quality Case Control Study. Recommendation: Level II
Intracranial pressure	In severe TBI, ICP, clinical presentation, and brain CT should be used in consideration for ICP monitoring.	Class of Evidence: Poor Quality Randomized Controlled Trial. Recommendation: Level III

TABLE 21-2 Brain Trauma Foundation Evidence-Based Guidelines for Severe Traumatic Brain Injury (TBI)—cont'd

PARAMETER		CLASSIFICATION OF RECOMMENDATION AND LEVEL OF EVIDENCE
Cerebral perfusion pressure (CPP)	In severe TBI, aggressive administration of fluids and vasopressors should be avoided to maintain CPP at >70 mm Hg, as the risk of adult respiratory distress syndrome is increased.	Class of Evidence: Moderate Quality Randomized Controlled Trial, Good Quality Cohort Study, or Good Quality Case Control Study. Recommendation: Level II
Cerebral perfusion pressure (CPP)	In severe TBI, the goal CPP is between 50 and 70 mm Hg. CPP of <50 mm Hg is to be avoided.	Class of Evidence: Poor Quality Randomized Controlled Trial. Recommendation: Level III
Brain oxygen monitoring	In severe TBI, parameters for treatment of brain oxygenation include a jugular venous oxygen saturation (SjvO$_2$) of <50% or a brain tissue oxygenation (PbtO$_2$) <15 mm Hg.	Class of Evidence: Poor Quality Randomized Controlled Trial. Recommendation: Level III

TABLE 21-3 The Glasgow Coma Scale (GCS)

Eye Opening (E)

Spontaneous	4
To call	3
To pain	2
None	1

Motor response (M)

Obeys commands	6
Localizes pain	5
Normal flexion (withdrawal)	4
Abnormal flexion (decorticate)	3
Extension (decerebrate)	2
None (flaccid)	1

Verbal response (V)

Oriented	5
Confused conversation	4
Inappropriate words	3
Incomprehensible sounds	2
None	1

GCS sum score = (E + M + V); best possible score = 15; worst possible score = 3.

From Rengacharry SS, Ellenbogen RG: *Principles of neurosurgery*, ed 2, Philadelphia, 2005, Elsevier.

TABLE 21-4 **AHA/ASA Guidelines for Hemodynamic and Intracranial Parameters in Spontaneous Aneurysmal Subarachnoid Hemorrhage (aSAH)**

PARAMETER		CLASSIFICATION OF RECOMMENDATION AND LEVEL OF EVIDENCE
Systemic blood pressure	The following recommendation has been made to prevent rebleeding after aSAH: Prior to aneurysm obliteration, a continuous titratable intravenous medication should be used to control blood pressure, minimize the risk of rebleeding related to hypertension, and maintain adequate cerebral perfusion pressure.	Class I: Benefit much greater than risk. Level B evidence: Evidence based on limited patient populations, utilizing one randomized trial or more than one nonrandomized trials.
Systemic blood pressure	The following recommendation has been made to minimize the risk of rebleeding after aSAH: Although the extent of systemic blood pressure control is unknown with regard to minimizing the risk of rebleeding, a systolic blood pressure of <160 mm Hg is reasonable.	Class IIa: Benefit greater than risk. Level C evidence: Evidence based on very limited patient populations, utilizing expert consensus, case studies, and standards of care.
Intravascular volume	The following recommendation has been made to manage cerebral vasospasm and delayed cerebral ischemia: To prevent delayed cerebral ischemia, euvolemia and a normal circulating blood volume should be maintained.	Class I: Benefit much greater than risk. Level B evidence: Evidence based on limited patient populations, utilizing one randomized trial or more than one nonrandomized trials.
Intravascular volume	The following recommendation has been made to manage cerebral vasospasm and delayed cerebral ischemia: Systemic hypervolemia is not recommended in the prevention of vasospasm.	Class III: No benefit and possibly harmful. Level B evidence: Evidence based on limited patient populations, utilizing one randomized trial or more than one nonrandomized trials.
Systemic hypertension	The following recommendation has been made to manage cerebral vasospasm and delayed	Class I: Benefit much greater than risk. Level B evidence: Evidence

TABLE 21-4 **AHA/ASA Guidelines for Hemodynamic and Intracranial Parameters in Spontaneous Aneurysmal Subarachnoid Hemorrhage (aSAH)—cont'd**

PARAMETER		CLASSIFICATION OF RECOMMENDATION AND LEVEL OF EVIDENCE
	cerebral ischemia: Unless the baseline systemic blood pressure is elevated or the patient's cardiac status prohibits induction of systemic hypertension, induction of systemic blood pressure is recommended in patient with delayed cerebral ischemia.	based on limited patient populations, utilizing one randomized trial or more than one nonrandomized trials.
Intracranial pressure	The following recommendation has been made to manage hydrocephalus associated with aSAH: An external ventricular drain or lumbar drain (depending on intracranial pressure and risk of herniation) should be used to manage aSAH associated with acute aSAH hydrocephalus.	Class I: Benefit much greater than risk. Level B evidence: Evidence based on limited patient populations, utilizing one randomized trial or more than one nonrandomized trials.
Intracranial pressure	The need for permanent cerebrospinal fluid (CSF) diversion (ventricular shunt) is not decreased by weaning the external ventricular drain over 24 hours.	Class III: No benefit and possibly harmful. Level B evidence: Evidence based on limited patient populations, utilizing one randomized trial or more than one nonrandomized trials.
Intravascular volume	The following recommendation has been made regarding management of aSAH associated medical complications: Fluid restriction and use of large amounts of hypotonic fluids are not recommended in the management of aSAH.	Class III: No benefit and possibly harmful. Level B evidence: Evidence based on limited patient populations, utilizing one randomized trial or more than one nonrandomized trials.

Continued

TABLE 21-4   AHA/ASA Guidelines for Hemodynamic and Intracranial Parameters in Spontaneous Aneurysmal Subarachnoid Hemorrhage (aSAH)—cont'd

PARAMETER		CLASSIFICATION OF RECOMMENDATION AND LEVEL OF EVIDENCE
Intravascular volume, central venous pressure (CVP), pulmonary artery occlusion pressure (PAOP), and fluid balance	The following recommendations have been made regarding management of aSAH associated medical complications: Intravascular volume status may be monitored utilizing CVP, PAOP parameters, and fluid balance, and intravascular volume depletion may be treated with crystalloid or colloid.	Class IIa: Benefit greater than risk. Level B evidence: Evidence based on limited patient populations, utilizing one randomized trial or more than one nonrandomized trials.
Blood transfusion	The following recommendation has been made regarding management of aSAH association medical complications: Aneurysmal SAH patient with anemia and at risk for cerebral ischemia may reasonably be treated with packed red blood cells. The optimal hemoglobin is not currently known.	Class IIb: Benefit greater than or equal to risk. Level B evidence: Evidence based on limited patient populations, utilizing one randomized trial or more than one nonrandomized trials.

TABLE 21-5   AHA/ASA Guidelines for Hemodynamic and Intracranial Parameters in Spontaneous Intracerebral Hemorrhage (ICH)

PARAMETER		CLASSIFICATION OF RECOMMENDATION AND LEVEL OF EVIDENCE
Systemic blood pressure, intracranial pressure, and cerebral perfusion pressure	The following recommendations have been made in regard to blood pressure, intracranial pressure, and cerebral perfusion pressure management for spontaneous ICH: 1. If the ICH patient's systemic blood pressure is >200 mm Hg or the mean arterial blood pressure is >150 mm Hg, blood pressure should be reduced with a continuous intravenous infusion of an antihypertensive agent with monitoring of blood pressure every 5 minutes.	Class IIb: Benefit greater than risk. Level C evidence: Evidence based on very limited patient populations, utilizing expert consensus, case studies, and standards of care.

TABLE 21-5   AHA/ASA Guidelines for Hemodynamic and Intracranial Parameters in Spontaneous Intracerebral Hemorrhage (ICH)—cont'd

PARAMETER		CLASSIFICATION OF RECOMMENDATION AND LEVEL OF EVIDENCE
	2. If the ICH patient's systemic blood pressure is >180 mm Hg or the mean arterial blood pressure is >130 mm Hg, and the ICP may be increased, consider utilizing ICP monitoring along with systemic blood pressure monitoring and decrease the systemic blood pressure with an intermittent or continuous intravenous infusion of an antihypertensive agent while also maintaining a CPP of 60 mm Hg. 3. If the ICH patient's systemic blood pressure is >130 mm Hg and no evidence of increased ICP, a goal blood pressure of 160/90 mm Hg or a MAP of 110 mm Hg utilizing intermittent or continuous intravenous antihypertensive medication may be used with reassessment every 15 minutes.	
Systemic blood pressure	4. If the spontaneous ICH patient's systolic blood pressure is 150–220 mm Hg, a decrease in the systemic blood pressure to 140 mm Hg is likely safe.	Class IIa: Benefit greater than risk. Level B evidence: Evidence based on limited patient populations, utilizing one randomized trial or more than one nonrandomized trials.
Intracranial pressure and cerebral perfusion pressure	The following recommendation has been made in regard to intracranial pressure and cerebral perfusion pressure management for spontaneous ICH: ICP monitoring and management should be considered for spontaneous ICH patients with (a) Glasgow Coma Scale <8; (b) evidence of transtentorial herniation; or (c) significant intraventricular hemorrhage or hydrocephalus. CPP of 50–70 mm Hg is a reasonable goal, depending on the patient's cerebral autoregulation status.	Class IIb: Benefit greater than risk. Level C evidence: Evidence based on very limited patient populations, utilizing expert consensus, case studies, and standards of care.
Intracranial pressure and cerebral perfusion pressure	If the spontaneous ICH patient has a decreased level of consciousness in the presence of hydrocephalus, ventricular drainage is reasonable.	Class IIa: Benefit greater than risk. Level B evidence: Evidence based on limited patient populations, utilizing one randomized trial or more than one nonrandomized trials.

TABLE 21-6 **AHA/ASA Guidelines for Hemodynamic and Intracranial Parameters in Acute Ischemic Stroke**

PARAMETER		CLASSIFICATION OF RECOMMENDATION AND LEVEL OF EVIDENCE
Systemic blood pressure	The following recommendation has been made regarding blood pressure after acute ischemic stroke in patients eligible for intravenous recombinant tissue plasminogen activator (rtPA): Systemic blood pressure should be lowered to systolic blood pressure <185 mm Hg and diastolic blood pressure <110 mm Hg before rtPA is given. Systemic blood pressure of less than 180/105 mm Hg must be maintained the first 24 hours after rtPA is given.	Class I: Benefit much greater than risk. Level B evidence: Evidence based on limited patient populations, utilizing one randomized trial or more than one nonrandomized trials.
Systemic blood pressure	The following recommendation has been made regarding blood pressure after acute ischemic stroke in patients eligible for other (non-IV rtPA) recanalization procedures (e.g., intra-arterial thrombolysis): Systemic blood pressure should be lowered to systolic blood pressure <185 mm Hg and diastolic blood pressure <110 mm Hg before rtPA is given. Systemic blood pressure of less than 180/105 mm Hg must be maintained the first 24 hours after rtPA is given.	Class I: Benefit much greater than risk. Level C evidence: Evidence based on very limited patient populations, utilizing expert consensus, case studies, and standards of care.
Systemic blood pressure	The following recommendation has been made regarding blood pressure after acute ischemic stroke in patients not receiving fibrinolysis: Systemic blood pressure may be safely lowered by 15% within the first 24 hours after acute ischemic stroke. Antihypertensives should be held until systolic blood pressure is >220 mm Hg or diastolic blood pressure is greater than 120 mm Hg.	Class I: Benefit much greater than risk. Level C evidence: Evidence based on very limited patient populations, utilizing expert consensus, case studies, and standards of care.

TABLE 21-6   **AHA/ASA Guidelines for Hemodynamic and Intracranial Parameters in Acute Ischemic Stroke—cont'd**

PARAMETER		CLASSIFICATION OF RECOMMENDATION AND LEVEL OF EVIDENCE
Intravascular volume	The following recommendation has been made regarding blood pressure after acute ischemic stroke: Correct hypovolemia with intravenous normal saline.	Class I: Benefit much greater than risk. Level C evidence: Evidence based on very limited patient populations, utilizing expert consensus, case studies, and standards of care.
Systemic blood pressure	The following recommendation has been made regarding blood pressure after acute ischemic stroke: Antihypertensive such as intravenous labetalol, nicardipine (Cardene), hydralazine (Apresoline), enalaprilat (Vasotec) are reasonable choices to lower systemic blood pressure, based on expert consensus. Data regarding the optimal choice of medications to achieve a lower blood pressure in acute ischemic stroke are lacking.	Class IIa: Benefit greater than risk. Level C evidence: Evidence based on very limited patient populations, utilizing expert consensus, case studies, and standards of care.
Systemic blood pressure	The following recommendation has been made regarding blood pressure after acute ischemic stroke: Optimal management is not completely known. Research to date is conflicting or inconclusive. Treatment of systemic hypertension in acute ischemic stroke has not been established. Malignant hypertension or other comorbidities negatively impacted by hypertension in acute ischemic stroke should be treated aggressively.	Class IIb: Benefit greater than risk. Level C evidence: Evidence based on very limited patient populations, utilizing expert consensus, case studies, and standards of care.
Systemic blood pressure	The following recommendation has been made regarding blood pressure after acute ischemic stroke: In rare instances, when systemic hypotension is result in neurologic sequelae, a vasopressor may be administered to improve cerebral blood flow.	Class I: Benefit much greater than risk. Level C evidence: Evidence based on very limited patient populations, utilizing expert consensus, case studies, and standards of care.

Continued

TABLE 21-6 **AHA/ASA Guidelines for Hemodynamic and Intracranial Parameters in Acute Ischemic Stroke—cont'd**

PARAMETER		CLASSIFICATION OF RECOMMENDATION AND LEVEL OF EVIDENCE
Intravascular volume and cerebral blood flow	The following recommendation has been made regarding blood pressure after acute ischemic stroke: The efficacy of high dose intravenous albumin for most patients with acute ischemic stroke is not well established.	Class IIb: Benefit greater than risk. Level B evidence: Evidence based on limited patient populations, utilizing one randomized trial or more than one nonrandomized trials.
Cerebral blood flow	The following recommendation has been made regarding blood pressure after acute ischemic stroke: The use of technology to augment cerebral blood flow in AIS is not substantiated.	Class IIb: Benefit greater than risk. Level B evidence: Evidence based on limited patient populations, utilizing one randomized trial or more than one nonrandomized trials.
Systemic blood pressure	The following recommendation has been made regarding blood pressure after acute ischemic stroke: The efficacy of vasopressor-induced systemic hypertension is not well established in acute ischemic stroke.	Class IIb: Benefit greater than risk. Level B evidence: Evidence based on limited patient populations, utilizing one randomized trial or more than one nonrandomized trials.
Intravascular volume	The following recommendation has been made regarding blood pressure after acute ischemic stroke: Volume expansion to achieve hemodilution after acute ischemic stroke is not recommended.	Class III: No benefit and possibly harmful. Level C evidence: Evidence based on very limited patient populations, utilizing expert consensus, case studies, and standards of care.
Intracranial pressure	The following recommendation has been made regarding malignant edema following a large hemispheric stroke: Decompressive craniectomy is strongly recommended. It is effective and may be life saving.	Class I: Benefit much greater than risk. Level B evidence: Evidence from single randomized trial or nonrandomized studies.
Intracranial pressure	The following recommendation has been made regarding intracranial pressure related to hydrocephalus following an acute ischemic stroke: Insertion of a ventricular drain is helpful in patient with acute ischemic stroke presenting with hydrocephalus.	Class I: Benefit much greater than risk. Level C. Only expert opinion, case studies, or standards of care.

Setup

Preparation of the drainage system with zeroing of the transducer is preferable before insertion of the ventricular catheter. The drainage system and the external strain gauge transducer are attached to each other and all connections tightened. While preparing the drainage system, the clinician wears a mask, and care is taken not to contaminate the connections.

The transducer and drainage system are primed with sterile, preservative-free normal saline prior to attaching the system to the ventricular catheter. The system may be zeroed and leveled prior to attachment to readily obtain an ICP reading once the insertion of the ventricular catheter is completed. The level of the transducer is placed approximately at the level of the foramen of Monro. The external reference for the foramen of Monro varies from source to source and institution to institution and may be measured at the external auditory meatus (EAM), the tragus of the ear, and in alignment with the outer canthus of the eye to the ear.[36] Whichever reference point is used, it must remain consistent for a particular patient and preferably for an institution.

Neurologic Baseline Before Intracranial Pressure Monitoring and Cerebrospinal Fluid Drainage

Prior to the insertion of the ventricular catheter and immediately after insertion, a neurologic assessment should be performed. The level of the drip chamber and an order for continuous or intermittent drainage must be prescribed on insertion and the drainage system adjusted accordingly. The character of the CSF is noted at this time as well. Once the catheter is attached to the external transducer, the system is set-up and patency is confirmed, the ICP and MAP are obtained to determine CPP.

Simultaneous determination of drainage and accurate ICP is not possible. When the drainage system is open to drainage, artifact on the waveform makes it impossible to obtain an accurate ICP value. The drainage system must be turned off to drainage to obtain an accurate ICP reading.[2,36,42] A corresponding waveform will appear with the numerical value when the drainage system is off to drainage. ICP is a mean value. The appearance of the waveform is noted at this time.

Normally, the ICP waveform has P1, P2, and P3 components, with the amplitude in descending order, specifically P1 > P2 > P3. An increase in P2 > P1 may be indicative of decreased intracranial compliance[36,42] as shown in Figure 21-13. However, an elevated P2 and decreased compliance do not always correspond clinically. Additional changes in ICP and waveform morphology are noted in Table 21-7.[36,42] Lundberg A and B waves are not easily captured on the typical bedside monitor, since the monitor may not allow visualization of trends over 5 minutes or more[37–39] (Figure 21-14).

Assessment

After leveling and zeroing the transducer and establishing a baseline, the drainage system and the patient are assessed at least every hour. The patient's neurologic status, ICP, CPP, and the amount and character of the drainage are noted and documented. Any drainage from the insertion site is documented as well. Complications related to

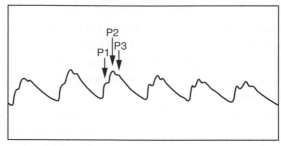

FIGURE 21-13 Abnormal intracranial pressure (ICP) waveform, as P2 > P1 is associated with decreased intracranial compliance. (From Kirkness CJ, Mitchell PH, Burr RI, et al.: Intracranial pressure waveform analysis: clinical and research implications, *J Neurosci Nurs* 32(5): 273, 2000.)

TABLE 21-7   Intracranial Pressure (ICP) Changes Related to Differing Physiologic Conditions

CONDITION	ICP CHANGES
Rapidly expanding mass lesion	• Increase in mean ICP • Increase ICP waveform amplitude
Increase or decrease in cerebrospinal fluid (CSF) volume	• Increase or decrease in mean ICP • Increase or decrease in ICP waveform amplitude • Little change in ICP waveform configuration
Several arterial hypotension	• Decrease in mean ICP • Decrease in ICP waveform amplitude, especially P1
Several arterial hypertension	• Increase in mean ICP • Increase in ICP waveform amplitude
Severe hypercapnia and hypoxia	• Increase in mean ICP • Increase in ICP waveform amplitude • Rounding of ICP waveform due to increase in later waveform components
Hyperventilation	• Decrease in mean ICP • Decrease in ICP waveform amplitude P2 and to a lesser degree P3, with little change in P1
Jugular vein compression	• Increase in mean ICP • Increase in ICP waveform amplitude mainly P2 and P3

From Kirkness CJ, Mitchell PH, Burr RI, et al.: Intracranial pressure waveform analysis: clinical and research implications, *J Neurosci Nurs* 32(5):273, 2000.

the insertion or ventricular drainage must be recorded, including underdrainage or overdrainage, and new intracranial hemorrhage. The rate of CSF drainage must be assessed prior to leaving the external ventricular catheter open initially with frequent observations because of the potential for under or overdrainage.[36]

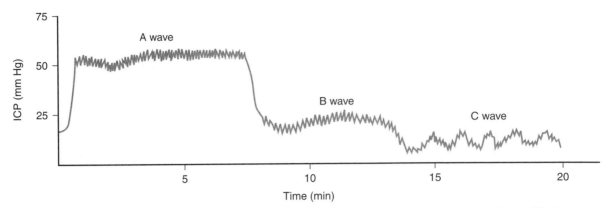

FIGURE 21-14 Intracranial pressure (ICP) waveforms with trend recording. (From Ellenbogen RG, Abdulrauf SI, Sekhar LN: *Principles of neurological surgery*, ed 3, Philadelphia, 2012, Elsevier.)

The MAP value that is most often used in the calculation of CPP is an arterial line with the transducer at the phlebostatic axis or a blood pressure cuff at the heart level. The arterial line must have an optimal waveform as evidenced by an acceptable square waveform test (see Figure 4-5 in Chapter 4). The same method of blood pressure measurement is used consistently. Some clinicians advocate for measurement of the "cerebral mean arterial pressure" by leveling the arterial line transducer with the foramen of Monro to calculate CPP.[37] However, this is controversial and has not gained widespread acceptance.[43]

Maintenance

Maintenance of an external ventricular catheter includes ongoing assessment of CSF output and ICP and CPP measurements. The hourly CSF drainage rate is generally recommended to approximate the amount of CSF production in an hour for an adult, or approximately 20 milliliters (mL) an hour. Overdrainage may cause headache, formation of a subdural hematoma, development of pneumocephalus, or herniation. Underdrainage may result in deterioration in neurologic status, increased ICP, hydrocephalus, and herniation.[36]

Leveling of the reference zero on the drainage system with the anatomic reference point (foramen of Monro), is required when the patient's position changes. Rezeroing is indicated per institutional policy and with each disconnect of the transducer from the bedside monitor cable. High and low pressure alarm limits are set. If the external ventricular catheter is open continuously, alarms may reflect trends but must not be interpreted as the actual ICP value.

Troubleshooting

Among the most common issues with a ventriculostomy catheter is decreased CSF drainage. Gradual slowing of the drainage without an increase in the height of the burette level must be noted before complete blockage and dangerously high ICPs occur. The drainage system may be assessed for patency by slightly lowering the burette—for a very short period—to determine the rate of drainage. Maneuvers that may restore patency include stimulating the patient to cough or repositioning the patient. Depending on institutional policy, the nurse may flush away from the head or change the drainage system if the underdrainage is related to the obstruction in the drainage system and not in the catheter. In some institutions, staff nurses, advanced practice nurses or physicians may have a protocol to flush into the CSF drain with a prescribed small amount of preservative-free sterile normal saline in emergency situations to restore patency. Loss of the ICP waveform may indicate blockage, loose system connections, or possibly transducer failure. A numeric value without a corresponding waveform is of no value.[36]

Patient Safety

- The external ventricular drain is the gold standard for ICP monitoring; however, it also presents the greatest safety concerns.

- Underdrainage, overdrainage, and infection are the biggest problems.

- Strategies to prevent infection include consistent sterile technique when inserting or accessing the catheter or drainage system and during dressing change; use of antibiotic-impregnated catheters; tunneling the catheter; and early identification and management of CSF infections.

- Routine exchange of the ventricular catheter and the drainage system has not been proven effective in decreasing the risk of infection.

- The best dressing for the insertion site is not currently known.

Patient Comfort

- Prior to insertion, immediately after insertion, and at removal of the external ventricular catheter, the patient's pain or potential for pain must be considered.

- Overdrainage, underdrainage, or infection, with the appearance of meningeal signs, may also require additional pain or comfort measures.

- Generally, awake patients do not complain of discomfort from the external ventricular catheter days after insertion.

Patient Education

- Education of the family and the patient who is awake and capable of understanding about the external ventricular catheter is mandatory.

- The patient and family are instructed to call the nurse for assistance with repositioning, including raising or lowering the head of the bed.

> **Patient Education—cont'd**
>
> - Failure of the patient or family to follow instructions may cause permanent neurologic deterioration or death.
>
> - If necessary, activating the lock mechanism on the bed may be necessary to prevent changes in the position of the bed by the family or patient.

Transducer-Tipped Intracranial Pressure Catheters

ICP catheters with the transducer in the tip may be fiberoptic, strain gauge, or pneumatic. They are typically placed through cranial bolt into the parenchyma but may also be placed in the surgical site at the time of surgery (Figure 21-15). The fiberoptic transducer-tipped ICP catheters are zeroed prior to insertion and cannot be rezeroed once inserted. Leveling of the catheter and determining the patient's anatomic reference are not required. Transducer-tipped catheters are most typically attached to a specialized ICP-monitor that displays the patient's ICP waveform and mean value; a cable connects this monitor with the patient's bedside monitor for a central alarm and larger view of the waveform.

Two devices, one a pneumatic device, and the other, an electronic chip strain gauge device, may be directly attached to the bedside monitor without an additional ICP monitor. The pneumatic device may be periodically rezeroed after insertion, as needed. At least one manufacturer makes a hybrid-type catheter with a fiberoptic tip and CSF drainage capability. Because the distance between catheter drainage lumens sizes and sensors differ with various manufacturers, it is best practice to close off the ventriculostomy drain to ensure the most accurate ICP reading.

Disadvantages of fiberoptic transducer-tipped catheters include their expense, inability to recalibrate once inserted, easy breakage, inability to drain CSF, and drift, particularly after 5 days. Transducer-tipped catheters are said to be less reliable than an external ventricular catheter and are not MRI compatible.[29] In addition, an intraparenchymal ICP catheter placed in the noninjured hemisphere may not adequately reflect increased ICP until the patient's condition has deteriorated dramatically.[38]

Clinical Procedure

Although the risk of infection with an intraparenchymal transducer-tipped catheter is less than that of an external ventricular catheter, sterile technique must be maintained during insertion. As with the external ventricular catheter, the patient's hair may be clipped, skin prepared, and drapes applied before the skin incision. The intraparenchymal transducer-tipped fiberoptic catheter is typically placed through a bolt—a hollow cannula—screwed into a burr hole in the skull. The dura is surgically opened through the burr hole, and the catheter is passed through the bolt and dural opening

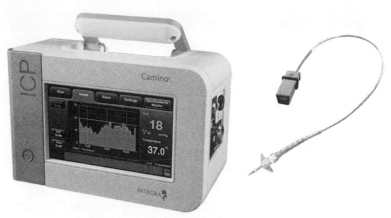

FIGURE 21-15 Fiberoptic Transducer-Tipped Intracranial Pressure (ICP) Monitoring System. (Permission granted by Integra LifeSciences Corporation, Plainsboro, New Jersey, USA.)

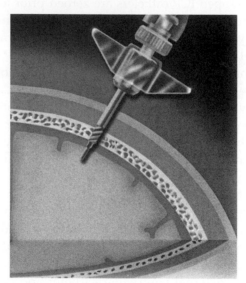

FIGURE 21-16 Fiberoptic transducer-tipped ICP catheter through bolt, and positioned in the cerebral cortex (gray matter). (Permission granted by Integra LifeSciences Corporation, Plainsboro, New Jersey, USA.)

and is positioned in the cerebral cortex (Figure 21-16). Prior to insertion, the catheter is zeroed to atmospheric pressure as indicated on the monitor. Markings on the outside of the catheter indicate the depth of the catheter. The catheter is secured at the desired depth in the bolt with a compression cap and sheath. Monitoring begins immediately. Another parameter that may be measured with the fiberoptic transducer-tipped catheters is brain temperature (T_{BR}), which will be discussed later in this chapter. The catheter, or the monitor that attaches to the catheter, may be connected to the bedside monitor to automatically calculate and display the CPP value, as part of a system of multimodal cerebral monitoring (Figure 21-17).

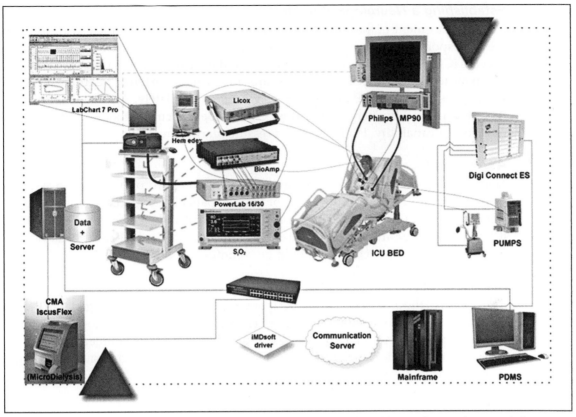

FIGURE 21-17 Multimodality monitoring with connection to bedside monitor, and a central alarm and display system. (Permission granted by Minerva Anesthesiologica.)

Indications

The indications for the transducer-tipped catheter are similar to those for the external ventricular catheter except that CSF drainage is not possible unless a hybrid catheter (external ventricular drain and transducer-tipped catheter) is inserted.[2]

Setup

The setup for the transducer-tipped catheter is less complicated than that for the external ventricular catheter. Steps include (1) gathering the equipment, including the monitor for the catheter; (2) assisting the physician to maintain sterile technique while attaching the catheter to the monitor cable; and (3) holding the cable while the physician zeros the catheter, prior to insertion. Once the catheter is in place, the nurse or physician may provide further protection of the catheter's position with tape and by attaching the cable to the patient's gown to prevent the catheter from sliding out of the bolt.

Establishing a Neurologic Baseline

Correct placement of the transducer-tipped catheter will yield an ICP waveform and the corresponding ICP number. A calibration step procedure may be required to connect the ICP monitor to the bedside monitor, and provide a larger display with a central alarm system.[10,44] The ICP waveforms are similar to the external ventricular catheter waveforms. ICP and CPP monitoring may begin immediately. Again, identification of the presence of Lundberg A and B waves will be difficult without additional trend monitoring capability. High and low pressure alarms must be set.[36,39]

Assessment

Neurologic assessment prior to the insertion and afterward provides some assurance that insertion did not cause any harm or that the patient did not deteriorate during the insertion procedure. With each neurologic assessment and observation of the patient's ICP numeric value and waveform, the nurse notes the depth of the catheter as indicated by the markings. Any changes should be communicated to the physician.

Maintenance

In addition to the assessment described above, the ICP monitor is plugged into the electrical wall current to maintain the battery charge, except during transport to radiology or to the operating room. Drift or inaccurate values may be encountered after 5 days after catheter insertion. Nursing care includes inspection of insertion site and change of dressing based on institutional policy.

Troubleshooting

A broken catheter may be indicated by an error message or loss of waveform on the ICP monitor. Other issues include malposition of the catheter. The nurse is responsible for assessing the position of the catheter based on the visible external markings. Even if the ICP catheter has a numeric display and an adequate waveform, the physician is to be alerted regarding the change in catheter position. The catheter may not be adequately reflecting the ICP at a particular location if it is no longer at the same depth. Loss of battery power or cable connections are common occurrences as well. In the absence of an obviously broken catheter, other options such as changing the ICP monitor or assessing the status of the bedside monitor must be explored prior to removing the catheter and inserting a new one.

Patient Safety

- Although less likely than with an external ventricular catheter and drain, the transducer-tipped ICP catheter may be a source of infection.

- In addition to monitoring the insertion site and using sterile technique to change the dressing, other indicators of infection such as an elevated white blood cell (WBC) count and fever must be noted as well.

Patient Safety—cont'd

- Regardless of the body region to be imaged, whether it is the brain or other body region, the catheter and the bolt are <u>not</u> MRI compatible.

- Failure to remove the catheter and bolt prior to MRI may result in heating of the fiberoptic-tipped catheter and bolt and result in thermal injury.[45]

- Failure to remove the catheter positioned in the surgical site prior to closure of the craniotomy may result in migration of the catheter with resultant brain injury.

- In some institutions, the nurse or the advanced practice nurse may remove the catheter and bolt with competency validation. This may be helpful in expediting transport to the magnetic resonance imaging (MRI) suite. Institutional policy must be followed.

Patient Comfort

Ensuring patient comfort is particularly important prior to insertion, immediately after insertion, and during and after removal of the transducer-tipped ICP catheter.

Patient Education

- Education for the patient and family includes the need for monitoring and remembering to call for assistance with patient position changes.

- Education of the family—and the patient as he or she is able to understand—includes a discussion about ICP monitoring being one of many aspects of neurologic assessment and not the only indicator of neurologic status.

Brain Oxygenation

Brain Tissue Oxygenation—PbtO$_2$ Catheter

Direct measurement of focal brain tissue oxygen or brain tissue oxygenation (PbtO$_2$) in a small area of brain tissue is accomplished with a catheter that has a polarographic Clarke-type microelectrode with a semipermeable membrane and electromagnetic features, or a catheter with optical luminescence. Currently, only the polarographic Clarke-type microelectrode catheter (Licox®), is commercially available in the United States to detect focal brain hypoxia.[10,44] The Licox brain tissue oxygen monitor triple bolt system is shown in Figure 21-18. The Clarke-type microelectrode catheter requires simultaneous temperature measurement for accurate measurement of the PbtO$_2$.[10,42] This particular catheter is available as a combination probe that allows simultaneous

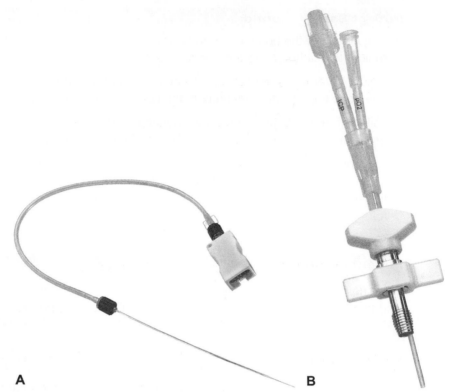

FIGURE 21-18 A, Licox brain tissue oxygen (PbtO$_2$) and brain temperature probe. **B,** Dual lumen bolt for placement of fiberoptic transducer-tipped ICP catheter and PbtO$_2$/brain temperature probe. (Permission granted by Integra LifeSciences Corporation, Plainsboro, New Jersey, USA.)

monitoring of PbtO$_2$ and brain temperature. Each catheter has its own calibration card, which must be placed in the monitor that connects to the catheter for accuracy.[46-48] (Figure 21-19).

The parameter itself, PbtO$_2$, has been questioned as to what it represents. The actual value has been demonstrated to be a strong indicator of diffusion of PaO$_2$ across the blood–brain barrier.[46] Patients with normal CPP and ICP have a PbtO$_2$ of 25 to 30 mm Hg.[47] A PbtO$_2$ of less than 20 mm Hg is typically considered low enough to require prompt recognition and intervention in the clinical setting, even though a PbtO$_2$ of 10 to 15 mm Hg has been cited as the critical value for ischemic damage.[47,48] A PbtO$_2$ of less than 10 mm Hg for greater than 30 minutes is associated with a higher mortality rate.[49,50] PbtO$_2$ of greater than 20 mm Hg has not been shown to result in better outcomes. As with transducer-tipped ICP catheters,[51] the PbtO$_2$ catheter is prone to drift, resulting in reduced accuracy after 5 days.[46-48]

Procedure

The PbtO$_2$ catheter is inserted under sterile conditions, either at the bedside in the critical care unit or in the operating room, similar to placement of the transducer-tipped

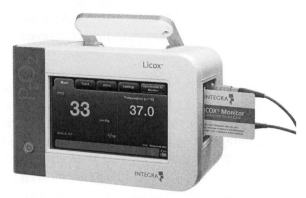

FIGURE 21-19 Licox brain tissue oxygen (PbtO$_2$) and brain temperature monitor and calibration "smart" card. (Permission granted by Integra LifeSciences Corporation, Plainsboro, New Jersey, USA.)

ICP catheter. The PbtO$_2$ catheter is most often placed through a cranial bolt adjacent to the ICP catheter and other monitoring devices such as a separate brain temperature catheter. Alternatively, the PbtO$_2$ catheter may be placed in the surgical site intraoperatively. The PbtO$_2$ catheter is typically positioned in the white matter of the brain, deeper than the positioning of the ICP catheter (Figure 21-18). Optimal placement is a matter of controversy. Placement options include (1) ipsilateral to the hemisphere with the greater area or potential area of injury but in normal tissue; (2) ipsilateral to the hemisphere with the greater area or potential area of injury, in the ischemic penumbra, the most vulnerable but potentially salvageable tissue; or (3) contralateral to hemisphere with the greater area or potential area of injury but in normal tissue.[42,47,52,53] Placement of the catheter itself causes some microtrauma and values obtained in that area may not be valid from 30 minutes up to 2 hours after placement.[47,48] The calibration card may be inserted in the monitor at any time, prior to, during, or immediately after insertion.

Once the PbtO$_2$ catheter is correctly positioned and secured, the catheter is connected to the monitor, which may also be attached to the bedside monitor for a central alarm capability. No waveform is associated with PbtO$_2$. While the clinician waits for the tissue microtrauma to resolve for an accurate PbtO$_2$ reading, the ICP is considered valid with an appropriate waveform.

Indications

Indications for PbtO$_2$ monitoring in the literature include severe TBI, aSAH, and, less frequently, brain tumor, as well as spontaneous ICH and normal pressure hydrocephalus. The Brain Trauma Foundation's *Guidelines for Severe Traumatic Brain Injury* have determined that a PbtO$_2$ of less than 15 mm Hg is a threshold for treatment (Level III of III, recommendation)[53] (see Table 21-2). The PbtO$_2$ catheter is not addressed in the AHA/ASA *Guidelines for Management of Spontaneous Aneurysmal Subarachnoid Hemorrhage*.[34] However, PbtO$_2$ monitoring is discussed in the Neurocritical Care Society's

Critical Care Management of Patient Following Aneurysmal Subarachnoid Hemorrhage Recommendations as one tool for the detection of delayed cerebral ischemia[35] (Table 21-8).

Setup

The setup for insertion of a $PbtO_2$ catheter is similar to the setup for a transducer-tipped ICP catheter but with the addition of the $PbtO_2$ monitor and cables. The Licox catheter must be stored in a refrigerator to maintain calibration until ready for use, and the corresponding calibration card, specific to that catheter and included in the packaging, is placed in the slot in the Licox monitor. The Licox monitor may be adjusted manually to body temperature for every hour $PbtO_2$ is obtained if the $PbtO_2$ catheter does not contain a T_{BR} sensor or a separate T_{BR} catheter is not placed adjacent to the $PbtO_2$ catheter and connected with a cable to the Licox monitor. Another cable may connect the Licox monitor to a pressure port in the bedside monitoring system for display of the $PbtO_2$ value and setting of alarms on the bedside monitor.

Neurologic Baseline Prior to Insertion

As stated previously, 30 minutes to 2 hours must pass before the $PbtO_2$ values are considered valid in relation to the microtrauma associated with the insertion.[48] If $PbtO_2$ remains low, the reason must be determined. First, the functionality of the catheter must be assessed. If the patient is not already on an FiO_2 of 1.0, increasing the FiO_2 to 1.0 for 5 minutes should result in an increase in $PbtO_2$. If an increase is not seen, the catheter may be damaged or positioned in blood clot or infarcted tissue. Assessment of the location of the probe with CT and repositioning may be necessary.

Low $PbtO_2$ indicates cerebral hypoxia; intracranial-specific reasons include increased ICP or decreased CPP and seizures. Systemic causes of low $PbtO_2$ include systemic hypoxia, hypotension, hypovolemia, anemia, fever, and agitation.[47–50] Rapid action must be taken to correct low $PbtO_2$ as soon as possible. However, prolonged periods of high oxygen delivery without a systemic need to maintain adequate $PbtO_2$ must be avoided to prevent acute lung injury. $PbtO_2$ must be assessed every hour along with neurologic status, ICP, and CPP.

Maintenance

Care must be taken to secure the catheter and the cables attached to the catheter. A sterile dressing is applied around the bolt at the insertion site and is changed according to institutional policy. Maintenance primarily involves continual assessment of the values and related interventions.

Troubleshooting

Troubleshooting continued low values has been addressed above. Other actions may include ensuring correct catheter and cable connections and changing the monitor before consideration of changing the catheter itself. If the Licox brand $PbtO_2$ catheter is used and the $PbtO_2$ monitor is changed, the calibration card for the catheter in the

TABLE 21-8 **Neurocritical Care Society Multidisciplinary Consensus Recommendation on Critical Care Management of Patients with Aneurysmal Subarachnoid Hemorrhage (aSAH)**

PARAMETER		CLASSIFICATION OF RECOMMENDATION AND LEVEL OF EVIDENCE
Systemic blood pressure	The following recommendation has been made to minimize the risk of rebleeding in aSAH with unsecured aneurysms: Moderate elevations in systemic blood pressure (mean arterial blood pressure <110 mm Hg) do not require management. Pre aSAH baseline systemic blood pressure should be used to adjust parameters. Systemic hypotension is to be avoided. Extreme systemic hypertension should be treated.	Low Quality Evidence: Additional research is highly likely to impact confidence in estimation of effect and is likely to impact estimation of the effect. Strong Recommendation
Intravascular volume status	The following recommendation has been made regarding monitoring of intravascular volume status after aSAH: Intravascular volume status monitoring may be beneficial.	Moderate Quality Evidence: Additional research is likely to impact confidence in estimation of effect and is likely to impact estimation of the effect. Weak Recommendation
Intravascular volume status	The following recommendation has been made regarding monitoring of intravascular volume status after aSAH: Attention to fluid balance should be the cornerstone for monitoring intravascular volume status. No specific invasive or noninvasive monitoring technology is recommended over clinical assessment.	Moderate Quality Evidence: Additional research is likely to impact confidence in estimation of effect and is likely to impact estimation of the effect. Weak Recommendation
Central venous pressure	The following recommendation has been made regarding monitoring of intravascular volume status after aSAH: Fluid management based entirely on central venous pressure measurement is not recommended. Central venous catheters should not be inserted exclusively to measure central venous pressure.	Moderate Quality Evidence: Additional research is likely to impact confidence in estimation of effect and is likely to impact estimation of the effect. Strong Recommendation

Continued

TABLE 21-8 **Neurocritical Care Society Multidisciplinary Consensus Recommendation on Critical Care Management of Patients with Aneurysmal Subarachnoid Hemorrhage (aSAH)—cont'd**

PARAMETER		CLASSIFICATION OF RECOMMENDATION AND LEVEL OF EVIDENCE
Pulmonary artery pressure	The following recommendation has been made regarding monitoring of intravascular volume status after aSAH: Routine placement of pulmonary artery catheters is not recommended. Pulmonary artery catheters are associated with unacceptable risk and lack of benefit.	Moderate Quality Evidence: Additional research is likely to impact confidence in estimation of effect and is likely to impact estimation of the effect. Strong Recommendation
Intravascular volume management	The following recommendation has been made regarding the management of intravascular volume status after aSAH: The goal for intravascular volume management should be euvolemia, not hypervolemia. Hypervolemia may result in harm related to aggressive fluid administration.	High Quality Evidence: Additional research is highly likely to impact confidence in estimation of effect and is likely to impact estimation of the effect. Strong Recommendation
Intravascular volume management	The following recommendation has been made regarding the management of intravascular volume status after aSAH: The preferred intravenous solution for volume replacement is isotonic crystalloid (e.g., normal saline).	Moderate Quality Evidence: Additional research is likely to impact confidence in estimation of effect and is likely to impact estimation of the effect. Weak Recommendation
Intravascular volume management	The following recommendation has been made regarding the management of intravascular volume status after aSAH: Fludrocortisone (Florinef) or hydrocortisone may be considered for the management of refractory negative fluid balance.	Moderate Quality Evidence: Additional research is likely to impact confidence in estimation of effect and is likely to impact estimation of the effect. Weak Recommendation
Intravascular volume	The following recommendation has been made regarding hemodynamic management after aSAH but with aneurysm repair: Maintenance of euvolemia, rather than induction of hypervolemia, should be the goal.	Moderate Quality Evidence: Additional research is likely to impact confidence in estimation of effect and is likely to impact estimation of the effect. Strong Recommendation

TABLE 21-8   Neurocritical Care Society Multidisciplinary Consensus Recommendation on Critical Care Management of Patients with Aneurysmal Subarachnoid Hemorrhage (aSAH)—cont'd

PARAMETER		CLASSIFICATION OF RECOMMENDATION AND LEVEL OF EVIDENCE
Intravascular volume and cerebral blood flow	The following recommendation has been made regarding hemodynamic management after aSAH but with aneurysm repair: Prior to other interventions, an intravenous bolus of saline should be administered to increase cerebral blood flow in areas of cerebral ischemia.	Moderate Quality Evidence: Additional research is likely to impact confidence in estimation of effect and is likely to impact estimation of the effect. Weak Recommendation
Systemic blood pressure	The following recommendation has been made regarding hemodynamic management after aSAH but with aneurysm repair: A trial of pharmacologically induced systemic hypertension should be undertaken for patients with suspected delayed cerebral ischemia.	Moderate Quality Evidence: Additional research is likely to impact confidence in estimation of effect and is likely to impact estimation of the effect. Strong Recommendation
Systemic blood pressure	The following recommendation has been made regarding hemodynamic management after aSAH but with aneurysm repair: The pharmacologic properties of the vasopressor, such as tachycardia or inotropy, should be considered in the choice of vasopressor.	Moderate Quality Evidence: Additional research is likely to impact confidence in estimation of effect and is likely to impact estimation of the effect. Strong Recommendation
Systemic blood pressure	The following recommendation has been made regarding hemodynamic management after aSAH but with aneurysm repair: To determine the optimal systemic blood pressure parameter, increases in blood pressure should be incremental changes with neurologic assessment at each mean arterial pressure level.	Low to Very Low Quality Evidence: Additional research is highly likely to impact confidence in estimation of effect and is likely to impact estimation of the effect. Strong Recommendation

Continued

TABLE 21-8 Neurocritical Care Society Multidisciplinary Consensus Recommendation on Critical Care Management of Patients with Aneurysmal Subarachnoid Hemorrhage (aSAH)—cont'd

PARAMETER		CLASSIFICATION OF RECOMMENDATION AND LEVEL OF EVIDENCE
Systemic blood pressure	The following recommendation has been made regarding hemodynamic management after aSAH: Nimodipine (Nimotop)-related systemic hypotension should be managed by changing the dosing to lower doses at more frequent intervals, i.e., from 60 mg every 4 hours to 30 mg every 2 hours. If systemic hypotension persists, the nimodipine should be stopped.	Low Quality Evidence: Additional research is highly likely to impact confidence in estimation of effect and is likely to impact estimation of the effect. Strong Recommendation
Systemic blood pressure	The following recommendation has been made regarding hemodynamic management after aSAH but with aneurysm repair: Inotropes may be considered in patients with delayed cerebral ischemia if the delayed cerebral ischemia does not improve with vasopressors.	Low Quality Evidence: Additional research is highly likely to impact confidence in estimation of effect and is likely to impact estimation of the effect. Strong Recommendation
Systemic blood pressure	The following recommendation has been made regarding hemodynamic management after aSAH but with aneurysm repair: Administration of beta-2 agonist properties, i.e., dobutamine may decrease the mean arterial pressure and the vasopressor dose may need to be increased.	High Quality Evidence: Additional research is highly likely to impact confidence in estimation of effect and is likely to impact estimation of the effect. Strong Recommendation
Cardiac output and systemic arterial blood flow	The following recommendation has been made regarding hemodynamic management after aSAH but with aneurysm repair: Intra-aortic balloon counter pulsation may be helpful in the augmentation of cardiac output and systemic blood flow.	Low Quality Evidence: Additional research is highly likely to impact confidence in estimation of effect and is likely to impact estimation of the effect. Weak Recommendation

TABLE 21-8 **Neurocritical Care Society Multidisciplinary Consensus Recommendation on Critical Care Management of Patients with Aneurysmal Subarachnoid Hemorrhage (aSAH)—cont'd**

PARAMETER		CLASSIFICATION OF RECOMMENDATION AND LEVEL OF EVIDENCE
Intravascular volume and cerebral blood flow	The following recommendation has been made regarding hemodynamic management after aSAH but with aneurysm repair: Other than patients with erythrocythemia, hemodilution should not be undertaken to improve cerebral blood flow.	Moderate Quality Evidence: Additional research is likely to impact confidence in estimation of effect and is likely to impact estimation of the effect. Strong Recommendation
Systemic blood pressure	The following recommendation has been made regarding hemodynamic management after aSAH but with unsecured aneurysm(s): In consideration of risk versus benefit, systemic blood pressure may be increased cautiously if the patient of an unsecured aneurysm develops delayed cerebral ischemia.	Low to Very Low Quality Evidence: Additional research is likely to impact confidence in estimation of effect and is likely to impact estimation of the effect. Strong Recommendation
Hemodynamic management	The following recommendation has been made regarding hemodynamic management after aSAH and securement of the ruptured aneurysm: Hemodynamic management should not be influenced by any unsecured aneurysms that have not ruptured (those not responsible for the aneurysmal SAH).	Moderate Quality Evidence: Additional research is likely to impact confidence in estimation of effect and is likely to impact estimation of the effect. Strong Recommendation
Intravascular volume	The following recommendation has been made regarding hemodynamic management after aSAH: Blood loss should be minimized blood sampling.	Low Quality Evidence: Additional research is highly likely to impact confidence in estimation of effect and is likely to impact estimation of the effect. Strong Recommendation
Intravascular volume	The following recommendation has been made regarding hemodynamic management after aSAH: The hemoglobin concentration should be maintained greater than 8-10g/dL.	Moderate Quality Evidence: Additional research is likely to impact confidence in estimation of effect and is likely to impact estimation of the effect. Strong Recommendation

Continued

TABLE 21-8 Neurocritical Care Society Multidisciplinary Consensus Recommendation on Critical Care Management of Patients with Aneurysmal Subarachnoid Hemorrhage (aSAH)—cont'd

PARAMETER		CLASSIFICATION OF RECOMMENDATION AND LEVEL OF EVIDENCE
Intravascular volume	The following recommendation has been made regarding hemodynamic management after aSAH: Patients with potential or actual delayed cerebral ischemia may benefit from higher hemoglobin levels; however, the benefit of transfusion is not known.	No Evidence: Research is extremely likely to impact confidence in estimation of effect and is likely to impact estimation of the effect. Strong Recommendation
Intravascular volume	The following recommendation has been made regarding hemodynamic management after aSAH: If vasopressin-receptor antagonists (e.g., Conivaptan) are used to manage hyponatremia, hypovolemia must be avoided.	Low to Very Low Quality Evidence: Additional research is highly likely to impact confidence in estimation of effect and is likely to impact estimation of the effect. Strong Recommendation
Intravascular volume	The following recommendation has been made regarding hemodynamic management after aSAH: Intravenous and enteral free water should be restricted.	Very Low Quality Evidence: Additional research is highly likely to impact confidence in estimation of effect and is likely to impact estimation of the effect. Strong Recommendation

patient's head must be placed in the new monitor and the value is considered accurate as soon as the $PbtO_2$ value stabilizes, usually in less than 5 minutes.

If the Licox brand $PbtO_2$ catheter itself is changed, a new calibration card that accompanies the new catheter must be inserted into the monitor, and 30 minutes to 2 hours must pass before the $PbtO_2$ values are considered valid. If the monitor indicates that the brain temperature is too high to obtain the $PbtO_2$ value, assess the patient's body temperature for comparison.

Patient Safety

- Prior to insertion and after insertion of the $PbtO_2$ catheter, the patient's neurologic status must be assessed to capture any neurologic deterioration.

- As with the transducer-tipped ICP catheter and bolt, sterile technique must be used during insertion, removal, and dressing change.

> **Patient Safety—cont'd**
>
> - The physician should be notified if CSF leak occurs while the catheter is in place or on discontinuation.
> - The $PbtO_2$ catheter and bolt are <u>not</u> MRI compatible and must be removed prior to MRI.
> - The bolt is larger than the bolt for the transducer-tipped ICP catheter, and the $PbtO_2$ catheter is placed deeper into the brain than the ICP catheter and is not typically removed by nurses.
> - As with all devices, coagulation parameters must be within normal limits and the site assessed after removal for bleeding or hematoma formation.

> **Patient Comfort**
>
> Ensuring patient comfort is particularly important prior to insertion, immediately after insertion, and during and after removal of the $PbtO_2$ catheter.

> **Patient Education**
>
> - Education of the patient—as able—and the family includes the rationale for monitoring and instruction to call for assistance with positioning, as the catheters and cable may break or move out of position during turning in the bed.
> - Education of the family—and patient if able to understand—includes a discussion about ICP monitoring being one of many aspects of neurologic assessment and not the only indicator of neurologic status.

Retrograde Jugular Bulb Catheter

Similar to the $PbtO_2$ catheter, the retrograde jugular bulb catheter measures brain oxygenation. However, its placement in the bulb of the internal jugular vein allows measurement of global, rather than focal, brain oxygenation.[47,48] The oximetric fiberoptic catheter placed in the dominant internal jugular vein measures $SjvO_2$ (Figure 21-20). $SjvO_2$ represents the balance between oxygen supply and demand after the brain has extracted the oxygen from the cerebral circulation as the venous blood returns to the heart.[47,52] The fiberoptic catheter attaches to a monitor that allows continuous monitoring of the $SjvO_2$.[44] If a fiberoptic catheter and compatible monitor are not available for continuous display, $SjvO_2$ may be obtained intermittently from an intravenous catheter inserted in a retrograde manner in the internal jugular bulb.[47,53,54] A pressurized normal saline bag is required to maintain patency. Unlike the systemic venous oxygen saturation catheters, the $SjvO_2$

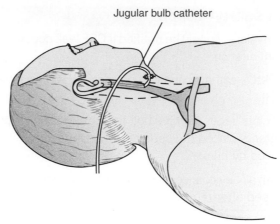

Jugular bulb catheter

FIGURE 21-20 Jugular venous oxygen saturation ($SjvO_2$) catheter in bulb of internal jugular vein. (Modified from Galla JD, McCullough JN, Ergin MA, et al.: Surgical techniques: Aortic arch and deep hypothermic circulatory arrest: real-life suspended animation, *Cardiology Clinics* 17(4): 767-778, 1999.)

catheter cannot be calibrated prior to insertion. Once inserted, correct positioning between the cervical vertebrae C1 and C2 at the jugular bulb is verified with a cervical spine film. The catheter must be calibrated in vivo by using an arterial and $SjvO_2$ blood draw and includes the patient's hemoglobin or hematocrit values.[42–44,52] The results of an arterial and venous oximetry panel are used to update the monitor. A derived parameter—the arteriojugular venous oxygen difference ($AjvDO_2$)—may be calculated. Normal $SjvO_2$ is 55% to 70% and $AjvDO_2$ is 4 to 8 milliliters per deciliter (mL/dL).[47,52–54] $SjvO_2$ of less than 50% represents global cerebral ischemia and $SjvO_2$ of greater than 75% represents an absolute or relative global hyperemia that exceeds the brain's metabolic demand.[10] Both an $SjvO_2$ less than 50% or $SjvO_2$ greater than 75% have been associated with unfavorable outcomes.[54]

Procedure

The $SjvO_2$ catheter is most often inserted at the bedside. Insertion is somewhat analogous to inserting a central venous catheter except it is placed in a retrograde manner. The patient's neck is prepared and draped per institutional policy. Typically, the right internal jugular vein, being dominant in most people, is cannulated,[47,54] and a small size 4 French (Fr) introducer is inserted. Once cannulation of the internal jugular vein is confirmed, a smaller pediatric fiberoptic catheter (4 Fr) is inserted through the introducer with the sheath in place, that will cover the catheter and allow repositioning of the catheter, as needed. Placement of the catheter in the internal jugular bulb is confirmed with a cervical spine film. The distance from the tip of the catheter to insertion site is noted for future confirmation of position. A pressure bag with normal saline at 300 mm Hg pressure is attached to the fiberoptic catheter to maintain patency. If the introducer has a side port, it must be capped with a "Do Not Use for Infusions" label to prevent inadvertent administration of intravenous solutions into the internal jugular bulb.

After successful placement, the catheter is calibrated using jugular venous blood from the stopcock closest to the fiberoptic catheter. A waste is drawn first followed by a specimen into an arterial blood gas (ABG) syringe. The blood is drawn slowly to minimize the risk of contamination from the facial vein. The signal quality intensity (SQI) is ideally 1 to 2 on the $SjvO_2$ monitor. The SQI is verified prior to drawing the specimen and with each assessment of $SjvO_2$. If not optimal, repositioning or other maneuvers such as turning the patient or suctioning to elicit a cough may improve the SQI. $SjvO_2$ is assessed hourly and as needed. Changes in $SjvO_2$ are validated with additional laboratory analysis of internal jugular venous and systemic arterial blood samples.[48]

Indications

Indications for $SjvO_2$ monitoring include risk for global hypoxia, in severe TBI, aSAH, and intraoperative monitoring during cardiac bypass.[48,52] Similar to the recommendation about thresholds for the $PbtO_2$ catheter, the Brain Trauma Foundation recommends the use of $SjvO_2$ monitoring and related management as a Level III recommendation based on lowest-quality of evidence[53] (see Table 21-2). The threshold for treatment is $SjvO_2$ of less than 50%.[53] $SjvO_2$ monitoring is particularly helpful in monitoring and managing severe TBI in the patient who is thought to have cerebral hyperemia and refractory ICP issues. With the use of $SjvO_2$ and $AjvDO_2$, hyperemia may be determined and the patient's $PaCO_2$ lowered with controlled hyperventilation while monitoring $SjvO_2$ to minimize the risk of global cerebral ischemia. By decreasing $PaCO_2$, CBF may be decreased to effectively reduce intracranial volume and ICP.[52,53]

Setup

The setup for the placement of the $SjvO_2$ catheter is similar to that for a central line. In addition, the $SjvO_2$ monitor (which is usually the SvO_2 and $ScvO_2$ monitor as well) is required along with a pressure bag with normal saline, the pediatric-size fiberoptic catheter, sheath, and introducer. Unlike the SvO_2 catheter, the $SjvO_2$ catheter must be calibrated in vivo, not prior to insertion.

Neurologic Baseline Prior to Insertion

The baseline for $SjvO_2$ and the derived parameter, $AjvDO_2$, is established at the time of insertion and placement confirmation with laboratory analysis of a blood sample from the $SjvO_2$ catheter. The formula for the determination of $AjvDO_2$ is:

$$[1.34 \, (SaO_2 - SjvO_2) \, \text{hemoglobin}] \div 100$$

Or, it is arterial oxygen content minus venous ($SjvO_2$) oxygen content and requires both arterial and venous blood:[55]

$$[CaO_2(mL/dL) - CjvO_2(mL/dL)]$$

Low $SjvO_2$ and high $AjvO_2$ are diagnostic for ischemia;[44,45] and high $SjvO_2$ and low $AjvDO_2$ may represent hyperemia, CBF, and $CMRO_2$ mismatch, or severe brain injury with inability of the brain tissue to extract the oxygen from the circulating blood.[37,44,45]

Assessment

Hourly assessment of the $SjvO_2$ value is accompanied by assessment of catheter placement, the SQI, and the patient. Recalibration is performed typically every 12 to 24 hours and as needed, according to institution policy. The pressure bag is assessed for maintenance of 300 mm Hg and reinflated, as needed. No waveform is monitored or assessed.

Maintenance

A priority in the maintenance of the $SjvO_2$ catheter is patency. With each assessment, the fast-flush device on the pressure tubing may be used. However, it should be squeezed and released in a pulsed-type action while continuously observing ICP as the fast-flush is activated. If ICP increases, the flushing is stopped until ICP returns to baseline. If a clot in the catheter is suspected, the clot is aspirated before flushing. A kink in the catheter may also cause resistance to flushing and may require removal and replacement of the tubing if still indicated. The catheter is dressed similar to a central venous catheter.

Troubleshooting

Troubleshooting issues typically involve the position of the catheter and patency. Those actions have been described above.

Patient Safety

- Similar to a central venous catheter, infection is a potential concern.

- The $SjvO_2$ catheter should be removed as soon as it is no longer needed.

- If an intraluminal thrombus is suspected, pressure flushing should not be attempted.

- Removal of the thrombus by aspiration is attempted first, and patency is assessed by gentle flushing.

- Removal of the $SjvO_2$ catheter may be performed by a staff nurse at the bedside in some institutions.

- No resistance should be encountered while removing the catheter. If any resistance is detected, the attempt to remove is stopped, and the physician is notified.[56]

- The Edwards LifeScience 4-Fr fiberoptic catheter is MRI compatible; unlike the SvO_2 catheter, it does not include an MRI-incompatible thermistor.[57]

Patient Comfort

Ensuring patient comfort is particularly important prior to insertion, immediately after insertion, and during and after removal of the $SjvO_2$ catheter. The patient may experience some discomfort with turning their head.

Patient Education

- Education is mostly provided to the family, as the patient may be too impaired or sedated to participate in the education process.

- An explanation regarding the catheter and the information it provides is included.

Near-Infrared Spectroscopy

Brain oxygenation can also be assessed using transcranial near-infrared spectroscopy (NIRS). This technology uses fiberoptic light transmitted through the skull to the frontal cerebral cortex. NIRS measures tissue oxygen saturation of hemoglobin in the arterial, venous, and capillary blood vessels. Proximal and distal electrodes are imbedded in two adhesive sensors that are attached to the forehead, one on the left and one on the right. The proximal electrode determines the amount of light absorbed by hemoglobin in the extracranial tissues of the face and skull; the distal electrode determines the amount of light absorbed by the extracranial and intracranial hemoglobin. The monitor that attaches to the adhesive sensors calculates the difference as the ratio of oxygenation hemoglobin to the total hemoglobin to provide the transcranial cerebral oxygen saturation, also known as the regional oxygen saturation (rSO_2) value[47] (Figure 21-21). Only one NIRS—the INVOS (Covidien)—is approved by the U.S. Food and Drug Administration (FDA) and commercially available in the United States. Because NIRS is limited to a tissue depth of 2 to 3 centimeters (cm) below the cortex, it may not detect deeper ischemia in the frontal lobes or more posteriorly.[48] In addition, extracranial hemorrhage and cerebral infarction may confound the data

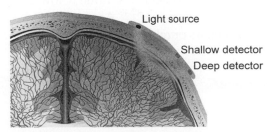

FIGURE 21-21 Extracranial and intracranial detection of infrared light absorption with INVOS near-infrared spectroscopy (NIRS) transcranial cerebral oxygen, or regional oxygen saturation (rSO_2), monitor. (Copyright © 2013 Covidien. All rights reserved. Reprinted with permission of Covidien.)

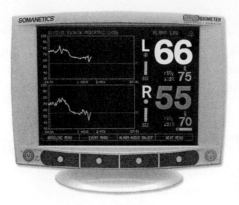
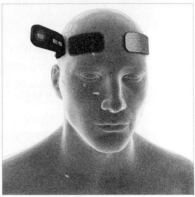

FIGURE 21-22 A, An INVOS near-infrared spectroscopy (NIRS) Transcranial Cerebral Oxygen, or regional oxygen saturation (rSO_2), monitor. **B,** Placement of somasensors. (Copyright © 2013 Covidien. All rights reserved. Reprinted with permission of Covidien.)

obtained. The reliability of NIRS has been questioned and limitations are still being debated.[47,58-61]

Procedure, Setup, Neurologic Baseline, and Maintenance

The NIRS sensors are placed on the frontal temporal forehead left and right of the midline (Figure 21-22). Adult sensors or patches must be used on adults, and pediatric sensors must be used on pediatric patients. The sensors are not reusable. The cable from the sensors is attached to the monitor, and the value obtained is considered the baseline. CT may be obtained to verify optimal placement.

Indications

NIRS has been used in severe TBI, aSAH, and acute ischemic stroke, intraoperatively during carotid endarterectomy, during cardiac surgery, and in seizures, cesarean section, and systemic hemorrhage with transfusion.

Assessment and Troubleshooting

Loose or nonadherent sensors are changed. A change in the rSO_2 of 20% from baseline is a cause for concern. A value below 50% is indicative of hypoxia and associated with a poor prognosis.[47,48] Assessment is hourly or more frequently as needed. If a change of sensors or relocation does not improve the signal, connections should be checked.

Patient Safety

- NIRS is noninvasive and has a low risk of injury.

- As with all electrical patient monitoring equipment, NIRS requires routine clinical engineering review, and any electrical interference with other patient care equipment must be addressed.

Patient Safety—cont'd

- As with other adhesive electrodes, the skin around and underneath the sensors is assessed to prevent irritation or breakdown.

Patient Comfort

Removal of the sensors may feel like adhesive tape being removed from the forehead, but the discomfort is brief.

Patient Education

Family and patient education—when the patient is able to understand—about the information gained by monitoring with NIRS is explained.

Cerebral Blood Flow

Transcranial Doppler

Transcranial Doppler (TCD) uses ultrasound technology to measure CBF velocity, which is an indirect measure of CBF.[62] A probe is placed at naturally thin areas of the skull (anatomic windows) or sometimes surgical defects in the skull to insonate the vessels that comprise the circle of Willis. The four anatomic windows include the transtemporal, transorbital, transforaminal, and submandibular areas (Figure 21-23). Not everyone has anatomic windows, and insonation may not always be possible.[62–66] Also, not everyone has a complete circle of Willis.[67,68] The angle of the probe, the

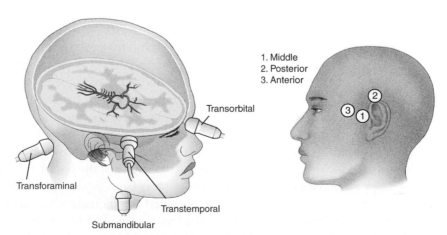

FIGURE 21-23 Four windows of transcranial Doppler insonation. (From Alexandrov AW: Transcranial doppler monitoring. In Wiegand DM, editor: *AACN procedure manual for critical care*, ed 6, St. Louis, 2011, Elsevier.)

TABLE 21-9 **Depth, Direction, and Main Flow Velocities for Circle of Willis Arteries***

ARTERY	DEPTH (mm)	FLOW DIRECTION†	MFV FOR ADULTS
M1 MCA	45-65	Toward	32-82 cm/sec
A1 ACA	62-75	Away	18-82 cm/sec
ICA siphon	60-64	Bi-directional	20-77 cm/sec
OA	50-62	Toward	Variable
PCA	60-68	Bi-directional	16-58 cm/sec
BA	80-100	Away	12-66 cm/sec
VA	45-80	Away	12-66 cm/sec

A1 ACA, First segment of the anterior cerebral artery; *BA*, basilar artery; *cm/sec*, centimeters per second; *ICA*, internal carotid artery; *M1 MCA*, first segment of the middle cerebral artery; *MFV*, mean flow velocity; *mm*, millimeters; *OA*, ophthalmic artery; *PCA*, posterior cerebral artery; *VA*, vertebral artery.
*Depth and MFV ranges may vary slightly between reference studies.
†Toward the probe indicates a positive (+) waveform; away from the probe indicates a negative (−) waveform.
From Alexandrov AW: Transcranial doppler monitoring. In Lynn-McHale Wiegand DJ, Wiegand DM, editor: *AACN procedure manual for critical care*, ed 6, St. Louis, 2011, Elsevier.

known depth of insonation, and the range of normal mean flow velocity for each cerebral vessel has been validated[63-67] (Table 21-9). The arterial waveform resembles an arterial line waveform, and the flow velocity is measured in centimeters per second (cm/sec). If the CBF is toward the probe, the TCD waveform is above the baseline; if the CBF is away from the probe, the waveform is below the baseline (Figure 21-24). If the blood flow is bi-directional (e.g., at the bifurcation), the waveform alternates both above and below the baseline[67] as illustrated in the last waveform in Figure 21-24.

Procedure

The TCD machine is placed next to the bed, and the probe is manually positioned over a cranial window (Figure 21-23). The ultrasound power is set at 100% to best identify the vessel except at the transorbital cranial window, where the power is limited to 10% to minimize risk of eye damage from ultrasound. The probe is held at an angle specific to a particular blood vessel within the circle of Willis, and the estimated depth of the vessel in millimeters (based on validated values) is entered into the machine. A waveform is obtained, similar to an arterial waveform as shown in the first waveform in Figure 21-24. The signal is followed out the length of the vessel, from shallow to deeper. A "signal envelope" with a maximum shift from peak-systolic to end-diastolic flow with every cardiac cycle, may be obtained for increased accuracy.[66,67] The position of the waveform, above or below the baseline is used to confirm vessel identification. The mean flow velocity of the cerebral vessel is primarily used in the clinical setting. Other values that are of clinical interest include the pulsatility index and middle

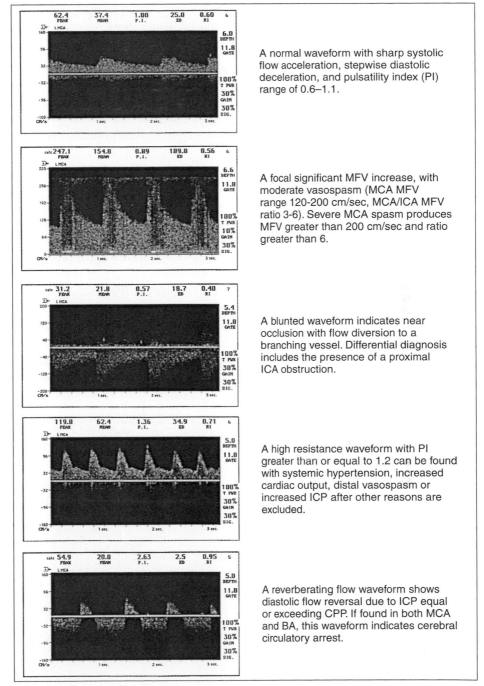

A normal waveform with sharp systolic flow acceleration, stepwise diastolic deceleration, and pulsatility index (PI) range of 0.6–1.1.

A focal significant MFV increase, with moderate vasospasm (MCA MFV range 120-200 cm/sec, MCA/ICA MFV ratio 3-6). Severe MCA spasm produces MFV greater than 200 cm/sec and ratio greater than 6.

A blunted waveform indicates near occlusion with flow diversion to a branching vessel. Differential diagnosis includes the presence of a proximal ICA obstruction.

A high resistance waveform with PI greater than or equal to 1.2 can be found with systemic hypertension, increased cardiac output, distal vasospasm or increased ICP after other reasons are excluded.

A reverberating flow waveform shows diastolic flow reversal due to ICP equal or exceeding CPP. If found in both MCA and BA, this waveform indicates cerebral circulatory arrest.

FIGURE 21-24 Typical middle cerebral artery waveforms. *BA,* Basilar artery; *cm/sec,* centimeters per second; *CPP,* cerebral perfusion pressure; *ICA,* internal carotid artery; *ICP,* intracranial pressure; *MCA,* middle cerebral artery; *MFV,* mean flow volume; *PI,* pulsatility index. (From Wiegand DM, editor: *AACN procedure manual for critical care,* ed 6, St. Louis, 2011, Elsevier.)

cerebral artery to internal carotid artery (MCA:ICA), Lindegaard, or hemispheric ratio. The pulsatility index (PI) is calculated using flow velocity (FV) in the following equation;

$$PI = (systolic\ FV - diastolic\ FV) \div mean\ FV$$

The PI has clinical significance as an indirect indicator of ICP.[47] A headband that holds bilateral probes at the level of the middle cerebral artery may also be used for hands-free bilateral monitoring of the right and left middle cerebral arteries.[65,66]

Indications

TCD is most frequently used in the diagnosis of cerebral vasospasm associated with aSAH but may also be used to detect traumatic SAH vasospasm (Box 21-1). TCD is used in the diagnosis and to guide management in acute ischemic stroke and cerebral emboli from carotid or vertebral dissection, or a patent foramen ovale, sickle cell disease, impaired cerebrovascular autoregulation following severe TBI, and brain cerebral circulatory arrest (brain death).

Agitated saline may be injected intravenously as the contrast media during TCD examination to detect emboli from a patent foramen ovale. Microemboli can be heard and seen from the TCD machine as they move into cerebral circulation from the heart.

Both static and dynamic pressure autoregulation testing can be performed with TCD. In static measurement, systemic blood pressure and CBF mean flow velocity may be obtained at baseline and then obtained again with pharmacologic increase

---

BOX 21-1   Criteria for a Normal Transcranial Doppler (TCD)

1. Optimal windows of insonation, permitting identification of all proximal arterial segments.
2. Direction of flow and depths consistent with criteria in Table 21-9.
3. Side-to-side difference between flow velocities in homologous arteries in 30% or less.
4. Presence of a normal flow velocity ratio: middle cerebral artery (MCA) greater than or equal to anterior cerebral artery (ACA), greater than or equal to internal carotid artery (ICA), siphon greater than or equal to posterior cerebral artery (PCA), greater than or equal to basilar artery, greater than or equal to vertebral artery.
5. Positive end-diastolic flow velocity of 20% to 50% of the peak systolic velocity values.
6. Low-resistance flow pattern, with pulsatility index (PI) between 0.6 and 1.1 in all intracranial arteries when partial pressure of arterial carbon dioxide ($PaCO_2$) is between 35 and 45 mm Hg.
7. High-resistance flow pattern with PI greater than or equal to 1.2 in the ophthalmic artery only.
8. High-resistance flow patterns with PI greater than or equal to 1.2 in all arteries during hyperventilation or elevated blood pressure.

(From Alexandrov AW: Transcranial doppler monitoring. In DJ Lynn-McHale Wiegand, editor: *AACN procedure manual for critical care*, ed 6, St. Louis, 2011, Elsevier.)

of the systemic blood pressure with vasopressors such as norepinephrine (Levophed) and neosynephrine (Phenylephrine).[2] Dynamic autoregulation testing may be performed at the bedside with TCD using thigh cuffs. Baseline TCD results are obtained. Then, the thigh cuffs are inflated and quickly deflated, and the decrease in systemic blood pressure and CBF mean flow velocity is noted; finally, the time required for these values to return to baseline is measured.[66,67,69]

Setup

Setup for TCD monitoring requires preparation of the patient, including supine positioning; medical record review for clinical data that may impact results such as reason for TCD, ICP, the presence of the external ventricular catheter, hematocrit, $PaCO_2$, and the presence of missing bone (decompressive craniectomy or large cranial defect).[66,67] (Criteria for a normal TCD are listed in Box 21-1). Acoustic transmission gel is required to conduct the signal. A sterile plastic cover of the probe is indicated if the probe will be placed over a cranial incision, or an area of bloody or CSF drainage. Mild analgesia may be required if the pressure from the probe impacts the patient's ability to lie quietly during the test.

Neurologic Baseline

Establishing a baseline is preferable in certain clinical scenarios, for example, within the first 24 hours after aSAH, before cerebral vasospasm occurs (see Figure 21-8). Also, a baseline is needed prior to initiating management of sickle cell crisis and when hemodynamic management such as fluids and red blood cell exchanges would be beneficial. Ideally the same sonographer performs the TCD evaluation for the same patient each day to ensure consistency in the performance and interpretation of the test. In most clinical settings, TCD is performed once daily, or less often, unless the bedside nurse or advanced practice nurse has competency validation to perform the examination when TCD sonographers are not available. Factors that influence flow velocity values related to vasospasm following subarachnoid hemorrhage are listed in Box 21-2.

Assessment and Troubleshooting

TCD sonography requires knowledge and skill validation. Competency is best achieved by frequent practice overseen by a skilled TCD sonographer. Clinical application for the posterior circulation is believed to be of less value than anterior circulation by some clinicians. A middle cerebral artery mean flow velocity of greater than 120 cm/sec and a middle cerebral artery to internal carotid artery (MCA:ICA) ratio of greater than 3 is consistent with mild vasospasm; middle cerebral artery mean flow velocity of greater than 200 cm/sec and an MCA:ICA ratio of greater than 6 is consistent with severe vasospasm.[60] An elevated MCA:ICA ratio must be present in addition to an elevated middle cerebral artery mean flow velocity to differentiate middle cerebral artery vasospasm from hyperdynamic or hyperemic flow (Figure 21-1).[42] Vasospasm for other cerebral blood vessels has been reported but has not been validated adequately. A PI of greater than 1.2 is associated with increased ICP but may also be associated with increased cardiac output or systemic

---

BOX 21-2   Factors that Influence Flow Velocity Values Related to Vasospasm Following Subarachnoid Hemorrhage

Anatomic Factors
- Individual variation in the circle of Willis: *normal physiologic and pathophysiologic*
- Arterial diameter at rest
- Aberrancy in vessel path
- Location(s), extent, and severity of vasospasm
- Coexisting hemodynamic impacting vascular lesions proximal to the area of vasospasm such as:
  - Extracranial common carotid or internal carotid artery high-grade stenosis or occlusion
  - Intracranial internal carotid artery stenosis or cerebral vasospasm
- Artifact from aneurysm clips or coils

Intracranial Physiologic Factors
- Increased intracranial pressure: focal or diffuse
- Hydrocephalus

Systemic Physiologic Factors: Cardiovascular
- Cardiovascular: blood pressure, cardiac output, volume status, cardiac arrhythmias

- Metabolic/Hematologic: Partial pressure of arterial carbon dioxide ($PaCO_2$), blood viscosity (hematocrit, fibrinogen), temperature

Effects of Therapeutic Interventions
- Hypertensive hypervolemic hemodilution, especially pharmacologically induced hypertension
- Calcium channel blockers (e.g., nimodipine, nicardipine)
- Transluminal angioplasty
- Intra-arterial injections of vasodilators (papaverine, nicardipine)

Technical Factors
- Sonographer interrater reliability and individual knowledge and experience
- Adequacy of acoustic windows in the skull
- Patient cooperation
- Adequacy of Doppler angle

Any Combination of the Factors Included in this Box

---

hypertension.[66,67] A reverberating (forward-to-backward) flow pattern, or absent flow signals in the middle cerebral artery and basilar arteries for 30 minutes is associated with near or probable cerebral circulatory arrest.[67] (See last waveform of Figure 21-24.)

Patient Safety

- A clean probe must be used for each patient. If the probe is in contact with a neck, head, or face incision, a sterile probe cover should be used.

- Although ultrasonography is generally considered safe, the ALARA (as low as reasonably achievable) principle is practiced, especially when insonating over the eyelid.

Patient Safety—cont'd

- Patient safety includes proper education and competency validation of the sonographer.

- In some institutions, the bedside nurse or advanced practice nurse performs transcranial Doppler (TCD) examinations. Competency validation is difficult to maintain if TCD is not performed on a regular basis.

Patient Comfort

- The patient may experience slight discomfort when the probe is held close to an incision.

- Mild analgesia may be needed to help the patient to not move their head because of slight discomfort when the probe is held adjacent to a wound or incision.

- Families and patients may be reassured that ultrasonography is not a painful procedure.

Patient Education

Families and patients (as able) should be informed that the technology used with TCD is ultrasonography, which is the same as that used during pregnancy. The patient does not receive any ionizing radiation.

Thermal Diffusion Flowmetry and Laser Doppler Flowmetry

Technical Considerations

Though less commonly used in the critical care setting compared with the technologies described above, direct CBF monitoring may be conducted with thermal diffusion flowmetry and laser Doppler flowmetry. Inserted through a burr hole, thermal diffusion flowmetry (TDF) uses a probe on the surface of the cerebral cortex or in the parenchyma to quantitatively measure cerebral blood flow. CBF is measured in milliliters per 100 grams per minute (mL/100 g/min).[63] CBF rates in the cerebral cortex (gray matter) and parenchyma (white matter) differ. A probe with two metal plates, called *thermistors*, detect the temperature difference related to CBF at two different areas of the cortex or two different areas of the parenchyma, depending on the manufacturer.[70–72]

Currently, one thermal diffusion flowmetry system, the Hemedex Bowman Perfusion Monitor, is commercially available in the United States[10,44] (Figure 21-25). The Bowman Perfusion Monitor (BPM) uses an intraparenchymal probe that contains two thermistors. One thermistor measures the baseline temperature and the second thermistor measures CBF by heat transfer to the capillaries. The thermistor at the tip of the probe measures perfusion in a 20-30 mm^3 brain volume.[71–72] The tip of the probe

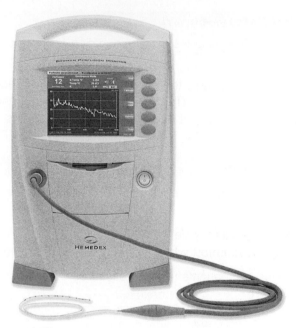

FIGURE 21-25 Thermal diffusion flowmetry: Hemedex Bowman Perfusion Monitor. (Courtesy of Hemedex, Inc.)

is heated 2°C above the brain temperature. The second thermistor 8 mm away from the tip of the probe detects and adjusts for changes in the baseline tissue temperature to determine CBF. The higher the CBF, the greater the heat loss from the tip to the proximal sensor and the greater the power required to maintain the 2°C temperature elevation from the tip to the proximal end 8 mm away.[73] The probe tip must be positioned 25 mm below the dura in the capillary bed away from pulsating vessels to operate effectively.[73]

Laser diffusion flowmetry provides continuous measurement of red blood cell velocity in the cerebral capillaries to determine cortical CBF. The laser diffusion flowmetry probe may be inserted into the brain parenchyma or placed on the cerebral cortex. Unlike thermal diffusion flowmetry, laser diffusion flowmetry does not quantify CBF absolutely but provides a measure of relative change in flow in a small brain volume of 1-2 mm^3.[10,44,72]

Procedures

The thermal diffusion flowmetry probe is inserted through a cranial bolt inserted into a burr hole, through a burr hole next to a craniotomy, or through an open craniotomy site, and is connected to a monitor that provides the numeric CBF, a graphical display of CBF, and a continuous numerical display of the changes in temperature.[70,73] Data is stored in the monitor and may be downloaded to a multimodality recording system. As with other invasive monitors, sterile technique must be used for insertion and the insertion site covered with a sterile dressing. The probe and bolt must be removed prior to MRI.

Indications

Thermal diffusion flowmetry and laser diffusion flowmetry have been used intraoperatively and in severe TBI and aSAH vasospasm.[10] As with the PbtO$_2$ catheter, both these physiologic methods depend on optimal placement because they only measure CBF in a local area. Laser diffusion flowmetry measures CBF in a brain volume of only 1 to 2 mm^3. [37,71]

Correlation between thermal diffusion flowmetry, CBF, and PbtO$_2$ was confirmed in one TBI study to occur 90% of the time.[72] However, in a study on aSAH vasospasm, the correlation between TCD, mean flow velocities, and laser diffusion flowmetry CBF was poor.[71] Additional research is needed to validate the accuracy of this technology. Laser diffusion flowmetry is affected by movement artifact.

Setup, Neurologic Baseline, and Maintenance

Following insertion of the probe and connection to the monitor, the thermal diffusion flowmetry monitor begins some routine calibration and temperature stabilization before CBF is displayed. The probe may be used for up to 10 days.[73] Among the limitations of thermal diffusion flowmetry are autocalibration interrupting continuous measurement every 30 minutes and loss of data when the brain temperature is greater than 39°C.[2,42,73]

Patient Safety

- As with any intracranial monitoring device, risk of infection exists.
- Sterile technique should be used during site care.
- The physician should be notified about any CSF leakage.
- Patients who require CBF probes may require chemical or mechanical restraints to prevent dislodgement of the probes.

Patient Comfort

Ensuring patient comfort is particularly important prior to insertion, immediately after insertion, and during and after removal of thermal diffusion flowmetry and laser diffusion flowmetry probes.

Patient Education

- Families and patients—as they are able to understand—should be informed that they will require assistance during turning and repositioning to prevent dislodgement of the thermal diffusion flowmetry or laser diffusion flowmetry probes.
- Families and patients are educated about the purpose of this monitoring device.

Cerebral Microdialysis

Cerebral microdialysis involves a semipermeable dialysis catheter placed through a cranial bolt or into the surgical site of the brain to obtain small amounts of interstitial brain fluid. A microvial is attached at the distal end of the catheter to collect interstitial brain fluid (Figure 21-26). One collection of the specimen is completed every hour. The sample is placed into an analyzer at the bedside to determine biomarkers of cerebral ischemia. An empty microvial replaces the one just removed for analysis. At the proximal end of the catheter, the dialysate, which is similar to CSF, is exchanged through the semipermeable membrane to obtain interstitial fluid (Figure 21-27). Interstitial fluid is typically analyzed for biomarkers of cerebral ischemia, including lactate, pyruvate, glycerol, glutamate, and glucose.[70,74] The microdialysate does not equal the actual extracellular fluid concentration, but a proportion of what is actually in extracellular brain fluid.[74] Cerebral microdialysis has generally been considered a research tool, but as more medical centers gain microdialysis experience, it may become more mainstream in neurocritical care.[74]

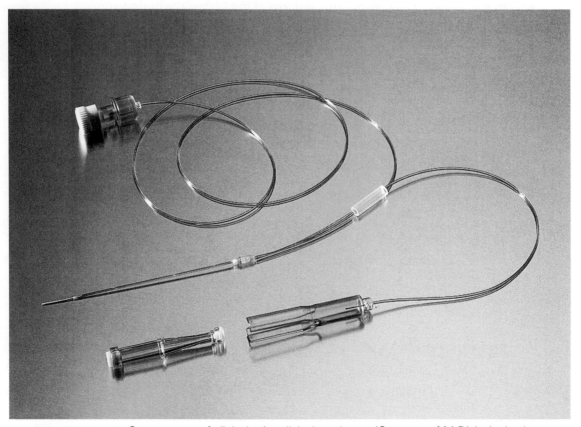

FIGURE 21-26 Components of clinical microdialysis catheter. (Courtesy of M Dialysis, Inc.)

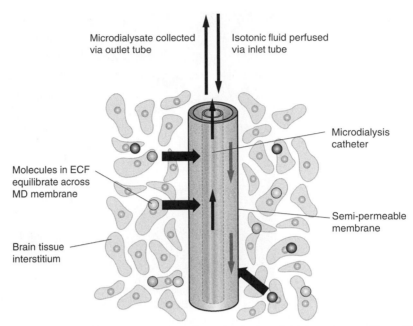

FIGURE 21-27 Schematic representation of cerebral microdialysis catheter. (From Tisdall MM, Smith M: Cerebral microdialysis: research technique or clinical tool, *Br J Anaesth* 97(1): 18-25, 2006.)

Procedure

Cerebral microdialysis is labor intensive. If the catheter is placed at the bedside, sterile technique must be used. The catheter is typically placed adjacent to the ICP and $PbtO_2$ catheters through the bolt. The bedside analyzer must be calibrated with control solutions before sample analysis can begin (Figure 21-28). The vials must then be exchanged and the interstitial fluid analyzed on a regular basis, typically hourly. The results are recorded with particular attention to trends.

Indications

Cerebral microdialysis has primarily been used in severe TBI and aSAH vasospasm to detect cerebral ischemia. In patients with TBI, the microdialysis substrates may be used to guide CPP goals and management with hyperventilation. Decreased brain glucose and an increased lactate-to-pyruvate ratio signifies metabolic derangement.[47,54] A lactate to pyruvate ratio of greater than 20 to 25 is associated with a poor prognosis.[2,74] In aSAH, an increase in the lactate-to-pyruvate ratio preceded by elevations in glutamate or followed by increases in glycerol, may be diagnostic for delayed cerebral ischemia associated with vasospasm.[54,70] In both TBI and aSAH, changes in the microdialysate may be an earlier predictor of neurologic deterioration compared with other assessment tools, and certainly earlier than bedside assessment.[54,74]

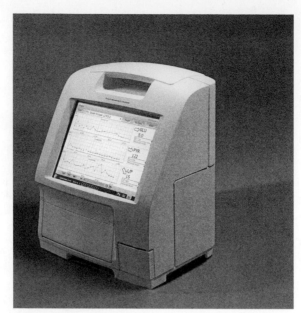

FIGURE 21-28 Microdialysis analyzer. (Courtesy of M Dialysis, Inc.)

Setup, Neurologic Baseline, and Maintenance

Setup of cerebral microdialysis involves insertion of the catheter, followed by calibration of the analyzer by analyzing control solutions of known quantities of the metabolites to be measured from interstitial fluid. The analyzer is also attached to a computer that assists in the monitoring of trends. A baseline analysis is conducted as soon as possible, followed by hourly analysis of the microdialysate. Cerebral microdialysis is not monitored in isolation and should be considered in the context of other measurement methods such as ICP and CPP, $PbtO_2$, $SjvO_2$, and TCD mean flow velocities.[52] Routine controls must be completed to ensure quality.

Patient Safety

- In addition to the labor intense nature of cerebral microdialysis, the patient's bedside examination and other clinical parameters must be closely monitored.

- Sterile technique in maintaining the microdialysis catheter and specimen collection is imperative.

Patient Comfort

Ensuring patient comfort is particularly important prior to insertion, immediately after insertion, and during and after removal of the microdialysis catheter.

Patient Education

- The family and patient—as able to understand—should be educated about the purpose of the microdialysis monitoring device.
- The family is educated that cerebral microdialysis is one of many parameters used to assess the patient.

Adjunctive Measurements

A number of other measurement tools are valuable in the care of the critically ill neuroscience patient. Three of them will be briefly discussed: temperature, $PetCO_2$ monitoring, and pupillometry.

Temperature

Systemic temperature values for monitoring the critically ill neuroscience patient may be obtained from any of the following: pulmonary artery, esophageal, bladder, rectal, temporal artery, tympanic membrane, oral, axilla, or groin. Some sites are considered more accurate than others, specifically core temperature obtained from a pulmonary artery catheter thermistor, a urinary drainage catheter with a bladder temperature sensor, or an esophageal probe at a depth of 32 to 38 cm.[76]

Another consideration in the brain injured patient is direct monitoring of brain temperature (T_{Br}). Catheters to monitor T_{Br} are commercially available and are used in combination with ICP and $PbtO_2$ catheters. T_{Br}, compared with rectal temperature, is usually 0.3 to 2.0°C higher.[75] However, exceptions exist. If the probe is located in an area of decreased CBF, T_{Br} may be lower than systemic temperature and could be an indicator of low CBF.[77] Use of T_{Br} for temperature management of the critically ill neuroscience patient has not been widely accepted. Clinicians continue to rely on traditional systemic temperature to guide management.

Patient Safety

- Brain temperature and systemic temperature do not necessarily correlate. In general, systemic temperature is the more widely acceptable parameter for temperature management.
- Correct positioning of any temperature monitoring device is essential.
- Indwelling urinary catheters with a temperature sensory may be inaccurate if the urine output is low.

Patient Comfort

- The patient undergoing continuous invasive temperature monitoring may experience minimal discomfort.

- Routine assessment of skin is essential to prevent tissue breakdown from temperature probes.

Patient Education

The family should be informed that brain and systemic temperatures are some of the many parameters used to assess the patient. The goal for temperature management (normothermia versus hypothermia) in the critically ill neuroscience patient is controversial.

End-Tidal Carbon Dioxide Monitoring

The partial pressure of end-tidal carbon dioxide ($PetCO_2$) monitoring, also called continuous $ETCO_2$ monitoring, has a role in management of the critically ill neuroscience patient (see Chapter 8). In addition to its usual roles—confirmation of endotracheal tube placement, transport safety, and effectiveness of chest compression during cardiopulmonary arrest, $PetCO_2$ is also valuable to monitor the $PetCO_2$ trends to manage ICP. $PetCO_2$ devices may be placed directly into the breathing circuit of the mechanical ventilator (see Figure 8-2). A bi-nasal $PetCO_2$ cannula is available for the spontaneously breathing patient (see Figure 8-8 in Chapter 8). Although $PetCO_2$ does not correspond exactly to $PaCO_2$, noting $PetCO_2$ at the time of obtaining an ABG sample allows the difference between $PaCO_2$ and $PetCO_2$ to be calculated. $PetCO_2$ can then be used for trending as an indirect indicator of the $PaCO_2$. This is vital because $PaCO_2$ is a cerebral vasodilator. As $PaCO_2$ rises, the cerebral vessels dilate, allowing increased CBF and increased ICP. The $PetCO_2$ monitor may be used to guide controlled hyperventilation with a goal $PaCO_2$ of 35 to 40 mm Hg to control ICP.[78,79]

Patient Safety

- The patient's $PaCO_2$ from an arterial blood gas (ABG) sample should be determined as a reference for the patient's exhaled partial pressure of end-tidal carbon dioxide ($PetCO_2$) value, because the values will not be exactly the same. Once the difference between $PaCO_2$ and $PetCO_2$ in mm Hg is calculated, the continuous noninvasive $PetCO_2$ value can be trended.

- $PetCO_2$ may be markedly different from $PaCO_2$ with underlying lung pathology.

- $PaCO_2$ of 35 to 40 mm Hg is recommended in patients with increased ICP.

- High $PetCO_2$, as a surrogate of $PaCO_2$, may contribute to increased ICP and a decreased level of consciousness.

- Low $PetCO_2$, as a surrogate of the $PaCO_2$, may contribute to secondary neuronal injury related to vasoconstriction and cerebral ischemia.

Patient Comfort

The spontaneously breathing patient who is being monitored with PetCO$_2$ via nasal cannula is assessed for discomfort at the nares, face, or behind the ears (see Figure 8-8).

Patient Education

- The purpose of the end-tidal CO$_2$ device is explained to the patient and the family.

- The family and the patient may need to be educated about airway secretions that may obstruct the PetCO$_2$ tubing, impede accurate carbon dioxide detection, and cause an alarm. In this situation, a change in device may be needed.

Pupillometry

Subtle pupil changes are often an indicator of increased ICP. Pupils are difficult to assess in some patients and interrater reliability, even among experienced neuroscience clinicians, has been demonstrated to be poor.[80] The pupillometer is a battery-powered hand-held device that allows quantitative measurement of pupil size and rate of reactivity (NeurOptics, Irvine, CA) (Figure 21-29). A proprietary parameter—the Neurological Pupil Index (NPi)—includes consideration of pupil size, constriction velocity, dilation velocity, and latency.[81] Available commercially in the United States for approximately a decade, the pupillometer uses infrared technology. A headrest attaches to the front of the pupillometer to ensure correct and consistent placement of the device in front of the patient's eye. A single measurement has a duration of 3.2 seconds, and the tracking of the pupil occurs at 30 frames each second. One prospective study consisting of 134 patients found that the NPi identified the inverse relationship between pupil reactivity and increased ICP.[80] Additional research is needed to fully determine the pupillometer's usefulness to detect early change in pupil size related to increased ICP before neurologic deterioration.[82]

Patient Safety

- The pupillometer must be cleaned between use on different patients. The pupillometer may be covered with plastic when the patient is in isolation without interference in the technology.

- The headrest is single patient use but may be used repetitively on the same patient.

- The pupillometer is best used as a trending device. It is not necessarily a replacement for pupil assessment with a penlight.

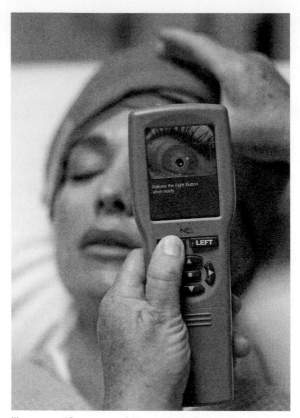

FIGURE 21-29 Pupillometer. (Courtesy of Neuroptics, Inc.)

Patient Comfort

- The patient may need assistance in holding the eyes open and the head still to achieve optimal measurements.

- The headrest should not be used if the pad is not on the headrest.

- The pupillometer may be turned 90 or 180 degrees, as needed, to obtain measurements and to avoid other monitoring and care devices or wounds.

Patient Education

The family and the patient—as they are able to understand—should be informed that the pupillometer is an additional device to look at the size and reactivity of the pupils. The device takes a number of pictures of the pupil in rapid succession and is most valuable as a trending device. It will not harm the eyes.

Hemodynamics and Intracranial Dynamics Monitoring in Selected Neurologic Injury and Illness

Severe Traumatic Brain Injury

Much of the discussion around hemodynamic management of the patient with severe TBI involves management of systolic blood pressure, MAP, and CPP in relationship to the usual intracranial parameters such as ICP, $PbtO_2$, and $SjvO_2$. The Brain Trauma Foundation *Guidelines for the Management of Severe Traumatic Brain Injury* do not address systemic hemodynamic monitoring other than reference to close attention to blood pressure.[83] The initial section states that even one prehospital episode of systemic hypotension has been associated with a worse outcome in severe TBI.[83]

Systemic hypotension is defined as a systolic blood pressure of less than 90 mm Hg. Avoidance of hypotension, with a systolic blood pressure below 90 mm Hg is a Level II of III recommendation.[83] A CPP threshold of 50 to 70 mm Hg is recommended (Level III of III recommendation)[11] (see Table 21-2).

Although the Brain Trauma Foundation *Guidelines* primarily summarize the research up to 2007, more recent discussion in the literature has focused on the complexity of decision making with the multimodal data.[10,84] Fortunately, these data are often available to the clinician caring for the patient with severe TBI.[4,10,84] Although sufficient evidence is lacking for one best way to work with multiple parameters, one hierarchical approach has been developed.[84] This hierarchical approach has its theoretical framework in the Brain Trauma Foundation *Guidelines*. Tiered interventions with regard to possible ICP and $PbtO_2$ scenarios are available[85] An example of a tiered therapy approach used in a major medical center is presented in Figure 21-30.

Possible ICP and $PbtO_2$ combinations include (1) normal ICP and normal $PbtO_2$; (2) high ICP and normal $PbtO_2$; (3) normal ICP and high $PbtO_2$; and (4) high ICP and high $PbtO_2$. Interventions include pharmacologic and nonpharmacologic treatments. As with other traumatic injuries, once the patient has been fully fluid resuscitated, vasoactive agents may be indicated to maintain CPP within the recommended goal of 50 to 70 mm Hg.[83] In a recent retrospective analysis of vasopressors used following severe TBI ($n = 114$), vasopressors used in descending order were phenylephrine (Neosynephrine); 43%; norepinephrine (Levophed); 30%; dopamine; 22%; and vasopressin; 5%.[85] Patients who received phenylephrine had a higher MAP and CPP compared with those who received dopamine or norepinephrine, respectively.

Phenylephrine (Neosynephrine), a selective alpha-1 adrenergic agonist is a preferential vasoconstrictor of the systemic vessels in the management of intracranial pathologies. The cerebral vessels contain less alpha-1 receptors, whereas the peripheral blood vessels have more alpha-1 receptors, which results in effective

Intracranial Hypertension

FIGURE 21-30 Traumatic brain injury protocol. (From Harborview Medical Center, Seattle, WA. Traumatic Brain Injury Algorithm. Management of Severe TBI: A Pocket Guide. 2008, Plainsboro, New Jersey; Permission granted by Integra LifeSciences Corporation, Plainsboro, New Jersey, USA.)

The algorithm chart shows a 2×2 matrix:
- Columns: Intracranial Hypertension — NO / YES
- Rows: Cerebral Ischemia — NO / YES

A (Ischemia NO, Hypertension NO): No interventions needed
B (Ischemia NO, Hypertension YES): Interventions directed at lowering ICP
C (Ischemia YES, Hypertension NO): Interventions directed at increasing $P_{bt}O_2$
D (Ischemia YES, Hypertension YES): Interventions directed at lowering ICP and increasing $P_{bt}O_2$

*Harborview Medical Center Algorithm

■ **A. Patient requires no further therapy**

■ **B. Treatments directed at lowering ICP**

TIER 1

- Head of the bed to 30° (if not at that level already)
- Maintain temperature < 37.5°C
- Adjust analgesia and sedation
- CSF drainage (if EVD available)
- Hypertonic saline bolus or continuous infusion
- Standard dose Mannitol (0.25-0.5 g/kg)

TIER 2

- Lower PCO_2 to 32-35 mm Hg
- High dose Mannitol I g/kg, or repeated dosing of standard dose Mannitol
- Neuromuscular blockade

Consider:

- Repeat CT to determine if increased size of intracranial mass lesions
- Placing EVD if one not available
- Continuous EEG to rule out seizure activity when using neuromuscular blockade

TIER 3

- Decompressive craniectomy
- Pentobarbital coma
- Induced hypothermia

■ **C. Treatment directed at increasing $P_{bt}O_2$**

- Consider jugular venous oxygen and lactate monitoring for confirmation
- Consider cerebral blood flow studies to determine generalizability of LICOX® ($P_{bt}O_2$) data

TIER 1

- Adjust head of the bed to 30°
- Check for detrimental influence on ICP/CPP
- Maintain temperature < 37.5°C
- Increase CPP to > 60 mm Hg
- Use fluids in preference to pressors until CVP > 8 cm H_2O, then employ vasopressors

TIER 2

- Increase FiO_2 to 0.60
- Increase PCO_2 to 45-50 mm Hg
- Transfuse pRBCs to Hgb > 10 g/dL

TIER 3

- Increase FiO_2 to 1.0
- Consider increasing PEEP to increase PaO_2 if FiO_2 is 1.0
- Decrease ICP to < 10 mm Hg
- CSF drainage
- Increase sedation
- Manipulation of serum osmolarity

■ **D. Treatment directed at lowering ICP and increasing $P_{bt}O_2$**

TIER 1

- Elevate head of the bed to 30°
- Maintain temperature < 37.5°C
- Adjust analgesia and sedation
- CSF drainage (if EVD available)
- Increase CPP to > 60 mm Hg
- Hypertonic saline bolus or continuous infusion
- Standard dose Mannitol (0.25-0.5 g/kg), to be administered as bolus infusion
- Consider placing EVD if one is not available

TIER 2

- High dose Mannitol I g/kg, or repeated dosing of standard dose Mannitol
- Increase FiO_2 to 0.60
- Transfuse to Hgb > 10 g/dL
- Neuromuscular blockade (1 hour trial of effect)

Consider:

- Repeat CT to determine if increased size of intracranial mass lesions
- Continuous EEG to rule out seizure activity when using neuromuscular blockade

TIER 3

- Increase FiO_2 to 1.0
- Consider increasing PEEP to increase PaO_2 if FiO_2 is 1.0
- Decompressive craniectomy
- Pentobarbital coma
- Induced hypothermia

■ **Reassess the patient**

- ICP still > 20 mm Hg:
- Consider consultation with a TBI specialist or transfer of the patient to a head injury center if advanced therapies are required
- If patient remains unresponsive to all interventions and GCS is 3-4, consider the possibility of organ donation and consult the local Organ Procurement Agency. (*)

*The Mandatory Donation Request Act established in 1987 requires health care providers in the United States to approach next of kin about organ donation. It is usually best for the request to be made by someone other than a direct caregiver in order to avoid the appearance of a conflict of interest.

constriction of the peripheral vessels to increase blood flow from the periphery to the cerebral blood vessels without excess constriction of the cerebral blood vessels themselves.[86,87]

Norepinephrine (Levophed) has both alpha and beta (cardiac) receptor action.[86,88] Three tiers of interventions are described. Not every intervention in every tier has to be implemented, but some interventions from the lower tiers must be implemented before advancing to the next tier.[85] Third tier interventions include decompressive craniectomy, pentobarbital coma, and therapeutic hypothermia, although the improved outcomes for therapeutic hypothermia have not been substantiated in multicenter prospective randomized controlled trials.[89]

In addition to the complexity inherent in severe TBI alone, not every patient with severe TBI has a single system injury, and not every severe TBI patient is in good health prior to the injury. Also, the neurologic injury may induce cardiopulmonary compromise. Therefore, extracranial injuries may necessitate additional hemodynamic monitoring, including use of a pulmonary artery catheter, arterial pulse contour and waveform analysis, continuous cardiac output monitoring, volume status, and fluid responsiveness assessment.[84]

Aneurysmal Subarachnoid Hemorrhage

Prior to surgical clipping or endovascular coiling of the ruptured aneurysm, a major goal is prevention of rebleeding. The primary systemic physiologic parameters of interest are systolic blood pressure and MAP. The AHA/ASA *Guidelines for the Management of Spontaneous Aneurysmal Subarachnoid Hemorrhage* do not recommend specific blood pressure parameters initially after aSAH, only that blood pressure must be monitored and controlled (a Class I of III recommendation, based on the highest quality of evidence).[34] The Neurocritical Care Society *Critical Care Management of Patients Following Aneurysmal Subarachnoid Hemorrhage* guidelines recommend a target MAP of greater than 110 mm Hg (low quality evidence but strongly recommended).[35]

Vasodilators may be required to control systemic hypertension. No preference for vasodilators is given in the guidelines. A nicardipine (Cardene) infusion is often used. Others agents include an esmolol (Brevibloc) infusion, and intravenous boluses of metoprolol (Lopressor), hydralazine (Apresoline), and clonidine (Klonopin). A ventriculostomy catheter, often referred to as an external ventricular drain (EVD), is typically inserted in the management of hydrocephalus, to prevent increased ICP and inadequate CPP.

Once the aneurysm is secured, vasospasm, a known risk in delayed cerebral injury, and ultimately secondary cerebral infarction, is of concern. For many years, a cornerstone in the prevention and management of vasospasm has been hypertensive hypervolemic hemodilution, also referred to as *HHH* or *triple H therapy*. A typical protocol for the patient receiving HHH therapy is to increase the intravascular volume to prescribed parameters with the use of crystalloid and perhaps even colloid on the basis of the amount of vasospasm, using the CVP, or less frequently the pulmonary artery occlusion pressure (PAOP) as a guide for management. The greater the vasospasm, the higher is the target CVP or PAOP parameter. In addition, a vasopressor is used to increase the systemic blood pressure depending on the amount of vasospasm. The greater the vasospasm, the higher is the blood pressure goal. Typical vasopressors might include phenylephrine or norepinephrine. Finally, hematocrit or hemoglobin parameters are often chosen to achieve hemodilution with a transfusion trigger (e.g., only transfuse if hemoglobin falls below 7 grams/dL).

Institutional variation in HHH therapy is significant. Despite its widespread use and inclusion in the AHA/ASA *Guidelines* as a Class II of III recommendation[34] (Table 21-10), HHH therapy has never been proven to improve patient outcomes. A number of negative sequelae have been associated with HHH therapy, including pulmonary edema and iatrogenic injury from the pulmonary artery catheter. What is known with some degree of certainty is that the patient with aSAH is at increased risk of delayed cerebral ischemia or secondary stroke, when in a hypovolemic state.[34,35]

Within the past 5 years, a number of clinicians have begun to investigate the value of HHH therapy, not only the whole concept, but also the individual components. Although some form of HHH therapy continues to be used across neuroscience centers, the literature, expert clinicians, and clinical researchers have all started to formally question its utility, particularly the role of hypervolemia and the best way to monitor volume status during cerebral vasospasm. Controlled hypertension has been postulated to be the most important component.[90–95]

The Neurocritical Care Society recently published multidisciplinary recommendations on *Critical Care Management of Patients Following Aneurysmal Subarachnoid Hemorrhage* (see Table 21-8). From the Neurocritical Care Society international multi-disciplinary consensus conference the following is recommended: (1) Monitoring intake and output may be beneficial; (2) the best method to monitor fluid balance is clinical assessment by documenting intake and output; (3) a central venous catheter is not indicated simply to obtain CVP measurements, nor should fluid management be based only on CVP measurements; and (4) pulmonary artery catheters are not routinely recommended; they are not without risk, and evidence of benefits are lacking.[35]

Again, certain patients will be outliers related to neurogenic stunned myocardium or myocardial infarction or premorbid heart disease. In those instances, systemic hemodynamic monitoring with the pulmonary artery catheter and newer modalities such as arterial waveform and pulse pressure analysis and transpulmonary thermodilution monitoring may be of value.[96] Additional agents to provide inotropic support for the heart may include dobutamine and milrinone.

Acute Ischemic Stroke

Blood pressure is the main hemodynamic parameter of concern in acute ischemic stroke. If the patient with acute ischemic stroke is admitted to the critical care unit,

TABLE 21-10 AHA/ASA Guidelines for Hemodynamic and Intracranial Parameters in the Management of Spontaneous Aneurysmal Subarachnoid Hemorrhage (aSAH)

PARAMETER		CLASSIFICATION OF RECOMMENDATION AND LEVEL OF EVIDENCE
Systemic blood pressure	The following recommendation has been made to prevent rebleeding after aSAH: Prior to aneurysm obliteration, a continuous titratable intravenous medication should be used to control blood pressure, minimize the risk of rebleeding related to hypertension, and maintain adequate cerebral perfusion pressure.	Class I: Benefit much greater than risk. Level B evidence: Evidence based on limited patient populations, utilizing one randomized trial or more than one nonrandomized trials.
Systemic blood pressure	The following recommendation has been made to minimize the risk of rebleeding after aSAH: Although the extent of systemic blood pressure control is unknown with regard to minimizing the risk of rebleeding, a systolic blood pressure of <160 mm Hg is reasonable.	Class IIa: Benefit greater than risk. Level C evidence: Evidence based on very limited patient populations, utilizing expert consensus, case studies, and standards of care.
Intravascular volume	The following recommendation has been made to manage cerebral vasospasm and delayed cerebral ischemia: To prevent delayed cerebral ischemia, euvolemia and a normal circulating blood volume should be maintained.	Class I: Benefit much greater than risk. Level B evidence: Evidence based on limited patient populations, utilizing one randomized trial or more than one nonrandomized trials.
Intravascular volume	The following recommendation has been made to manage cerebral vasospasm and delayed cerebral ischemia: Systemic hypervolemia is not recommended in the prevention of vasospasm.	Class III: No benefit and possibly harmful. Level B evidence: Evidence based on limited patient populations, utilizing one randomized trial or more than one nonrandomized trials.
Systemic hypertension	The following recommendation has been made to manage cerebral vasospasm and delayed cerebral ischemia: Unless the baseline systemic blood pressure is elevated or the patient's cardiac status prohibits induction of systemic hypertension, induction of systemic blood pressure is recommended in patient with delayed cerebral ischemia.	Class I: Benefit much greater than risk. Level B evidence: Evidence based on limited patient populations, utilizing one randomized trial or more than one nonrandomized trials.

Continued

TABLE 21-10 **AHA/ASA Guidelines for Hemodynamic and Intracranial Parameters in the Management of Spontaneous Aneurysmal Subarachnoid Hemorrhage (aSAH)—cont'd**

PARAMETER		CLASSIFICATION OF RECOMMENDATION AND LEVEL OF EVIDENCE
Intracranial pressure	The following recommendation has been made to manage hydrocephalus associated with aSAH: An external ventricular drain or lumbar drain (depending on intracranial pressure and risk of herniation) should be used to manage aSAH associated with acute aSAH hydrocephalus.	Class I: Benefit much greater than risk. Level B evidence: Evidence based on limited patient populations, utilizing one randomized trial or more than one nonrandomized trials.
Intracranial pressure	The need for permanent CSF diversion (ventricular shunt) is not decreased by weaning the external ventricular drain over 24 hours.	Class III: No benefit and possibly harmful. Level B evidence: Evidence based on limited patient populations, utilizing one randomized trial or more than one nonrandomized trials.
Intravascular volume	The following recommendation has been made regarding management of aSAH associated medical complications: Fluid restriction and use of large amounts of hypotonic fluids are not recommended in the management of aSAH.	Class III: No benefit and possibly harmful. Level B evidence: Evidence based on limited patient populations, utilizing one randomized trial or more than one nonrandomized trials.
Intravascular volume, central venous pressure, pulmonary occlusive wedge pressure, and fluid balance	The following recommendations have been made regarding management of aSAH associated medical complications: Intravascular volume status may be monitored utilizing central venous pressure, pulmonary artery occlusive wedge pressure parameters and fluid balance and intravascular volume depletion may be treated with crystalloid or colloid.	Class IIa: Benefit greater than risk. Level B evidence: Evidence based on limited patient populations, utilizing one randomized trial or more than one nonrandomized trials.
Blood transfusion	The following recommendation has been made regarding management of aSAH associated medical complications: Aneurysmal SAH patient with anemia and at risk for delayed cerebral ischemia may reasonably be treated with packed red blood cells. The optimal hemoglobin is not currently known.	Class IIb: Benefit greater than risk. Level B evidence: Evidence based on limited patient populations, utilizing one randomized trial or more than one nonrandomized trials.

the primary focus may well be blood pressure management. The AHA/ASA *Guidelines for the Early Management of Acute Ischemic Stroke* have liberalized blood pressure guidelines to minimize risk of secondary ischemia from attempts to normalize and excessively lower the blood pressure.[41] Many patients with acute ischemic stroke are hypertensive prior to their stroke, and consequently their cerebral autoregulation shifts to the right, because of the need for a higher blood pressure compared with the normotensive patient to perfuse the brain.[97,98] Blood pressure parameters for individuals not eligible for thrombolytic therapy include a systolic pressure less than 220 mm Hg and a diastolic pressure less than 120 mm Hg.

Thrombolytic candidates pre-tPA (tissue plasminogen activator) administration require a systolic pressure less than 185 mm Hg and/or a diastolic pressure of less than 110 mm Hg.[41,98] Following tPA administration, systolic blood pressure must be maintained at less than 180 mm Hg and diastolic pressure at less than 105 mm Hg.[41,98] An arterial catheter is not recommended if thrombolytics are to be administered because of the risk of hemorrhage at the insertion site. Some clinicians prefer a manual blood pressure cuff rather than an automatic one to minimize trauma from the blood pressure cuff inflation during and after tPA administration (see Table 21-6).

A few patients with acute ischemic stroke may require critical care monitoring for hypotension. If fluid boluses are not successful in raising the systolic blood pressure, or the patient cannot tolerate fluid boluses because of other medical conditions, a vasopressor may be required. As with severe TBI and aSAH, phenylephrine, an alpha-1 agonist, is most often the vasopressor of choice. The cerebral blood vessels have fewer alpha-1 receptors compared with the peripheral blood vessels, and the peripheral blood vessels will constrict effectively to propel blood toward the cerebral circulation without compromising cerebral blood flow.[98] As with other catastrophic neurologic injuries, most patients with acute ischemic stroke only require additional hemodynamic monitoring when other comorbidities are present.

Spontaneous Intracerebral Hemorrhage

Blood pressure, and CPP (MAP minus ICP) are the major parameters of concern in spontaneous ICH. Avoiding an increase in the size of the hemorrhage yet maintaining adequate CPP is the goal. The AHA/ASA *Guidelines for the Management of Spontaneous Intracerebral Hemorrhage* state that lowering systolic blood pressure to 140 mm Hg is probably not too low (Class IIa of III recommendation)[40] (see Table 21-5). Although not a recommendation, systolic blood pressure is also discussed in the guideline with regard to patients with ICH with elevated ICP. In those instances, the goal is a CPP above 60 mm Hg. If the systemic blood pressure and ICP are elevated, a MAP of 110 mm Hg or systolic and diastolic blood pressure of 160/90 are the goal parameters.[40] Best blood pressure management in spontaneous ICH remains controversial and has not been definitively determined.[99] Surgical removal of the hemorrhage, particularly if the hemorrhage is deep, may not be possible or has not been shown to improve outcome. A ventriculostomy catheter with external drain (EVD) may be useful to remove intraventricular blood and control and monitor ICP.[40]

Case Study

A 56-year-old female presents to the Emergency Department with the worst headache of her life. A noncontrast CT of the head shows extensive SAH, classified as a Hunt-Hess Grade 3 of 5. She is somnolent, confused, with medium focal deficits and a Fisher Grade III of IV with a dense collection of blood (>1 mm thick in the vertical plane or 5×3 mm in the longitudinal or transverse dimension).

Hunt-Hess Classification of Subarachnoid Hemorrhage

GRADE	CLINICAL DESCRIPTION
0	Unruptured
1	Asymptomatic or mild headache and slight nuchal rigidity
2	Moderate to severe headache, nuchal rigidity, no neurologic deficit other than cranial nerve palsy
3	Mild focal deficit, lethargy, confusion
4	Stupor, hemiparesis
5	Coma, extensor rigidity

From LeRoux PD, Winn HR, Newell DW: *Management of cerebral aneurysms*, Philadelphia, 2004, Saunders.

Fisher Subarachnoid Hemorrhage Grade

GRADE	CLINICAL DESCRIPTION
Grade I	No detectable blood on CT
Grade II	Diffuse thin subarachnoid hemorrhage on CT. Vertical layers <1 mm thick
Grade III	Local clot or thick subarachnoid hemorrhage. Vertical layers >1 mm thick
Grade IV	Intracerebral or intraventricular blood

From Le Roux PD, Winn HR, Newell, DW: *Management of cerebral aneurysms*, Philadelphia, 2004, Saunders.

Case Study—cont'd

On cerebral angiography, two anterior communicating aneurysms (ACoA) are seen, one has ruptured.

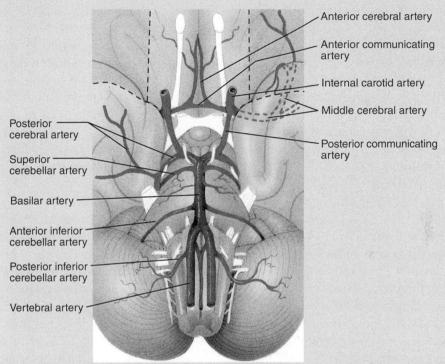

(Image from Lundy-Ekman L: *Neuroscience: fundamentals for rehabilitation*, ed 4, St. Louis, 2013, Elsevier.)

On routine ECG, ST segment depression is noted in V3-V5 leads. A rise in serum troponin is noted as well. The patient is intubated and is placed on FiO_2 of 0.40 (40%). The CVP is 14 mm Hg. Her systolic blood pressure is 150 mm Hg. A continuous infusion of nicardipine (Cardene) is started to achieve a systolic goal of less than 120 mm Hg to decrease the risk of aneurysmal rebleeding.

On day 1, the ruptured ACoA is coiled in interventional neuroradiology; the second aneurysm at the Anterior communicating artery (ACoA) cannot be coiled. A baseline transcranial Doppler (TCD) is obtained; mean flow velocities are within normal limits. Computed tomography perfusion (CTP) scan reveals decreased perfusion in the right frontal and temporal lobes. Troponin peaks around 7.04. During the day, the patient has decreased movement of her left lower extremity.

On day 2, an aneurysm clip is placed on the second ACoA aneurysm in surgery. She remains mechanically ventilated after surgery. Her CVP is stable at 8 mm Hg.

On day 3, the patient's FiO_2 requirements increase to 0.50. Her troponin has decreased to normal at this time. TCD shows severe vasospasm of the basilar artery and moderate

Continued

Case Study—cont'd

vasospasm of the right middle cerebral artery (MCA) and right internal carotid artery (ICA). The patient stops following commands. Triple H (HHH) therapy goals are set at a systolic blood pressure 160 to 180 mm Hg, CVP 8 to 10 mm Hg, and total hourly intravenous fluids at 200 mL/hr. Norepinephrine is started to increase the systemic blood pressure. The patient's CVP is now 9 mm Hg. The patient is taken to interventional neuroradiology for angioplasty of the vasospastic vessels. However, the neuroradiology interventionalist is unable to reach the distal vasospastic branches with the angioplasty catheter. Nicardipine (Cardene) is administered through the catheter to vasodilate the distal branches.

On day 4, the patient's blood pressure remains below goal (160–180 mm Hg) on norepinephrine. Phenylephrine is added, but no improvement is seen. Dopamine and dobutamine are trialed, but the addition of these agents increases the heart rate, so they are discontinued. The patient's highest achievable systolic blood pressure is 100 to 110 mm Hg. Her SpO_2 is 80%. The patient stops moving her left side. Oxygen requirements are now FiO_2 1.0 (100%) with a positive end-expiratory pressure (PEEP) of 15 centimeters of water (cm H_2O). Chest radiography reveals bilateral opacities. Transthoracic echocardiography shows an ejection fraction of 21% and severe cardiac wall abnormalities, termed "cardiomyopathy." A bronchoscopy is attempted but aborted with a fall in systolic blood pressure to 60 mm Hg each time. Pulse pressure variation (PPV) and stroke volume variation (SVV) are obtained with the LiDCO. Both values are less than 10%, indicating that the patient is not fluid responsive. The LiDCO is then calibrated, using the patient's arterial catheter to obtain a cardiac index of 2.7 L/min/m^2 and systemic vascular resistance (SVR) of 1400 dynes·sec/cm^5. The best obtainable systolic blood pressure is 150 mm Hg. The patient is continued on norepinephrine and phenylephrine. A cardiology consult is obtained, and intra-aortic balloon pump (IABP) is considered but held because the patient's neurologic status has improved. She is moving her left side again.

On day 5, the patient has numerous episodes of tachycardia up to 200 beats per minute, interpreted as atrial fibrillation or multifocal atrial tachycardia. The rhythm is unresponsive to adenosine but responds to cardioversion (100 joules). However, the patient requires five cardioversions that day. She is started on an infusion of amiodarone (Cordarone) and remains on norepinephrine and phenylephrine. Her highest achievable systolic blood pressure is 140 mm Hg. A pulmonary artery catheter is inserted. PAOP is 30 mm Hg; CVP 16 to 18 mm Hg; CI 1.8 L/min/m^2; SVR 1800 dynes·sec/cm^5; and SvO_2 48%. In addition, the patient's brain natriuretic peptide (BNP) is 1200 nanograms per milliliter (ng/mL). The dilemma is that the patient needs afterload reduction and inotropic support but also needs phenylephrine and norepinephrine to raise her blood pressure to combat the cerebral vasospasm. Milrinone (Primacor) is started to support her failing heart. The goal systolic blood pressure is greater than 140 mm Hg. Prostacyclin (Flolan) is administered for pulmonary

Case Study—cont'd

hypertension and pulmonary edema. The patient is diagnosed with takotsubo cardiomyopathy, which has been associated with aSAH (see Figure 21-11).

On day 6, the milrinone dose is increased, and the patient is eventually weaned off amiodarone. PAOP decreases to 24 mm Hg; CVP decreases to 14 mm Hg; SVR decreases to 1400 dynes·sec/cm^5; and SvO_2 increases to 55%.

On day 7, TCD right MCA and ICA mean flow velocity (MFV) remain high but are improving. Neurologically, the patient is noted to move her left extremities with increased strength.

Over days 7 to 11, her CVP, PAOP, cardiac index, and SVR continue to trend toward normal.

By day 12, the patient's TCDs are normal, and her deficits are primarily some left-sided weakness and left neglect. However, she is able to follow commands and is eventually weaned off all vasoactive agents and mechanical ventilation. Following some days in acute care, the patient is discharged to rehabilitation, where her left-sided weakness and perceptual deficits are the focus for her rehabilitation. ∎

Clinical Reasoning Pearl

- Changes in neurologic assessment should be investigated regardless of the data obtained from the monitoring devices. There is no substitute for a well-performed neurological assessment.

- Intracranial monitoring equipment is one aspect of neurologic monitoring. The information obtained from bedside monitoring equipment and from clinical assessment must be integrated to provide the best possible care.

- Brain injury impacts the entire body just as other illnesses may impact the brain. Attention to other systems is paramount to providing optimal care to the brain. Failure to provide optimal care to other systems will negatively impact the brain.

- Across all neurologic illnesses and injuries, management of systemic blood pressure remains among the most important factors. Blood pressure parameters must be maintained and the provider notified immediately when blood pressure parameters are above or below those prescribed.

- For some patients with unstable intracranial dynamics, routine awakening to perform a neurologic assessment may be more harmful than not awakening the patient if quality multimodality monitoring is in place.

Conclusion

Care of the critically ill neuroscience patient requires knowledge and skill in both hemodynamics and intracranial dynamics. The critical care nurse must know (1) key physiologic concepts; (2) measurement methods and the technology available to obtain those measurements; and (3) current best practice in caring for this complex patient population. Familiarity with evidence-based guidelines from such organizations as the Brain Trauma Foundation, AHA/ASA, the Neurocritical Care Society, American Association of Critical Care Nurses, and the American Association of Neuroscience Nurses can provide support in clinical decision making. Finally, the obvious need for additional collaborative research in hemodynamics and intracranial dynamics is a call for all nurses to use their knowledge and skills to participate in research and further the science in the care of the critically ill neuroscience patient.

References

1. Rosengart MR: Critical care medicine: landmarks and legends, *Surg Clin North Am* 86:1305–1321, 2006.
2. Feyen BF, Sener S, Jorens PG, et al.: Neuromonitoring in traumatic brain injury, *Minerva Anestesiol* 78(8):949–958, 2012.
3. Padayachy LC, Figaju AA, Bullock MR: Intracranial pressure monitoring for traumatic brain injury in the modern era, *Childs Nerv Syst* 26:441–452, 2010.
4. Wartenberg KE, Schmidt JM, Mayer SA: Multimodality monitoring in neurocritical care, *Crit Care Clin* 23:507–538, 2007.
5. March K: Intracranial pressure concepts, cerebral blood flow, and metabolism. In Bader MK, Littlejohns LR, editors: *AANN core curriculum for neuroscience nursing*, 5 ed., Glenview, IL, 2010, American Association of Neuroscience Nursing, pp 79–86.
6. Bershad EM, Humphries WE, Suarez JI: Intracranial hypertension, *Semin Neurol* 28:690–702, 2008.
7. Czosnyka M, Smielewski P, Timofeev I, et al.: Intracranial pressure: more than a number, *Neurosurg Focus* 22(5):E10, 2007.
8. Coles JP, Fryer TD, Coleman MR, et al.: Hyperventilation following head injury: effect on ischemic burden and cerebral oxidative metabolism, *Crit Care Med* 35(2):568–578, 2007.
9. Oertel M, Kelly DF, Lee JN: Efficacy of hyperventilation, blood pressure elevation, and metabolic suppression therapy in controlling intracranial pressure after head injury, *J Neurosurg* 97(5):1045–1053, 2002.
10. Hemphill JC, Andrews P, De Georgia M: Multimodal monitoring and neurocritical care bioinformatics, *Nat Rev Neurol* 7:451–460, 2011.
11. Bratton SL, Chesnut RM, Ghajar J, et al.: Cerebral perfusion thresholds. In The Brain Trauma Foundation's Guidelines for the management of severe traumatic brain injury, ed 3, *J Neurotrauma* 24(Suppl 1):S59–S64, 2007.
12. Howells T, Elf K, Jones PA, et al.: Pressure reactivity as a guide in the treatment of cerebral perfusion pressure in patients with brain trauma, *J Neurosurg* 102:311–317, 2005.
13. Andrews PJD: Cerebral perfusion pressure and brain ischaemia: can one size fit all? *Crit Care* 9 (6):638–639, 2008.
14. Kirkness CJ: Cerebral blood flow monitoring in clinical practice, *AACN Clin Issues* 16 (4):476–487, 2005.

15. Philip S, Udomphorn Y, Kirkham FJ, Vavilala MS: Cerebrovascular pathophysiology in pediatric traumatic brain injury, *J Trauma* 67:S128–S134, 2009.

16. Vivilala M, Lam A: Cerebral blood flow and vascular physiology, *Anesthesiol Clin North America* 20:247–264, 2002.

17. Paulsen OB, Strandgaard S, Devinsson L: Cerebral autoregulation, *Cerebrovasc Brain Metab Rev* 2:161–191, 1990.

18. Vergouwen MDI: The Participants in the International Multi-disciplinary Consensus Conference on the Critical Care Management of Subarachnoid Hemorrhage. Vasospasm versus delayed cerebral ischemia as an outcome event in clinical trials and observational studies, *Neurocrit Care* 15:308–311, 2011.

19. Wartenberg KE: Critical care of poor-grade subarachnoid hemorrhage, *Curr Opin Crit Care* 17:85–93, 2011.

20. Rabenstein AA, Friedman JA, Weigand SD, et al.: Predictors of cerebral infarction in aneurysmal subarachnoid hemorrhage, *Stroke* 35:1862–1866, 2004.

21. Fergusen S, Macdonald RL: Predictors of cerebral infarction in patients with aneurysmal subarachnoid hemorrhage, *Neurosurgery* 60:658–667, 2007.

22. Vergouwen MDI, Ilodigwe D, Macdonald RL: Cerebral infarction after subarachnoid hemorrhage contributes to poor outcome by vasospasm-dependent and -independent effects, *Stroke* 42:942–949, 2011.

23. Baumann A, Audibert G, McDonnell J, Mertes PM: Neurogenic pulmonary edema, *Acta Anaesthesiol Scand* 51:447–455, 2007.

24. Muroi C, Keller M, Pangalu A, et al.: Neurogenic pulmonary edema in patients with subarachnoid hemorrhage, *J Neurosurg Anesthesiol* 20(3):188–192, 2008.

25. Sedy J, Zicha J, Junes J, et al.: Mechanisms of neurogenic pulmonary edema development, *Physiol Res* 57:499–506, 2008.

26. Gahart BL, Nazareno AR: *Dobutamine hydrochloride 2014 Intravenous Medications,* ed 30, St. Louis, MO, 2014, Mosby.

27. Nguyen H, Zaroff JG: Neurogenic stunned myocardium, *Curr Neurol Neurosci Rep* 8:486–491, 2009.

28. Lee VH, Oh JK, Mulvagh SL, Wijdicks EF: Mechanism in neurogenic stress cardiomyopathy after aneurysmal subarachnoid hemorrhage, *Neurocrit Care* 5:243–249, 2006.

29. Bratton SL, Chesnut RM, Ghajar J, et al.: Intracranial pressure monitoring technology. Guidelines for the management of severe traumatic brain injury, ed 3, *J Neurotrauma* 24(Suppl 1):S45–S54, 2007.

30. Hebl JR: The importance and implications of aseptic techniques during regional anesthesia, *Reg Anesth Pain Med* 31:311–323, 2006.

31. Bratton SL, Chesnut RM, Ghajar J, et al.: Indications for intracranial pressure monitoring. Guidelines for the management of severe traumatic brain injury, 3rd ed, *J Neurotrauma* 24(Suppl 1):S37–S44, 2007.

32. Farahvar A, Huang JH, Papdakos PJ: Intracranial monitoring in traumatic brain injury, *Curr Opin Anesthesiol* 24:209–213, 2011.

33. Leeper B, Lovasik D: Cerebrospinal drainage systems: external ventricular and lumbar drains. In *AACN-AANN protocols for practice: monitoring technologies in critically ill neuroscience patients,* Boston, MA, 2011, Jones and Bartlett, pp 71–101.

34. Connolly ES, Rabinstein AA, Carhuapoma JR, et al.: Guidelines for the management of aneurysmal subarachnoid hemorrhage: a guideline for healthcare professionals from the American Heart Association/American Stroke Association, *Stroke* 43(6):1711–1737, 2012.

35. Diringer MN, Bleck TP, Hemphill JC, et al.: Critical care management of patients following aneurysmal subarachnoid hemorrhage: recommendations from the Neurocritical Care Society's multidisciplinary consensus conference, *Neurocrit Care* 15:211–240, 2011.

36. Slazinski T, Anderson TA, Cattell E, et al.: *Care of the patient undergoing intracranial pressure monitoring/external ventricular drainage or lumbar drainage,* Glenview, IL, 2011, American Association of Neuroscience Nurses, AANN clinical practice guidelines series.

37. Wartenberg KE, Schmidt JM, Mayer SA: Multimodality monitoring in neurocritical care, *Crit Care Clin* 23:507–538, 2007.

38. Lavinio A, Menon DK: Intracranial pressure: why we monitor it, how we monitor it, what we do with the number and what's the future? *Curr Opin Anesthesiol* 24:117–123, 2011.

39. March K, Madden L: Intracranial pressure management. In *AACN-AANN protocols for practice: monitoring technologies in critically ill neuroscience patients,* Boston, MA, 2011, Jones and Bartlett, pp 35–69.

40. Morgenstern LB, Hemphill JC, Anderson C, et al.: Guidelines for the management of spontaneous intracerebral hemorrhage: a guideline for healthcare professionals from the American Heart Association/American Stroke Association, *Stroke* 41:2108–2129, 2010.

41. Jauch EC, Saver JL, Adams HP, et al.: Guidelines for the early management of patients with acute ischemic stroke: a guideline for healthcare professionals from the American Heart Association/American Stroke Association, *Stroke* 44(3):870–937, 2013.

42. Le Roux P: Physiological monitoring of the severe traumatic brain injury patient in the intensive care unit, *Curr Neurol Neurosci Rep* 13(3):331, 2013.

43. Jones HA: Arterial transducer placement and cerebral perfusion pressure monitoring: a discussion, *Nurs Crit Care* 14(6):303–310, 2009.

44. Barazangi N, Hemphill JC: Advanced cerebral monitoring in neurocritical care, *Neurol India* 56(4):405–414, 2008.

45. Tanaka R, Yumoto T, Shiba N, et al.: Overheated and melted intracranial pressure transducer as cause of thermal brain injury during magnetic resonance image, *J Neurosurg* 117(6):1100–1109, 2012.

46. Rosenthal G, Hemphill JC, Sorani M, et al.: Brain tissue oxygen tension is more indicative of oxygen diffusion than oxygen delivery and metabolism in patients with traumatic brain injury, *Crit Care Med* 36(6):1917–1924, 2008.

47. Rao GSU, Durga P: Changing trends in monitoring brain ischemia: from intracranial pressure to cerebral oximetry, *Curr Opin Anesthesiol* 24:487–494, 2011.

48. Blissitt PA: Brain oxygen monitoring. In *AACN-AANN protocols for practice: monitoring technologies in critically ill neuroscience patients,* Boston, MA, 2011, Jones and Bartlett, pp 103–144.

49. Valadka AB, Gopinath SP, Contant CF, et al.: Relationship of brain tissue PO_2 to outcome after severe head injury, *Crit Care Med* 25(9):1576–1581, 1998.

50. Rose JC, Neill TA, Hemphill JC: Continuous monitoring of the microcirculation in neurocritical care: an update on brain tissue oxygenation, *Curr Opin Crit Care* 12:97–102, 2006.

51. Wijayatilake DS, Shepherd SJ, Sherren PB: Updates in the management of intracranial pressure in traumatic brain injury, *Curr Opin Anesthesiol* 25(5):540–547, 2012.

52. Schell RM, Cole DJ: Cerebral monitoring: jugular venous oximetry, *Anesth Analg* 90(3):559–566, 2000.

53. Bratton SL, Chesnut RM, Ghajar J, et al.: Brain oxygen monitoring and thresholds. Trauma Foundation's guidelines for the management of severe traumatic brain injury, ed 3, *J Neurotrauma* 24(Suppl 1):S65–S70, 2007.

54. Kirkman MA, Smith M: Multimodal intracranial monitoring: Implications for clinical practice, *Anesthesiol Clin* 30(2):269–287, 2012.

55. March KS, Olson D, Arbour R: Technology. In Bader MK, Littlejohns LR, editors: *AANN core curriculum for neuroscience nursing,* 5 ed., Glenview, IL, 2010, American Association of Neuroscience Nursing, pp 185–216.

56. Slazinski T: Jugular venous oxygen saturation monitoring: Insertion (assist), patient care, troubleshooting, and removal. In DJ Lynn-McHale Wiegand, editor: *AACN procedure manual for critical care*, 6 ed., Philadelphia, 2011, Elsevier, pp 816–821.

57. Edwards LifeSciences: *MRI compatibility of 4 French fiberoptic catheter*, Personal Communication (Letter) Irvine, CA, 2009, Edwards LifeSciences.

58. Steiner LA, Andrews PJD: Monitoring the injured brain: ICP and CBF, *Br J Anaesth* 97(1):26–38, 2006.

59. Oddo M, Filla F, Citerio G: Brain multimodality monitoring: an update, *Curr Opin Crit Care* 18 (2):111–118, 2012.

60. Springborg JB, Frederiksen HJ, Eskesen V, Olsen NV: Trends in monitoring patients with aneurysmal subarachnoid hemorrhage, *Br J Anaesth* 94(3):259–270, 2005.

61. Ghosh A, Elwell C, Smith M: Cerebral near-infrared spectroscopy in adults: a work in progress, *Anesth Analg* 115(6):1373–1383, 2012.

62. Kirkness C: Cerebral blood flow monitoring. In *AACN-AANN protocols for practice: monitoring technologies in critically ill neuroscience patients*, Boston, MA, 2011, Jones and Bartlett, pp 145–174.

63. Kassah MY, Majid A, Farooq Fu, et al.: Transcranial Doppler: an introduction for the primary care physician, *J Am Board Fam Med* 20:65–71, 2007.

64. Mopphet IJ, Mahajan RP: Transcranial Doppler ultrasonography in anaesthesia and intensive care, *Br J Anaesth* 93:710–724, 2004.

65. Sloan MA, Alexandrov AV, Tegeler CH, et al.: Assessment: transcranial Doppler ultrasonography: report of the therapeutics and Technology Assessment Subcommittee of the American Academy of Neurology, *Neurology* 62(9):1468–1481, 2004.

66. Alexandrov AW: Transcranial Doppler. In DJ Lynn-McHale Wiegand, editor: *AACN procedure manual for critical care*, ed 6, St. Louis, MO, 2010, Saunders, pp 849–860.

67. Nicoletto H: Transcranial Doppler series part II: performing a transcranial Doppler, *Am J Electroneurodiagnostic Technol* 49(1):14–27, 2009.

68. Eftekhar B, Dadmehr M, Ansari S, et al.: Are the distributions of variations of circle of Willis different in different populations? Results of an anatomical study and review of the literature, *BMC Neurol* 6:22, 2006.

69. White H, Venkatesh B: Applications of transcranial Doppler in the ICU: a review, *Intensive Care Med* 32(7):981–994, 2006.

70. Smith M: Perioperative uses of transcranial perfusion monitoring, *Anesthesiol Clin* 25:557–577, 2007.

71. Jaeger M, Soehle M, Schuhmann MU, et al.: Correlation of continuously monitored regional cerebral blood flow and brain tissue oxygen, *Acta Neurochir (Wien)* 56:147–151, 2005.

72. Bhatia J, Gupta AK: Neuromonitoring in the intensive care unit. I. Intracranial pressure and cerebral blood flow monitoring, *Intensive Care Med* 33:1263–1271, 2007.

73. Hemedex Inc.: *Bowman Perfusion Monitor (BPM) Neuromonitoring guide*. http://www.promedics.de/Downloads/HEMEDEX/BPM%20Neuromonitoring%20Guide%20rel%205%2011.pdf. Accessed November 22, 2014.

74. Tisdall MM, Smith M: Cerebral microdialysis: research technique or clinical tool, *Br J Anaesth* 97:18–25, 2006.

75. Polderman KH, Herold I: Therapeutic hypothermia and controlled normothermia in the intensive care unit: practical considerations, side effects, and cooling methods, *Crit Care Med* 37 (3):1101–1120, 2009.

76. Mamood MA, Zwiefler RM: Progress in shivering control, *J Neurol Sci* 261:47–54, 2007.

77. Kuo J-R, Lo C-J, Wang CC, et al.: Measuring brain temperature while maintaining brain normothermia in patients with severe traumatic brain injury, *J Clin Neurosci* 18(8):1059–1063, 2011.

78. Donald MJ, Paterson B: End tidal carbon dioxide monitoring in prehospital and retrieval medicine: a review, *Emerg Med J* 23:728–730, 2006.

79. Kim S, McNames J, Goldstein B: Intracranial pressure variation associated with changes in end-tidal CO_2, *Conf Proc IEEE Eng Med Biol Soc* 1:9–12, 2006.

80. Wilson SF, Amling JK, Floyd SD, McNair ND: Determining interrater reliability of nurses' assessments of pupillary size and reaction, *J Neurosci Nurs* 20(3):189–192, 1988.

81. Chen JW, Gombart ZJ, Rogers S, et al.: Pupillary reactivity as an early indicator of increased intracranial pressure: the introduction of the Neurological Pupil Index, *Surg Neurol Int* 2:82, 2011.

82. Fountas KN, Kapsalaki EZ, Machinis TG, et al.: Clinical implications of quantitative infrared pupillometry in neurosurgical patients, *Neurocrit Care* 5:55–60, 2006.

83. Bratton SL, Chesnut RM, Ghajar J, et al.: Blood pressure and oxygenation. In the Brain Trauma Foundation's guidelines for the management of severe traumatic brain injury, ed 3, *J Neurotrauma* 24(Suppl 1):S7–S13, 2007.

84. Lazaridis C: Advanced hemodynamic monitoring: principles and practice in neurocritical care, *Neurocrit Care* 16(1):163–169, 2012.

85. Chesnut RM: Care of the central nervous system injuries, *Surg Clin North Am* 87(1):119–156, 2007.

86. Sookplung P, Siriussawakul A, Malakouti A, et al.: Vasopressor use and effect on blood pressure after severe adult traumatic brain injury, *Neurocrit Care* 15(1):46–54, 2011.

87. Wartenberg KH: Critical care of poor-grade subarachnoid hemorrhage, *Curr Opin Crit Care* 17(2):85–93, 2011.

88. Stead LG, Bellolio F, Gilmore RM, et al.: Pharmacologic elevation of blood pressure in acute brain ischemia, *Neurocrit Care* 8(2):259–261, 2008.

89. Sydenham E, Roberts I, Alderson P: Hypothermia for traumatic brain injury (Review), *Cochrane Database Syst Rev* (3):2, 2009. Art No: CD001048, http://dx.doi.org/10.1002/14651858.CD001048.pub-4.

90. Muench E, Horn P, Bauhuf C, et al.: Effects of hypervolemia and hypertension on regional cerebral blood flow, intracranial pressure, and brain tissue oxygenation after subarachnoid hemorrhage, *Crit Care Med* 35(8):1844–1851, 2007.

91. Hoff RG, van Dijk GW, Algra A, et al.: Fluid balance and blood volume measurement after aneurysmal subarachnoid hemorrhage, *Neurocrit Care* 8:391–397, 2008.

92. Treggiari MM, Deem S: Which H is the most important in triple-H therapy for cerebral vasospasm? *Curr Opin Crit Care* 15:83–86, 2009.

93. Dankbaar JW, Slooter AJC, Rinkel GJE, van der Schaaf IC: Effect of different components of triple-H therapy on cerebral perfusion in patients with aneurysmal subarachnoid hemorrhage: a systematic review, *Crit Care* 14:R23, 2010.

94. Martini RP, Deem S, Brown M, et al.: The association between fluid balance and outcomes after subarachnoid hemorrhage, *Neurocrit Care* 17(2):191–198, 2012.

95. Gress DR: The participants in the International Multi-disciplinary Consensus Conference on the Critical Care Management of Subarachnoid Hemorrhage, *Neurocrit Care* 15(2):270–274, 2011.

96. Mutoh T, Kazaumata K, Ishikawa T, Terasaka S: Performance of bedside transpulmonary thermodilution monitoring for goal-directed hemodynamic management after subarachnoid hemorrhage, *Stroke* 40:2368–2374, 2009.

97. Stead LG, Bellolio F, Gilmore RM, et al.: Pharmacologic elevation of blood pressure for acute brain ischemia, *Neurocrit Care* 8:259–261, 2008.

98. Owens WB: Blood pressure control in acute cerebrovascular disease, *J Clin Hypertens* 13(3):205–211, 2011.

99. Elliott J, Smith M: The acute management of intracerebral hemorrhage, *Anesth Analg* 110:1419–1427, 2010.

Goal-Directed Hemodynamics

22

Barbara McLean

Despite improvements in resuscitation and supportive care, progressive organ dysfunction occurs in a large proportion of patients with acute, life-threatening illnesses and those undergoing major surgery. It has been proposed that the multi-organ dysfunction syndrome of the critically ill is a consequence of tissue hypoxia due to inadequate oxygen delivery, often exacerbated by a microcirculatory injury, increased tissue metabolic demands, and shock.

Shock is a potentially reversible life-threatening physiologic state characterized by end-organ dysfunction resulting from an imbalance in oxygen delivery (DO_2) and tissue demand (VO_2). Independent of its etiology, untreated shock precipitates a cascade of pro-inflammatory mediators causing cellular damage. Once circulatory shock has resulted in inadequate tissue perfusion manifesting as hyperlactatemia and metabolic acidosis, end-organ dysfunction and injury are already occurring.

Heart

A low cardiac output is seen in hypovolemic shock, cardiogenic shock, and obstructive shock (Figure 22-1).

Volume

Guidelines for administration of fluid are often based on static hemodynamic targets such as central venous pressure (CVP), and delayed volume status indexes such as blood pressure, heart rate, capillary refill, and urine output. Traditional fluid management protocols also rely on estimates of fluid deficit, intravascular fluid volume status, fluid loss, and basal fluid requirements to guide perioperative fluid administration. Recent advances in hemodynamic monitoring have produced sophisticated dynamic measures of volume status such as stroke volume variation (SVV) and pulse pressure variation (PPV), which may serve as functional indexes for fluid administration.[1] Volume administration is a concern in the perioperative environment because a limited cardiopulmonary reserve is a major risk factor for increased morbidity and mortality, when patients cannot meet the increased oxygen demand incurred during major surgery (Figure 22-1).

Vascular Tone

Bedside assessments of cardiorespiratory status and evolving systemic processes such as sepsis, acute lung injury, and hemorrhage are always masked by the body's own compensatory mechanisms until the pathology is so advanced that the patient decompensates. There are multiple processes that are activated, depending on the clinical cause: hemorrhage, associated with a low cardiac output and impaired cardiovascular reserve; ischemic cardiomyopathy associated with cardiac pump failure; and pulmonary hypertension associated with pulmonary obstruction. All are associated with increased sympathetic tone, increased vasoconstriction, and tachycardia. Vasodilated states such as sepsis and spinal shock also increase sympathetic tone, causing tachycardia, although sympathetic output is insufficient to overcome the dilated peripheral vasculature.[2]

The literature on the role of hemodynamic monitoring in improving outcomes for critically ill medical and surgical patients provides two constant suggestions: (1) implementation of treatment protocols with specific hemodynamic targets and early initiation of resuscitation, before significant oxygen debt is incurred, and (2) application of treatment protocols as early as possible in the disease process. The target goals should have multiple endpoints that, together, ensure tissue perfusion (Figure 22-1). Avoid the use of a single static endpoint.

Goal-Directed Therapy

Goal-directed therapy is a term generally used to predefine resuscitation endpoints, which guide the use of inotropic, volume, and vasopressor therapies. Historically, goals have

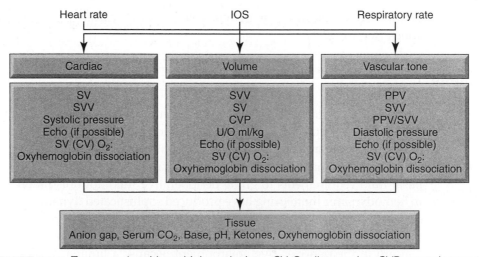

FIGURE 22-1 Target goals with multiple endpoints. *CV,* Cardiovascular; *CVP,* central venous pressure; *IOS,* index of suspicion; *PPV,* pulse pressure variation; *SV,* stroke volume; *SVV,* stroke volume variation; *U/O,* urine output.

been driven by mean arterial pressure (MAP), urine output, and central venous pressure (CVP) or pulmonary arterial occlusion (wedge) pressure (PAOP). Fluid therapy is considered the first step in the resuscitation of most patients with hypotension and shock. Uncorrected hypovolemia, leading to inappropriate infusions of vasopressor agents, may increase organ hypoperfusion and ischemia. However, overzealous fluid resuscitation has been associated with increased complications, increased length of stay in the critical care unit in the hospital, and increased mortality.[3–5]

Hemodynamic measures are frequently based on the components of cardiac output (heart rate and stroke volume) as well as the balance of oxygen delivery and consumption. Dynamic changes in pulse pressure, stroke volume, or plethysmographic variability index (PVI) to assess perfusion, together with echocardiographic assessment of left ventricular (LV) function and size, provide useful information for assessing preload and preload responsiveness; however, these techniques do not allow for the detection and quantification of fluid excess or deficit.

CVP and PAOP are poor measures of volume status and cannot be used reliably to detect volume overload.[6] Radiographic and clinical signs of pulmonary edema are also late signs of volume overload and provide a poor endpoint for fluid resuscitation.

Without a doubt, having a goal, which directs daily practice and intervention, is reasonable, but identifying the specific components of that goal remains controversial.[7] The target endpoints should afford protection of the mitochondria, perfusion of the cells, and modulation of organ dysfunction.

Historical Milestones

In 2001, Rivers and colleagues redefined the focus of resuscitation for patients with septic shock. They demonstrated that early, target-focused interventions reduced mortality in sepsis.[8] The 2001 study was critiqued for its single-center design and for the use of a specialized catheter to measure saturation of central venous oxygen (ScvO$_2$). In addition, there was significant concern regarding the learning curve required for monitoring central venous oxygen in the emergency department.

In recent years, the terms *early* and *goal-directed* have been applied to the care of the perioperative patient,[9,10] the patient with pancreatitis, survivors of cardiac arrest, patients with sepsis, and those with brain injury. However, the lack of consensus regarding early endpoint definitions continues to be problematic.[11]

Shock and Oxygen Delivery

All types of shock develop along a continuum. A simple continuum merely displays the difference between "early" (compensated) and "late" (decompensated) shock. This continuum underscores the concept well known to those in trauma as the "golden hour." Compensated shock may be veiled while the internal compensatory mechanisms sustain blood pressure, and support the circulating volume and metabolism via a series of neuroendocrine events. The golden hour of shock is based on appropriate evaluation and intervention before the oxygen debt is too large to be repaid. Patients with limited cardiopulmonary reserve are at particular risk of mortality and morbidity.

Early augmentation of the oxygen delivery index (DO_2I) with intravenous fluids and inotropes, also known as early goal-directed therapy (EGDT) has been shown to reduce postoperative mortality and morbidity in high-risk patients. Concerns regarding cardiopulmonary complications associated with fluid challenges and inotropes may deter clinicians from using goal-directed therapy interventions. Normal ranges that may be used as target values are listed in Table 22-1.

Of the various forms of circulatory shock, three distinct groups can be defined. Group 1 exhibits low stroke volume, or an inadequate cardiac output based on tissue demand, which profoundly impacts arterial oxygen delivery (DaO_2) and mixed venous oxygenation (SvO_2). Low stroke volume is a hallmark sign of hypovolemic, cardiogenic, and obstructive shock.

TABLE 22-1   Early Goal-Directed Therapy Target Values

PARAMETER	NORMAL	MEASURES	SIGNIFICANCE OF ABNORMAL VALUES
Cardiac output	4.0–8.0 L/min	Cardiac output measures volume of blood pumped by the left ventricle in 1 min	Indicator of volume status and left ventricular function. Most often used for goal-directed therapy in combination with measures of fluid-responsive hypovolemia such as stroke volume variation.
Cardiac index	2.5–4.0 L/min/m^2	Cardiac index is an individual measure of cardiac output normalized for body surface area (BSA)	• If cardiac index is decreased (↓) and SVV is ↑, fluid is administered to optimize cardiac index. • If cardiac index is decreased (↓) and SVV is ↓, positive inotropes are administered to optimize cardiac index.
Stroke volume	60–100 mL	Stroke volume measures volume of blood pumped by the left ventricle in one heartbeat.	Indicator of volume status and left ventricular function. Primary goal of many goal directed therapeutic strategies is to maximize stroke volume or stroke volume index by administering blood or crystalloid (depending on hematocrit concentration) until stroke volume or stroke volume index no longer increases by ≥10% in response to fluid therapy.
Stroke volume index	30–65 mL/beat/m^2	Stroke volume index is an individual measure of stroke volume normalized for BSA	

TABLE 22-1	Early Goal-Directed Therapy Target Values—cont'd		
PARAMETER	**NORMAL**	**MEASURES**	**SIGNIFICANCE OF ABNORMAL VALUES**
Stroke volume variation (SVV)	13%–15%	Variation in stroke volume during controlled positive pressure ventilation; calculated by various methods including esophageal Doppler monitoring measurements or pulse contour analysis of area beneath arterial waveform curve	Indicator of volume status; ↑ SVV indicates fluid-responsive hypovolemia.
Central venous oxygen saturation ($ScvO_2$)	65%–85%		An $ScvO_2$ value of 50% is considered critical, see Table 22-2.
Mixed venous oxygen saturation (SvO_2)	60%–80%		An SvO_2 value of 50% is considered critical, see Table 22-2.
Oxygen delivery Oxygen delivery index	DO_2: 1000 mL/min DO_2I: 500–600 mL/min/m^2	Calculated value that combines inputs. Cardiac output or cardiac index and content of oxygen (hemoglobin [saturation × 1.34]) to provide an individualized BSA-based indicator of oxygen delivery adequacy	Indicator of oxygen delivery; ↓ DO_2I indicates ↓ tissue perfusion. Most often used for goal-directed therapy in combination with those inputs that comprise it and with measures of fluid-responsive hypovolemia. • If, for example, DO_2I is ↓ and SVV is ↑, fluid is given to optimize DO_2I. • If DO_2I is↓ and SVV is ↓, inotropes or vasopressors are administered to optimize DO_2I. • If DO_2I remains ↓, hemoglobin is evaluated and optimized
Lactic acid	<1.5		Elevated values signify the failure of aerobic mechanisms or the ability to excrete lactate.

>, Greater than; <, less than; ↑, increased; ↓, decreased; *BSA*, body surface area.

Group 2 has difficulty maintaining vascular tone and may have inappropriate flow. Low blood flow affects tissue perfusion pressure and may increase shunting, which, in turn, impairs organ perfusion. Loss of vascular tone occurs in septic, anaphylactic, and neurogenic shock.

Group 3 is identified by a failure to utilize oxygen, despite adequate delivery, as seen in severe sepsis and septic shock, where metabolic cellular defects impair the uptake and utilization of oxygen.

The role of a protocol is to provide a roadmap for clinicians to respond early and appropriately. In group 1 shock, low stroke volume is the problem. The vascular tone is generally responsive to endogenous and exogenous stimulants, depressants, and hormones. If the global problem is corrected by intravenous fluid administration, improvement in myocardial function, or relief of the obstruction, the peripheral tissue consequences of prolonged inadequacy of global oxygen delivery may not develop.

In group 2 shock, the failure of sympathetic nervous system activation, or the local opposition of mediators, promotes a widespread vasodilation that requires exogenous alpha activation and possibly neuroendocrine support. If treatment is delayed or ineffective, shock progresses to an anaerobic state, and organ failure rapidly follows.

Group 3 is the late-stage group, where manipulation of the "global" or delivery components of oxygen alone will be ineffective. Prompt effective treatment of "early" shock or compensated shock, may prevent progression to "late" shock or decompensated shock and organ failure.

Volume Resuscitation Assessment

Debate exists as to the optimal method of assessing volume responsiveness. The EGDT algorithm, adopted by the Surviving Sepsis Campaign (see Figure 20-1 in Chapter 20), relies heavily on CVP, MAP, and ScvO$_2$ measurements. Other researchers have compared this algorithm against newer technologies to identify best patient outcomes.[12–15]

> ### Clinical Reasoning Pearl
>
> For assessment of acute volume responsiveness, a passive leg raise maneuver, combined with ultrasound assessment of vena cava collapsibility, or percentage of stroke volume variation (SVV) / pulse pressure variation (PPV), should be performed prior to volume loading.

Bouferrache and associates (2013) compared use of transesophageal echocardiography with the recommendations in the Surviving Sepsis Campaign guidelines for consensus about when to administer fluid volume and inotropes in 46 mechanically ventilated patients with septic shock.[12] Only a limited agreement existed between the two methods. Fluid loading was initiated when the index of collapsibility of the superior vena cava was more than 36%, and inotropic support was initiated when the LV fractional area change was less than 45% without collapse of the vena cava or increased vasopressor support. Only 70% of patients responded to volume resuscitation. In the remaining 30%, fluid loading did not lead to volume expansion, even though the CVP was less than 12 mm Hg. Transesophageal echocardiography demonstrated that 30% of the patients had poor LV function and received inotropes, whereas only 9% of the patients would have been started on an inotrope if the Surviving Sepsis Campaign guidelines were applied.[12]

Keller and colleagues retrospectively studied whether PPV coupled with CVP and PAOP impacted identification of fluid responsiveness of cardiac surgery patients under general anesthesia.[13] Only 67% (31 of 46 patients) responded to fluid therapy. Neither CVP nor PAOP was a helpful predictor of fluid responsiveness, either alone or combined with PPV.

Broch and colleagues prospectively studied 92 patients undergoing coronary artery bypass surgery.[14] The global end-diastolic volume index and respiratory variations in LV outflow tract velocity were analyzed and compared against PPV and SVV. The PiCCO system monitor, transesophageal echocardiography, and CVP measurements were obtained in all patients. Fluid responsiveness was identified by a greater than 15% increase in the stroke volume index in response to a passive leg raise test. In this study, both PPV and SVV were highly accurate in determining fluid responsiveness.[14]

Salzwedel and associates used a hemodynamic goal-directed algorithm incorporating PPV, cardiac index, and MAP in a prospective study of 160 patients undergoing major abdominal surgery. Compared with control, use of an algorithm decreased postoperative complications.[15]

Velissaris and associates examined whether $ScvO_2$ values were associated with fluid responsiveness in 65 critically ill patients with severe sepsis. In this study, baseline $ScvO_2$ was not related to fluid responsiveness.[16]

At least 10 randomized controlled trials have demonstrated that hemodynamic strategies based on PPV or SVV monitoring are associated with a significant reduction in postsurgical complications and hospital length of stay.[17] An algorithm for stroke volume optimization is shown in Figure 22-2. Ongoing controversies about optimal volume assessment include the use of CVP-guided fluid management,[18,19] the use of blood products to augment oxygen delivery,[20,21] and vasopressor selection for the augmentation of MAP.[22–25]

PPV and SVV are increasingly used to guide fluid therapy in both the operating suite and critical care units. This was confirmed by peer-reviewed surveys that reported an increase in the use of dynamic parameters from 1% in 1998[26] to 45% in 2012.[27] The use of minimally invasive hemodynamic monitoring technologies is understandably of great interest. The technologies may augment or replace traditional monitoring systems.

Oxygen Delivery and Oxyhemoglobin Dissociation

Tissue hypoxia is the central pathophysiologic process in shock and an important cofactor in the development of organ dysfunction. The fundamental principle that

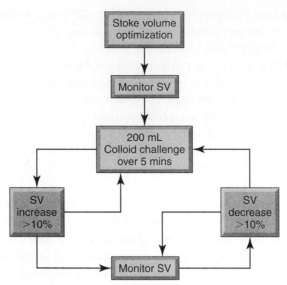

FIGURE 22-2 Stroke volume (SV) optimization. (Used with permission, Mervyn Singer, MB, BS, MD, FRCP(Lon), FRCP(Edin), FFICM, University College London.)

BOX 22-1   Properties of Oxygen Delivery

1. Cardiac output (CO)
   CO = Heart rate × stroke volume
2. Total hemoglobin (oxygen-carrying capacity: hemoglobin [HgB; 1.34])
3. Saturation of hemoglobin (SaO_2)

   Calculated as: CO (HgB × SaO_2)(1.34) ÷ 100 (only divide by 100 when expressing saturation in % [90%] rather than as a fraction [0.9])

---

underlies goal-directed therapy is optimization of tissue perfusion. Mixed venous oxygen saturation (SvO_2) is a sensitive indicator of the adequacy of whole-body tissue oxygenation. $ScvO_2$ reflects the adequacy of oxygenation in the brain and upper part of the body and differs from SvO_2 as discussed in detail in Chapters 6 and 7.

Recognition of inadequate global oxygen delivery (DO_2) may be difficult in the early stages because the clinical features are often nonspecific. These features include progressive metabolic acidosis, hyperlactatemia, and falling venous oxygen saturation ($ScvO_2$), as well as organ specific features such as oliguria and impaired level of consciousness.

An increase in cardiac output is the first line compensatory mechanism. Thus, the first step in any goal-directed program is to ensure an effective and efficient stroke volume. If goals are not reached after preload optimization, therapy with positive inotropes may be indicated. A full discussion of inotropes and vasopressors is presented in Chapter 9.

TABLE 22-2 **Mixed Venous Oxygen (SvO$_2$) and Central Venous Oxygen (ScvO$_2$) Values**

SvO$_2$	OXYGENATION STATUS
>75%	Normal O$_2$ extraction Oxygen delivery (DO$_2$) increased tissue demand (VO$_2$)
75%–50%	Increasing VO$_2$ or decreasing DO$_2$ Compensatory O$_2$ extraction
50%–30%	Exhaustion of O$_2$ extraction Beginning of lactic acidosis
30%–25%	Severe lactic acidosis
<25%	Cellular death

>, Greater than; <, less than.

Venous oxygen saturation differs among organ systems because individual organs extract different amounts of oxygen as shown in Figures 1-10 and 7-11 (see Chapters 1 and 7). In general, low values of SvO$_2$ or ScvO$_2$ indicate a mismatch between oxygen delivery and tissue oxygen need. The measurement of SvO$_2$ requires the insertion of a pulmonary artery catheter. The measurement of ScvO$_2$ requires a slightly less invasive central venous catheter, inserted into the subclavian vein or jugular vein. The ScvO$_2$ fiberoptic catheter measures the saturation of blood from the upper body only. By contrast, the pulmonary artery contains a mixture of blood from both the superior vena cava, and from the inferior vena cava, which receives venous blood from the metabolically active abdominal organs. Consequently, the mixed venous (SvO$_2$) value is about 7.5% below the upper body central venous (ScvO$_2$) value, when measured in the same patient, at the same time.[28] Many consider the overall trend of the SvO$_2$ and ScvO$_2$ measurements to be more important than how similar individual percentage measurements are.[29–32]

During cardiogenic and hypovolemic shock, blood flow to the mesentery and kidneys decreases accompanied by an increase in oxygen extraction. During septic shock, regional oxygen consumption by the gastrointestinal tract increases to a greater extent than does blood flow. In both situations, the blood in the inferior vena cava is more desaturated, and the SvO$_2$ value is lower than the ScvO$_2$. Thus, in shock states, a low ScvO$_2$ implies an even lower SvO$_2$.[28] An ScvO$_2$ value of 50% is considered critical as noted in Table 22-2.

Goal-Directed Therapy and Protocols

Goal-directed therapy utilizes flow-based hemodynamic monitoring to guide therapeutic interventions to a predefined hemodynamic and oxygenation endpoint. Goal-directed algorithms also standardize treatment, especially in high-risk situations.

Several studies have examined the impact of goal-directed therapy in the perioperative environment.

Hamilton and colleagues published a systematic review and meta-analysis of 29 randomized controlled trials published between 1995 and 2008.[33] The 29 trials enrolled 4805 patients who received a variety of pre-emptive hemodynamic interventions, depending on the individual study. Overall mortality was 7.6%. The meta-analysis showed mortality and surgical complications to be lower in the algorithm-guided groups.[33] Interestingly, overall mortality in the control group also declined over time.[33]

Arulkumaran and associates examined the impact of goal-directed therapy on cardiac complications in a meta-analysis of 22 studies with 2129 high-risk surgical patients. Use of perioperative goal-directed therapy was associated with a reduction in cardiovascular complications.[34]

Goal-Directed Therapy and Sepsis

Many clinicians recommend the use of minimally invasive monitoring in conjunction with a goal-directed protocol to achieve the most benefit.[35] Adherence to the bundles developed and supported by the Surviving Sepsis Campaign continues to demonstrate a positive impact on mortality and morbidity.[36] Recent evidence has shown that compliance with sepsis bundles leads to significant improvement in mortality rates.[37]

The results of the recently published ProCESS (Protocolized Care in Early Septic Shock) trial suggest that much of the benefit of sepsis therapy may be derived from early identification and intervention, rather than a specific endpoint involving hemodynamic treatments targeted to tissue perfusion.[7] The ProCESS trial was conducted in 31 Emergency Departments in the United States and enrolled 1341 patients with severe sepsis. Emergency department clinicians used specific identification criteria, early antibiotics and fluid resuscitation, based on a high index of suspicion to treat sepsis. The ProCESS investigators propose that awareness of treatment goals is as important, if not more important, than a protocol with targeted endpoints.[7] However, concerns about whether EGDT treatment was initiated before enrollment into the ProCESS trial in some patients, have been raised.[38] The ProCESS study is discussed in detail in the sepsis chapter (Chapter 20).

Another large study that evaluated the impact of EGDT in sepsis just published strikingly similar results to the ProCESS trial. The Australasian Resuscitation In Sepsis Evaluation (ARISE) randomized controlled trial took place in 51 Emergency Departments, predominantly in Australia and New Zealand.[39] Almost 1600 patients with sepsis were enrolled, half received protocol-EGDT therapy, and half were in the usual care (control) group. In both groups the first dose of antibiotics was administered in just over an hour, with a range of 38–114 minutes. In general, patients in the EGDT group received slightly more fluid, vasopressors, red-cell transfusions, and dobutamine. However, there was no difference between the groups in outcome, including length of hospital stay, duration of organ support, in-hospital mortality or 90-day survival.[39]

When discussing these results, the ARISE trial authors questioned the benefit of protocol-EGDT to treat sepsis.[39] As with the ProCESS trial the essential elements appear to be early recognition, early interventions and early administration of antibiotics.

The Protocolized Management in Sepsis (ProMISe) trial is ongoing in the United Kingdom (UK).[40] Approximately 48 Emergency Departments in the UK will be involved.[40] The ProMISe trial also compares EGDT with usual care for patients with severe sepsis. There will be considerable interest in the ProMISe trial results, as to whether their findings resemble those of the ProCESS and ARISE trials previously discussed. All three studies used a serum lactate level of greater than 4 mg/dL for a patient to be enrolled into the study.[40] This value was selected to match the original 2001 EGDT single-center study criteria.[8]

A minimum level of awareness regarding global oxygen delivery and perfusion pressure in the critically ill patient with signs and symptoms of shock sets the stage for therapeutic interventions. Treatment methodologies will be customized, especially as the perils of overly aggressive fluid resuscitation are recognized.[41] The large-volume fluid bolus approach for patients in septic shock has been questioned,[42] and smaller boluses with earlier use of vasopressors have shown some success in Australia and New Zealand.

Conclusion

Early detection and correction of tissue hypoxia is essential if progressive organ dysfunction and death are to be avoided. Whether choosing a known protocol, or selecting invasive or minimally invasive endpoints for a therapy target, particular attention must be placed on early and rapid identification of patients at risk.

Hemodynamic monitoring plays an important role in the management of today's acutely ill patient. Hemodynamic monitoring can be helpful in two key settings. The first is when a problem has been recognized and the clinician connects the pathophysiology to appropriate forms of therapy. The second is a preventive setting, with monitoring allowing pre-emptive actions to be performed before a significant problem arises. Research has shown the latter scenario to be helpful for the perioperative patient where monitoring can be used to detect hypovolemia or low oxygen delivery at an early stage, enabling timely corrective therapy to be initiated.[43]

A conclusive answer is not yet known; however, it is clear that a goal for perfusion and evidence-based practice initiatives must guide management of critically ill patients. Goal-directed therapy typically includes the use of fluid loading and inotropes, to optimize the preload, contractility, and afterload of the heart while maintaining an adequate coronary perfusion pressure. Despite the observed benefits, it remains a challenge to implement this management because of difficulties in identifying these patients, skepticism, and lack of critical care resources.

References

1. Mayer J, Boldt J, Mengistu AM, et al.: Goal-directed intraoperative therapy based on autocalibrated arterial pressure waveform analysis reduces hospital stay in high risk surgical patients: a randomized controlled trial, *Crit Care* 14(1):R18, 2010.
2. Pinsky MR, Dubrawski A: Gleaning knowledge from data in the ICU, *Am J Respir Crit Care Med* 190(6):606–610, 2014.
3. Vincent JL, Sakr Y, Sprung CL, et al.: Sepsis in European intensive care units: results of the SOAP study, *Crit Care Med* 34:344–353, 2006.
4. The ARDSNet Group: Comparison of two fluid-management strategies in acute lung injury, *N Engl J Med* 354:2564–2575, 2006.
5. Shoemaker WC, Appel PL, Waxman K, et al.: Clinical trial of survivors' cardiorespiratory patterns as therapeutic goals in critically ill postoperative patients, *Crit Care Med* 10:398–403, 1982.
6. Marik PE, Baram M, Vahid B: Does the central venous pressure predict fluid responsiveness? A systematic review of the literature and the tale of seven mares, *Chest* 134:172–178, 2008.
7. The ProCESS Investigators: A randomized trial of protocol-based care for early septic shock, *N Engl J Med* 370(18):1683–1693, 2014.
8. Rivers E, Nguyen B, Havstad S, et al.: Early Goal-Directed Therapy Collaborative Group: Early goal-directed therapy in the treatment of severe sepsis and septic shock, *N Engl J Med* 345:1368–1377, 2001.
9. Kapoor PM, Kakani M, Chowdhury U, et al.: Early goal-directed therapy in moderate to high-risk cardiac surgery patients, *Ann Card Anaesth* 11:27–34, 2008.
10. Pearse R, Dawson D, Fawcett J, et al.: Early goal-directed therapy after major surgery reduces complications and duration of hospital stay. A randomised, controlled trial [ISRCTN38797445], *Crit Care* 9:R687–R693, 2005.
11. Gattinoni L, Carlesso E: Supporting hemodynamics: what should we target? What treatments should we use? *Crit Care* 17(Suppl 1):S4, 2013.
12. Bouferrache K, Amiel JB, Chimot L, et al.: Initial resuscitation guided by the Surviving Sepsis Campaign recommendations and early echocardiographic assessment of hemodynamics in intensive care unit septic patients: a pilot study, *Crit Care Med* 40:2821–2827, 2012.
13. Keller G, Sinavsky K, Desebbe O, Lehot JJ: Combination of continuous pulse pressure variation monitoring and cardiac filling pressure to predict fluid responsiveness, *J Clin Monit Comput* 26:401–405, 2012.
14. Broch O, Renner J, Gruenewald M, et al.: Variation of left ventricular outflow tract velocity and global end-diastolic volume index reliably predict fluid responsiveness in cardiac surgery patients, *J Crit Care* 27:325, e7–e13.
15. Salzwedel C, Puig J, Carstens A, et al.: Perioperative goal-directed hemodynamic therapy based on radial arterial pulse pressure variation and continuous cardiac index trending reduces postoperative complications after major abdominal surgery: a multi-center, prospective, randomized study, *Crit Care* 17:R191, 2013.
16. Velissaris D, Pierakkos C, Scolletta S, et al.: High mixed venous oxygen saturation levels do not exclude fluid responsiveness in critically ill septic patients, *Crit Care* 15(4):R177, 2011 (6 pages).
17. Michard F: Long live dynamic parameters! *Crit Care* 18:413, 2014.
18. Marik PE: Surviving sepsis: going beyond the guidelines, *Ann Intensive Care* 1:17, 2011.
19. Marik PE, Baram M, Vahid B: Does central venous pressure predict fluid responsiveness? A systematic review of the literature and the tale of seven mares, *Chest* 134:172–178, 2008.
20. Reade MC, Huang DT, Bell D, et al.: Variability in management of early severe sepsis, *Emerg Med J* 27:110–115, 2010.

21. Parsons EC, Hough CL, Seymour CW, et al.: Red blood cell transfusion and outcomes in patients with acute lung injury, sepsis and shock, *Crit Care* 15:R221, 2011.
22. De Backer D, Aldecoa C, Njimi H, Vincent JL: Dopamine versus norepinephrine in the treatment of septic shock: a meta-analysis, *Crit Care Med* 40:725–730, 2012.
23. De Backer D, Biston P, Devriendt J, et al.: Comparison of dopamine and norepinephrine in the treatment of shock, *N Engl J Med* 362:779–789, 2010.
24. Sakr Y, Reinhart K, Vincent JL, et al.: Does dopamine administration in shock influence outcome? Results of the Sepsis Occurrence in Acutely Ill Patients (SOAP) Study, *Crit Care Med* 34:589–597, 2006.
25. Varpula M, Tallgren M, Saukkonen K, et al.: Hemodynamic variables related to outcome in septic shock, *Intensive Care Med* 31:1066–1071, 2005.
26. Boldt J, Lenz M, Kumle B, Papsdorf M: Volume replacement strategies on intensive care units: results from a postal survey, *Intensive Care Med* 24:147–151, 1998.
27. Srinivasa S, Kahokehr A, Soop M, et al.: Goal-directed fluid therapy—a survey of anaesthetists in the UK, USA, Australia and New Zealand, *BMC Anesthesiol* 13:5, 2013.
28. Reinhart K, Kuhn HJ, Hartog C, Bredle D: Continuous central venous and pulmonary artery oxygen saturation monitoring in the critically ill, *Intensive Care Med* 30:1572–1578, 2004.
29. Reinhart K, Rudolph T, Bredle D, et al.: Comparison of central-venous to mixed-venous oxygen saturation during changes in oxygen supply/demand, *Chest* 95:1216–1221, 1989.
30. Dueck M, Klimek M, Appenrodt S, et al.: Trends but not individual values of central venous oxygen saturation agree with mixed venous oxygen saturation during varying hemodynamic conditions, *Anesthesiology* 103:249–257, 2005.
31. Ladakis C, Myrianthefs P, Karabinis A, et al.: Central venous and mixed venous oxygen saturation in critically ill patients, *Respiration* 68:279–285, 2001.
32. Turnaoglu S, Tugrul M, Camci E, et al.: Clinical applicability of the substitution of mixed venous oxygen saturation with central venous oxygen saturation, *J Cardiothorac Vasc Anesth* 15:574–679, 2001.
33. Hamilton MA, Cecconi M, Rhodes A: A systematic review and meta-analysis on the use of preemptive hemodynamic intervention to improve postoperative outcomes in moderate and high-risk surgical patients, *Anesth Analg* 112(6):1392–1402, 2011.
34. Arulkumaran N, Corredor C, Hamilton MA, et al.: Cardiac complications associated with goal-directed therapy in high-risk surgical patients: a meta-analysis, *Br J Anaesth* 112:648–659, 2014.
35. Cecconi M, Bennett D: Should we use early less invasive hemodynamic monitoring in unstable ICU patients? *Crit Care* 15:173, 2011.
36. van Zanten AR, Brinkman S, Arbous MS, et al.: Guideline bundles adherence and mortality in severe sepsis and septic shock, *Crit Care Med* 42(8):1890–1898, 2014.
37. Gao F, Melody T, Daniels DF, et al.: The impact of compliance with a six hour and twenty four hour sepsis bundles on hospital mortality in patients with severe sepsis: a prospective observational study, *Crit Care* 9(6):764–770, 2005.
38. Surviving Sepsis Campaign: *Surviving sepsis campaign responds to the ProCESS trial.* http://www.survivingsepsis.org/SiteCollectionDocuments/SSC-Responds-Process-Trial.pdf. Updated May 19, 2014. Accessed September 15, 2014.
39. ARISE Investigators and ANZICS Clinical Trials Group: Goal-directed resuscitation for patients with early septic shock, *N Engl J Med* 371(16):1496–1506, 2014.
40. The ProCESS/ARISE/ProMISe Methodology Writing Committee: Harmonizing international trials of early goal directed resuscitation for severe sepsis and septic shock: methodology of ProCESS, ARISE, and ProMISe, *Intensive Care Med* 39:1760–1775, 2013.

41. Boyd J, Forbes J, Nakada T, et al.: Fluid resuscitation in septic shock: a positive fluid balance and elevated central venous pressure are associated with increased mortality, *Crit Care Med* 39 (2):259–265, 2011.

42. Hilton AK, Bellomo R: A critique of fluid bolus resuscitation in severe sepsis, *Crit Care* 16:302, 2012.

43. Vincent JL, Rhodes A, Perel A, et al.: Clinical review: update on haemodynamic monitoring—a consensus of 16, *Crit Care* 15:229–237, 2011.

Hemodynamic Equations and Normal Values

NAME	EQUATIONS	NORMAL RANGE AND UNITS	REFERENCE TABLE / BOX
Cardiovascular			
Cardiac Output (CO)	$SV \times HR$	4.0-8.0 L/min	Table 1-2 Box 5-2 Table 5-4
Cardiac Index (CI)	$CO \div BSA$	2.5-4.0 L/min/m^2	Table 1-2 Table 5-4
Ejection Fraction (EF%)	Stroke Volume (SV) / End diastolic volume (EDV) Multiply by 100 to convert to %		Table 1-2
Mean Arterial Pressure (MAP)	$MAP = DBP + 1/3(SBP - DBP)$	70-100 mm Hg	Table 1-2 Table 5-4
Mean Pulmonary Artery Pressure (mean PA)	mean $PA = PAD + 1/3(PAS - PAD)$	8-15 mm Hg	Table 5-4
Pulmonary Vascular Resistance (PVR)	$PVR = \dfrac{(\text{mean PA} - \text{mean PAOP})}{CO} \times 80$	<250 dynes·sec/cm^5	Table 1-2 Box 5-2 Table 5-4
Systemic Vascular Resistance (SVR)	$SVR = \dfrac{(MAP - CVP)}{CO} \times 80$	800-1200 dynes·sec/cm^5	Table 1-2 Box 5-2 Table 5-4
Stroke Volume (SV) in milliliters (mL)	$SV = (CO \times 1000) / HR$	60-100 mL/beat	Box 5-2 Table 5-4
Stroke Volume Index (SVI)	$SI = (CI \times 1000) / HR$	30-65 mL/beat/m^2	Box 5-2 Table 5-4

Stroke Volume Variation (SVV)	$SVV = (SV\,max - SV\,min) /$ Mean SV over 20–30 seconds Multiply by 100 to convert to %	10%-15%	Table 12-3
Pulse Pressure Variation (PPV)	Maximum PP – Minimum PP / Mean PP over a respiratory cycle Multiply by 100 to convert to %	13%-15%	Table 12-3

Oxygenation: Venous and Arterial

Arterial Oxygen Content (CaO_2)	$CaO_2 = Hgb \times 1.38 \times SaO_2 + PaO_2 \times 0.0031$	16-22 mL/dL	Table 7-1
Oxygen Delivery (DO_2)	$DO_2 = Hgb \times 1.38 \times SaO_2 \times CO \times 10$	1000 mL/min	Table 7-1
Oxygen Delivery Index (DO_2I)	$DO_2I = Hgb \times 1.38 \times SaO_2 \times CI \times 10$	500-600 mL/min/m^2	Table 7-1
Venous Oxygen Content (CvO_2)	$CvO_2 = Hgb \times 1.38 \times SvO_2 \times CO \times 10$	750 mL/min	Table 7-1
Oxygen Consumption (VO_2)	$VO_2 = CO\,(SaO_2 - SvO_2) \times Hgb \times 1.38 \times 10$	200-250 mL/min	Table 7-1
Oxygen Consumption Index (VO_2I)	$VO_2I = CI\,(SaO_2 - SvO_2) \times Hgb \times 1.38 \times 10$	120-160 mL/min/m^2	Table 7-1

Neurologic

Cerebral Perfusion Pressure (CPP)	$CPP = MAP - ICP$	60-160 mm Hg	Table 21-1

<, Indicates less than; >, indicates greater than; *Hgb,* hemoglobin; *HR,* heart rate; *min,* minute; *mm Hg,* millimeters of mercury; *PA,* pulmonary artery; *PaO$_2$,* partial pressure of arterial oxygen; *PAOP,* pulmonary artery occlusion pressure; *PP,* pulse pressure.

Index

Note: Page numbers followed by "*b*" indicate boxes, "*f*" indicate figures and "*t*" indicate tables.

Case Studies and Case Examples

CASE STUDY	HEMODYNAMIC FOCUS	CHAPTER	PAGE/BOX
Acute heart failure	Physical assessment	2	Pages 51-52 Case Study
Pulmonary embolus and hypotension	Management guided by patient symptoms and arterial pressure values	3	Pages 83-84 Case Study
Sepsis	Management guided by sepsis EGDT protocol, including central venous pressure values	4	Pages 107-109 Case Study
Acute decompensated heart failure	Hemodynamic management of heart failure, including use of pulmonary artery catheter	5	Pages 142-143 Case Study
Hypercapnia post-anesthesia	Challenges of monitoring only with SpO_2	6	Page 162 Box 6-4
Hypoxemia	Arterial-alveolar (a-A) oxygen ratio	6	Page 168 Box 6-9 and Box 6-10
Oxygenation	P/F ratio and oxygenation index	6	Pages 167 and 170 Box 6-7 and Box 6-11
Respiratory and metabolic acidosis	Assessment of blood glucose, oxygenation, acid–base, and mechanical ventilation	6	Pages 198-199 Case Study #1
Hypoxemia, ARDS post-trauma	Facial trauma, difficult intubation, mechanical ventilation	6	Pages 199-202 Case Study #2
Low cardiac output following cardiac surgery	Use of SvO_2	7	Pages 225-227 Case Study #1
Occult bleeding following cardiac surgery	Use of SvO_2	7	Page 227 Case Study #2
Esophageal intubation— atelectasis and mucus plug	Use of capnography during intubation and mechanical ventilation	8	Page 252 Case Study
Pneumonia and septic shock	Treatment with fluid, antibiotics, vasoactive medications, and mechanical ventilation	9	Pages 274-277 Case Study

Child with septic shock	Assessment with transcutaneous Doppler	10	Pages 302-303 Case Study
Dilated cardiomyopathy	Assessment with bedside ultrasound	11	Pages 333-334 Case Study #1
Pericardial effusion	Assessment with bedside ultrasound	11	Page 335 Case Study #2
Tension pneumothorax	Assessment with bedside ultrasound	11	Page 336 Case Study #3
Trauma with free fluid in the abdomen	Assessment with bedside ultrasound	11	Page 337 Case Study #4
Cardiac surgery—coronary artery bypass graft	Management guided by dynamic parameters—SV and SVV	12	Pages 363-364 Case Study
ARDS post-trauma	Mechanical ventilation management	14	Pages 417-419 Case Study
Left ventricular assist device	Hemodynamic and MCS management	15	Pages 461-463 Case Study
Cardiac surgery—aortic valve replacement	Hemodynamic management	16	Pages 488-489 Case Study
Acute decompensated heart failure	Hemodynamic management	17	Pages 520-521 Case Study #1
Dilated cardiomyopathy—IABP and LVAD	Hemodynamic and MCS management	17	Pages 522-524 Case Study #2
Acute myocardial infarction (STEMI) with right heart dysfunction	Hemodynamic and medication management	18	Pages 544-545 Case Study #1
Pulmonary hypertension	Medication management	18	Pages 565-566 Case Study #2
Trauma—bleeding and hypovolemia	Hemodynamic, fluid, and mechanical ventilation management	19	Pages 573-574 Case Study
SIRS and severe sepsis	Treatment with fluid, antibiotics, vasoactive medications, and mechanical ventilation	20	Pages 626-628 Case Study
Ruptured aneurysm and subarachnoid hemorrhage— Takotsubo syndrome	Neurocritical care management	21	Pages 704-707 Case Study

ARDS, Acute respiratory distress syndrome; *EGDT*, early goal directed therapy; *IABP*, intra-aortic balloon pump; *MCS*, mechanical circulatory support; *P/F ratio*, PaO_2/FIO_2 ratio; *SpO_2*, pulse oximetry saturation; *STEMI*, ST elevation myocardial infarction; *SV*, stroke volume; *SvO_2*, mixed venous oxygen saturation; *SVV*, stroke volume variation.